ATHLETIC INJURY ASSESSMENT

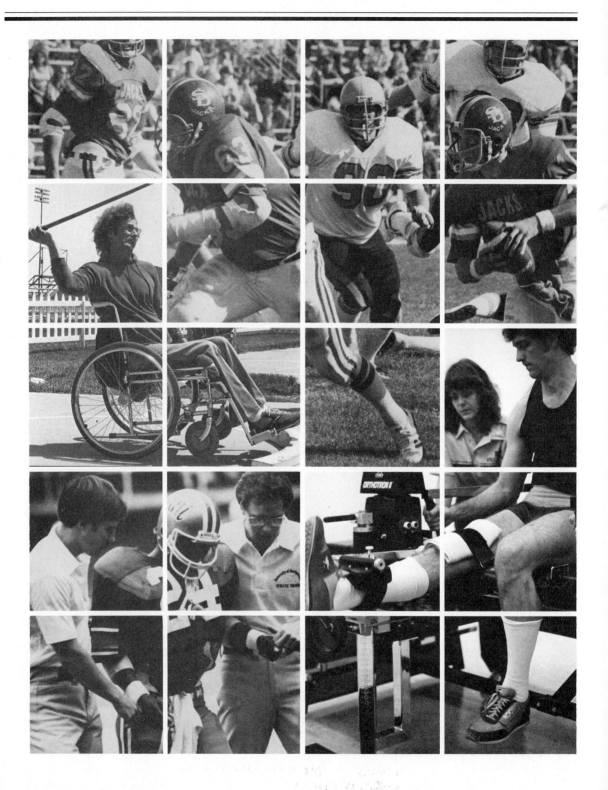

Athletic Injury Assessment

JAMES M. BOOHER, Ph.D., A.T.,C., R.P.T.

Professor, Department of Health, Physical Education, and Recreation,
South Dakota State University,
Brookings, South Dakota

GARY A. THIBODEAU, Ph.D.

Professor, Department of Biology,
South Dakota State University,
Brookings, South Dakota

With 776 Illustrations

TIMES MIRROR/MOSBY College Publishing

St. Louis • Toronto • Santa Clara   1985

This book is based on research, recommendations, and suggestions of athletic trainers, physicians, and other health professionals currently active in the field of sports medicine. The authors and publisher disclaim responsibility for any adverse effects or consequences resulting from the misapplication or injudicious use of the information contained within this text.

Editor: Nancy K. Roberson
Developmental Editor: Michelle Turenne
Manuscript Editor: Mark Spann
Designer: Kay M. Kramer
Cover designer: Diane Beasley
Production: Linda R. Stalnaker, Mary Stueck, Margaret B. Bridenbaugh

A division of The C.V. Mosby Company
11830 Westline Industrial Drive
St. Louis, Missouri 63146

Printed in the United States of America

Library of Congress Cataloging in Publication Data

Booher, James M.
  Athletic injury assessment.

  Includes index.
  1. Sports—Accidents and injuries—Diagnosis.
2. Physical diagnosis. I. Thibodeau, Gary A.,
1938-   II. Title.
RD97.B65   1985   617'.1027   84-14896
ISBN 0-8016-0711-6

A/VH/VH   9 8 7 6 5 4   05/C/610

FOREWORD

Having attempted to teach injury assessment courses at a number of universities, I have always been plagued by the task of providing appropriate texts or references. If one truly attemps to supply the best references, those benefiting most would be the campus book store and the library copying service because the material is scattered among multiple disciplines and a variety of texts and periodicals. The difficulty in finding appropriate references seems to be the result of three factors: (1) the material is too discipline-specific, (2) too disease-specific, or (3) assumes too much on the part of the reader.

The problem with discipline specificity is its inherent limited perspective. The physiologist views the world at a cellular or subcellular level, emphasizing normal or supranormal function, and views disease states as annoyances. At the other end of the spectrum is the surgeon, viewing nothing but a diseased environment. No one describes the reasonably normal person who suffers relatively minor diseases—the stuff of which clinical sports medicine is made.

A disease- or injury-specific orientation presents much the same problems. Whereas the most authoritative material regarding athletic injuries deals with single-disease entities, as a rule this type of treatment fails to yield any global perspective of how important that particular problem is in the athletic world. For example,

having read and digested all the information pertaining to anterior cruciate ligament injuries of the knee, you would find that this knowledge is of little value when assessing over three quarters of the knee problems presented by athletes. Likewise, extensive knowledge of the dynamics of the body's management of heat dissipation will be of little value if an athlete's leg cramps are the result of an injured and inadequately rehabilitated muscle.

Finally, a majority of the sports medicine literature assumes too much. Like the child being told to "look it up in the dictionary" after asking how to spell a word, the seeker of injury assessment information might reply, "if I knew what was wrong I wouldn't need to look it up." Material dealing with anatomy assumes the reader already knows what can go wrong with that anatomy. Material dealing with surgical treatment assumes the reader can make the diagnosis. Material dealing with diagnostic tests assumes the reader knows what to do if the test is positive.

Unfortunately, few of us are able to put all of this in perspective because we deal only with bits and pieces of the athlete. Not so the athletic trainer, who deals with the whole athlete, sick or well, on a daily basis. Who then should be in a better position to know what is important and realistic?

Athletic Injury Assessment offers something I

have not seen before: a format of presenting a useful and scientifically accurate discussion of anatomy and physiology, the pathologic potential, a scheme for discovering salient points in the history, a step-by-step description of the physical examination, and a list of circumstances under which you should seek help. This material is supplemented by boxes of key points, appropriate illustrations and pictures, and a complete bibliography. This is all accomplished in a manner that is highly useful to the sports medicine novice as well as the sports medicine specialist.

Athletic Injury Assessment provides not only a single source textbook of injury assessment for athletic trainers but also an equally appropriate resource for anyone dealing with injured athletes.

James G. Garrick, M.D.
San Francisco

PREFACE

Assessment of athletic injuries is one of the most vital skills required of the athletic trainer. Yet its significance has not been given adequate attention in athletic training textbooks currently available. Dramatic changes have occurred in the profession during the past decade, and the athletic trainer is now viewed as one of the most important members of the sports medicine–health care team. Ensuring timely and accurate assessment of injury is one of the most important elements in any successful athletic training program. Professionally, more is expected of the athletic trainer in the area of assessment than ever before.

To adequately prepare students to enter the athletic training profession, academic curricula have been expanded, and increased emphasis is being placed on clinical or practical experience. Development of assessment skills is now treated as a separate course or as a major area of emphasis in most athletic training curricula. *This text is intended to fill the need for a comprehensive text in assessment, specifically designed for use in athletic training curricula. It should also be of value to other health professionals and to coaches and others in the field of health, physical education, and recreation. It provides a reliable, ready reference and explanation of assessment skills required to evaluate athletic injuries.*

In the past, teachers and students alike were forced to glean the necessary information required for an assessment course from many sources. Frequently, use of multiple sources can be confusing to students because information on a single assessment topic is presented differently in terms of level of complexity or sequencing of material. For example, textbooks or other materials on assessment procedures designed for the emergency medical technician, physical therapist, or practicing physician may be inappropriate in certain circumstances for use by the athletic trainer. This book is not intended to make diagnosticians of athletic trainers. Instead, it aims to provide the athletic trainer with the best possible skills so that athletic injuries can be accurately and quickly recognized and proper treatment or referral initiated without delay. This text was written in response to a demand for specialized information not currently available for use in the rapidly maturing and increasingly sophisticated area of athletic training. The content, organization, and sequencing of material in this text clearly address that need.

Content features

In Unit I the professional identity of the athletic trainer is clearly established and the necessary review of basic body structure is addressed. In addition, the early chapters stress the importance of viewing the body in its entirety during assessment, and the student is reminded of the importance of using appropriate anatomic terminology. Chapters 3, 4, and 5 provide an overview of three areas of primary concern to the athletic trainer: the structure and function of the skeletal, articular, and muscular systems.

Unit II is concerned with how the body responds to detrimental traumas or stresses associated with athletic activity and the development of related signs and symptoms. Recognizing and evaluating the signs and symptoms associated with athletic trauma is the basis of assessment. Chapter 6 discusses the body's basic responses to trauma and environmental conditions, and Chapter 7 deals with specific athletic injuries.

The athletic injury assessment process is discussed in Unit III. Athletic trainers are continually evaluating and re-evaluating athletic-related trauma, and the more highly skilled they become in the assessment process, the more accurate and successful they become in managing athletic injuries. Chapter 8 discusses various factors related to the evaluation of athletic injuries; Chapter 9 presents a rational approach to the athletic injury assessment process.

The final three units of this text are concerned with athletic injuries occurring to various areas of the body. Unit IV discusses athletic injuries of the axial region, which includes the head, spine, and torso. This area of the body was presented first because of the vital organs within this region and the possibility that injuries involving these organs can be life-threatening. Unit V is concerned with athletic injuries to the most frequently injured area of the body, the lower extemities. The final section of this text, Unit VI, is concerned with athletic injuries occurring to the upper extremities.

Learning aids

Some of the unique pedagogic features incorporated into each chapter of this text include:

1. Brief introductory outlines. These provide an overview of the topics to be examined.
2. Prolific use of illustrations (line drawings, photographs, and photographic sequences) provide the student with a visual review of the procedures, functional tests, and assessment techniques discussed.
3. Each chapter covering athletic injuries to an area of the body provides:
    A review of regional anatomy
    Common mechanisms of injury
    Athletic injuries and the associated signs and symptoms
    The sequence for assessment of athletic injuries
    An evaluation of findings with a list of conditions that indicate when an athlete should be referred for medical assistance
    An athletic injury assessment checklist outlining the process

Additionally, many photographs of specific athletic injuries and related types of trauma are included to provide a broad base of exposure to the real world of sports medicine.

4. Key terms are highlighted in **_boldface italics_** and defined clearly and concisely within the chapter and again at the end of each chapter to reinforce learning.

5. Suggested Readings in each chapter provide the most complete and up-to-date resources available to allow the reader to gain further information.

6. A glossary is located at the end of the text for convenient access to important terms and to provide an additional method of review.

Acknowledgments

Throughout the writing of this text we have been fortunate indeed to have the benefit of the experience and counsel of Drs. John Billion and Bruce Lushbough. The critical suggestions, provocative questions, and enthusiastic support of many physicians, athletic trainers, and health professionals active in the field has helped immeasurably in making this text a reality. We are grateful to Ernest W. Beck for the use of several illustrations appearing in Chapters 4, 5, 7, 11, 12, 13, and 17 and which were originally prepared for _Textbook of Anatomy and Physiology_.

For their thoughtful suggestions and constructive criticism, we would like to thank the publisher's reviewers: John G. Baynes, M.Ed., A.T.,C., Northeastern University; Linda S. Arnold, A.T.,C., Memphis State University; Gary Delforge, Ed.D., A.T.,C., University of Arizona; William F. Joy, A.T.,C., Eastern New Mexico University; Sally A. Perkins, M.S., A.T.,C., Southern Illinois University—Carbondale; Michelle E. Piette, A.T.,C., Arizona State University; John W. Powell, Ph.D., A.T.,C., The Pennsylvania State University; Ronald Stefancin, M.S.Ed., A.T.,C., James Madison University; Clint Thompson, M.A., A.T.,C., Michigan State University; Karen R. Toburen, Ed.D., A.T.,C., University of Wisconsin—La Crosse. Our special thanks go to Barbara Moran who, as an extremely conscientious teacher and researcher in the athletic training profession, provided constant support, encouragement, and assistance during the development and writing of this text. We also extend our appreciation to the students enrolled in our athletic curriculum, who gave freely of their time as subjects and photographers throughout the preparation of this text.

James M. Booher
Gary A. Thibodeau

CONTENTS

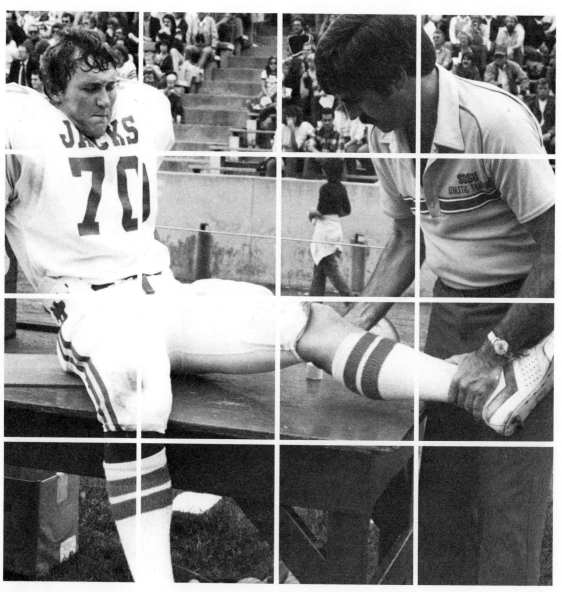

Athletic trainer assessing a knee injury.

O N E

Introduction and anatomic basis for athletic injury assessment

Athletic injury assessment is the comprehensive evaluation of an athletic injury. Assessment skills are necessary for all who are responsible for the medical care of athletes. Competency and proficiency in assessing athletic injuries requires many skills, including knowledge, technique, and experience. This unit provides an introduction to the profession of athletic training and the importance of athletic injury assessment (Chapter 1) as well as a basic review of the essential anatomic characteristics of the human body as they relate to athletic injury assessment.

Chapter 1 introduces the student to the concept of athletic injury assessment. In addition to material covered in Chapter 1 and the development in Chapter 2 of an appreciation for the physical characteristics of the whole body, this unit highlights the anatomy of the three major organ systems of most direct importance to those interested in athletics and the assessment of athletic injuries—bones, articulations (joints), and muscles.

1   Introduction to athletic injury assessment

2   The body as a whole

3   Osteology

4   Arthrology

5   Myology

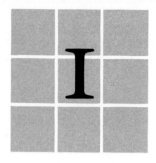

I Introduction to athletic injury assessment

Sports medicine

Athletic training
   Prevention
   Assessment
   Management and treatment
   Rehabilitation
   Organization and administration
   Education and counseling

It is inevitable that injuries will always be associated with physical activity and athletics. The risk of injury is much higher in some sports, such as those requiring contact or collision, but is inherent to all athletic activity. Although the majority of athletic injuries are relatively minor, the potential for serious and possibly life-threatening injuries is constantly present. The incidence of serious and life-threatening conditions associated with athletic activity has decreased over the last several years as a result of the delineation of causative factors and subsequent rule modifications in many sports and vast improvements and increased sophistication in all facets of sports medicine and athletic training. In spite of this increased sophistication, there has been an overall increase in the number of athletic injuries; this is primarily the result of an increase in the number of participants, the intensity of modern training techniques, and the expansion of athletic activities.

Today a wider selection of athletic activities, physical fitness programs, and sports are available to a larger cross-section of the population than ever before. Interest in physical activities and athletics continues to increase and participation is no longer limited to high school, college, amateur, and professional athletes. A greater number of organized athletic programs are available to children in junior high school and upper elementary grades. Youth sports competition, recreational programs, intramural activities, and sports for the handicapped and all age groups are increasing in popularity. The number of participants in all areas continues to increase dramatically. The development of many women's athletic programs is another factor that has greatly changed the number of sports activities and opportunities for participation. Because of all these developments, there are greater opportunities for persons of all ages to participate in recreational and competitive activities.

People are becoming more health and fitness conscious than ever before. This awareness has produced an increased interest in the benefits of physical fitness. More people than ever before are participating in life-time activities such as walking, jogging, bicycling, swimming, golf, and tennis. People today have more leisure time available as a result of many factors, including shorter work weeks, mechanization, and time-saving devices. Many people are using this additional leisure time to participate in recreational activities requiring some degree of physical exertion.

Whatever the reason for the dramatic increase in the number of participants and activities available, injuries are a reality at every level of participation and in every type of program. Participants in all forms of athletic activity are subjected to many stresses and forces that can result in injury. It is important to remember that injuries to athletes are essentially no different from those suffered by nonathletes. A sprained ankle can result in the same severity of damage whether it is sustained by a competitive athlete or a weekend jogger. However, the demands in terms of evaluation, treatment, rehabilitation, and return to activity are usually significantly greater for the competitive athlete.

SPORTS MEDICINE

Just as there have been tremendous increases in participation and interest in athletics, there have been corresponding increases in interest, knowledge, and understanding concerning all aspects of the medical management of athletes and athletic injuries. A new phrase has been coined to describe this vast network of medical management: *sports medicine.* Sports medicine encompasses all phases of medical concerns relating to the athlete: biomechanical, psychologic, nutritional, environmental, pathologic, and physiologic. The field of sports medicine has seen phenomenal development in recent years, as evidenced by the professional associations designating sports medicine as a subspeciality, the vast amounts of literature, research, and educational experiences now available, and the number of medical clinics specializing in sports medicine emerging throughout the country. Sports medicine is a rapidly growing, dynamic field.

The knowledge and techniques gained are benefiting not only competitive athletes and the vast legion of fitness buffs but also everyone else involved in athletic and nonathletic activities. Sports medicine includes all medical and paramedical professionals who are concerned with and provide expertise aimed at improving the performance and the health care of athletes. One of the subspecializations of sports medicine is athletic training.

ATHLETIC TRAINING

As a sports medicine subspeciality, *athletic training* provides a wide array of health care support services for athletes. Athletic training as defined by the National Athletic Trainers' Association (NATA) is "the art and science of prevention and management of injuries at all levels of athletic activity." The provider of athletic training services is an *athletic trainer.* The profession of athletic training and the position of the athletic trainer on the sports medicine team have developed to meet a demand for someone highly skilled in the evaluation, management, and care of athletic injuries. As long as there has been athletics, there has generally been someone designated to manage or care for athletes who become injured. In the past this position of responsibility was generally filled by a coach, teacher, student, or other interested person. Now many of these positions at the collegiate and professional levels are being filled by a qualified athletic trainer. However, much of the responsibility for the medical care of athletes, particularly at the high-school level, remains with the coach and will continue as such until the need for highly skilled athletic trainers is recognized. There appears to be a need for an increase in the number and availability of qualified athletic trainers nationally.

As compared with other allied health professions, athletic training is quite young. NATA was founded in 1950. The qualifications and requirements to become an athletic trainer have become more stringent over the years. In 1969 a procedure was developed for those institutions

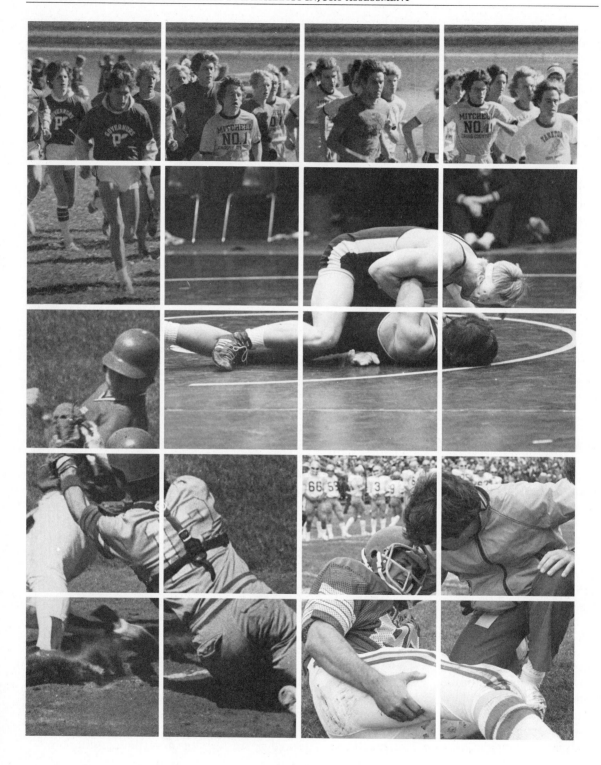

offering athletic training curricula to obtain NATA approval. At that time only two schools were selected that met all requirements for approval. Today there are over 70 schools offering NATA-approved curricula. In 1970 a certifying procedure for athletic trainers was established and has been continually upgraded and improved. To become an athletic trainer a person must possess a college degree that fulfills specific educational and practical requirements. On successful completion of these requirements the candidate must then take a national certifying examination designed to ensure that he or she meets the minimal standards and competencies required to become an athletic trainer. In addition to obtaining the initial certification, athletic trainers must also earn a designated number of continuing educational units to maintain their certified status.

Today's athletic trainer is more than just a technician designated to tape ankles, apply bandages, or "rub down" athletes. Athletic training is becoming more scientific, and athletic trainers are more knowledgeable about the many aspects of health care for athletes. The athletic trainer has become a vital member of the sports medicine team. In addition to the athletic trainer, this team includes the team physician, coach, and other professionals involved in providing health care for athletes. It is the athletic trainer's responsibility to coordinate the health care services available.

In 1982 a role delineation study conducted by the NATA classified the duties or functions of an athletic trainer into six major categories: (1) prevention, (2) assessment, (3) treatment, management, and disposition, (4) rehabilitation, (5) organization and administration, and (6) education and counseling of injured athletes. Each of these areas is important and all are interrelated. The athletic trainer must develop knowledge and competency in each category to provide athletes with optimal medical care. The athletic trainer must be able to combine medical and scientific information in the areas of anatomy, physiology, kinesiology, psychology, physiology

of exercise, health, physics, nutrition, and first aid with a wide array of complex practical skills. In addition, he or she must also have a sincere interest in athletics and in working with athletes and must possess communication and leadership skills. The athletic trainer is no longer a "jack of all trades, master of none." He or she is a professional who must be proficient in many varied skills. The primary skills or proficiencies necessary for each of these functions are listed in Table 1-1.

Prevention

The best method of managing and caring for athletic injuries is to prevent them from occurring; thus much of the athletic trainer's time and effort is devoted to preventing injuries. Numerous factors briefly discussed in this section are important in the prevention of athletic injuries. A thorough preparticipation evaluation does not guarantee that an athlete will participate injury free but it does affirm that there is no discernible clinical reason to preclude participation. Proper conditioning is the preventive medicine of athletics. Athletic trainers often work in conjunction with coaches in establishing preseason, inseason, and postseason conditioning programs. Another facet of athletic injury prevention in which the athletic trainer is involved is the selection, fitting, and maintenance of protective equipment. An athletic trainer may also be responsible for checking the safety of facilities and apparatus required for athletic activity.

More familiar preventive tasks performed by athletic trainers include the application of protective taping, padding, bandaging, braces, and other devices. Athletic trainers must also constantly observe their athletes. If recognized early, minor problems can often be treated with minimal inconvenience to the athlete and no significant decrease in performance. Early recognition and effective treatment prevent most minor injuries from becoming more severe and disabling. An injury that is properly recognized and managed effectively generally does not become more severe, and the potential for reinjury is less. In

Table 1-1. Functions of an athletic trainer

Prevention	Assessment	Treatment and management
Preparticipation examination	Primary survey	Immediate first aid
Medical history	Airway	Ice
Physical examination	Breathing	Compression
Fitness screening	Circulation	Elevation
Proper conditioning	Secondary survey	Rest
Protective equipment	History	Follow-up treatment
Selection	Observation	Therapeutic modalities
Fitting	Palpation	Exercise programs
Maintenance	Stress tests	Protective techniques
Safety supervision	Evaluation of findings	Taping
Facilities	Medical referral	Splinting
Equipment	Treatment applica-	Padding
Preventive techniques	tion	Supporting
Taping		Immobilizing
Padding		Assessment techniques
Bandaging		Evaluation of the effects of treat-
Bracing		ment procedures on signs and
Observing athletes		symptoms
Recognize problems and minor		
injuries		
Hygiene		
Rest		
Diet		
Assessment techniques		
Recognizing injury		
Determining severity of injury		
Observe when returned to activity		
Emergency care procedures		
Supplies		
Plan of action		
Immediate care		
Rehabilitation strategies		
Prevent reinjury		
Strengthen previously injured area		
Monitoring environmental conditions		

addition, athletic trainers are often asked to counsel athletes and coaches in the areas of diet, rest, and sanitation.

Assessment

Athletic trainers must possess a high level of proficiency in assessment skills to accurately recognize and evaluate the nature and severity of an athletic injury. Athletic trainers are normally at the location or playing field where an injury occurs and will have to handle the emergency care. They must be able to recognize and deal with such conditions as severe head or spine injuries, hemorrhaging, shock, heat illness, or choking. Athletic trainers must be prepared to administer cardiopulmonary resuscitation, apply emergency splinting, or supervise the transportation of an injured athlete.

Rehabilitation	Organization and administration	Education and counseling
Range of motion	Maintain records	Previous injuries and present status
Muscular strength	Injuries	Medical history
Muscular endurance	Treatment	Requirements of each sport
Coordinated movements	Facilities	Health topics
Functional activities	Inspection	Knowledge of health education
Cardiovascular endurance	Safety	Social and personal problems
Assessment techniques	Sanitation	Knowledge of available professionals
Evaluation of effects of re-	Equipment and supplies	Knowledge of situation requiring
habilitation program	Purchasing	consultation
	Maintaining	Referral procedures
	Health care services	Knowledge of team or family physician
	Organize	Instructing student trainers
	Communication	Continuing education
	Policies and procedures	
	Emergency support services	

The athletic injury assessment process is based on a scientific method that involves (1) recognition and statement of the problem, (2) collection of data about the problem, and (3) creation and testing of hypotheses to solve the problem. An athletic trainer's initial assessment creates the foundation or data base for the ensuing procedures. It begins with the collection of data related to the injury through the systematic steps of history, observation, palpation, and stress maneuvers. From the data collected, the athletic trainer must determine and initiate the appropriate course of action. This includes emergency medical care, follow-up treatment procedures, transportation, medical referral, rehabilitation strategies, or return to athletic activity. Once action has been taken, the athletic trainer must continually evaluate the results of this action. Is the athlete getting better or worse? Why? What can be done to improve or enhance the athlete's recovery? The athletic trainer should then modify or adjust the plan of action accordingly. Assessment and reassessment are ongoing processes in athletic training. The assessment process is discussed in more detail in Unit Three, and assessment procedures are discussed throughout this text.

Management and treatment

Athletic trainers must be skilled in various management and treatment procedures. These include (1) administering immediate first aid, (2) providing therapy to promote healing and recovery, (3) applying protective techniques to support and protect an injured area, and (4) referring an injured athlete for other medical assistance when necessary. Athletic trainers can have a dramatic effect on the overall recovery of an injured athlete by the proper use of treatment procedures. The goal is to return the injured athlete to activity as soon as possible without risking further injury. The treatment of an athletic injury is a three-step process: (1) examination of the signs and symptoms, (2) application of treatment routines, and (3) assessment of the effects of these techniques on the signs and symptoms of the injury. This cycle continues throughout the treatment process; that is, assessment, treatment, and reassessment. If an athlete is to return to optimum physical activity in a minimal amount of time, there can be no delay in an accurate assessment and a properly instituted treatment program.

Rehabilitation

Rehabilitation is the restoration of normal form and function after an injury. Athletic *rehabilitation* is the reconditioning of an injured athlete to his or her highest level of function in the shortest possible time. This level of function is generally higher than that of a nonathlete. Athletic trainers must be skilled in developing programs to effectively rehabilitate an athlete in a minimal amount of time. Depending upon the

nature and the conditions surrounding the injury, rehabilitation requires a progressive, systematic program that develops range of motion, muscular strength and endurance, coordinated movements, functional activities, and circulorespiratory endurance. Although each of these phases overlap, maximal development of any phase requires prior development of the preceding phases. During rehabilitation there should be repeated assessment techniques performed to evaluate progress and indicate appropriate follow-up care.

Organization and administration

Often overlooked aspects of an athletic trainer's responsibilities are the organization and administration of the athletic training program. Athletic trainers must plan, organize, evaluate, and implement procedures and policies necessary to provide their athletes with the most effective health care available. To aid in efficient health care delivery, athletic trainers must maintain accurate and detailed records to document injuries and treatments and other services rendered to the athletes under their care. Selecting, purchasing, maintaining, and instructing others in the use of equipment and supplies necessary for operation of a training room are also the athletic trainer's responsibilities.

Education and counseling

The last function of an athletic trainer to be discussed is the role of education and counselor to the athlete and student athletic trainer. Athletic trainers need to have the skill and knowledge necessary to instruct students in the competencies required to become professional athletic trainers. This responsibility requires that the athletic trainer keep abreast of current sports medicine issues and also be able to convey this information to others. Another facet of education and counseling skills required is the athletic trainer's ability to recognize situations requiring consultation with other health care professionals regarding an athlete's social or personal problem. This involves skill in assessing an athlete's need for professional consultation and referral of the athlete to the appropriate professional. To be effective in this area, an athletic trainer must possess effective communication skills. These communication skills enable the athletic trainer to interact with athletes, parents, coaches, administrators, physicians, and other professionals concerning various health-related topics.

To summarize, athletic trainers must develop knowledge and competency in each of these duties or functions to provide optimal medical care to athletes. Note that assessment or evaluation skills are listed and discussed under each of these categories. Athletic injury assessment is a necessary and extremely important skill for anyone who has medical responsibilities for athletes. Indeed, planning an athlete's medical care based on an accurate assessment is the foundation of current athletic training practices. Athletic injury assessment affects each of the other major duties or functions of an athletic trainer (Fig. 1-1). This

textbook specifically addresses this important function of athletic training.

KEY TERMS

athletic trainer Provider of athletic training services, which can be divided into six major functions: (1) prevention, (2) assessment, (3) management and treatment, (4) rehabilitation, (5) organization and administration, and (6) education and counseling

athletic training Sports medicine subspecialty that provides a wide array of health care support services for athletes

rehabilitation Restoration of optimal form and function after an injury in the shortest possible time

sports medicine Field encompassing all medical concerns of the athlete: biomechanical, psychologic, nutritional, environmental, pathologic, and physiologic

SUGGESTED READINGS

Emerick, C.E., and Schrader, J.W.: Back to reality: athletic training at the high school level, Athletic Training **16**:180-181, 1981.

Fig. 1-1. Effect of an athletic injury on performance.

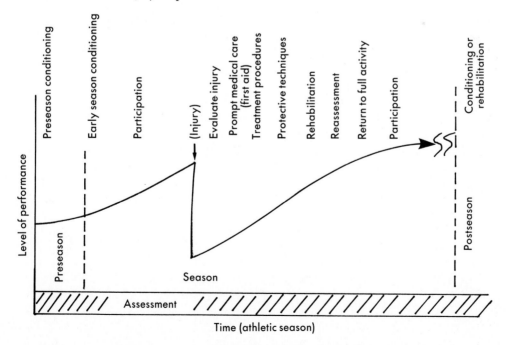

Gieck, J.: The athletic trainer and counselor education, Athletic Training **12**:58-60, 1977.

Hage, P.: Medical care for athletes: are coaches getting the message? Physician Sportsmedicine **10**:159-164, 1982.

Hage, P., and Moore, M.: Medical care for athletes: what is the coaches role? Physician Sportsmedicine **9**:140-151, 1981.

Kegerreis, S.: Health care for student athletes, JOPER **50**:78-79, 1979.

Kelley, E.J., and Miller, S.J.: The need for a certified athletic trainer in the junior-senior high schools, Athletic Training **11**:180-183, 1976.

National Athletic Trainers' Association: Professional preparation in athletic training, Champaign, Ill., 1982, Human Kinetics, Inc.

National Athletic Trainers' Association: 1982 Role delineation study of the entry-level athletic trainer, 1982, The Association.

O'Shea, M.E.: A history of the national athletic trainers' association, 1980, National Athletic Trainers' Association.

Powers, H.W.: The organization and administration of an athletic training program, Athletic Training **11**:14-16, 1976.

Redfearn, R.W.: Are high school athletes getting good health care? Physician Sportsmedicine **3**:34-39, 1975.

Vinger, P.F., and Hoerner, E.F.: Sports injuries; the unthwarted epidemic, Boston, 1982, John Wright–PSG, Inc.

Walker, B., and Muenchen, J.: Policies and procedures are necessary in the training room, Athletic Training **13**:211, 1978.

Yearger, B.: Medical care for young athletes: pretty barbaric, but that's the way it is, Physician Sportsmedicine **2**:75-80, 1974.

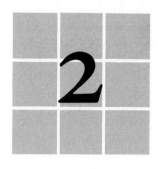

2 The body as a whole

Proficiency and knowledge in athletic injury assessment procedures depend on much more than good technique and a thorough understanding of anatomy in the area of injury. Assessment begins with systematic and deliberate observations of the person as a whole. Athletes are certainly more than the sum of their parts, and the old adage "know your athlete" is as important to the athletic trainer as to the coach.

In studying and perfecting the techniques for assessment of an athletic injury to specific body parts or areas it is all too easy to think of each part in isolation from the body as a whole. Always remember that you are dealing with an injured person and not just an injured knee, elbow, or shoulder. Having a complete and detailed information base or profile on an athlete before an injury will be of immense help in making an accurate assessement of an injury should the need arise. Information presented in this chapter is intended to help you view the athlete, healthy or injured, as a whole person. Material covered includes a brief introduction to the concept of body type (somatotype) and some generalizations on the organization of the body and the language of anatomy.

SOMATOTYPE

Athletes come in many different shapes and sizes. "Somatotyping" describes a system of classifying body build or physique. The most widely accepted technique, first described by Sheldon, identifies three main body types according to dominant morphologic traits or components. These traits or components are called *endomorphy, mesomorphy* and *ectomorphy*. By studying the body build of a large number of athletes, Sheldon and others have found that these basic components of physique occur in varying degrees in every person. Indeed, most persons display physiques that are obvious intermixtures of all three components. Fig. 2-1 illustrates the extremes of the three somatotype components. A seven-point rating scale is used to reflect the dominance of each of the three primary components of physique. A rating of 1 indicates the minimal component manifestation, whereas 7 indicates the maximal manifestation. The number 4 is used to indicate the manifestation of a particular component that is judged to

be halfway between 1 and 7. Thus the physique of any person can be described by a series of three numerals indicating, in order, the dominance of endomorphy, mesomorphy, or ectomorphy. This number, which is the patterning of morphologic traits, is called the *somatotype* of the person. The somatotype designation is read as three separate numerals and not as a three-digit number. For example, a 117 somatotype should be read as "one-one-seven" and not as "one hundred and seventeen."

Each body type in Fig. 2-1 illustrates the result of almost total dominance by a single somatotype component. Such physiques are extremely rare. For example, the 117 body type represents an extremely ectomorphic physique with mini-

Fig. 2-1. Examples of the extreme somatotypes. Note the almost total dominance of a single somatotype component in each type of physique.

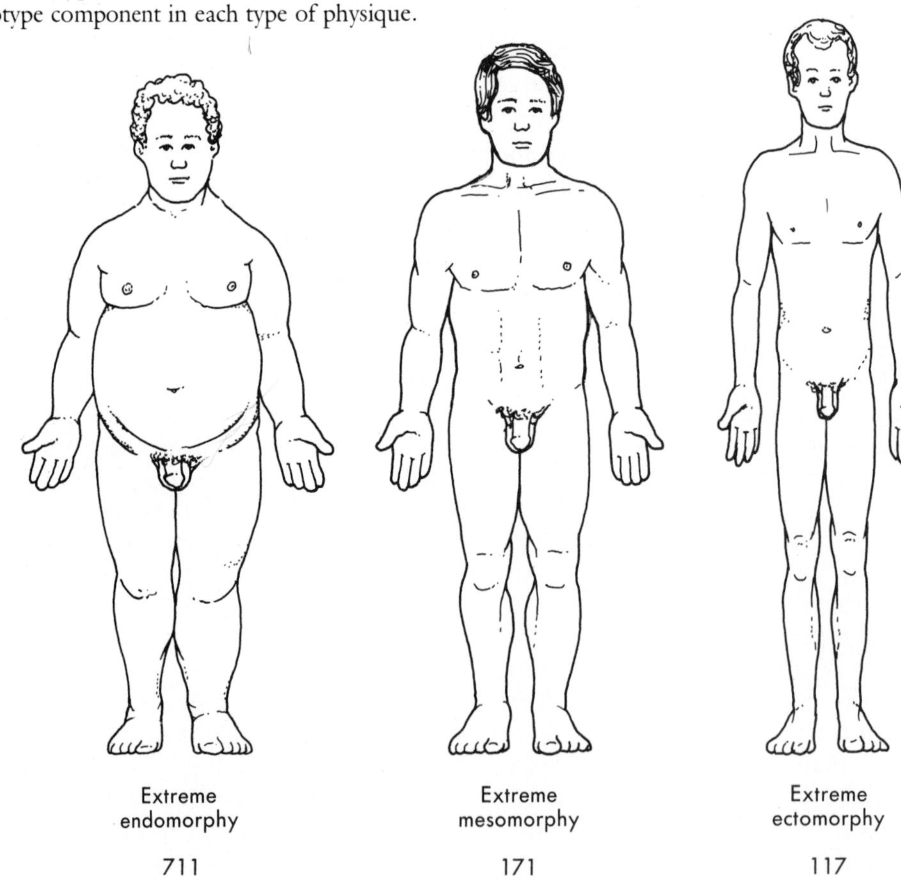

Extreme endomorphy	Extreme mesomorphy	Extreme ectomorphy
711	171	117

mal amounts of the other two components. Note how the 117 somatotype almost totally lacks any of the plump, round, and smooth characteristics of the endomorph or the defined muscularity of the typical mesomorph.

Body type can be a predisposing factor in many types of athletic injuries. In addition, environmental factors such as temperature and humidity can selectively influence the performance and well-being of athletes of one body type when compared with another under otherwise similar conditions. Endomorphs, for example, are notoriously susceptible to heat-related injuries; ectomorphs, because of their large body surface area in relation to body weight and lack of insulating fat, are often prone to heat-loss problems associated with cold weather.

Endomorphy

Endomorphy, the first component in the somatotype, indicates the relative predominance of roundness and softness of body. Endomorphic persons tend to be fat. Typically, they have a heavy torso with a protruding abdomen and slightly smaller thorax. Smoothness of contours caused by accumulation of fat under the skin all but eliminates muscle definition. In the extreme endomorph (rating 711) the neck is short and the head is almost always large and spherical. The limbs are short, with tapering and rounding of the thighs and upper arms. There is some breast development (fat deposition) in the male endomorph. In addition, the buttocks are full and round and show no lateral dimpling.

Mesomorphy

Mesomorphy, the second component of the somatotype (rating 171), describes a relative preponderance of muscle, bone, and connective tissue. Mesomorphs are heavily muscled and have large, prominent bones. The distal segments of the arms and legs are prominent and massive. The shoulders of a mesomorphic person usually project laterally from the torso. In addition, the thoracic segment of the trunk predominates over the abdominal segment, and the waist is low. A muscular dimpling is common at the lateral margins of the buttocks (Fig. 2-2).

Ectomorphy

Ectomorphy, the third component of the somatotype (rating 117), indicates relative predominance of linearity (height) over fat or muscle. These persons tend to be tall and thin. Typically, they have a relatively short trunk, long limbs, and poorly developed musculature. A shoulder droop is common in ectomorphs. Unlike endomorphy, the distal segments of the arms and legs tend to be relatively long and thin. The neck is long and slender, and the face is small, with sharp, fragile features.

Distribution of somatotypes

The distribution of somatotypes among athletes is remarkably diverse. Differences in body build are apparent not only between athletes engaged in different sports but also between individual participants in a single sport competing at different positions or weight classes. In general, when one of the somatotype components is represented to a high degree in an athlete, it precludes high scores in the others. Thus a somatotype of 262 is possible, whereas one of 737 is not.

Fig. 2-2. Example of muscular dimpling at the lateral margins of the buttocks in a male athlete characterized as a mesomorph.

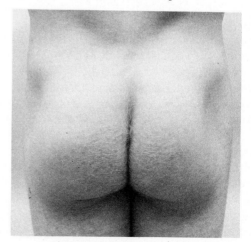

Table 2-1. Descriptive and numerical classification of selective somatotype categories

Descriptive classification	Numeric somatotype designation
Extreme endomorph	711
Mesomorphic endomorph	621, 631, 532
Endomorphic mesomorph	361, 462, 372
Extreme mesomorph	171
Ectomorphic mesomorph	162, 253, 154
Mesomorphic ectomorph	345, 235, 126
Extreme ectomorph	117
Endomorphic ectomorph	435, 326, 415
Ectomorphic endomorph	524, 612, 623

Table 2-1 lists the nine categories or descriptive somatotype classifications most frequently referred to in the training literature and gives an example of numeric somatotypes that might be included in each group. If you learn to correlate each one of the descriptive somatotype designations (for example, ectomorphic mesomorph) with a specific numeric somatotype (for example, 154), you will quickly develop the ability to mentally quantify otherwise subjective physical characteristics—an ability that will prove valuable in development of assessment skills.

Somatotyping technique

Somatotyping is accomplished by a trained person carefully studying the precisely posed athlete in anterior, lateral, and posterior views. After analyzing each view, an estimate is made of the approximate strength of each component in the somatotype for the body as a whole. Before that somatotype is assigned, the three-digit estimate is compared with somatotypes that are common to persons having the same height/weight index as the athlete in question. This height/weight index is known as ***Ponderal index.*** It is calculated by dividing the height in inches by the cube root of the weight in pounds. The Ponderal index can provide a relatively reliable estimate of the somatotype of a college-age athlete. Standard charts showing the relationship between Ponderal index and expected somatotype are readily available. In addition to somatotyping, an understanding of the Ponderal index is valuable to the athletic trainer involved in nutrition counseling, cardiovascular conditioning, or rehabilitation programs.

Actual assignment of a formal numeric somatotype designation is a complex and time-consuming process seldom employed by the athletic trainer except in a research setting. However, exposure to the basic concept of somatotyping can make you a more critical observer of the body as a whole and more aware of the complex interrelationships of its component parts. When viewing an athlete for the first time, make a mental estimate of numeric somatotype and then try to refine it with time. Keep in mind that up to a certain point repeated contact with an athlete will produce corrections of estimates originally made even by an experienced observer. Most students find that conscious attempts to identify and separate somatotype components in a person quickly sharpen their observational skills. For example, they often report that subtle differences in muscle symmetry and definition tend to become more apparent.

BODY COMPOSITION

Athletic trainers skilled in somatotyping are frequently called on to evaluate an athlete's body composition. Such information is valuable in setting a realistic and safe minimum weight for athletes in sports such as wrestling and boxing, monitoring the progress of a weight loss or gain program, or identifying those athletes who need to reduce their fat weight. Athletes will frequently turn to age/weight tables to determine "optimal" body weight. Because these tables are based on only one skeletal dimension, height, and do not differentiate between lean body weight and fat body weight, they may be misleading. In many cases athletes may be overweight according to these tables but not overfat. As with somatotyping there are numerous methods used to determine body density. One of the most frequently used methods is the skinfold measurement technique, (Fig. 2-3), which involves pinching the body at various sites and measuring the thickness of the skin and its underlying adipose tissue. By inserting these data into appropriate mathematic equations, the athlete's body density and percentage of body fat can be estimated.

Extensive checklists of inspection criteria for identifying each somatotype component or details of formal somatotyping or body composition techniques are beyond the scope of this text. Students wishing such information are referred to the literature.

GENERALIZATIONS ABOUT BODY STRUCTURE
Bilateral symmetry

Bilateral symmetry is one of the most obvious of the external organizational features in humans. To say that humans are bilaterally symmetric simply means that the right and left sides of the body are mirror images of each other (Fig. 2-4). One of the most important features of bilateral symmetry is balanced proportions. There is a remarkable correspondence in size and shape when comparing similar anatomic parts or areas on opposite sides of the body.

Assessment of injury, especially to an extremity, often requires careful comparison of the injured with the noninjured side. Minimal swelling or deformity on one side of the body is often apparent only to the trained observer who routinely compares a suspected area of injury with its corresponding part on the opposite side of the body. The term *contralateral* means "opposite" and is used to designate an anatomic part or region on the uninjured or opposite side of the body. If the right knee were injured, the left knee would be designated as the contralateral knee. The term *ipsilateral,* on the other hand, means "on the same side" and refers to a body part or area situated on the same side of the body as the injury. For example, if reference is made to ipsilateral muscle spasms in the thigh after an injury to the right knee, those spasms would be in the right thigh.

Body regions

The body as a whole can be divided into *axial* and *appendicular* divisions. These primary divisions are subdivided as follows and should be reviewed in Fig. 2-5.

Axial	Appendicular
Head	Upper extremity
Skull (cranium)	Shoulder
Face	Arm
Neck	Elbow
Trunk	Forearm
Thorax	Wrist
Upper Back	Hand and fingers
Lower Back	Lower extremity
Abdomen	Buttocks
Pelvis	Thigh
	Knee
	Lower leg
	Ankle
	Foot and toes

Fig. 2-3. Obtaining skinfold measurement data.

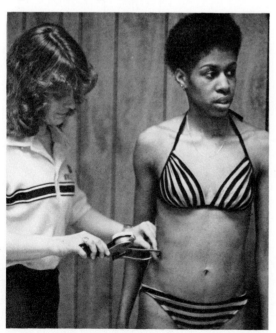

Anatomic position

In assessing an athletic injury it is necessary to use precise terms to describe body parts or areas and the relationships that exist between them. To avoid misunderstanding when using terms that describe direction or location on the body, a standardized anatomic position has been adopted. In the *anatomic position* the body is erect and facing forward, as in Fig. 2-5, *A*. Note the position of the arms at the side of the body with the palms of the hands turned forward (forearms supinated).

Directional terms

When the body is in the anatomic position, the following directional terms can be used to describe the location of one body part with respect to another. Refer often to Fig. 2-5.

Superior: Toward the head end of the body; upper (the eyes are superior to the mouth)

Inferior: Away from the head; lower (the bladder is inferior to the stomach)

Anterior (ventral): Front (the eyes are located on the anterior surface of the head)

Posterior (dorsal): Back (the shoulder blades are located on the posterior side of the body)

Medial: Toward the midline of the body (the great toe is located at the medial side of the foot)

Lateral: Away from the midline of the body (the little toe is located at the lateral side of the foot)

Proximal: Nearer the point of attachment of an extremity to the trunk or the point of origin of a part (the elbow is proximal to the wrist)

Distal: Farther from the point of attachment of an extremity to the trunk or the point of origin of a part (the hand is located at the distal end of the forearm)

Superficial: Nearer the surface (the skin of the arm is superficial to the muscles below it)

Deep: Farther from the body surface (the humerus of the arm is deep to the muscles that surround it)

Fig. 2-4. Bilateral symmetry. As a result of this organizational feature the right and left sides of the body are mirror images of each other.

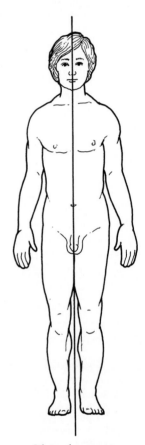

Bilateral symmetry

Fig. 2-5. The anatomic position showing axial and appendicular subdivisions. **A,** Anterior view; **B,** posterior view. Directional terms are used in describing a number of body regions.

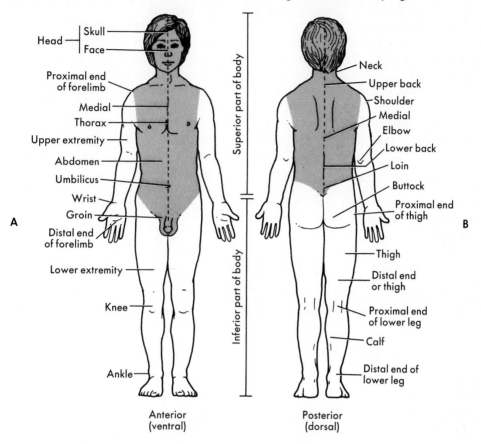

A

B

Anterior
(ventral)

Posterior
(dorsal)

Body planes (sections)

To visualize the internal organs, it is necessary to cut, or section, the body into component parts for study. The body is a three-dimensional structure and as such can be divided by three standard planes or sections of reference (Fig. 2-6). Each plane is oriented at right angles to the two remaining planes as they pass through the body.

The *coronal (frontal) plane* (Fig. 2-6, *A*) runs from side to side. It cuts the body or any of its parts into anterior and posterior (front and back) portions.

The *midsaggital plane* (Fig. 2-6, *B*) runs from front to back. This lengthwise plane divides the body into right and left halves that are mirror images of each other.

The *transverse (horizontal) plane* (Fig. 2-6, *C*) is a crosswise cut or section that divides the body or any of its parts into superior and inferior (upper and lower) portions.

Fig. 2-6. Body planes or sections.

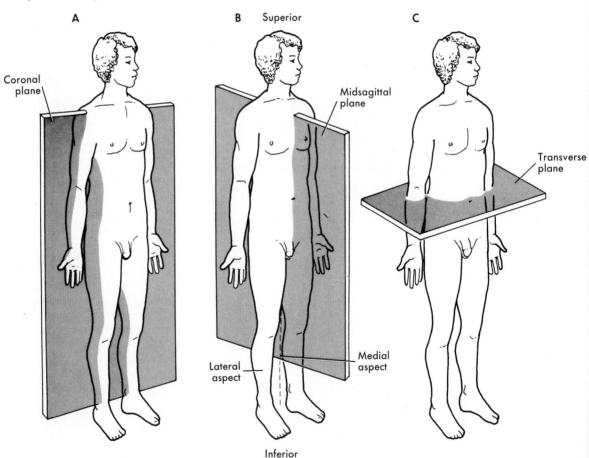

Abdominopelvic quadrants and regions

Clinicians and other allied health personnel generally divide the abdominal area into quadrants (Fig. 2-7) to more easily describe and locate organs in the abdominopelvic cavity. To accomplish this, the umbilicus is intersected by two planes or sections. The midsagittal plane is intersected at the umbilicus by a horizontal or transverse section or cut. As a result, the two sections divide the abdomen into right and left superior (upper) quadrants and right and left inferior (lower) quadrants. Anatomists often use a more precise method of locating organs in the abdominal cavity by dividing the area into nine regions.

Surface anatomy

The study of human anatomy often begins with visual inspection of the form and markings of the body surface. An appreciation of body form and symmetry is critically important in athletic injury assessment, and the need to sharpen observational skills cannot be overemphasized. With that end in mind, carefully inspect and compare the male and female forms in Fig. 2-8. Differences in body form between men and women are strikingly evident. Note, however, that the axial and appendicular portions of the body and the divisions of each region are easily identifiable in both sexes.

The smooth, more rounded contours of the female form result in large part from accumulation of more fat below the skin surface of the body as a whole than is typical of the male form. In addition, the bony framework is generally smaller and more delicate in women. In areas such as the buttocks, breasts, hips, flanks, and outer thighs, accumulation of fatty tissue is particularly noticeable in the female. In women the gluteal fat merges into the fat of the loin area so that the buttocks appear to extend almost to the waist (Fig. 2-9). As a result, women tend to have a relatively large abdominal surface area and a lower center of gravity than men.

Carefully note and compare differences in appearance of the extremities. In the female the arm is more cylindric, in the male, flatter from side to side. The female thigh tends to be shorter and more conical than the male thigh. Note the obvious difference in definition of the calf muscles between the sexes in Fig. 2-10. Even in women with powerfully developed musculature, the even layer of fatty tissue just below the skin surface tends to confer a smoother form and appearance.

Fig. 2-7. Subdivision of the abdominal area into four quadrants. Midsagittal and transverse planes intersect at right angles at the umbilicus.

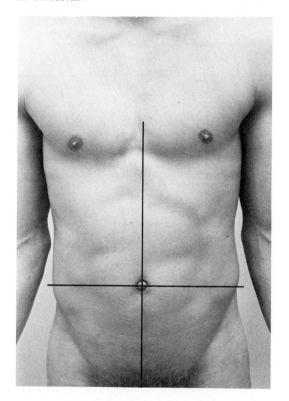

Fig. 2-8. The human body viewed from the front.

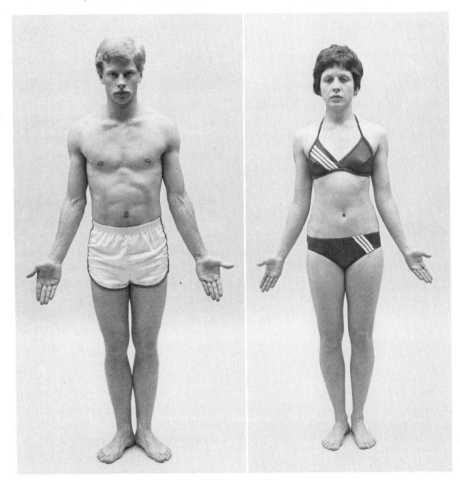

Fig. 2-9. The human body viewed from behind. Note the differences in fat distribution. In the female loin area, fat extends from the buttocks to the waist.

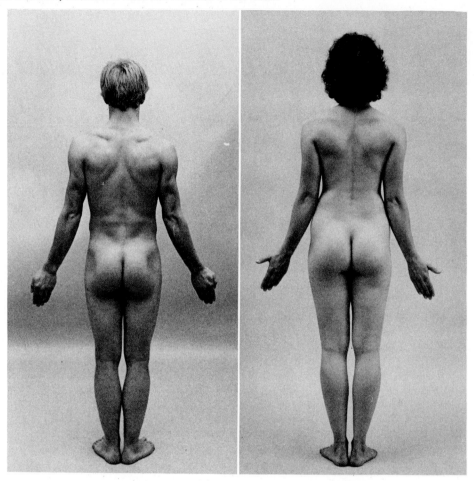

Fig. 2-10. Comparing the differences in definition of calf musculature between a male and a female athlete.

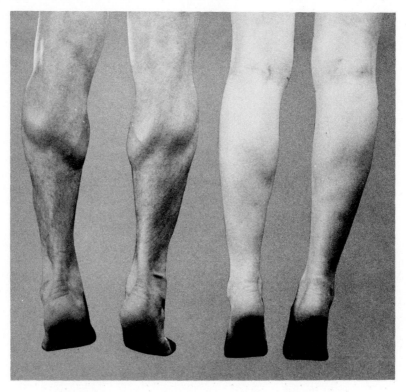

KEY TERMS

anatomic position Position in which the body is upright, with the feet parallel and palms of the hands facing forward

anterior (ventral) Front

appendicular Pertaining to the appendages of a structure—in the body this refers to the upper and lower extremities

axial Pertaining to the axis of a structure—in the body this refers to the head, neck, and trunk

contralateral Pertaining to the opposite side

coronal (frontal plane) Plane that runs from side to side and divides the body into front and back halves

deep Away from the body surface

distal Farther from the point of attachment of an extremity to the trunk or the point of origin of a part

ectomorphy Type of body build in which there is a relative predominance of linearity over fat and muscle

endomorphy Type of body build in which there is a relative predominance of roundness and softness of the body

inferior Away from the head; lower

ipsilateral Pertaining to the same side

lateral Away from the midline of the body

medial Toward the midline of the body

mesomorphy Type of body build in which there is a relative predominance of muscle, bone, and connective tissue

ponderal index Height/weight index in which height in inches is divided by the cube root of the weight in pounds $\dfrac{\text{height (inches)}}{\sqrt[3]{\text{weight (pounds)}}}$

posterior (distal) Back

proximal Nearer the point of attachment of an extremity to the trunk or the point of origin of a part

sagittal plane Plane that runs from front to back and divides the body into right and left halves

somatotype Particular category of body build, determined on the basis of certain morphologic traits

somatotyping System of objectively classifying body build or physique

superficial Near the surface

superior Toward the head end of the body

transverse (horizontal plane) Crosswise plane that divides the body into upper and lower halves

SUGGESTED READINGS

Anthony, C.P., and Thibodeau, G.A.: Textbook of anatomy and physiology, ed. 11, St. Louis, 1983, The C.V. Mosby Co.

Carter, J.E.L.: The Health-Carter somatotype method, San Diego, 1972, San Diego State College.

Damon, A., and others: Predicting somatotype from body measurements, Am. J. Phys. Anthropol. 20:461-475, 1962.

Goss, C.M., editor: Gray's anatomy, ed. 29, Philadelphia, 1980, Lea & Febiger.

Hollinshead, W.H.: Textbook of anatomy, ed. 3, New York, 1974, Harper & Row, Publishers, Inc.

Lohman, T.G., and others: relationships of somatotype to body composition in college-aged men, Ann. Hum. Biol. 5:174-180, 1978.

McMinn, R.M.H., and Hutchings, R.T.: Color atlas of human anatomy, Chicago, 1984, Year Book Medical Publishers, Inc.

Sheldon, W.H., and others: The varieties of human physique, New York, 1940, Harper Brothers.

Spalteholz, W.: Atlas of human anatomy, ed. 16, New York, 1967, F.A. Davis Co. (Revised and re-edited by R. Spanner.)

Tanner, J.M.: The reliability of anthropometric somatotyping, Am. J. Phys. Anthropol. 12:257-265, 1954.

Vannini, V., and Pogliana, G., editors: The color atlas of human anatomy, New York, 1981, Crown Publishers, Inc.

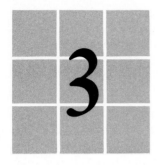

3

Osteology

A thorough understanding of the underlying anatomy of an injured area is an absolute prerequisite for the successful assessment of athletic injuries. Therefore an adequate review of appropriate anatomy will always precede discussion of specific assessment techniques introduced in subsequent chapters of the text. The intent is to provide the necessary anatomic detail required to understand and execute specific assessment procedures immediately before practical application of that information. Chapters 3, 4, and 5 are intended only to provide a general overview of

bones, joints, and muscles, the body areas most often involved in athletic injuries.

The human skeleton is a joined framework of living organs called bones. The skeleton lies buried within the muscles and other soft tissues, thus providing a support structure for the body.

The adult skeleton is composed of 206 separate bones. Rare variations in the total number of bones present in the body may occur as a result of certain anomalies such as extra ribs or from failure of certain small bones to fuse in the course of development.

FUNCTIONS OF THE SKELETON

The skeleton has five principal functions. The first three listed below are of particular interest to athletic trainers.

Protection

Bones protect vital and delicate soft tissue structures from injury. Obvious examples include the brain encased within the skull or the heart and lungs protected by the rib cage.

Support

The skeleton provides the support necessary to safely maintain upright posture. A number of unique skeletal support mechanisms, for example, make it possible to run or jog without subjecting the body to undue stress and potential injury.

Movement

Bones serve as points of attachment for muscles. As the muscles contract and shorten, force is applied to bones, which then act as levers. It is the joints or articulations between bones that serve as pivot points or fulcrums that permit actual movement to occur.

Mineral storage

The skeleton serves as a massive storage reservoir for minerals, especially the salts of calcium and phosphorus. In the event of increased demand or inadequate intake of calcium or phosphorus the body can activate complex regulatory mechanisms that result in transfer of one or both of these important salts from bone (osseous) tissue to the blood. Maintaining a normal blood level of calcium is particularly important because of calcium's role in blood clot formation, muscle contraction, and nerve impulse conduction.

Hemopoiesis

Hemopoiesis is the process of blood cell formation. It occurs in red bone marrow found in the sternum and ribs, in the bodies of the vertebrae, and in the proximal ends of the femur and humerus.

CLASSIFICATION OF BONES

Bones may be divided into five groups for study purposes.

Long bones

Long bones of the body often serve as levers. If pulled by contracting muscles, these bones make movement of the body possible. Examples of long bones are the humerus, radius, and ulna of the arm and the femur, tibia, and fibula of the leg.

Short bones

The carpal bones of the wrist are typical short bones. As a group, short bones tend to be cube shaped and are generally found in areas in which only very limited motion is required. Their principal function is to provide strength.

Flat bones

Flat bones consist of parallel, platelike layers of hard or compact bone separated by a thin layer of spongy or cancellous bone tissue. These bones provide large areas for muscle attachment and in general serve a protective function. The bones of the skull (such as frontal and parietal) and the shoulder blades (scapulae) are good examples of flat bones.

Irregular bones

Bones that have obvious peculiarities in their shape are placed in this classification. Unique in their appearance and function, these bones must be studied individually. Examples include the pelvic bones, certain bones of the skull such as the ethmoid, and the ossicles of the ear.

Sesamoid bones

The patella, or kneecap, is the largest and most definitive of the sesamoid bones. As a group, these small and rounded or triangular bones develop within the substance of tendons or fascial tissue and are found adjacent to joints. They are named for their fancied resemblance to sesame seeds.

FEATURES OF A TYPICAL BONE

Every bone in the skeleton is a unique organ—a distinct structural unit. However, as a group, long bones uniformly possess many of the features of bones in general. For this reason, the major anatomic features of a "typical" long bone are often described before the study of individual bones in the skeleton. A long bone consists of the following structures visible to the naked eye: diaphysis, or shaft, epiphyses, articular cartilage, periosteum, medullary (marrow) cavity, and endosteum. Identify each of these parts in Fig. 3-1 as you read the following paragraphs.

Diaphysis

The *diaphysis* is the long, shaftlike portion of the bone. The hollow, cylindric shape of the diaphysis provides strong support without cumbersome weight. Functionally, it can be compared to a length of strong metal tubing. The walls of the diaphysis are formed from hard, dense, compact bone.

Epiphyses

The *epiphyses* are the extremities or ends of long bones. They enter into the formation of joints and, because of their somewhat bulbous shape, provide generous space for muscle attach-

Fig. 3-1. Schematic diagram of the structural features of a typical long bone. **A,** Longitudinal section. **B,** Cutaway section.

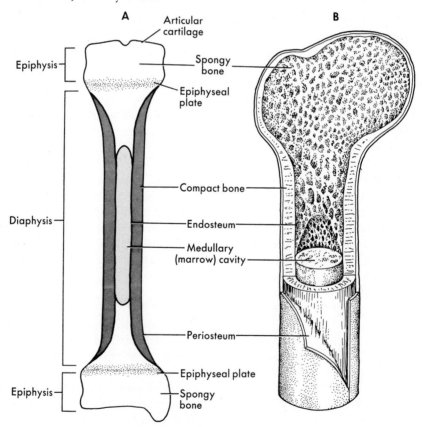

ments. Note the appearance of the bone in the epiphysis in Fig. 3-1, *B*. Like a sponge, it is permeated by innumerable small spaces—hence its name, spongy or cancellous bone. Because of the porous nature of this bone and because the epiphyses have only a thin layer of dense, compact bone over their outer surface, they are lightweight structures for their size. A thin plate of cartilage separates the diaphysis from each epiphysis in growing bones. These plates of cartilage are called *epiphyseal (growth) plates.* They are replaced by bone at maturity, at which time the epiphyses are said to be closed. Marrow fills the spaces of cancellous bone—yellow marrow in most adult epiphyses but red marrow in the proximal epiphyses of the humerus and femur. It must be remembered that epiphyseal plates in growing children are the weakest links along the bone and therefore may be involved in an athletic injury. Young athletes must be evaluated carefully for epiphyseal involvement, especially after traumatic injury to long bones.

Articular cartilage

A thin layer of *hyaline,* or *articular, cartilage* covers the joint surfaces of epiphyses. This layer of gristlelike material is firmly fixed to the thin layer of compact bone that covers the epiphyses. Resiliency of the articular cartilage cushions jars and blows that might otherwise erode or damage opposing epiphyseal bone surfaces in joints.

Periosteum

The *periosteum* is a dense, fibrous membrane that covers the outer surface of long bones except at the joint surfaces of the epiphyses, where articular cartilage forms the covering. The periosteal membrane is composed of an outer fibrous layer and a deep, more cellular layer close to the bone surface. Many of the periosteum's outer fibers (Sharpey's fibers) penetrate the underlying bone, welding these two structures together. In addition, muscle tendon fibers interlace with periosteal fibers, thereby anchoring muscles firmly to bone. The deep cellular layer of the periosteum contains numerous blood vessels and bone-forming cells called osteoblasts. These specialized cells are essential for normal bone growth and for repair of bones after an injury. Blood vessels pass from the deep cellular layer of the periosteum to supply nutrients to both bone and marrow. This fact helps explain the very serious nature of periosteal avulsion injuries. If the periosteum is stripped from bone as a result of injury, the resulting decrease in blood supply may cause death of underlying and adjacent bone. Such injuries are often more serious in terms of potential for bone loss than fractures.

Marrow (medullary) cavity

The *marrow cavity* is a tubelike hollow in the diaphysis of long bones. In the adult it contains yellow or fatty marrow.

Endosteum

The endosteum is a fibrous membrane that lines the marrow cavity of long bones. Specialized bone-destroying cells, called osteoclasts, are found in this membrane. During the growth years, maintenance of appropriate shape and proportion in long bones is possible only by constant remodeling. Concomitant activity of bone-building (osteoblast) cells in the periosteum and bone-destroying (osteoclast) cells in the endosteum is required. As osteoblasts add bone to the diaphysis under the periosteum, osteoclasts excavate the marrow cavity proportionately. The result is maintenance of a relatively constant relationship between the circumference of the shaft and the diameter of the marrow cavity.

BONE MARKINGS

All bones exhibit surface markings that, if identified correctly, can provide a wealth of useful and functional information. Bone markings are functional in the sense that they provide information concerning the relationships that exist between bones, joints, muscles, tendons, blood vessels, nerves, and the body as a whole. Examples include markings that help to join one bone to another, to provide for attachment of muscles, or to serve as passageways for blood vessels or nerves. Bone markings that can be felt or palpated through the skin are especially useful to the athletic trainer in assessment of injury.

In many cases the location of a specific "externally palpable bony landmark" is one of the first steps in the assessment process. Instruction in the location and identification of these unique skeletal landmarks will occur as assessment techniques are presented in subsequent chapters of the text. The medial and lateral condyles at the lower end of the femur are good examples of such landmarks. Both condyles articulate with the tibia to form the knee joint and often serve as points of reference during assessment of injury in this area.

Although the anatomic terms used to describe bone markings are not always consistent, they

Table 3-1. Bone markings

Marking	Description	Example
PROCESSES (including elevations and projections)		
Processes that form joints		
Head	A rounded projection beyond a narrow neckline	Head of femur
Condyle	A rounded projection that usually articulates with another bone	Medial or lateral condyle of femur
Facet	A small flat or nearly flat surface	Articular facet of a vertebra
Processes to which muscles, tendons, or ligaments attach		
Tubercle	A small, rounded projection	Rib tubercles
Tuberosity	A large, rounded projection	Ischial tuberosity of hipbone
Trochanter	A very large projection	Greater trochanter of femur
Spine (spinous process)	A sharp, slender projection	Spinous process of vertebra
Epicondyle	A projection located above a condyle	Medial epicondyle of humerus
Crest	A prominent, narrow, ridgelike projection on a bone	Iliac crest of hipbone
Line	A ridge of bone less prominent than a crest	Linea aspera of femur
Process	Any prominent projection	Mastoid process of temporal bone
Suture	A line of union between bones	Sagittal suture between parietal bones of skull
Cavities (depressions) (including openings and grooves)		
Fossa	A hollow or depression	Mandibular fossa of temporal bone
Sinus	A cavity or hollow space within a bone	Frontal sinus
Foramen	A hole in a bone	Foramen magnum in base of skull
Meatus	A tubelike passageway within a bone	External auditory meatus of temporal bone
Sulcus (groove)	A furrow or groovelike depression on a bone	Intertubercular groove of humerus
Fovea	A very small pit or depression	Fovea capitis of femur

can be divided into two groups: (1) *processes* (including elevations and projections), and (2) *cavities* or depressions (including openings and grooves). Table 3-1 describes and gives examples of many terms in common use.

If available, an articulated skeleton will prove to be especially useful as you complete this chapter. If skeletal material is not routinely available for study, ready access to a well-illustrated reference textbook of anatomy is recommended.

ORGANIZATION OF THE SKELETON

The 206 bones of the adult skeleton are grouped into two subdivisions, namely, the axial skeleton (80 bones) and the appendicular skeleton (126 bones). The axial skeleton includes 6 tiny middle ear bones and the 74 bones that form the upright axis of the body, including the skull, vertebral column, and thorax (sternum and ribs). The 126 bones of the appendicular skeleton form the appendages and girdles that attach them to the axial skeleton. Included are the bones in the shoulder girdles, arms, wrists, and hands and the bones in the hip girdles, legs, ankles, and feet. Bones in each component of the axial and appendicular subdivisions of the skeleton are listed in Tables 3-2 and 3-3.

Locate as many of the major bones of the axial and appendicular subdivisions of the skeleton listed in Tables 3-2 and 3-3 as you can in Figs. 3-2 and 3-3.

Table 3-2. Bones in the axial division of the skeleton

Area	Number of bones
Skull	
Cranium	8
Face	14
	22
Vertebral column	
Cervical vertebrae	7
Thoracic vertebrae	12
Lumbar vertebrae	5
Sacrum	1 (5 fused bones)
Coccyx	1 (3 to 5 fused bones)
	26
Sternum	1 (3 fused bones)
Manubrium	
Body	
Xiphoid process	
Ribs	12 pairs
Hyoid	1
Ear ossicles	
Malleus	2
Incus	2
Stapes	2
	6
TOTAL	80 Bones

Table 3-3. Bones in the appendicular division of the skeleton

Area	Number of bones
Shoulder girdle	
Clavicle	2
Scapula	2
	4
Upper extremities	
Humerus	2
Ulna	2
Radius	2
Carpals	16
Metacarpals	10
Phalanges	28
	60
Hip girdle	
Os coxae	2
Lower extremities	
Femur	2
Fibula	2
Tibia	2
Patella	2
Tarsals	14
Metatarsals	10
Phalanges	28
	60
TOTAL	126 Bones

Fig. 3-2. Skeleton, anterior view.

Fig. 3-3. Skeleton, posterior view.

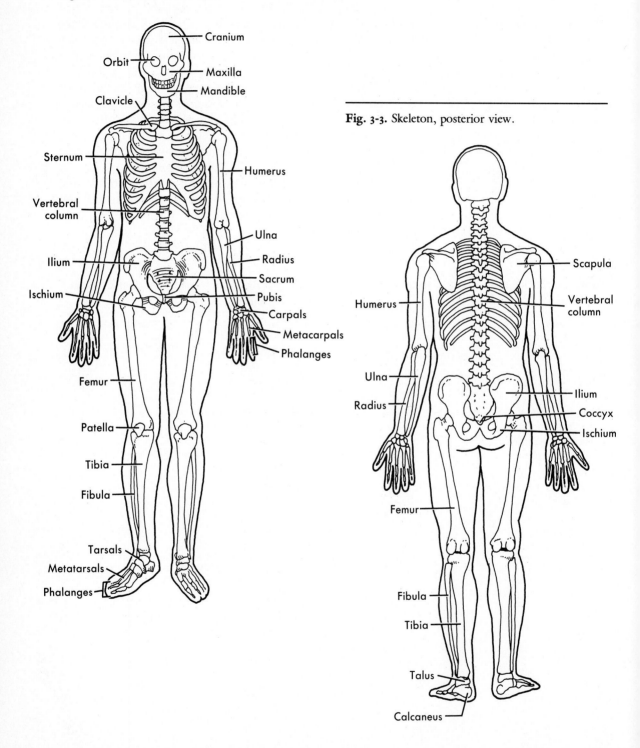

Fig. 3-4. Skull viewed from the front.

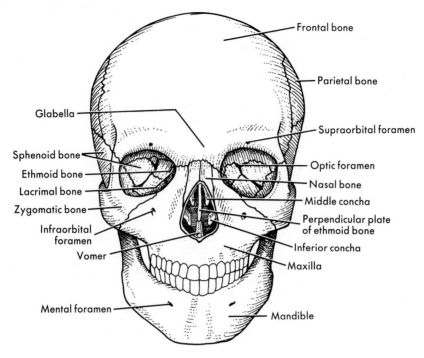

Frontal bone

Parietal bone

Glabella

Supraorbital foramen

Sphenoid bone

Optic foramen

Ethmoid bone

Nasal bone

Lacrimal bone

Middle concha

Zygomatic bone

Perpendicular plate of ethmoid bone

Infraorbital foramen

Inferior concha

Vomer

Maxilla

Mental foramen

Mandible

Fig. 3-5. Skull viewed from the right side.

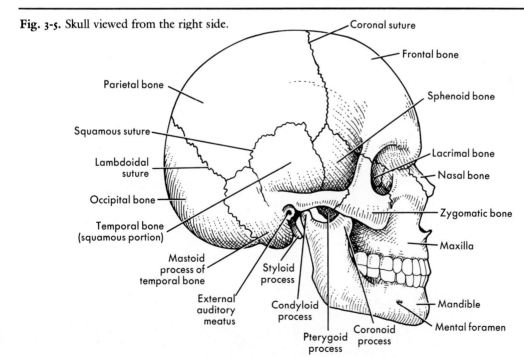

Coronal suture

Frontal bone

Parietal bone

Sphenoid bone

Squamous suture

Lacrimal bone

Lambdoidal suture

Nasal bone

Occipital bone

Zygomatic bone

Temporal bone (squamous portion)

Maxilla

Mastoid process of temporal bone

Styloid process

External auditory meatus

Condyloid process

Mandible

Mental foramen

Pterygoid process

Coronoid process

Axial skeleton

Skull

Twenty-two bones form the skull (Figs. 3-4 to 3-6). It consists of two major divisions: the cranium or brain case (8 bones) and the face (14 bones). For convenience the six ear ossicles are classified in Table 3-2 as part of the axial skeleton. They are, however, generally considered by anatomists as a separate group of bones rather than as a component of the skull proper. The single, U-shaped hyoid bone lies just below the skull, imbedded in the musculature of the tongue. The hyoid is the only bone in the body that does not articulate with any other bone. Names, locations, and brief descriptions of the cranial bones, face bones, ear ossicles, and hyoid are given in Table 3-4.

Fig. 3-6. Floor of the cranial cavity.

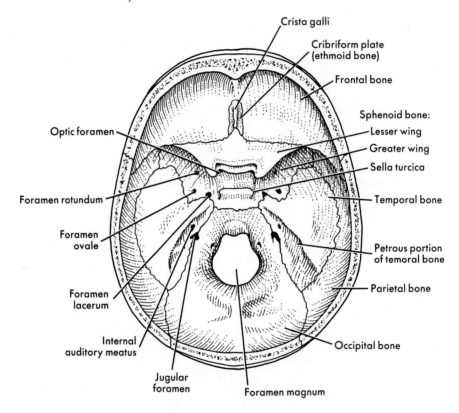

Table 3-4. Bones of the skull, including ear ossicles and hyoid bone

Name	Number	Description
CRANIAL BONES		
Frontal	1	Forehead bone; also forms front part of floor of cranium and most of upper part of eye sockets; cavity inside bone above upper margins of eye sockets (orbits) called *frontal sinus;* lined with mucous membrane
Parietal	2	Form bulging topsides of cranium
Temporal	2	Form lower sides of cranium; contain *middle* and *inner ear structures; mastoid sinuses* are mucosa-lined spaces in *mastoid process,* the protuberance behind ear; *external auditory canal* is tube leading into temporal bone
Occipital	1	Forms back of skull; spinal cord enters cranium through large hole *(foramen magnum)* in occipital bone
Sphenoid	1	Forms central part of floor of cranium; pituitary gland located in small depression sphenoid called sella turcica *(Turkish saddle)*
Ethmoid	1	Complicated bone that helps form floor of cranium, side walls and roof of nose and part of its middle partition (nasal septum), and part of orbit; contains honeycomb-like spaces, the *ethmoid sinuses; superior* and *middle turbinate bones* (conchae) are projections of ethmoid bone; form ledges along side wall of each nasal cavity
FACIAL BONES		
Nasal	2	Small bones that form upper part of bridge of nose
Maxillary	2	Upper jawbones; also help form roof of mouth, floor, and side walls of nose and floor of orbit; large cavity in maxillary bone is *maxillary sinus*
Zygoma (malar)	2	Cheek bones; also help form orbit
Mandible	1	Lower jawbone
Lacrimal	2	Small bone; helps form medial wall of eye socket and side wall of nasal cavity
Palatine	2	Form back part of roof of mouth and floor and side walls of nose and part of floor of orbit
Inferior turbinate	2	Form curved "ledge" along inside of side wall of nose, below middle turbinate
Vomer	1	Forms lower, back part of nasal septum
EAR OSSICLES		
Malleus	2	Malleus, incus, and stapes are tiny bones in middle ear cavity in temporal bone; malleus means "hammer"—shape of bone
Incus	2	Incus means "anvil"—shape of bone
Stapes	2	Stapes means "stirrup"—shape of bone
HYOID BONE	1	U-shaped bone in neck at base of tongue

Vertebral column

The vertebral column (backbone or spine) of an adult consists of 26 separate bony segments or vertebrae. They form a strong, flexible, curved column that extends from the base of the skull above to the bony pelvis below. Individual vertebrae are named and numbered according to their location (Fig. 3-7). There are seven cervical vertebrae in the neck region, twelve thoracic vertebrae behind the chest or thorax, five lumbar vertebrae in the small of the back, and a single sacrum and coccyx. The cervical, thoracic, and lumbar vertebrae are often called "true" or movable vertebrae, whereas the sacral and coccygeal portions of the spine are referred to as "false" or fixed vertebrae.

Note in Fig. 3-7 that four curves can be identified in the normal vertebral column when it is viewed from the side. Located in the cervical, thoracic, lumbar, and sacral regions of the spine, these curves increase both the strength and resilience of the column and help to maintain balance in the upright position. In addition to serving as an axis for bearing weight, the vertebrae surround and protect the spinal cord and emerging spinal nerves (Table 3-5).

Thorax (sternum and ribs)

The thorax (Fig. 3-8) is a bony, cagelike structure that resembles a flattened cone in shape, being broad below and quite narrow on top. It is formed by the sternum and costal cartilages anteriorly, the ribs laterally, and the thoracic vertebrae posteriorly. The floor of the thorax is formed by the diaphragm. The thorax encloses and protects the lungs, heart, and other life-sustaining structures of the chest cavity. It also supports the bones of both shoulder girdles and the upper extremities (Table 3-5).

Sternum. The dagger-shaped sternum (Fig. 3-8) consists of three parts: the upper "handle" portion or manubrium; the middle "blade" portion, the body or gladiolus; and a lower tip called the xiphoid process.

Ribs. There are 12 pairs of ribs in humans (Fig. 3-8). The first seven pairs (1 through 7) are called true or *vertebrosternal* ribs because they articulate *directly* with the sternum through their costal cartilages. The remaining five pairs of ribs (8 through 12) are called false ribs. The eighth, ninth, and tenth rib pairs are also referred to as *vertebrochondral* ribs because they articulate with the sternum *indirectly* by fusion of their costal cartilages to the cartilages of the rib pairs above them. The eleventh and twelfth rib pairs do not articulate in any way with the sternum. They are called "floating ribs."

Fig. 3-7. Lateral view of the vertebral column.

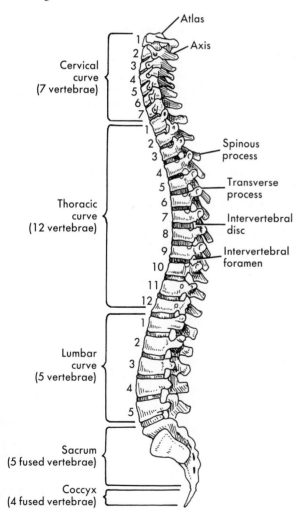

Atlas

Axis

Cervical curve (7 vertebrae)
1
2
3
4
5
6
7

Thoracic curve (12 vertebrae)
1
2
3
4
5
6
7
8
9
10
11
12

Spinous process

Transverse process

Intervertebral disc

Intervertebral foramen

Lumbar curve (5 vertebrae)
1
2
3
4
5

Sacrum (5 fused vertebrae)

Coccyx (4 fused vertebrae)

Table 3-5. Bones of the vertebral column and thorax

Name	Number	Description
VERTEBRAL COLUMN		
Cervical vertebrae	7	Upper seven vertebrae, in neck region; first cervical vertebra called *atlas;* second called *axis*
Thoracic vertebrae	12	Next twelve vertebrae; ribs attach to these
Lumbar vertebrae	5	Next five vertebrae; those in small of back
Sacrum	1	In child, five separate vertebrae; in adult, fused into one
Coccyx	1	In child, three to five separate vertebrae; in adult fused into one
THORAX		
True ribs	14	Upper seven pairs; attach to sternum by way of *costal cartilages*
False ribs	10	Lower five pairs; lowest two pairs do not attach to sternum, therefore, called *floating ribs;* next three pairs attach to sternum by way of costal cartilage of seventh ribs
Sternum	1	Breastbone; shaped like a dagger; piece of cartilage at lower end of bone called *xiphoid process*

Fig. 3-8. Anterior view of the thorax.

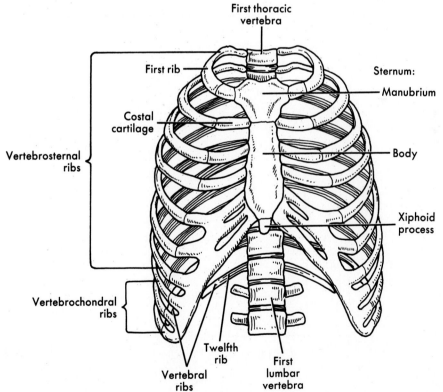

Appendicular skeleton
Shoulder girdle and upper extremities

The shoulder girdles are formed by two pairs of bones, the clavicles (collar bones) in front and the scapulae (shoulder blades) behind. Together, these bones serve to attach each upper extremity to the axial skeleton. The mechanism of attachment that exists between the shoulder girdles, upper extremities and axial skeleton provides for maximal mobility. As you learn to assess injury in this area, the price paid for this high degree of mobility (frequent fractures and joint disarticulations) will become apparent. It should be stressed that the articulation between clavicle and sternum (sternoclavicular joint) is the only bony joint that exists between the shoulder girdle and the axial skeleton (Fig. 3-9). For the athletic trainer this is an extremely important and practical anatomic fact. It helps to explain the high incidence of clavicular fractures in contact sports, especially those that occur when an athlete uses the arm to break a fall.

Each upper extremity is attached to the shoulder girdle by articulation between the head of the humerus and the scapula. There is no direct bony articulation between the axial skeleton and the upper extremities. Each upper extremity contains 30 bones and consists of the humerus (brachium or upper arm), radius and ulna (fore-

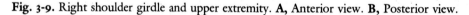

Fig. 3-9. Right shoulder girdle and upper extremity. **A,** Anterior view. **B,** Posterior view.

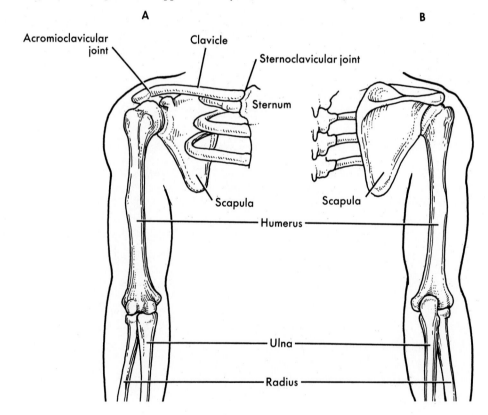

Table 3-6. Bones of the upper extremities

Name	Number	Description
UPPER EXTREMITIES		
Clavicle	2	Collarbones; only joints between shoulder girdle and axial skeleton are those between each clavicle and sternum
Scapula	2	Shoulder bones; scapula plus clavicle forms *shoulder girdle; acromion process*—tip of shoulder that forms joint with clavicle; *glenoid cavity*—arm socket
Humerus	2	Upper arm bone
Radius	2	Bone on thumb side of lower arm
Ulna	2	Bone on little finger side of lower arm; *olecranon process*—projection of ulna known as elbow or "funny bone"
Carpal bones	16	Irregular bones at upper end of hand; anatomic wrist
Metacarpals	10	Form framework of palm of hand
Phalanges	28	Finger bones; three in each finger, two in each thumb

Fig. 3-10. Right humerus and elbow joint in **A,** anterior view and **B,** posterior view.

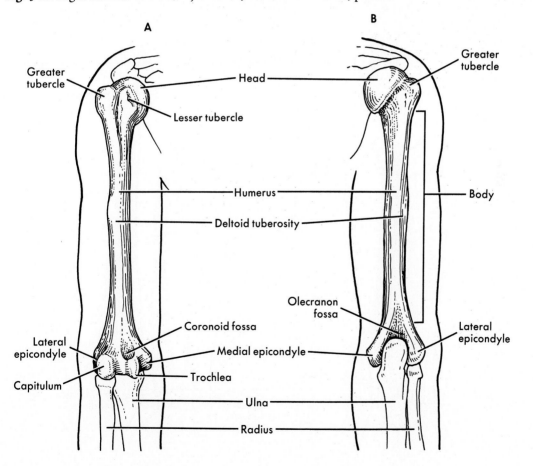

arm), carpals (wrist), metacarpals (palm), and phalanges (fingers and thumb). Table 3-6 includes the name, location, and a brief description of these bones.

Humerus (Fig. 3-10). The humerus is the largest and longest bone of the upper extremity. It forms the bony framework of the upper arm (brachium). The humerus articulates with the scapula proximally and with both the radius and ulna distally.

Radius and ulna (Fig. 3-11). The radius is located on the thumb or lateral side of the forearm. It articulates with the humerus proximally and with the carpals of the wrist distally. Its companion, the ulna, is found on the little finger or medial side of the forearm. It also articulates with the humerus proximally but distally it articulates with a fibrocartilaginous disc and not with the carpal bones of the wrist directly.

Carpals, metacarpals, and phalanges (Fig. 3-12). The eight carpal or wrist bones are arranged in two irregular rows, each containing four bones. Only the pisiform is easily identifiable. It projects posteriorly from the little finger or medial side of the wrist. The pisiform is a good example of an externally palpable bony landmark.

In the anatomic position the arms are at the sides, with the palms of the hands turned forward (Fig. 2-5). In this position the five metacarpals that make up the framework of the palm

Fig. 3-11. Right ulna and radius. **A,** Anterior view and **B,** posterior view.

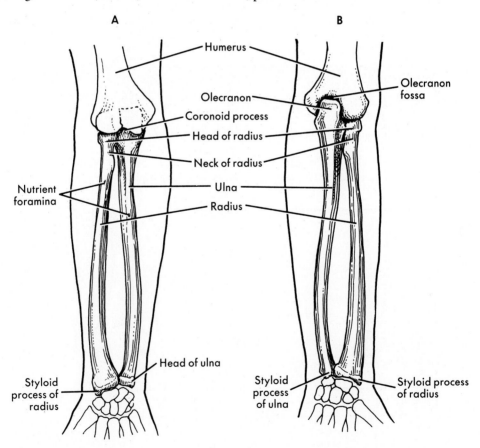

of the hand are numbered in ascending order. Metacarpal number 1 is found on the most lateral or thumb side of the hand; metacarpal number 5 is the most medial and articulates with the little finger. The phalanges form the bony framework of the fingers and thumb. There are 14 phalanges in each hand—three in each finger and two in the thumb.

Hip girdle and lower extremities (Fig. 3-13)

Strong ligaments bind the right and left hip bones (os coxae or innominate bones) together to form the hip or pelvic girdle. The hip girdle is a circular base that supports the trunk and, unlike the shoulder girdle, serves as a very stable point of attachment for the lower extremities. Although athletic trainers deal with shoulder disarticulations all too frequently, a dislocated hip is seldom seen as a result of athletic injury. The mechanism of attachment that exists between the hip girdle, lower extremities, and axial skeleton provides for *maximum stability*. The lower extremities are very firmly attached to the hip girdle on each side by articulation between the head of the femur and a deep, cup-shaped depression in each innominate (hip) bone called the acetabulum.

Each lower extremity contains 30 bones and consists of the femur (thigh or leg bone), patella (kneecap), tibia and fibula (lower leg), tarsals

Fig. 3-12. Right wrist and hand. **A,** Dorsal view and **B,** palmar view.

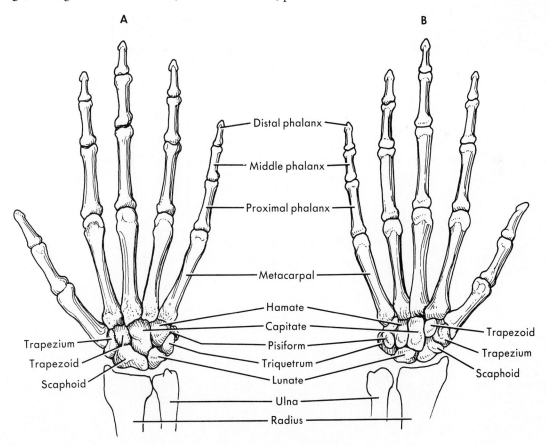

A

B

Distal phalanx

Middle phalanx

Proximal phalanx

Metacarpal

Hamate
Capitate
Pisiform
Triquetrum
Lunate
Ulna
Radius

Trapezium
Trapezoid
Scaphoid

Trapezoid
Trapezium
Scaphoid

(ankle), metatarsals (foot), and phalanges (toes). Table 3-7 includes names, locations, and brief descriptions of these bones.

Femur (Fig. 3-14). The thighbone, or femur, is the longest and one of the strongest bones in the skeleton. Located between the hip and knee, it articulates above with the acetabular socket in each innominate and below with the tibia and patella, or kneecap.

Tibia and fibula (Fig. 3-15). The tibia, or shin bone, is the larger, stronger, and more medially and superficially located of the two lower leg bones. Because of its superficial location, the tibia is often subjected to painful "bone bruises."

Fig. 3-13. Right pelvic girdle and lower extremity. **A,** Anterior view; **B,** posterior view.

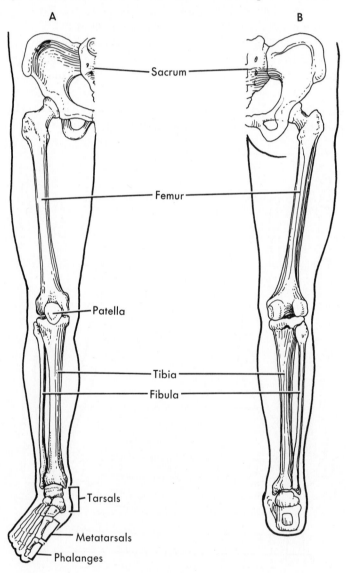

A   B

- Sacrum
- Femur
- Patella
- Tibia
- Fibula
- Tarsals
- Metatarsals
- Phalanges

The upper (proximal) end or epiphysis of the tibia expands to form two condyles that articulate with and bear the weight transmitted by the femur. The fibula is parallel with the tibia but does not enter into formation of the knee joint and is not a weight-bearing bone of the lower leg. The distal epiphysis of the fibula projects downward into a pointed process called the lateral malleolus. It is this process that forms the prominent outer surface of the ankle.

Tarsals, metatarsals, and phalanges (Fig. 3-16). The basic structure of the ankle and foot is similar in many ways to that of the wrist and hand. The most prominent structural differences noted in the ankle and foot are adaptations that increase stability or provide a strong base for support of weight. The largest and strongest of the seven tarsal bones is called the calcaneus, or heel bone. It is the calcaneus that transmits the weight of the body to the ground. The bones of the feet are held together in such a way as to form springy lengthwise and crosswise arches. Strong ligaments and leg muscle tendons normally hold the foot bones firmly in these arched positions. Unfortunately, these arches sometimes weaken, causing a condition aptly called fallen arches or flatfeet.

Note in Fig. 3-16 that the tarsal bones consist of cuneiforms (three), navicular, talus, cuboid, and calcaneus. The five metatarsals of the foot are numbered from medial to lateral, with the first metatarsal extending to the base of the great toe. The tarsals and metatarsals play the major role in the function of the foot as a supporting structure, with the phalanges being relatively unimportant. The reverse is true for the hand. Recall that in the hand, manipulation (mobility) is the main function rather than support; consequently, the phalanges are of primary importance, the carpals and metacarpals being secondary.

DIFFERENCES BETWEEN MALE AND FEMALE SKELETONS

Both general and specific differences exist between male and female skeletons. The general difference is one of size and weight, the male skeleton being larger and heavier. Examples of

Table 3-7. Bones of the lower extremities

Name	Number	Description
LOWER EXTREMITIES		
Pelvic bones	2	Hipbones; *ilium*—upper flaring part of pelvic bone; *ischium*—lower back part; *pubic bone*—lower front part; acetabulum—hip socket; *symphysis pubis*—joint in midline between two pubic bones; pelvic inlet—opening into *true pelvis,* or pelvic cavity; if pelvic inlet is misshapen or too small, infant skull cannot enter true pelvis for natural birth
Femur	2	Thigh or upper leg bones; *head of femur*—ball-shaped upper end of bone; fits into acetabulum
Patella	2	Kneecap
Tibia	2	Shinbone; *medial malleolus*—rounded projection at lower end of tibia commonly called inner anklebone
Fibula	2	Long slender bone of lateral side of lower leg; *lateral malleolus*—rounded projection at lower end of fibula commonly called outer anklebone
Tarsal bones	14	Form heel and back part of foot; anatomic ankle
Metatarsals	10	Form part of foot to which toes attach; tarsal and metatarsal bones so arranged that they form three arches in foot; *inner longitudinal arch* and *outer longitudinal arch,* both of which extend from front to back of foot, and transverse or *metatarsal arch* that extends across foot
Phalanges	28	Toe bones; three in each toe, two in each great toe

Fig. 3-14. Right femur showing proximal (hip) and distal (knee) articulations. **A,** Anterior view; **B,** posterior view.

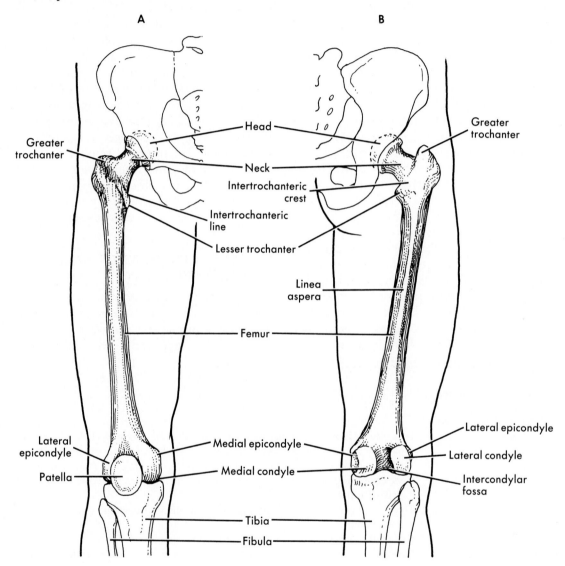

Fig. 3-15. Right tibia and fibula. **A,** Anterior view; **B,** posterior view.

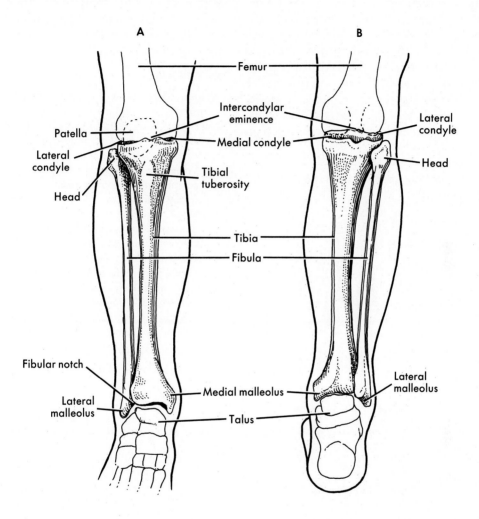

A

B

Femur

Intercondylar eminence

Lateral condyle

Patella

Medial condyle

Head

Lateral condyle

Head

Tibial tuberosity

Tibia

Fibula

Fibular notch

Medial malleolus

Lateral malleolus

Lateral malleolus

Talus

specific differences include the angle of articulation between certain bones in the extremities and the angle of attachment of the extremities as a whole to their respective girdles. There are also marked sex differences in the pelvis. The male pelvis is deep and funnel-shaped, whereas the female pelvis is shallow, broad, and flaring. The wider pelvis in the female results in a greater inward slant of the thighs from the hips to the knees. In general, the bones of the lower extremity in the male tend to be longer than in a female with a torso of the same length. Those skeletal differences important to mastering assessment techniques are highlighted and explained in subsequent chapters.

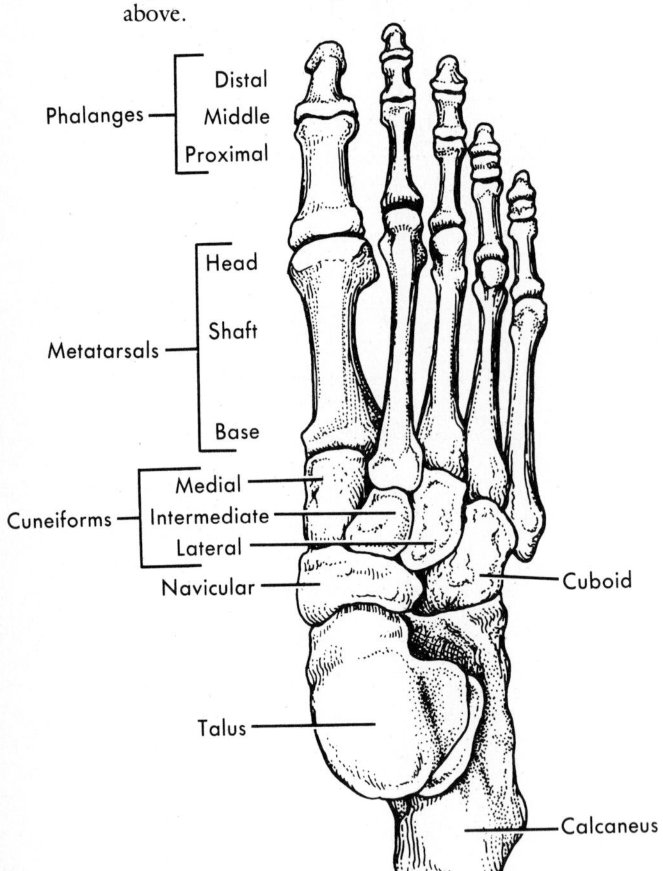

KEY TERMS

cavities Depressions, openings, and grooves within bones

diaphysis Long shaftlike portion of a bone

endosteum Fibrous membrane that lines the marrow cavity of long bones

epiphyseal (growth) plates Thin plates of cartilage separating the diaphysis from each epiphysis in growing bones

epiphyses Extremities or ends of long bones

hemopoiesis Process of blood cell formation

hyaline (articular) cartilage Thin layer of gristle-like material firmly fixed to layer of compact bone covering joint surfaces of epiphyses

marrow (medullary) cavity Tubelike hollow in diaphysis of long bones

periosteum Dense fibrous membrane covering outer surface of long bones except at joint surfaces

processes Prominences and projections on bones

SUGGESTED READINGS

Beck, E.W.: Mosby's atlas of concise functional human anatomy, St. Louis, 1982, The C.V. Mosby Co.

Bourne, G.W., editor: The biochemistry and physiology of bone, ed. 2, New York, 1972, Academic Press, Inc.

Crafts, R.C.: A textbook of human anatomy, ed. 2, New York 1979, Wiley-Interscience.

Evans, F.G., editor: Studies in the anatomy and function of bones and joints, New York, 1966, Springer-Verlag New York, 1979, Wiley-Interscience.

Garn, S.: Bone loss and aging. In Garn, S.: The physiology and pathology of human aging, New York, 1975, Academic Press, Inc.

Hogan, L., and Beland, I.: Cervical spine syndrome, Am. J. Nurs. **76:**1104-1107, 1976.

Romanes, G.J.: Cunningham's textbook of anatomy, ed. 12, London, 1981, Oxford University Press.

Zuidema, G.D., editor: The Johns Hopkins atlas of human functional anatomy, ed. 2, Baltimore, 1980, The Johns Hopkins University Press.

Fig. 3-16. Bones of right foot viewed from above.

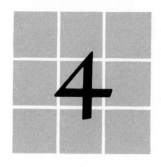

4 Arthrology

Arthrology is a specialized area of anatomy that deals with the study and description of joints or articulations. By definition a joint or articulation exists where two or more skeletal components, whether bone or cartilage, come together or meet. For the athletic trainer the practical importance of acquiring a basic understanding of arthrology cannot be overemphasized. This information is important in understanding how joints normally function and in providing a basis for understanding the nature of joint injuries. Athletes are almost universally characterized by an ability to execute complex, highly coordinated, and purposeful movements. Without joints between bones the controlled and graceful movement of the athlete would be impossible; the body would be a rigid, immobile

hulk. Simply stated, it is the existence of joints between bones that makes movement of body parts possible. This chapter provides an overview of the classification, structure, and function of joints or articulations. The anatomy of individual joints is presented in subsequent chapters of the text and precedes discussion of techniques employed in the assessment of specific joint injuries.

CLASSIFICATION OF JOINTS

Joints are classified into three major groups or types using either structural features or potential for movement as distinguishing criteria (Table 4-1). For the athletic trainer, a system of joint classification using degree of movement is clearly the more functional and appropriate method.

On this basis, three joint classes can be identified: *synarthroses* (immovable joints), *amphiarthroses* (slightly movable joints), and *diarthroses* (freely movable joints). If structural criteria are used for classification, these three joint classes are called, in the same order, fibrous, cartilaginous, and synovial.

Synarthroses

There are three basic types of synarthrotic, or immovable, joints (Fig. 4-1).

Syndesmosis

This type of synarthrotic joint is characterized by the presence of a dense fibrous membrane

Table 4-1. Primary joint classification

Functional name	Structural name	Degree of movement permitted	Example
Synarthroses	Fibrous	Immovable	Sutures of skull
Amphiarthroses	Cartilaginous	Slightly movable	Pubic symphysis
Diarthroses	Synovial	Freely movable	Shoulder joint

Fig. 4-1. Types of synarthrotic joints. **A,** Suture (coronal suture); **B,** Gomphosis (root of tooth in socket); **C,** Syndesmosis (distal tibiofibular articulation).

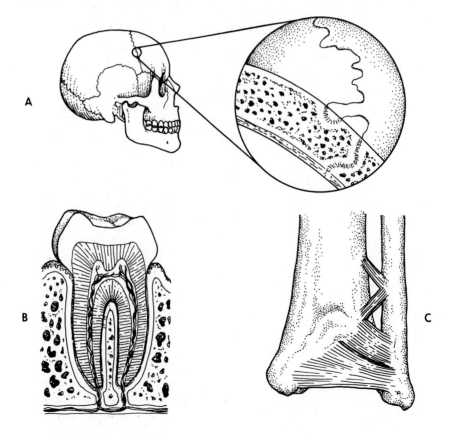

that binds the articular bone surfaces very closely and tightly to each other. Ligaments play an important role in restriction of movement in these joints. The articulation between the distal ends of the tibia and fibula is a good example of a syndesmosis.

Suture

True sutures are found only in the skull. As a group, sutures are not characterized by the substantial fibrous membranes or dense ligaments seen in syndesmoses. Instead, the adjoining bone margins are united into rigid, immovable joints by a series of jagged, interlocking processes. The sagittal suture between the two parietal bones of the skull is a good example of this joint type.

Gomphosis

By definition a gomphosis is a synarthrotic or fibrous joint in which a conical peg or projection fits into a socket. Articulations between the roots of the teeth and sockets of the jaw bones are the only examples of this type of joint in the body. The fibrous type of membrane found between the root of the tooth and its socket is called the *peridontal membrane.* Successful replacement of teeth that have been knocked out as a result of injury is possible if this membrane remains relatively undamaged.

Amphiarthroses

Slightly movable joints, or *amphiarthroses,* have a pad of either hyaline or fibrocartilage located between adjoining bony surfaces. There are two types of amphiarthrotic joints (Fig. 4-2).

Synchrondrosis

In this type of joint a pad of hyaline cartilage joins one bone to another. Examples of synchondroses are the joints between rib pairs 1 through 10 and the sternum.

Fig. 4-2. Types of amphiarthrotic joints. **A,** Synchondroses (articulation between true ribs and sternum); **B,** Symphyses (symphysis pubis).

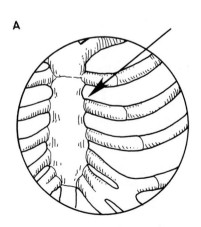

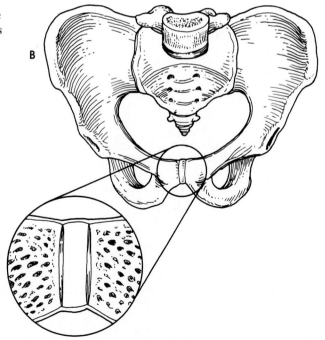

Symphysis

Symphyses are articulations, generally located in the midline of the body, that have a pad of fibrocartilage between opposing bone surfaces. The pubic symphysis, the midline joint between the two hipbones in front (anteriorly), is an example of this type of joint.

Diarthroses

Diarthrotic (freely movable) joints are often called *synovial joints* because they are characterized by the presence of a closed cavity, called the synovial or joint cavity, between the bones. As a group, the diarthrotic or synovial joints include by far the majority of the body's articulations. Because they are the most mobile of the three types of joints, they are functionally the most important. They also have the most complex structure and are most vulnerable to athletic injuries.

Structural features

Refer to Fig. 4-3 to identify the following structural features of synovial joints.

Fibrous joint capsule

In movable joints a tough but flexible sleeve-like structure called the joint capsule helps to hold the articulating bones together. The capsule encloses a space or cleft that exists between the opposing bone surfaces. Note in Fig. 4-3 that the joint capsule consists of two layers: a tough, fibrous, outer layer called the fibrous capsule of the joint and a more cellular inner layer called the synovial membrane. Fibers in the outer layer of the joint capsule run in different directions to form a dense tubular structure that connects the periosteal membrane of one bone in the joint to that of the other. The resulting fibrous layer of the capsule has great tensile strength that completely encases the ends of the bones and binds them to each other. This structure is uniquely constructed to resist shearing forces that would otherwise result in dislocation (luxation) of opposing bone surfaces at the joint. The term "subluxation" is sometimes used to describe partial dislocations that occur if the capsule is stretched but not torn. At points of recurring stress in the capsule, fibers may become ori-

---

Fig. 4-3. Section through diarthrotic joints, **A,** without, and **B,** with an intervening articular disc in the joint cavity.

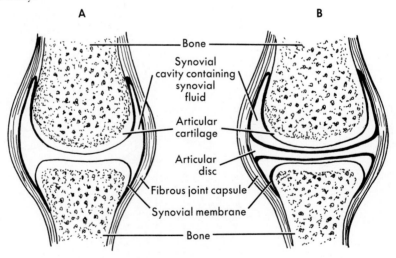

A   B

Bone
Synovial cavity containing synovial fluid
Articular cartilage
Articular disc
Fibrous joint capsule
Synovial membrane
Bone

ented in definite parallel bands to form *intracapsular ligaments*. These structures provide additional stability and help bind the bones together.

Synovial membrane

The deep, or cellular, layer of the joint capsule forms the moist and slippery synovial membrane. It lines the joint space between opposing bones and, as Fig. 4-3 shows, attaches to the margins of the articular cartilage. Functionally, the synovial membrane secretes synovial fluid, or synovia, which serves to lubricate the joint and provide nourishment for the articular cartilage. The term "synovial" is from the Latin word meaning "with egg" because it resembles egg white in consistency and appearance. Synovial fluid will vary in amount from less than 0.1 ml to over 3.0 ml in different joints of the body. Quantity depends on both joint size and potential for movement.

Articular cartilage

In Chapter 3 the presence of a specialized type of articular cartilage was included as one of six anatomic features common to long bones as a group. Articular, or *hyaline,* cartilage (Fig. 4-4) is a unique type of connective tissue. It consists of specialized cells called *chondrocytes* and a firm, gellike intercellular matrix. Note in Fig. 4-4 that very few fibers are present in hyaline cartilage and that the chondrocytes reside in little spaces called *lacunae.* The intercellular matrix that surrounds the chondrocytes is similar to a fairly firm, smooth, plastic and, if kept lubricated, is superbly adapted for coating the articulating ends (epiphyses) of bones in movable joints. Tough collagenous fibers anchor articular cartilage to the underlying bone and adjacent periosteal membrane.

It is important to note that no blood vessels penetrate the gellike matrix of hyaline (articular) cartilage. It is said to be *avascular.* For cells in cartilage tissue to survive without a direct blood supply, nutrients and oxygen must pass through the matrix bed by diffusion from synovial fluid. Diffusion over such distances is a slow and generally inefficient way to transfer nutrients to cells. Indeed, in tissues other than cartilage it is

Fig. 4-4. Micrograph of hyaline cartilage. Note the absence of blood vessels in the gel-like matrix of this unique avascular tissue.
(From Anthony, C.P., and Thibodeau, G.A.: Textbook of anatomy and physiology, ed. 11, St. Louis, 1983, The C.V. Mosby Co.)

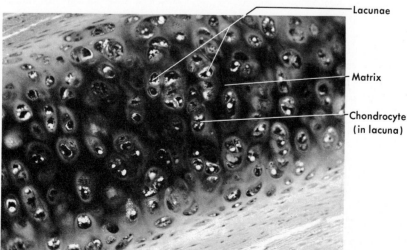

Lacunae

Matrix

Chondrocyte (in lacuna)

not possible to sustain cell life if the normal blood supply is cut off. It is the unique diffusion mechanism of nutrient transfer in cartilage, however, that explains how bits of this tissue that detach from articulating bone surfaces by injury not only survive but also grow and increase in size. These small but sometimes troublesome bits of cartilage derive their nutrients by diffusion from the synovial fluid in the joint space.

In addition to the thin layer of hyaline cartilage that covers the articulating bone surfaces in movable joints, pads of fibrocartilage may lie between the bones and divide the joint cavity (Fig. 4-3, *B*). These pads of fibrocartilage are called **articular discs,** or **menisci.** They provide an additional "cushion" between the articulating ends of the bones and help stabilize the joint. Fibrocartilage, as the name implies, contains a large number of collagenous fibers imbedded in the matrix than is typical of hyaline. The direct blood supply to fibrocartilage is little better, however, than that of the hyaline variety. Torn or damaged fibrocartilage in a joint quite often does not heal properly and must be removed by surgery. In most instances, only the damaged portion must be removed, thus saving as much of the structure as possible.

Types of diarthroses

Diarthrotic (synovial) joints are grouped or subdivided on the basis of (1) the kind of movement each joint is capable of performing and (2) the shape of the surfaces of the adjacent articulating bones. Table 4-2 lists the six types of diarthroses that can be grouped into three categories according to axial movement.

Uniaxial joints. Uniaxial joints (Fig. 4-5) permit movement in only one plane and around a single axis. There are two types of uniaxial joints: *hinge* and *pivot.*

Hinge joints such as the elbow permit movement only about one axis, which passes through the joint from side to side. Only flexion and extension occur in hinge joints. Because they allow movement in only one plane, hinge joints are those most often involved in athletic injuries.

Typically, the single axis of *pivot* joints is vertical. In this type of uniaxial joint, movement is limited to rotation. In pivot joints a type of bony ring on one bone rotates around a pivot point on another bone. For example, the first cervical vertebra, or atlas, acts as a bony ring that rotates around a conical pivot process called the **dens** on the second cervical vertebra, or axis. This joint permits you to turn (rotate) your head from side to side.

Biaxial joints. In biaxial joints (Fig. 4-6), movement occurs in two planes and around two axes that are at right angles to each other. Flexion and extension are allowed around one axis and abduction and adduction around the second axis. There are two types of biaxial joints: *saddle* and *condyloid.*

The articular surface of one bone in a *saddle* joint is concave in one direction and convex in the other, whereas the articular surface of the remaining bone is exactly the opposite (Fig. 4-9, *A*). The opposing saddle-shaped surfaces fit neatly together, permitting flexion and extension around one axis and abduction and adduction around the other. The carpometacarpal joint at the base of the thumb is the only saddle joint in the body. Articulation occurs between

Table 4-2. Classification of diarthrotic or synovial joints

Axes of movement	Shape of articulating bone surfaces	Example
Uniaxial	Hinge	Elbow joint
	Pivot	Proximal radioulnar joint
Biaxial	Saddle	Joint between first (thumb) metacarpal and trapezium of wrist
	Condyloid	Joint between distal end of radius and carpal bones
Multiaxial	Ball-and-socket	Hip joint
	Gliding	Joints between carpal bones

Fig. 4-5. Uniaxial joints.
A, Hinge (elbow); **B,** Pivot
(atlantoaxial joint).

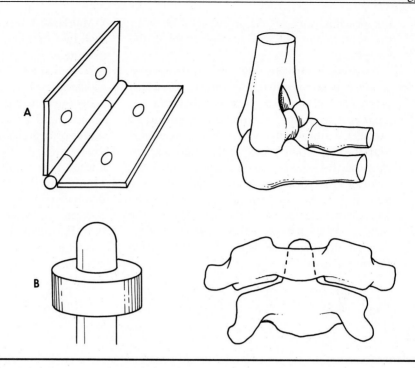

Fig. 4-6. Biaxial joints. **A,** Saddle (joint between first metacarpal and trapezium of wrist).
B, Condyloid (joint between distal end of radius and carpal bones).

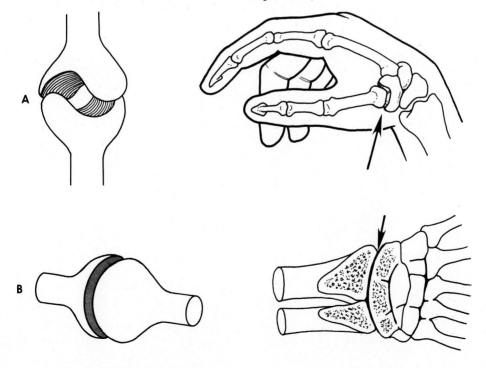

the proximal end of the metacarpal bone of the thumb and the carpal bone named the trapezium.

Condyloid joints are those in which an oval condyle fits into an elliptic socket or cavity. This type of articular surface permits angular movement in two planes, but no axial rotation. In short, it permits biaxial movement. The radius joins the carpal bones (scaphoid, lunate, and triquetrum) by means of a condyloid joint. Movements in the frontal plane are called radial and ulnar flexion. ***Radial flexion*** is movement at the wrist of the thumb side of the hand toward the forearm. ***Ulnar flexion*** is movement at the wrist of the little finger side of the hand toward the forearm.

Multiaxial joints. Multiaxial joints (Fig. 4-7) have two or more axes of rotation and permit movement in three or more planes. There are two types of multiaxial joints: *ball-and-socket* and *gliding*.

Ball-and-socket joints are those in which a ball-shaped head of one bone fits into a concave socket or depression of another bone. Of all the joints in our bodies, ball-and-socket joints permit the widest and freest range of movements in almost any direction or plane. Movements in this type of joint include flexion, extension, abduction, adduction, rotation, and circumduction. Examples are the shoulder and hip joints.

Gliding joints are numerous and almost always small. Articular surfaces in these joints are

Fig. 4-7. Multiaxial joints. **A,** Gliding (joints between carpal bones) and **B,** ball-and-socket (hip).

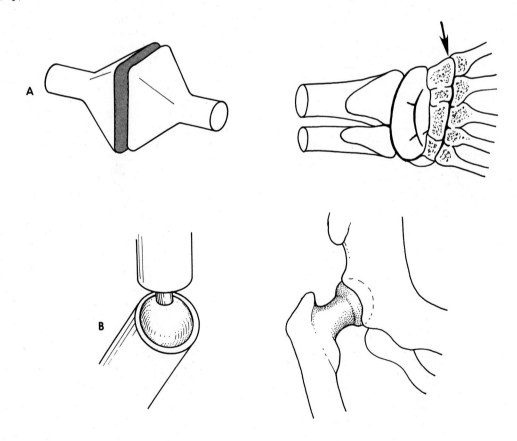

either flat, nearly flat, or slightly curved. They include most of the joints between both the carpal and tarsal bones and also all the joints between the articular processes of the vertebrae. These joints allow only the simplest kind of slight displacement motion between their articular surfaces. Gliding movements occur in all planes.

Range and type of movement in diarthroses
Range of motion (ROM)

Diarthrotic, or synovial, joints are often referred to as "freely movable joints." Such a description, of course, applies only to the normal direction and range of motion (ROM) available at any particular joint. Even for the most supple athlete there are distinct and necessary limitations to joint mobility.

In Chapter 9, four basic types of stress maneuvers, called active, resistive, passive, and functional movements, are discussed and included in the necessary sequence of steps required in assessment of joint injury. Correct interpretation of these important assessment steps requires knowledge of the normal type and range of motion available at the joint in the absence of injury.

The normal type and range of joint movements are influenced primarily by four factors: (1) the shape of the articular or joint surfaces; (2) the restraining effects of the joint capsule; (3) the number, type of attachment, and tautness of ligaments; and (4) the effect of muscles that may act as fixators to stabilize the joint. In addition, there is also frequent and sometimes considerable variation in the range of movement among individuals.

Repeated observations of ROM in both active and passive movements at a joint will prove helpful in visualizing the underlying anatomy. In active movements the athlete voluntarily moves a joint or body part through its pain-free ROM, and in passive movements the athletic trainer moves the part with the muscles relaxed. Normally, both active and passive range of motion maneuvers should be about equal.

Types of movement

Although we have the ability to perform a single movement at a single joint at one time, most coordinated types of body activity occur only as a result of simultaneous or successive movements at many joints. Articulating bones in synovial joints, acting in conjunction with other joints, are capable of moving in many directions, along different axes of rotation, and through different planes of reference in the body. The various types of combined joint movements that occur as a result of such activity can be categorized or grouped as follows (1) *angular* if there is a change in the angle between bones, (2) *rotation and circumduction* if there is movement of a bone around its own axis, (3) *gliding* if the only movement produced is simple displacement between articulating surfaces, and (4) *special* if the movement produced is so unique that it must be described individually.

Angular movements (Fig. 4-8)

Flexion decreases the size of the angle between the anterior or posterior surfaces of articulated bones. An exception to this definition is the shoulder joint. Shoulder flexion occurs as the arm is elevated forward in the sagittal plane. Flexing movements are bending or folding movements. Bending the head forward on the chest, for example, is flexion of the joint between the occipital bone at the base of the skull and the atlas, or first cervical vertebra. Bending the elbow, as when the forearm bends back on the arm, is another example of flexion.

Extension is the return from the flexed position and generally results in an increase of a joint angle. Whereas bending movements are flexion, straightening or stretching movements are extension. Most major joints are in extension when a person restores an extremity or body part from a flexed position to the anatomic position. Continuation of extension beyond the anatomic position is called *hyperextension.* Extension of the head, for example, means to return it to the upright anatomic position from the flexed position; hyperextension of the head would result in

Fig. 4-8. Examples of angular movements at synovial joints.

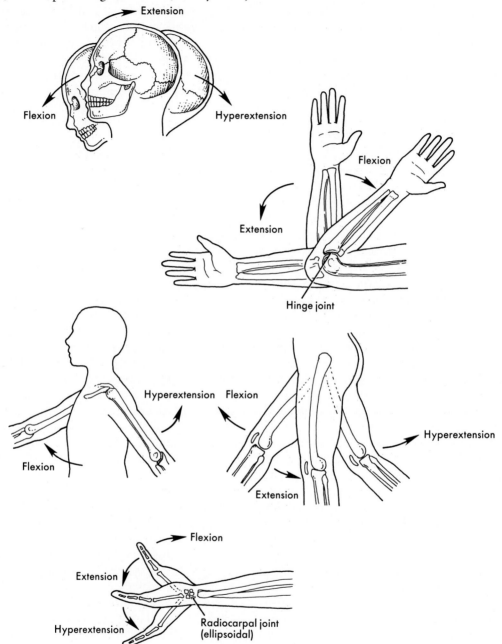

its being stretched backward from the upright position.

Flexion and extension of the ankle joint are termed plantar and dorsal flexion. ***Plantar flexion*** is movement of the sole of the foot downward, such as standing on your toes. ***Dorsiflexion*** is movement of the top (dorsum) of the foot upward.

Abduction is movement of a body part or extremity away from the midline or center of the body. An example of abduction is movement of the arm away from the body in the frontal plane. ***Horizonal abduction*** is movement of the upper limb through the transverse plane at shoulder level away from the midline of the body.

Adduction is the opposite of abduction. It moves the body part toward the midline or center of the body. An example would be bringing the arms back to the sides of the body from the abducted position. ***Horizontal adduction*** is movement of the upper limb through the transverse plane at shoulder level toward the midline of the body.

In discussing abduction and adduction of the fingers and toes the plane of reference is not the midline of the body but an imaginary line drawn through the midline finger or second toe. Movement of the fingers or toes away from these imaginary reference lines results in "spreading" movements or abduction. Movement of the fingers or toes toward these imaginary reference lines results in adduction.

Rotation and circumduction (Fig. 4-9)

Rotation is the pivoting of a bone on its own central or longitudinal axis, somewhat as a top turns on its axis. An example is holding your head in an upright position and turning it from one side to the other, as in saying no.

Circumduction is a composite movement that combines flexion, abduction, extension, and adduction. The result is rotational movement that causes the segment as a whole to describe a cone as it moves.

Gliding movements

Gliding is the simplest type of movement that can occur in movable joints and occurs to some degree in all of them. In some joints this type of slight relative displacement between adjoining bone surfaces is the only type of motion available. Gliding movements occur when one articulating bone surface in a joint moves over another, unaccompanied by angular or rotary movement. Movement between the carpal bones of the wrist is largely gliding in nature.

Fig. 4-9. Rotation and circumduction. **A,** Rotation at the atlantoaxial joint; **B,** circumduction at the shoulder.

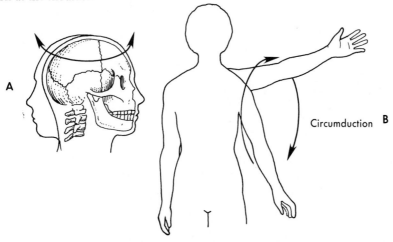

Circumduction **B**

Fig. 4-10. Examples of special movements at synovial joints. **A,** Pronation and supination; **B,** protraction and retraction; **C,** elevation and depression; **D,** inversion and eversion.

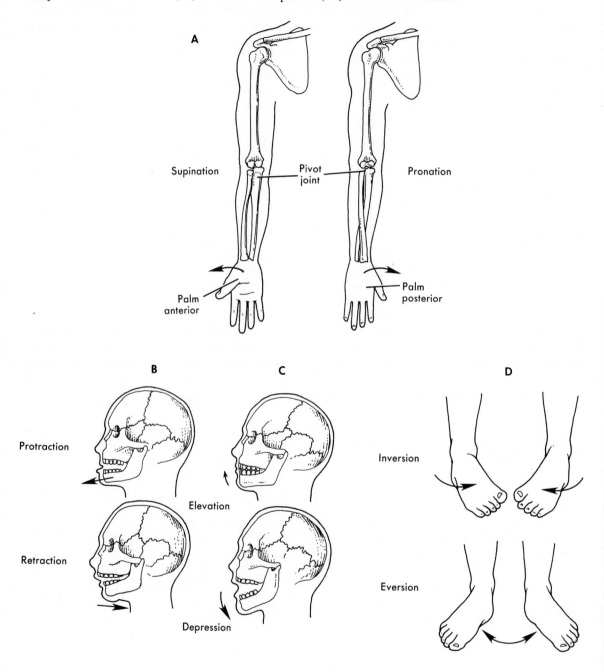

Special movements (Fig. 4-10)

Supination takes place at the radioulnar joint. In the anatomic position the hands and forearms are already supinated (palms forward). Note in Fig. 4-10 that the radius and ulna of the forearm are parallel and that the palm of the hand faces anteriorly in the supinated position. A handball serve involves supinating the hand.

Pronation describes the inward rotation or movement of the supinated forearm and hand, which causes the palm of the hand to face posteriorly. In pronation the radius crosses diagonally over the ulna in the forearm. The position of the hands when you do a push-up is an example of the hands and forearms in pronation.

In *inversion* the sole of the foot is turned inward and the inner (medial) margin of the foot is raised. This is the movement most commonly associated with a sprained ankle.

In *eversion* the foot is turned so that the sole faces outward (laterally) and its outer margin is raised (opposite of inversion). Inversion and eversion movements take place within the subtalar and transverse tarsal joints.

Elevation results in upward movement, whereas *depression* is a lowering of a body part or return from an elevated position. These terms are used most commonly to describe movements of the mandible and shoulder girdle.

Protraction refers to motion that moves a part forward. Reaching for an object involves protraction of the shoulder girdle. This is also known as scapula abduction.

Retraction is the motion that returns a protracted body part to its original or usual position. Retraction is also known as scapular adduction.

KEY TERMS

abduction   Movement of a body part away from the midline of the body

adduction   Movement of a body part toward the midline of the body

amphiarthroses   Slightly movable joints having a pad of either hyaline cartilage or fibrocartilage located between adjoining bony surfaces

avascular   Without bood vessels

chondrocytes   Cartilage cells

circumduction   Composite movement, combining flexion, abduction, extension, and adduction, in which the body segment describes a cone

dens   Conical pivot process that projects from the superior surface of the axis

depression   Return of movement from an elevated position

diarthroses   Freely movable joints, often called synovial joints

dorsiflexion   Movement of the top of the foot upward

elevation   Upward movement of the shoulder girdle

eversion   Sole of the foot is turned outward

extension   Return from the flexed position

flexion   Decreasing the size of the angle between the anterior or posterior surfaces of articulated bones

gomphosis   Type of synarthrotic joint in which a conical peg or projection fits into a socket

horizontal abduction   Movement of the upper limb through the transverse plane at shoulder level away from the midline of the body

horizontal adduction   Movement of the upper limb through the transverse plane at shoulder level toward the midline of the body

hyaline   Glossy, transparent cartilage

hyperextension   Continuation of extension beyond the anatomic position

inversion   Sole of the foot turned inward

lacunae   Small cavity in cartilage or bone

menisci   Crescent-shaped discs of fibrocartilage

periodontal membrane   Fibrous membrane located between the root of a tooth and its socket

plantar flexion   Movement of the sole of the foot downward

pronation   Palms-backward position

protraction   Motion moving a body part forward

radial flexion   Movement at the wrist of the thumb side of the hand toward the forearm

retraction Return of a protracted body part

rotation Pivoting of a body part on its own central or longitudinal axis

supination Palms-forward position

suture Type of synarthrotic joint united into rigid, immovable joints by a series of jagged, interlocking processes

symphysis Type of amphiarthrotic joint in which a pad of fibrocartilage joins one bone to another

synarthrosis Immovable joint

synchondrosis Type of amphiarthrotic joint in which a pad of hyaline cartilage joins one bone to another

syndesmosis Type of synarthrotic joint characterized by the presence of a dense fibrous membrane that binds the articular surfaces together

synovial joint Diarthrotic or freely movable joint

ulnar flexion Movement at the wrist of the little finger side of the hand toward the forearm

SUGGESTED READINGS

Clemente, C.D.: Anatomy: a regional atlas of the human body, ed. 2, Philadelphia, 1981, Lea & Febiger.

Hamilton, W.J., editor: Textbook of human anatomy, ed. 2, St. Louis, 1976, The C.V. Mosby Co.

Hencke, H.R.: Arthroscopy of the knee joint, Berlin, 1979, Springer-Verlag.

O'Connor, R.L.: Arthroscopy, Philadelphia, 1977, J.B. Lippincott Co.

Sonstegard, D.A., and others: The surgical replacement of the human knee joint, Sci. Am. **238**(1):44-51, 1978.

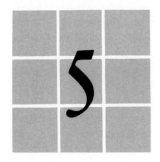

5 Myology

We have already reviewed the basic architectural plan of the body as a whole (Chapter 2), the skeletal system (Chapter 3), and the system of joints or articulations that make the potential for movement possible (Chapter 4). Regardless of body type, bones and joints cannot move themselves. They must be moved by the contraction of muscle tissue. This chapter discusses the 40% to 50% of our body weight that is skeletal muscle—those muscle masses that attach to bones and make movement possible. We will cover only muscles of particular functional significance, with emphasis on those that can be located externally either by palpation or by sight. If appropriate, additional details of individual muscle attachment and function will accompany actual assessment procedures in subsequent chapters.

The study of skeletal muscles is termed **_myology_.** Each of the over 600 skeletal muscles in the body can be thought of as a separate organ. Ordinarily, however, muscles act in coordinated groups and not as single units. They tend to occur and function in pairs, or in sets of three, four, or more muscles. Kinesiologists, for example, identify over 215 functional pairs of skeletal muscles. Each pair performs a unique and essential muscular action. Muscles vary significantly in size and shape. In addition, their individual fibers are arranged differently and attach in differing ways to the bones they move. They all have the same function, however, and behave in the same way; that is, they shorten. As muscle fibers shorten, their ends are pulled toward the center and contractile force or tension is developed in the muscle. The result is the basic ingredient of all physical activity—movement.

GENERAL FUNCTIONS

The essential functions of skeletal muscle include the following.

Movement

Skeletal muscle contractions produce movements either of the body as a whole (locomotion) or of its parts. Muscle tissue, because of its irritability, contractility, extensibility, and elasticity, is admirably suited to this function. The force of pull generated by the contraction of muscle tissue is generally applied through a leverage system of bones and joints. Whereas most of the systems of the body play some role in accomplishing movement, it is the skeletal and muscular systems acting together that actually produce movement.

Heat production

Muscle cells, like all cells, produce heat as a by-product during the catabolism of nutrients for energy. Because skeletal muscle cells are both highly active and numerous, they produce a major portion of total body heat. As a result, heat-related problems in athletes frequently occur as a result of muscular exertion in a hot or humid environment. In mild or cold environmental conditions, skeletal muscle contractions constitute one of the most important parts of the mechanism for maintaining homeostasis of temperature.

Posture, protection, and support

The continued partial contraction of many skeletal muscles makes possible standing, sitting, and other maintained positions of the body. In addition, skeletal muscle mass gives shape to the body and provides protection and support.

MUSCLES AND BONY LEVERS

Knowledge of both the mechanics of lever systems and the points of muscle attachment to bones gives the athletic trainer a basis for understanding not only body movements but also muscle strength and range of movement (ROM) at specific joints. Maximal muscle strength and maximal ROM at the same joint are mutually exclusive. This inverse relationship between strength of muscle contraction and range of motion at a given joint is a basic principle of leverage, or mechanical advantage, and is of practical importance. As a general rule, if two muscles of equal length cross and act on the same joint, the muscle that inserts (attaches) farther from the fulcrum (joint) will produce the more powerful contraction, and the muscle inserting closer to the joint will produce the greater range of movement.

Another basic of muscle action in a lever system is called the *optimum angle of pull.* Generally, the optimum angle of pull for any muscle is a right angle to the long axis of the bone to which it is attached. When the angle of pull departs from a right angle and becomes more parallel to the long axis, the strength of contraction decreases dramatically. Contraction of the brachialis muscle demonstrates this principle very well. The brachialis crosses the elbow from humerus to ulna. In the anatomic position, the elbow is extended and the angle of pull of the brachialis is parallel to the long axis of the ulna. Contraction of the brachialis at this angle is very inefficient. As the elbow is flexed and the angle of pull approaches a right angle, the contraction strength of the muscle is greatly increased. If asked to assess brachialis muscle strength, how would you position the forearm? It is this type of information that makes a rational approach to the correct assessment of many joint and muscle injuries possible.

Lever systems

A lever system is a simple mechanical device composed of four component parts: (1) a rigid rod or bar (bone), (2) a fixed pivot, or fulcrum, around which the rod moves (joint), (3) a weight, or resistance, that is moved, and (4) a force, or effort, that produces movement (muscle contraction). In Fig. 5-1 the fulcrum is symbolized as a circle, the resistance as a square, and the effort as *E*. Fig. 5-1 shows the three different types of lever arrangements that are categorized according to placement of the fulcrum, effort, and resistance. All three types are found in the human body.

Fig. 5-1. Classes of levers. Each class of lever is determined by the placement of fulcrum, effort, and resistance. **A,** First class lever, **B,** second class lever, and **C,** third class lever.

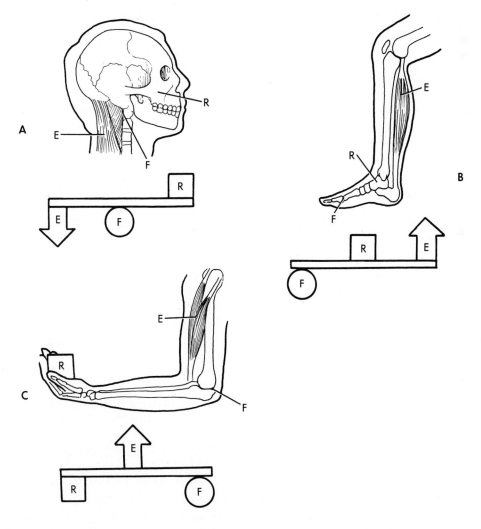

First-class levers

As you can see in Fig. 5-1, the placement of the fulcrum in a first-class lever lies between the effort and the resistance, as in a set of scales, a pair of scissors, or a child's see-saw. In the body, the head being raised or tipped backward on the atlas would be an example of a first-class lever in action. The facial portion of the skull is the resistance, the joint between the skull and atlas the fulcrum, and the muscles of the back, such as the splenius capitus, produce the effort. In the human body, first-class levers are not abundant. They generally serve as levers of stability.

Second-class levers

In second-class levers the weight, or resistance, lies between the fulcrum and the joint at which the pull, or effort, is exerted. The wheelbarrow is often used as an example. The presence of second-class levers in the human body is a controversial issue. Some authorities interpret the raising of the body on the toes as an example of this type of lever (Fig. 5-1). In this example the point of contact between the toes and the ground would be the fulcrum, the resistance would be located at the ankle, and effort would be exerted by the gastrocnemius muscle through the Achilles tendon. Opening the mouth against resistance (depression of the mandible) is also considered to be an example of a second-class lever.

Third-class levers

In a third-class lever the effort is exerted between the fulcrum and resistance or weight to be moved. Flexing of the forearm at the elbow joint is a frequently used example of this type of lever. Third-class levers permit rapid and extensive movement and are the commonest type found in the body. They allow insertion of a muscle very close to the joint that it moves.

ANATOMY OF SKELETAL MUSCLES
Size and shape

Each skeletal muscle is a separate organ consisting of skeletal muscle fibers plus important connective, nervous, and vascular tissue components. Individual skeletal muscles vary considerably in size and shape. They range from extremely tiny strands, such as the stapedius muscle of the middle ear, to large masses, such as the quadriceps femoris muscles of the thigh. Some skeletal muscles are broad in shape and some narrow. Some are long and tapering and some short and blunt. Some are triangular, some quadrilateral, and some irregular. Some form flat sheets and others bulky masses.

A typical muscle is often described as having a central fleshy, or meaty, contractile portion called the belly, or *gaster,* and two tendinous extremities by which the muscle is attached to bone. One attachment is called the **origin** and the other the **insertion.** The origin is the end that remains fixed or stationary when the muscle contracts. It is usually proximal to the joint. The insertion is the extremity that moves when the muscle contracts. It is distal to the joint and moves toward the origin when the muscle contracts.

Fiber arrangement

Arrangement of fibers varies among different muscles (Fig. 5-2). In some muscles, such as the rectus abdominis, the fibers are *parallel* to the long axis of the muscle. In the pectoralis major the fibers are said to be *radiate* in arrangement and converge from a broad area of origin to a narrow insertion. The deltoid exhibits a complex *multipennate* fiber arrangement resulting from the convergence of fibers in several muscular components. The long sartorius muscle has *longitudinally* arranged fibers, and the rectus femoris has a *bipennate* arrangement, with fibers directed obliquely from both sides of a central tendon. A *unipennate* arrangement exhibits fibers inserting diagonally on only one side of a similar tendon that runs the entire length of the muscle, much like the feathers in an old-fashioned plume pen. *Circular* fiber bundles are curved to encircle an opening and are typical in sphincter muscles such as the orbicularis oris. The direction of the fibers composing a muscle is significant because of its relationship to function. Bipennate and unipennate fiber arrangements, for example, produce the strongest contraction.

Connective tissue components

Every skeletal muscle contains a number of extremely important connective tissue elements (Fig. 5-3). It is interesting to note that most muscular injuries in athletics occur in the connective tissue element of the muscle. These noncontractile structures are intimately associated with muscle fibers, both anatomically and functionally. The contraction (shortening) of skeletal muscle cells cannot produce actual movement unless the cells are effectively attached to the structure to be moved. The connective tissue elements of skeletal muscle serve to "harness" the muscle to

the structures they pull on during contraction.

A fine meshwork of loose connective tissue fibers, the ***endomysium,*** surrounds each muscle fiber. Groups of 15 to 40 fibers are bound into bundles called ***fasciculi.*** Each fascicle is covered by a coarser and more fibrous connective tissue sheath called the ***perimysium.*** The perimysium partitions between fasciculi merge with the endomysium and ultimately extend to the surface of the muscle, where they become continuous with a thicker, outer connective tissue sheath, the ***epimysium,*** which covers the entire muscle.

The epimysium, perimysium, and endomysium of a muscle become continuous with fibrous tissue that extends from the muscles as a ***tendon,*** a strong, tough cord continuous at its other end with the fibrous covering of bone

Fig. 5-2. Types of muscle fiber arrangement.

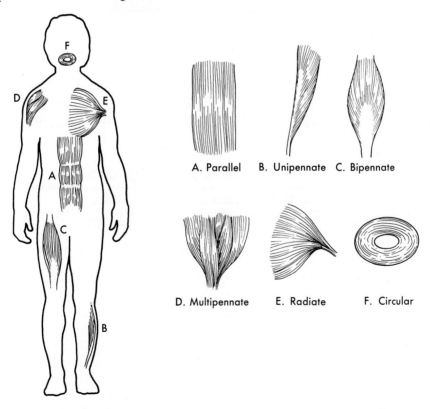

A. Parallel   B. Unipennate   C. Bipennate

D. Multipennate   E. Radiate   F. Circular

Fig. 5-3. Connective tissue and contractile components of skeletal muscle. Illustration shows the increasingly more detailed submicroscopic structure of a skeletal muscle fiber.

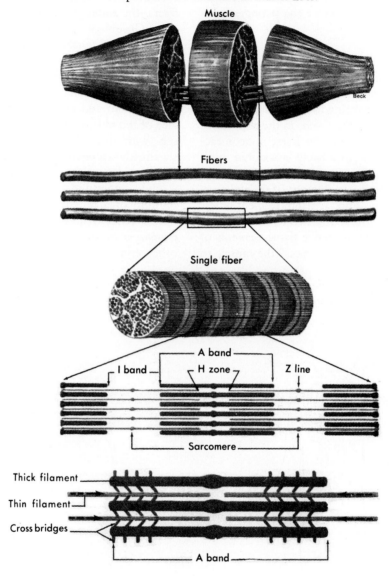

(periosteum). The fibrous wrapping of a muscle may also extend as a broad, flat sheet of connective tissue (aponeurosis) attaching it to adjacent structures, usually the fibrous wrappings of another muscle.

Tubular structures of fibrous connective tissue, called *tendon sheaths,* enclose certain tendons, notably those of the wrist, hand, ankle, and foot. Like the bursae, tendon sheaths have a lining of synovial membrane. Its moist, smooth surface enables the tendon to move easily, almost frictionlessly, in the tendon sheath.

You may recall that a continuous sheet of loose connective tissue known as the *superficial fascia* lies directly under the skin. Under this lies a layer of dense fibrous connective tissue, the *deep fascia.* Extensions of the deep fascia form the epimysium, perimysium, and endomysium of muscles and their attachments to bones and other structures and also enclose viscera, glands, blood vessels, and nerves.

Nerve tissue

Nerves containing both sensory and motor components enter skeletal muscles through the covering epimysium and course between the fasciculi in the perimysium. Ultimately each muscle fiber is innervated by a somatic *motoneuron.* One neuron plus the muscle fibers it innervates constitutes a *motor unit.* The single axon fiber of a motor unit, on entering the skeletal muscle, divides into a variable number of branches. Those of some motor units terminate in only a few muscle fibers, whereas others terminate in numerous fibers. Consequently, impulse conduction by one motor unit may stimulate only a half dozen or so muscle fibers to contract at one time, whereas conduction by another motor unit may activate a hundred or more fibers simultaneously. This fact bears a relationship to the function of the muscle as a whole. As a general rule, the fewer the number of fibers supplied by a skeletal muscle's individual motor units, the more precise the movements that muscle can produce. For example, in certain small muscles of the hand, each motor unit includes only a few muscle fibers, and these muscles produce precise finger movements. In contrast, motor units in large abdominal or thigh muscles that do not produce precise movements are reported to include more than a hundred muscle fibers each.

The area of contact between a nerve and muscle fiber is known as the *motor end-plate* or *neuromuscular junction.* When nerve impulses reach the ends of the axon fibers in a skeletal muscle, small vesicles in the axon terminals release a chemical called acetylcholine into the neuromuscular junction. Diffusing swiftly across this microscopic trough, acetylcholine contacts the sarcolemma of the adjacent muscle fibers, stimulating the fiber to contract. In addition to motor nerve ends, there are also many sensory nerve endings in skeletal muscles. The purpose of the sensory nerves is to transmit impulses to the central nervous system to convey information concerning body position, pain, and other types of sensation. Examples of sensory components include muscle spindles and Golgi tendon organs.

MICROSCOPIC ANATOMY

It is suggested that you review the basic microscopic anatomy of skeletal muscle in a textbook of anatomy and physiology or histology. Detailed information of this type lies beyond the scope of an assessment text but is useful in understanding cellular repair in muscle tissue after injury. In general, individual skeletal muscle cells (fibers) are multinucleated, elongated, and cylindric (Fig. 5-4). When viewed under the microscope they show very distinct cross-striations of alternating light and dark bands, which give the cell a striated or striped appearance. The cross-striations are produced by the repetitive or periodic arrangement and overlapping of interdigitating filaments. Individual contractile units are called *sarcomeres.* When adjacent sarcomeres contract simultaneously the entire fiber shortens and a measurable pulling force (contraction) is generated.

MUSCLE ACTION

It is the voluntary contraction of specific skeletal muscles that produce the types of diarthrotic joint movements described in Chapter 4. Some muscles abduct a joint, whereas others may be positioned to adduct or flex it. Generally, muscles span the joint at which movement occurs and attach to both articulating bones. In most cases the body of the muscle lies proximal to the part moved. Thus muscles that move the forearm lie proximal to it, in the upper arm.

In understanding muscle actions it is important to realize that skeletal muscles almost always act in groups rather than singly. In other words, most movements are produced by the coordinated action of several muscles. Some of the muscles in the group contract while others relax.

To identify each muscle's special function in the group, the following classification is used.

Prime movers, or agonists: Muscle or muscles whose contraction actually produces movement

Antagonists: One or more muscles that oppose the action of another group of muscles or the pull of gravity*

Synergists: Muscles that contract at the same time as the prime mover, assisting or sup-

---

*Antagonistic muscles have opposite actions and opposite locations. If the flexor lies anterior to the part, the extensor will be found posterior to it. For example, the pectoralis major, the flexor of the upper arm, is located on the anterior aspect of the chest, whereas the latissimus dorsi, the extensor of the upper arm, is located on the posterior aspect of the chest. The antagonist of a flexor muscle is obviously an extensor muscle and that of an abductor muscle, an adductor muscle. Some frequently used antagonists are listed in Table 5-2.

Fig. 5-4. A, Skeletal or striated voluntary muscle tissue. **B,** Skeletal (striated) muscle, higher magnification.

(Courtesy Dr. C.R. McMullen Department of Biology, South Dakota State University.)

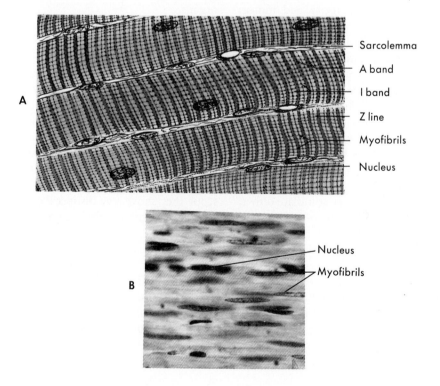

Sarcolemma
A band
I band
Z line
Myofibrils
Nucleus

Nucleus
Myofibrils

plementing a prime mover in producing a particular movement

Fixators: Muscles that serve to fix or stabilize a joint to augment the effectiveness of a prime mover

HOW SKELETAL MUSCLES ARE NAMED

Muscle names seem more logical and therefore easier to learn and remember when you understand the reasons for their use. Most muscles are named on the basis of one or more distinctive features or characteristics. It is possible for a student to learn much about a muscle just from its name. Characteristics used in naming muscles include the following:

Action or function: The name or part of the name indicates its function (such as flexor or extensor)

Direction of its fibers: For example, the external oblique muscle in the abdominal wall

Location: For example, the tibialis anterior muscle is located on the front of the leg

Number of divisions: Such as biceps, triceps, or quadriceps

Shape: Such as deltoid (triangular) or quadratus (square)

Size: Such as gluteus maximus and minimus

Points of attachment: The origin is the first part of the muscle's name and the insertion is last, as in brachioradialis—the brachium (arm or humerus) is the origin, and the radius is the insertion

A good way to start the study of a muscle is by trying to find out what its name means.

ORIGINS, INSERTIONS, FUNCTIONS, AND INNERVATIONS OF REPRESENTATIVE MUSCLES

Table 5-1 lists a number of important muscles grouped according to location on the body; Table 5-2 gives examples of muscles grouped according to function. Start by making yourself familiar with the names, shapes, functions, and general locations of the larger muscles. Refer often to illustrations and to a skeleton, if available, as you study individual muscles. Also, when possible, palpate each muscle on your own body. To understand muscle actions, you need first to know certain anatomic facts, such as which bones muscles attach to and which joints they pull across. If you relate these structural facts to functional assessment principles (for in-

Table 5-1. Muscles grouped according to location

Location	Muscles
Neck	Sternocleidomastoid
Back	Trapezius
	Latissimus
Chest	Pectoralis major
	Serratus anterior
Abdominal wall	External oblique
Shoulder	Deltoid
Upper arm	Biceps brachii
	Triceps brachii
	Brachialis
Forearm	Brachioradialis
	Pronator teres
Buttocks	Gluteus maximus
	Gluteus minimus
	Gluteus medius
	Tensor fascia latae
Thigh	
Anterior surface	Quadriceps femoris group
	Rectus femoris
	Vastus lateralis
	Vastus medialis
	Vastus intermedius
Medial surface	Gracilis
	Adductor group (brevis, longus, magnus)
Posterior surface	Hamstring group
	Biceps femoris
	Semitendinosus
	Semimembranosus
Leg	
Anterior surface	Tibialis anterior
Posterior surface	Gastrocnemius
	Soleus
Pelvic floor	Levator ani
	Levator coccygeus
	Rectococcygeus

Table 5-2. Muscles grouped according to function

Part moved	Example of flexor	Example of extensor	Example of abductor	Example of adductor
Head	Sternocleidomastoid	Semispinalis capitis		
Upper arm	Pectoralis major	Trapezius Latissimus dorsi	Deltoid	Pectoralis major with latissimus dorsi
Forearm	With forearm supinated: biceps brachii With forearm pronated: brachialis With semisupination or semipronation: brachioradialis	Triceps brachii		
Hand	Flexor carpi radialis and ulnaris Palmaris longus	Extensor carpi radialis, longus, and brevis Extensor carpi ulnaris	Flexor carpi radialis	Flexor carpi ulnaris
Thigh	Iliopsoas Rectus femoris (of quadriceps femoris group)	Gluteus maximus	Gluteus medius and gluteus minimus	Adductor group
Leg	Hamstrings	Quadriceps femoris group		
Foot	Tibialis anterior	Gastrocnemius Soleus	Evertors Peroneus longus Peroneus brevis	Invertor Tibialis anterior
Trunk	Iliopsoas Rectus abdominis	Sacrospinalis		

Table 5-3. Muscles that move shoulder

Muscle	Origin	Insertion	Function	Innervation
▪ Trapezius	**Occipital bone** (protuberance)	**Clavicle**	Raises or lowers shoulders and shrugs them	Spinal accessory, second, third, and fourth cervical nerves
	Vertebrae (cervical and thoracic)	**Scapula** (spine and acromion)	Extends head when occiput acts as insertion	
Pectoralis minor	Ribs (second to fifth)	Scapula (coracoid)	Pulls shoulder down and forward	Medial and lateral anterior thoracic nerves
▪ Serratus anterior	**Ribs** (upper eight or nine)	**Scapula** (anterior surface, vertebral border)	Pulls shoulder forward; abducts and rotates it upward	Long thoracic nerve

stance, those associated with lever systems), you will find your study of muscles more interesting and less difficult.

The object of this chapter is to provide you with a generalized overview of myology. Rote memorization of many minute details will be counterproductive. Such facts only "make sense" when they help explain the rationale that undergirds actual assessment techniques. Necessary anatomic details will be a part of each assessment technique described in subsequent chapters of the text. Use the information and illustrations in this chapter as a reference source.

Basic information about many muscles is given in Tables 5-3 to 5-15 and Figs. 5-5 to 5-18. Each table describes a group of muscles that move one part of the body. Muscles that, in our judgment, are the most important for students of athletic injury assessment to know are preceded by a block, and the origins and insertions so judged are set in boldface type. The actions listed for each muscle are those for which it is a prime mover. Remember, a single muscle contracting alone rarely accomplishes a given action. Instead, muscles act in groups as prime movers, fixators, synergists, and antagonists.

Table 5-4. Muscles that move upper arm

Muscle	Origin	Insertion	Function	Innervation
▪ Pectoralis major	**Clavicle** (medial half) **Sternum** **Costal cartilages of true ribs**	**Humerus** (greater tubercle)	Flexes upper arm Adducts upper arm anteriorly; draws it across chest	Medial and lateral anterior thoracic nerves
▪ Latissimus dorsi	**Vertebrae** (spines of lower thoracic, lumbar, and sacral) **Ilium** (crest) Lumbodorsal fascia	**Humerus** (intertubercular groove)	Extends upper arm Adducts upper arm posteriorly	Thoracodorsal nerve
▪ Deltoid	**Clavicle** **Scapula** (spine and acromion)	**Humerus** (lateral side about halfway down—deltoid tubercle)	Abducts upper arm Assists in flexion and extension of upper arm	Axillary nerve
Coracobrachialis	Scapula (coracoid process)	Humerus (middle third, medial surface)	Adduction; assists in flexion and medial rotation of arm	Musculocutaneous nerve
Supraspinatus	Scapula (supraspinous fossa)	Humerus (greater tubercle)	Assists in abducting arm	Suprascapular nerve
Teres major	Scapula (lower part, axillary border)	Humerus (upper part, anterior surface)	Assists in extension, adduction, and medial rotation of arm	Lower subscapular nerve
Teres minor	Scapula (axillary border)	Humerus (greater tubercle)	Rotates arm outward	Axillary nerve
Infraspinatus	Scapula (infraspinatus border)	Humerus (greater tubercle)	Rotates arm outward	Suprascapular nerve

Table 5-5. Muscles that move lower arm

Muscle	Origin	Insertion	Function	Innervation
▪ Biceps brachii	**Scapula** (supraglenoid tuberosity) **Scapula** (coracoid)	**Radius** (tubercle at proximal end)	Flexes supinated forearm Supinates forearm and hand	Musculocutaneous nerve
▪ Brachialis	**Humerus** (distal half, anterior surface)	**Ulna** (front of coronoid process)	Flexes pronated forearm	Musculocutaneous nerve
Brachioradialis	Humerus (above lateral epicondyle)	Radius (styloid process)	Flexes semipronated or semisupinated forearm; supinates forearm and hand	Radial nerve
▪ Triceps brachii	**Scapula** (infraglenoid tuberosity) **Humerus** (posterior surface—lateral head above radial groove; medial head, below)	**Ulna** (olecranon process)	Extends lower arm	Radial nerve
Pronator teres	Humerus (medial epicondyle) Ulna (coronoid process)	Radius (middle third of lateral surface)	Pronates and flexes forearm	Median nerve
Pronator quadratus	Ulna (distal fourth, anterior surface)	Radius (distal fourth, anterior surface)	Pronates forearm	Median nerve
Supinator	Humerus (lateral epicondyle) Ulna (proximal fifth)	Radius (proximal third)	Supinates forearm	Radial nerve

Table 5-6. Muscles that move hand

Muscle	Origin	Insertion	Function	Innervation
Flexor carpi radialis	Humerus (medial epi-condyle)	Second metacarpal (base of)	Flexes hand Flexes forearm	Median nerve
Palmaris longus	Humerus (medial epi-condyle)	Fascia of palm	Flexes hand	Median nerve
Flexor carpi ulnaris	Humerus (medial epi-condyle) Ulna (proximal two thirds)	Pisiform bone Third, fourth, and fifth metacarpals	Flexes hand Adducts hand	Ulnar nerve
Extensor carpi radialis longus	Humerus (ridge above lateral epi-condyle)	Second metacarpal (base of)	Extends hand Abducts hand (moves toward thumb side when hand supi-nated)	Radial nerve
Extensor carpi radialis brevis	Humerus (lateral epi-condyle)	Second, third meta-carpals (bases of)	Extends hand	Radial nerve
Extensor carpi ulnaris	Humerus (lateral epi-condyle) Ulna (proximal three fourths)	Fifth metacarpal (base of)	Extends hand Adducts hand (move toward little finger side when hand supinated)	Radial nerve

Table 5-7. Muscles that move thigh

Muscle	Origin	Insertion	Function	Innervation
▪ Iliopsoas (iliacus and psoas major)	**Ilium** iliac fossa) **Vertebrae** (bodies of twelfth thoracic to fifth lumbar)	**Femur** (small trochanter)	Flexes thigh Flexes trunk (when femur acts as origin)	Femoral and second to fourth lumbar nerves
▪ Rectus femoris	**Ilium** (anterior, inferior spine)	**Tibia** (by way of patellar tendon)	Flexes thigh Extends lower leg	Femoral nerve
▪ Gluteal group				
Maximus	**Ilium** (crest and posterior surface) Sacrum and coccyx (posterior surface) Sacrotuberous ligament	**Femur** (gluteal tuberosity) **Iliotibial tract**	Extends thigh—rotates outward	Inferior gluteal nerve
Medius	**Ilium** (lateral surface)	**Femur** (greater trochanter)	Abducts thigh—rotates outward; stabilizes pelvis on femur	Superior gluteal nerve
Minimus	**Ilium** (lateral surface)	**Femur** (greater trochanter)	Abducts thigh; stabilizes pelvis on femur Rotates thigh medially	Superior gluteal nerve
▪ Tensor fasciae latae	**Ilium** (anterior part of crest)	**Tibia** (by way of **iliotibial tract**)	Abducts thigh Tightens iliotibial tract	Superior gluteal nerve
Piriformis	Vertebrae (front of sacrum)	Femur (medial aspect of greater trochanter)	Rotates thigh outward Abducts thigh Extends thigh	First or second sacral nerves
▪ Adductor group				
Brevis	**Pubic bone**	**Femur** (linea aspera)	Adducts thigh	Obturator nerve
Longus	**Pubic bone**	**Femur** (linea aspera)	Adducts thigh	Obturator nerve
Magnus	**Pubic bone**	**Femur** (linea aspera)	Adducts thigh	Obturator nerve
Gracilis	Pubic bone (just below symphysis)	Tibia (medial surface behind sartorius)	Adducts thigh and flexes and adducts leg	Obturator nerve

Table 5-8. Muscles that move lower leg

Muscle	Origin	Insertion	Function	Innervation
▪ Quadriceps femoris group				
Rectus femoris	**Ilium** (anterior, inferior spine)	**Tibia** (by way of patellar tendon)	Flexes thigh Extends leg	Femoral nerve
Vastus lateralis	**Femur** (linea aspera)	**Tibia** (by way of patellar tendon)	Extends leg	Femoral nerve
Vastus medialis	**Femur**	**Tibia** (by way of patellar tendon)	Extends leg	Femoral nerve
Vastus intermedius	**Femur** (anterior surface)	**Tibia** (by way of patellar tendon)	Extends leg	Femoral nerve
▪ Sartorius	**Os innominatum** (anterior, superior iliac spines)	**Tibia** (medial surface of upper end of shaft)	Adducts and flexes leg Permits crossing of legs tailor fashion	Femoral nerve
▪ Hamstring group				
Biceps femoris	**Ischium** (tuberosity)	**Fibula** (head of)	Flexes leg	Branch of sciatic nerve
	Femur (linea aspera)	**Tibia** (lateral condyle)	Extends thigh	Branch of sciatic nerve
Semitendinosus	**Ischium** (tuberosity)	**Tibia** (proximal end, medial surface)	Extends thigh	Branch of sciatic nerve
Semimembranosus	**Ischium** (tuberosity)	**Tibia** (medial condyle)	Extends thigh	Branch of sciatic nerve

Table 5-9. Muscles that move foot

Muscle	Origin	Insertion	Function	Innervation
▪ Tibialis anterior	**Tibia** (lateral condyle of upper body)	**Tarsal** (first cuneiform) Metatarsal (base of first)	Flexes foot Inverts foot	Common and deep peroneal nerves
▪ Gastrocnemius	**Femur** (condyles)	**Tarsal** (calcaneus by way of Achilles tendon)	Extends foot Flexes lower leg	Tibial nerve (branch of sciatic nerve)
▪ Soleus	**Tibia** (underneath gastrocnemius) **Fibula**	**Tarsal** (calcaneus by way of Achilles tendon)	Extends foot (plantar flexion)	Tibial nerve
Peroneus longus	Tibia (lateral condyle) Fibula (head and shaft)	First cuneiform Base of first metatarsal	Extends foot (plantar flexion) Everts foot	Common peroneal nerve
Peroneus brevis	Fibula (lower two thirds of lateral surface of shaft)	Fifth metatarsal (tubercle, dorsal surface)	Everts foot Flexes foot	Superficial peroneal nerve
Tibialis posterior	Tibia (posterior surface) Fibula (posterior surface)	Navicular bone Cuboid bone All three cuneiforms Second and fourth metatarsals	Extends foot (plantar flexion) Inverts foot	Tibial nerve
Peroneus tertius	Fibula (distal third)	Fourth and fifth metatarsals (bases of)	Flexes foot Everts foot	Deep peroneal nerve

Table 5-10. Muscles that move head

Muscle	Origin	Insertion	Function	Innervation
▪ Sternocleido-mastoid	**Sternum Clavicle**	**Temporal bone** (mastoid process)	Flexes head (prayer muscle) One muscle alone, rotates head toward opposite side; spasm of this muscle alone or associated with trapezius called torticollis or wry-neck	Accessory nerve
Semispinalis capitis	Vertebrae (transverse processes of upper six thoracic, articular processes of lower four cervical)	Occipital bone (between superior and inferior nuchal lines)	Extends head; bends it laterally	First five cervical nerves
Splenius capitis	Ligamentum nuchae Vertebrae (spinous processes of upper three or four thoracic)	Temporal bone (mastoid process) Occipital bone	Extends head Bends and rotates head toward same side as contracting muscle	Second, third, and fourth cervical nerves
Longissimus capitis	Vertebrae (transverse processes of upper six thoracic, articular processes of lower four cervical)	Temporal bone (mastoid process)	Extends head Bends and rotates head toward contracting side	

Table 5-11. Muscles that move abdominal wall

Muscle	Origin	Insertion	Function	Innervation
▪ External oblique	**Ribs** (lower eight)	**Ossa coxae** (iliac crest and pubis by way of inguinal ligament) **Linea alba** by of an aponeurosis	Compresses abdomen Important postural function of all abdominal muscles is to pull front of pelvis upward, thereby flattening lumbar curve of spine; when these muscles lose their tone, common figure faults of protruding abdomen and lordosis develop	Lower seven intercostal nerves and iliohypogastric nerves
▪ Internal oblique	**Ossa coxae** (iliac crest and inguinal ligament) **Lumbodorsal fascia**	**Ribs** (lower three) **Pubic bone** **Linea alba**	Same as external oblique	Last three intercostal nerves; iliohypogastric and ilioinguinal nerves
▪ Transversalis	**Ribs** (lower six) **Ossa coxae** (iliac crest, inguinal ligament) **Lumbodorsal fascia**	**Pubic bone** **Linea alba**	Same as external oblique	Last five intercostal nerves; iliohypogastric and ilioinguinal nerves
▪ Rectus abdominis	**Ossa coxae** (pubic bone and symphysis pubis)	**Ribs** (costal cartilage of fifth, sixth, and seventh ribs) Sternum (xiphoid process)	Same as external oblique; because abdominal muscles compress abdominal cavity, they aid in straining, defecation, forced expiration, childbirth, etc.; abdominal muscles are antagonists of diaphragm, relaxing as it contracts and vice versa Flexes trunk	Last six intercostal nerves

Table 5-12. Muscles that move chest wall

Muscle	Origin	Insertion	Function	Innervation
External intercostals	Rib (lower border; forward fibers)	Rib (upper border of rib below origin)	Elevate ribs	Intercostal nerves
Internal intercostals	Rib (inner surface, lower border; backward fibers)	Rib (upper border of rib below origin)	Probably depress ribs	Intercostal nerves
▪ Diaphragm	**Lower circumference of thorax** (of rib cage)	**Central tendon of diaphragm**	Enlarges thorax, causing inspiration	Phrenic nerves

Table 5-13. Muscles of pelvic floor

Muscle	Origin	Insertion	Function	Innervation
Levator ani	Pubis (posterior surface) Ischium (spine)	Coccyx	Together form floor of pelvic cavity; support pelvic organs; if these muscles are badly torn at childbirth or become too relaxed, uterus or bladder may prolapse, that is, drop out	Pudendal nerve
Coccygeus (posterior continuation of levator ani)	Ischium (spine)	Coccyx Sacrum	Same as levator ani	Pudendal nerve

Table 5-14. Muscles that move trunk

Muscle	Origin	Insertion	Function	Innervation
▪ Sacrospinalis (erector spinae)			Extend spine; maintain erect posture of trunk Acting singly, abduct and rotate trunk	Posterior rami of first cervical to fifth lumbar spinal nerves
Lateral portion: Iliocostalis lumborum	Iliac crest, sacrum (posterior surface), and lumbar vertebrae (spinous processes)	Ribs, lower six		
Iliocostalis dorsi	Ribs, lower six	Ribs, upper six		
Iliocostalis cervicis	Ribs, upper six	Vertebrae, fourth to sixth cervical		
Medial portion: Longissimus dorsi	Same as iliocostalis lumborum	Vertebrae, thoracic ribs		
Longissimus cervicis	Vertebrae, upper six thoracic	Vertebrae, second to sixth cervical		
Longissimus capitis	Vertebrae, upper six thoracic and last four cervical	Temporal bone, mastoid process		
Quadratus lumborum (forms part of posterior abdominal wall)	Ilium (posterior part of crest) Vertebrae (lower three lumbar)	Ribs (twelfth) Vertebrae (transverse processes of first four lumbar)	Both muscles together extend spine One muscle alone abducts trunk toward side of contracting muscle	First three or four lumbar nerves
▪ Iliopsoas	See muscles that move thigh		Flexes trunk	

Table 5-15. Muscles of facial expression and of mastication

Muscle	Origin	Insertion	Function	Innervation
MUSCLES OF FACIAL EXPRESSION				
Epicranius (occipito-frontalis)	Occipital bone	Tissues of eyebrows	Raises eyebrows, wrinkles forehead horizontally	Cranial nerve VII
Corrugator supercilii	Frontal bone (superciliary ridge)	Skin of eyebrow	Wrinkles forehead vertically	Cranial nerve VII
Orbicularis oculi	Encircles eyelid		Closes eye	Cranial nerve VII
Orbicularis oris	Encircles mouth		Draws lips together	Cranial nerve VII
Platysma	Fascia of upper part of deltoid and pectoralis major	Mandible (lower border) Skin around corners of mouth	Draws corners of mouth down—pouting	Cranial nerve VII
Buccinator	Maxillae	Skin of sides of mouth	Permits smiling Blowing, as in playing a trumpet	Cranial nerve VII
MUSCLES OF MASTICATION				
Masseter	Zygomatic arch	Mandible (external surface)	Closes jaw	Cranial nerve V
Temporal	Temporal bone	Mandible	Closes jaw	Cranial nerve V
Pterygoids (internal and external)	Undersurface of skull	Mandible (mesial surface)	Grate teeth	Cranial nerve V

Fig. 5-5. Superficial muscles of the posterior surface of the trunk.

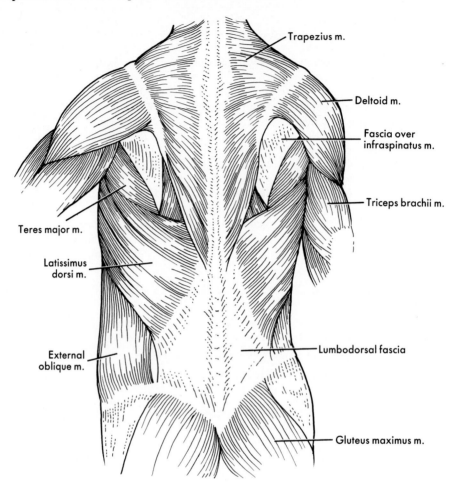

Fig. 5-6. Superficial muscles of the anterior surface of the trunk.

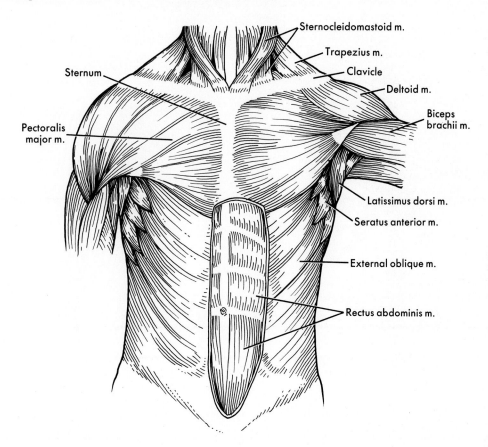

Sternocleidomastoid m.

Trapezius m.

Clavicle

Deltoid m.

Biceps brachii m.

Sternum

Pectoralis major m.

Latissimus dorsi m.

Seratus anterior m.

External oblique m.

Rectus abdominis m.

Fig. 5-7. Muscles of the flexor surface of the upper extremity.

Fig. 5-8. Muscles of the extensor surface of the upper extremity.

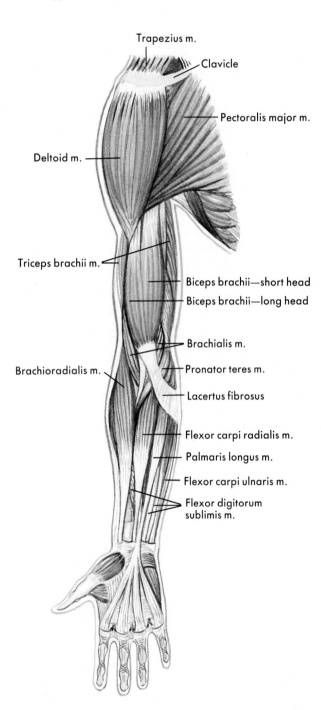

Trapezius m.

Clavicle

Pectoralis major m.

Deltoid m.

Triceps brachii m.

Biceps brachii—short head

Biceps brachii—long head

Brachialis m.

Brachioradialis m.

Pronator teres m.

Lacertus fibrosus

Flexor carpi radialis m.

Palmaris longus m.

Flexor carpi ulnaris m.

Flexor digitorum sublimis m.

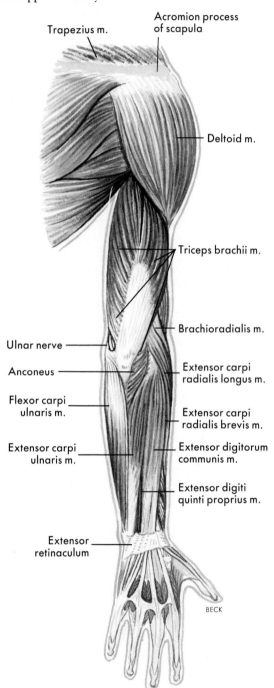

Trapezius m.

Acromion process of scapula

Deltoid m.

Triceps brachii m.

Brachioradialis m.

Ulnar nerve

Anconeus

Extensor carpi radialis longus m.

Flexor carpi ulnaris m.

Extensor carpi radialis brevis m.

Extensor carpi ulnaris m.

Extensor digitorum communis m.

Extensor digiti quinti proprius m.

Extensor retinaculum

BECK

Fig. 5-9. Biceps brachii muscle. *O*, Origin. *I*, Insertion.

Fig. 5-10. Brachialis muscle. *O*, Origin. *I*, Insertion.

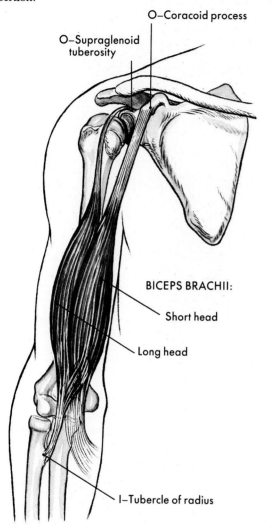

O–Coracoid process

O–Supraglenoid tuberosity

BICEPS BRACHII:

Short head

Long head

I–Tubercle of radius

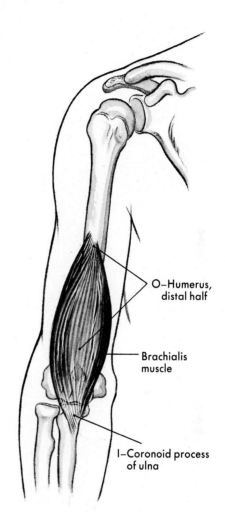

O–Humerus, distal half

Brachialis muscle

I–Coronoid process of ulna

Fig. 5-11. Triceps brachii muscle. *O*, Origin. *I*, Insertion.

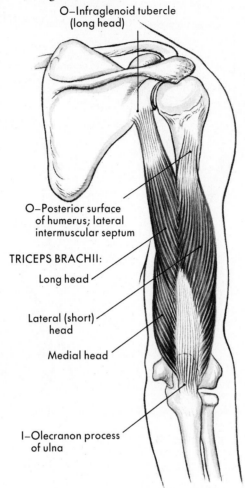

O—Infraglenoid tubercle
(long head)

O—Posterior surface
of humerus; lateral
intermuscular septum

TRICEPS BRACHII:

Long head

Lateral (short)
head

Medial head

I—Olecranon process
of ulna

Fig. 5-12. Superficial muscles of the right thigh and leg—anterior view.

Fig. 5-13. Superficial muscles of the right thigh and leg—posterior view.

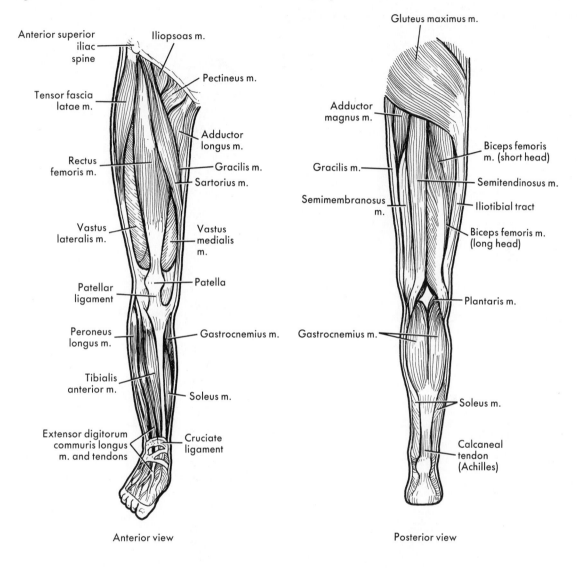

Anterior superior iliac spine

Iliopsoas m.

Pectineus m.

Tensor fascia latae m.

Adductor longus m.

Rectus femoris m.

Gracilis m.

Sartorius m.

Vastus lateralis m.

Vastus medialis m.

Patellar ligament

Patella

Peroneus longus m.

Gastrocnemius m.

Tibialis anterior m.

Soleus m.

Extensor digitorum commuris longus m. and tendons

Cruciate ligament

Anterior view

Gluteus maximus m.

Adductor magnus m.

Biceps femoris m. (short head)

Gracilis m.

Semitendinosus m.

Semimembranosus m.

Iliotibial tract

Biceps femoris m. (long head)

Plantaris m.

Gastrocnemius m.

Soleus m.

Calcaneal tendon (Achilles)

Posterior view

Fig. 5-14. Quadriceps femoris group of thigh muscles: rectus femoris, vastus intermedius, vastus medialis, and vastus lateralis.

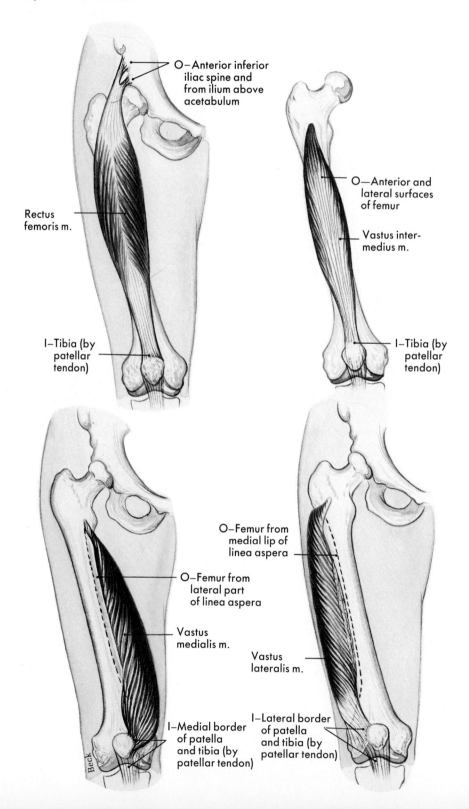

O—Anterior inferior iliac spine and from ilium above acetabulum

Rectus femoris m.

I—Tibia (by patellar tendon)

O—Anterior and lateral surfaces of femur

Vastus inter-medius m.

I—Tibia (by patellar tendon)

O—Femur from medial lip of linea aspera

O—Femur from lateral part of linea aspera

Vastus medialis m.

Vastus lateralis m.

I—Medial border of patella and tibia (by patellar tendon)

I—Lateral border of patella and tibia (by patellar tendon)

Beck

Fig. 5-15. Muscles that adduct the thigh.

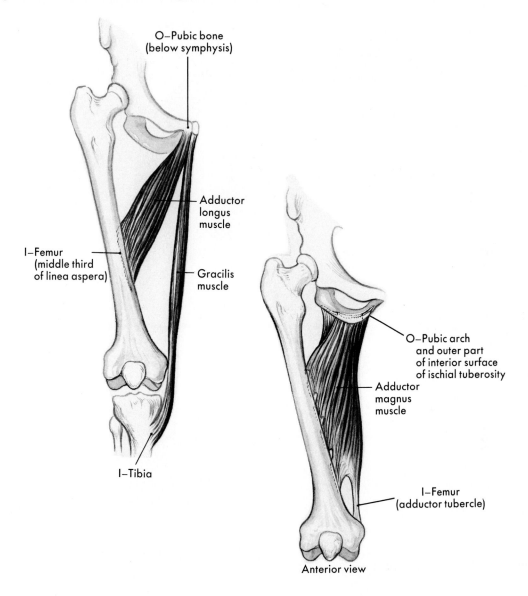

O—Pubic bone
(below symphysis)

Adductor
longus
muscle

I—Femur
(middle third
of linea aspera)

Gracilis
muscle

I—Tibia

O—Pubic arch
and outer part
of interior surface
of ischial tuberosity

Adductor
magnus
muscle

I—Femur
(adductor tubercle)

Anterior view

Fig. 5-16. Gluteus maximus muscle. *O*, Origin. *I*, Insertion.

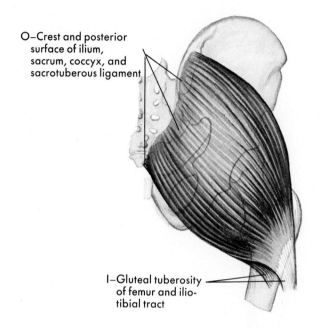

O–Crest and posterior
surface of ilium,
sacrum, coccyx, and
sacrotuberous ligament

I–Gluteal tuberosity
of femur and ilio-
tibial tract

Fig. 5-17. Hamstring group of thigh muscles: biceps femoris, semitendinosus, and semimembranosus.

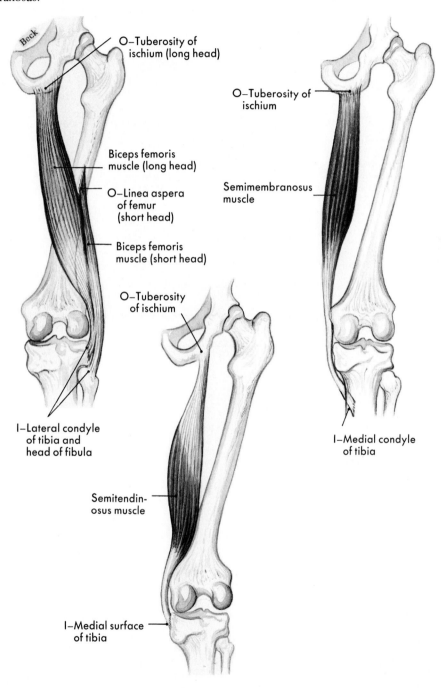

O–Tuberosity of ischium (long head)

O–Tuberosity of ischium

Biceps femoris muscle (long head)

Semimembranosus muscle

O–Linea aspera of femur (short head)

Biceps femoris muscle (short head)

O–Tuberosity of ischium

I–Lateral condyle of tibia and head of fibula

I–Medial condyle of tibia

Semitendinosus muscle

I–Medial surface of tibia

Fig. 5-18. Muscles of the head. These muscles make possible various facial expressions.

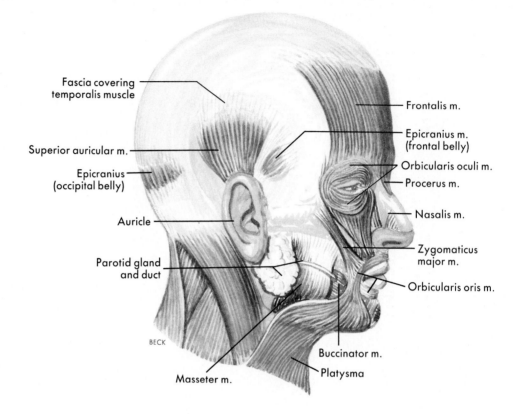

Fascia covering
temporalis muscle

Superior auricular m.

Epicranius
(occipital belly)

Auricle

Parotid gland
and duct

BECK

Masseter m.

Frontalis m.

Epicranius m.
(frontal belly)

Orbicularis oculi m.

Procerus m.

Nasalis m.

Zygomaticus
major m.

Orbicularis oris m.

Buccinator m.

Platysma

KEY TERMS

agonists (prime movers) Muscles whose contraction produces movement

antagonists Muscle or muscles that oppose action of other muscles or gravity

deep fascia Sheet of fibrous connective tissue investing the trunk, limbs, and muscles

endomysium Connective tissue between individual muscle fibers

epimysium Connective tissue sheath that envelops a skeletal muscle

fasciculi Groups of individual muscle fibers bound into discrete bundles

fixators Muscles that fix or stabilize joints to assist prime movers

gaster The central fleshy or "meaty" contractile portion of a muscle (belly)

insertion The more movable end of a muscle attachment

lever A mechanical device consisting of a bone (force arm), fulcrum (joint), weight arm (resistance), and force or effort movement (muscle contraction: **First-class lever**—lever system in which the fulcrum lies between the effort and resistance; **second-class lever**—lever system in which the resistance lies between a long force and a short weight arm; **third-class lever**—lever system in which the effort is exerted between the fulcrum and resistance

locomotion Movement of the body as a whole

motoneuron Nerve fiber that transmits nerve impulses away from the brain or spinal cord (to a muscle)

motor unit One neuron plus the muscle fibers it innervates.

myology The study of muscles

neuromuscular junction Area of contact between a nerve and muscle fiber

optimum angle of pull A right angle to the long axis of a bone to which a muscle is attached

origin The more fixed end of a muscle attachment

perimysium Connective tissue between bundles of muscle fibers

posture Position or attitude of the body

sarcomere Contractile unit of muscle tissue

superficial fascia Sheet of fibrous connective tissue just below the skin

synergists Muscles that assist prime movers

tendon Band or cord of fibrous connective tissue that attaches a muscle to a bone or other structure

SUGGESTED READINGS

Basmajian, J.V.: Grant's method of anatomy, ed. 10, Baltimore, 1980, The Williams & Wilkins Co.

Cohen, C.: The protein switch of muscle contraction, Sci. Am. 233(5):36-45, 1975.

Huxley, H.E.: The mechanism of muscular contraction, Sci. Am. 213(6):18-27, 1965. (Classic article.)

Margaria, R.: The sources of muscular energy, Sci. Am. 226(3):84-91, 1972.

Murray, J.M., and Weber, A.: The cooperative action of muscle proteins, Sci. Am. 230(2):59-71, 1974.

Quiring, D.P.: The head, neck, and trunk, Philadelphia, 1955, Lea & Febiger.

Quiring, D.P., and others: The extremities, Philadelphia, 1954, Lea & Febiger.

Snell, Richard S.: Atlas of clinical anatomy, Boston, 1978, Little, Brown & Co.

Sobotta, J., and Figge, F.H.J.: Atlas of human anatomy, ed. 8, New York, 1963, Hafner Publishing Co., Inc.

U N I T

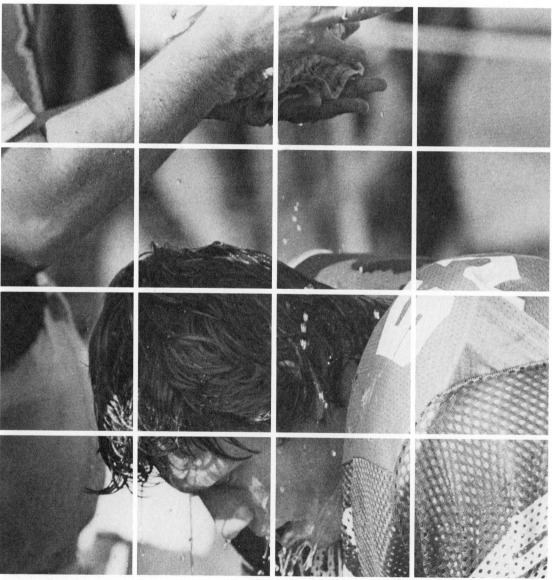

Helping an athlete cope with heat stress.
(Courtesy Argus Leader, Sioux Falls, S.D.)

T W O
Athletic-related trauma

To become competent and efficient in assessing athletic injuries, the athletic trainer must be familiar with the broad scope of athletic injuries or conditions and possess a fundamental knowledge of how the body responds to various types of traumas or stresses associated with athletic activity. Athletic injuries or conditions normally result from some type of physical trauma, but can be caused by other circumstances, such as infectious agents or exposure to hot or cold environments. The information in this unit will enable you to better understand the body's responses to athletic-related trauma and how the associated signs and symptoms can assist in the assessment process.

6   The body's response to trauma and environmental stress
7   Athletic injuries and related skin conditions

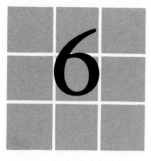

6

The body's response to trauma and environmental stress

When the body is subjected to injurious trauma or stress, it will usually respond in a systematic and predictable manner. Fortunately, when changes in normal body functions occur, they are manifested by signs or symptoms that provide important clues to assist in identifying underlying medical conditions. To adequately and effectively care for athletic injuries, it is necessary for the athletic trainer to have a fundamental knowledge of the anatomic and physiologic responses to an injury and to understand how di-

agnostic signs and symptoms develop. The incorporation of this knowledge into athletic injury assessment and management strategies can provide for a rational approach to both the initial evaluation and the subsequent care of an injured athlete. Poor management of an athletic injury can contribute to such circumstances as delayed healing, an unstable or weakened body area, an unsightly scar, or more seriously, permanent disability or possibly death. This chapter discusses some of the body's basic responses to

Fig. 6-1. Cycle of an athletic injury.

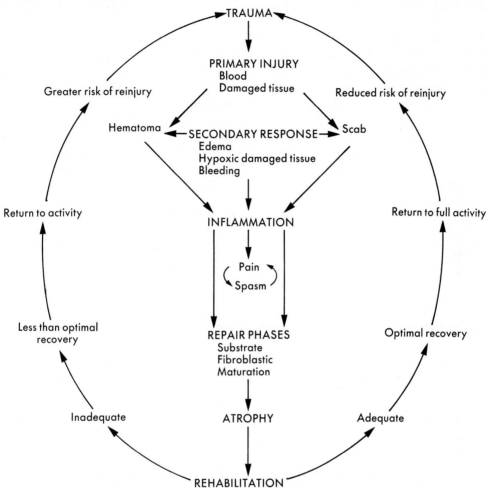

trauma resulting from athletic activity and adverse environmental conditions and the associated signs and symptoms. This chapter also briefly discusses procedures an athletic trainer can employ to positively affect and influence these body responses.

BODY'S RESPONSE TO PHYSICAL TRAUMA

The body's immediate and long-term responses to physical trauma are essentially the same for all types of athletic injuries; that is, the processes of inflammation and healing. Although these phenomena are not completely or clearly understood, the physiologic and anatomic changes that characterize each step are reliable and predictable indicators from which a trained observer can deduce a great deal of information about both the initial injury and the subsequent course of the recovery process. The body's basic response to a traumatic athletic injury is illustrated in Fig. 6-1. This cycle outlines the sequence of events following an injury through the inflammatory and healing processes. Ideally, the end result is optimal recovery. Of course, depending on the severity of the injury and the management procedures used, this cycle can vary greatly in its length and conclude in less-than-optimal recovery and possibly reinjury or permanent loss of function.

The majority of athletic injuries are caused by some type of trauma, such as a direct blow, rotational stress, forced abnormal motion and over-stretching or tearing forces. When these forces

TRAUMA
Direct blow
Rotational stress
Abnormal motion
Overstretching

are greater than the tissues can withstand, varying degrees of damage result. Athletic trauma frequently involves the skin, muscles, tendons, ligaments, bones or nerves. A certain amount of hemorrhaging or bleeding will also be present if capillaries or other blood vessels are damaged. This bleeding may be external, if there is an open wound, or internal, if there is no break in the continuity of the skin. The body responds to hemorrhage by activating the clotting mechanism in an attempt to control the bleeding. In this type of injury there is also at least some direct cell damage as a result of the trauma. Cells that are damaged or torn lose their nutrition and, as a result, the ability to maintain the necessary cellular activities required for normal function. The result is often cell death or **necrosis.** These necrotic tissue cells and the **extravasated** blood remaining outside the blood vessels as a result of hemorrhage will eventually develop into a mass called a **hematoma.** With open injuries, the blood and necrotic debris may form a thin blood clot, fill the apposed margins of the wounds, and subsequently form a scab on the surface.

The damaged tissue and extravasted blood resulting primarily from direct trauma are termed the initial insult or **pri-**

PRIMARY INJURY
Blood
Damaged tissue

mary injury. Other than initiating procedures to bring bleeding under control as quickly as possible, athletic trainers have little if any effect on the extent of primary injury. Although it is considered the end of damage directly caused by initial trauma, swelling and tissue damage may not cease with the control of bleeding. Frequently, additional damage will occur that is secondary to the initial trauma or primary injury. This is called the secondary response or **secondary injury** and is discussed along with the inflammatory process. Athletic trainers can greatly affect this phase of the athletic injury cycle.

Acute inflammatory process

The acute inflammatory process begins within minutes of the onset of injury. **Inflammation** is the basic response of vas-

SUBSTRATE PHASE
Vascular changes
Phagocytosis

cularized tissues to an injurious agent, whether the source is physical, bacterial, thermal, or chemical. The inflammatory process is a nonspecific response designed to be the body's defense mechanism against trauma, regardless of cause. In athletics the most frequent cause of inflammation is physical trauma. The goal of the inflammatory process is threefold: (1) to localize the extent of the injured area, (2) to rid both the body as a whole and the injury site of waste products resulting from the initial trauma and secondary response, and (3) to enhance healing.

Substrate phase

The initial phase of the acute inflammatory response is called the **substrate phase** and is characterized by localized vascular changes. Immediate vasoconstriction occurs first and is followed by vasodilation and increased vascular permeability. After the injury there is an immediate transient constriction of local blood vessels, resulting in a decreased blood flow to the injured area. The initial vasoconstriction may last from 5 to 10 minutes, providing sufficient time for initial evaluation of the injury and transportation of the athlete off the field or court if necessary. This decreased flow of blood reduces the amount of oxygen and nutrients being delivered to the injury site and surrounding area and may cause cells uninjured by the initial trauma to be damaged by *hypoxia.* Cells that undergo secondary hypoxic death add to the debris from the initial injury, increasing the size of the hematoma. As a result of cells undergoing hypoxic death, the extent of the injury may be greater than that caused by the initial insult.

Transient vasoconstriction at the time of injury is followed by active vasodilation of local blood vessels and increased blood flow to the trauma site. These changes are attributed to chemical substances released at the injury site, the most significant being histamine. Concurrent to this increased blood flow is congestion in the blood vessels and increased vascular permeability that allows the white blood cells (leukocytes), which have lined up along the vessel walls during vasoconstriction (a process called *margination*), to migrate toward the injury site. Physiologists refer to this amoeboid type of movement of leukocytes from the interior or lumen of blood vessels into the tissue spaces as *diapedesis.* The increased vascular permeability, and any actual structural damage to blood vessels resulting from the injury, allow plasma and plasma proteins to leak out or escape *(extravasate)* from the blood vessels. This contributes to the collection of an excessive amount of blood fluids in the tissue spaces surrounding the blood vessels at the point of injury. This protein-rich fluid is called *exudate.* This leakage of blood fluids accounts for much of the swelling *(edema)* associated with an injury and may continue for 24

SECONDARY RESPONSE
Edema
Hypoxic-damaged tissue
Additional blood

to 48 hours, causing the injury site to be more extensive than that caused by the initial trauma.

The inflammatory process is an important defense mechanism that occurs for a specific purpose, namely to protect and heal an injured area.

The four cardinal signs of inflammation, which were originally identified by Celsus in the first century AD, are (1) redness, (2) swelling, (3) heat, and (4) pain. A fifth sign, loss of function, has since been added. These signs and symptoms serve to remind an athlete that he or she has been injured and are present to prevent the athlete from exceeding safe limits of activity and reinjuring the area. To effectively manage an injury the athletic trainer must be able to recognize the signs and symptoms of inflammation and understand what they indicate. Following is a brief explanation of the signs and symptoms of inflammation and their causes:

INFLAMMA- TION
Redness
Swelling
Heat
Pain
Loss of function

Redness (rubor): Caused by dilation of arterioles and increased flow of blood to the injured area

Swelling (tumor): Caused by the accumulation of blood and damaged tissue cells in the primary injury area, as well as blood, hypoxic-damaged tissue debris, and edema resulting from the secondary reaction

Heat (calor): Caused by increased biochemical activity in the affected tissues and increased blood flow to the skin surface

Pain (dolor): Caused by direct injury to nerve fibers as well as pressure of the hematoma or area of edema on nerve endings

Loss of function (functio laesa): Caused by the resulting pain and swelling or the actual destruction of an anatomic structure, such as a fractured bone, ruptured ligament, or torn muscle

The primary function of the inflammatory process in the days following an injury is to rid the area of waste products resulting from the primary and secondary responses in preparation for the healing process. As the blood vessels become more permeable and allow blood cells to migrate into the tissues, leukocytes infiltrate the injured area and concentrate at the injury site. In the early stages of the acute inflammatory response, these leukocytes engage in *phagocytosis,* which is the injesting and disposing of unwanted substances, such as elements of the hematoma. During the later phases of acute inflammation, the predominant phagocyte is a macrophage type of cell that emigrates to the injury site in large numbers. After the debris is injested, these phagocytes reenter the blood stream or lymphatic system and are carried away from the injury site. The successful completion of this phagocytic activity usually marks the end of the acute inflammatory reaction. In most wounds not contaminated with bacteria or large amounts of foreign material, the acute inflammatory process subsides within several days, and the repair process continues to evolve.

Pain-spasm cycle

An additional response to trauma is the pain-spasm cycle. Generally, pain and muscle spasm of varying degrees accompany musculoskeletal injuries. Muscle spasm is a protective mechanism, designed to prevent further damage to an already injured area. The body attempts to splint the area surrounding the injured area through the involuntary contraction of muscles or groups of muscles. The resulting contraction is called muscle spasm. As the muscle spasm develops, there is increased pressure on the nerve endings, resulting in more pain. The body responds to the increased pain with increased muscle spasms, resulting in more pain, and so on; hence the name pain-spasm cycle.

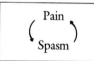

Psychologic responses to trauma

Another phenomenon athletic trainers must consider with any athletic injury is the psychologic responses of the athlete to physical trauma and pain. Athletes perceive physical trauma in different ways. Perceived changes in body habitus, gait, appearance, and functional ability all contribute to the psychologic reality of injury. Some may perceive an athletic injury as a disaster, whereas others may find it a welcome relief from poor performance, a losing season, or lack of playing time. Athletes can undergo a variety of psychologic reactions to an injury, such as anger, disbelief, denial, alienation, depression, isolation, resignation, or acceptance. In fact, an athlete may go through all of these reactions during a single injury situation. Some of these reactions can develop into a self-defeating attitude and become blocking forces to effective recovery and rehabilitation. Athletes may lack motivation to recover and wonder if they ever will completely recover and compete again. Although it is not the purpose of this text to discuss complex psychologic mechanisms of human behavior, athletic trainers must be aware that these factors can greatly affect the physiologic responses to trauma. Recovery depends on the proper psychologic attitude as well as on the physiologic processes involved. Athletic trainers should combine sound physiologic treatment techniques with a positive, encouraging attitude in an attempt to effectively treat the mind as well as the body. We recommend that athletic trainers continue to learn more about psychologic phenomenon associated with athletes and athletic injuries.

The process of wound healing

The process of wound healing begins with the acute inflammatory reaction and then accelerates when enough of the hematoma has been removed to permit the growth of new tissue. The formation of new tissue is required to replace tissues that were damaged by the injury. Most tissues involved in athletic injuries do not have the ability to regenerate their respective specialized cells, and instead undergo a relatively nonspecific repair process, that of scar formation. Our epidermis and bones, however, do have the ability to regenerate, or heal, with the same type of tissue that was damaged. Unfortunately, most soft tissues in the body heal with the formation of scar tissue,

> **REPAIR PHASES**
> Fibroplastic
>   Collagen fibers
> Maturation
>   Scar develops

which is less than an ideal replacement. Scar formation is virtually identical in all tissues of the body. However, the final appearance of a scar and its effect on function will vary, depending on the tissue involved and the treatment given. Treatment and rehabilitation procedures differ somewhat between various types of tissues injured. These procedures are briefly discussed on p. 100.

Fibroplastic phase. The removal of most of the necrotic debris from the injury site is followed by development of a dense network of capillaries early in the healing process. Along with the formation of this capillary network, *fibroblasts,* which are connective tissue cells that form the fibrous connective tissues in the body, proliferate in the damaged area. This phase of wound healing or scar formation is known as *fibroplasia.* These fibroblasts manufacture collagen, which is the main supportive protein in skin, tendon, bone, cartilage, and connective tissue. Significant amounts of collagen are laid down by the fourth or fifth day after an injury, so that a loose mesh of fibrous connective tissue occupies the injured area. This connective tissue is vascular and fragile. The phenomenon of fibroblast proliferation and collagen accumulation after injury usually continues for 2 to 4 weeks. During this time the vascularity of the new fibrous connective tissue continues to decrease, and the tensile strength increases. As a sufficient quantity of collagen is produced, the number of fibroblasts in the wound diminishes. The disappearance of these fibroblasts marks the end of the fibroplastic phase and the beginning of the *maturation phase.*

Maturation phase. During the maturation phase of wound healing, pronounced changes occur in the newly formed fibrous connective tissue. The scar that is formed during fibroplasia is an enlarged and dense but unorganized structure of collagen. The fibers of collagen are initially randomly arranged but in time will line up along lines of stress. The union between the damaged tissues is still moderately fragile. During the next several months, the strength of the scar continues to increase and the collagen fibers change to a more organized pattern. As the scar tissue matures, it shrinks and becomes avascular and acellular. This maturation process may continue for a year or longer.

It is important for athletic trainers to understand the basic fundamentals of wound repair and scar formation to gain optimum treatment results and achieve full recovery with injured athletes. It is the responsibility of the athletic trainer to localize the inflammatory response, promote the healing process, and ensure that athletes are not imposing undue stresses on healing tissue that is not mature or ready for strenuous activity.

Open wounds, those involving a break in the continuity of the skin, should be thoroughly cleansed to remove any foreign material, obvious necrotic tissue, or bacterial contaminants. Wound healing that occurs in the absence of infection is called *healing by first intention.* If infection with pus formation does occur, there will be little if any healing until the infection is overcome. This is called *healing by second intention.* Wound edges must be restored as closely as possible to normal anatomic relationships to minimize both the amount of fibroplasia required for healing to occur and the width of the resulting scar. Although this is primarily a physician's responsibility, the athletic trainer will be called on to protect the injured area when the athlete returns to activity and to inspect the wound periodically to ensure that it does not reopen or become infected. Remember, the epidermis is undergoing constant replacement by regeneration, and injuries involving only this outer layer of the skin will heal without scar formation. Epidermal wounds heal by migration and proliferation of epithelial cells originating in the margins of the wound.

Athletic injuries involving structures deep to the skin must be treated to heal in such a way that function of the involved anatomic part will be restored to an optimum level. In many instances, when a structure is ruptured or torn, it is desirable to repair it surgically. The goal of surgical repair is to bring the ruptured ends together so that a shorter distance has to be spanned by scar tissue. The injured area must be protected from abnormal stresses, which can interfere with the healing process and weaken, stretch, or tear the developing scar tissue and result in loss of function or instability. This protection or immobilization may be in the form of a cast, brace, splint, tape, or rest.

Rehabilitation procedures will differ, depending on the type of tissues injured. Injuries involving the contractile unit (muscles and tendons) are treated and managed differently than those involving noncontractile tissues such as ligaments. If muscles and tendons are allowed to heal without active early motion, it may be very difficult to restore full strength and range of motion. Range of motion exercises should be started as early as possible once swelling and tenderness have subsided to the point that exercises are not unduly painful. However, starting too early may impede the healing process, cause additional hemorrhage and swelling, and result in a bigger scar and possibly a limitation in function. Allowing the musculotendinous unit to heal in a shortened state will result in a loss of motion, requiring constant stretching and making the athlete more vulnerable to repeated strains. These contractile tissues may require a certain amount of support and protection when activity is resumed. Occasionally injuries to the contractile unit will result in the formations of fibrous *adhesions* that bind the tendon or muscle to surrounding tissues and interfere with normal movement.

Ligament injuries require a long period of time (possibly 6 months) to heal to the point of regaining near normal tensile strength. If ligaments are subjected to abnormal stresses early in the healing process, the developing scar tissue may elongate, resulting in some degree of permanent instability of the involved joint. External means of protection or immobilization, such as a cast, brace, or taping, are used until the healing ligament is moderately strong and the surrounding muscles can be rehabilitated to assist in the

support of the joint. In many cases the injured joint will require continued support and protection when athletic activity is resumed.

Another result of the injury cycle that an athletic trainer must be aware of is *atrophy*. Atrophy is the wasting away or deterioration of a tissue, organ, or part. During the healing process, if the injured area has been immobilized or otherwise inactive, atrophy will occur. In most cases the degree of atrophy is directly proportional to the amount and time of immobilization. Occasionally, changes in vascularity and innervation of a body area will also result in atrophy. Regardless of cause, an area of the body that has atrophied is more susceptible to reinjury, thus instigating repetition of the injury cycle. Therefore the injured athlete should not be returned to full athletic activity until the area has been rehabilitated to an optimal level.

The immediate care of athletic injuries

The standard procedures for the immediate care of athletic injuries are based on how the body responds to trauma and the acute inflammatory process. These initial

INITIAL TREATMENT
Ice
Compression
Elevation
Rest

treatment procedures are designed to control the swelling and minimize the magnitude of the hematoma, which allows the process of healing to begin earlier and proceed at a more rapid rate. The standard procedures for the initial care of an athletic injury are universally accepted and can be remembered by the acronym ICER. These letters stand for the steps of *I*ce, *C*ompression, *E*levation, and *R*est. Each of these steps is important and should not be overlooked when caring for an acute athletic injury.

Ice

The first step is to put some form of cold application on the injured area, whether it is an ice pack or cold immersion. Cold applied promptly after an injury can slow down or minimize some of the acute inflammatory reactions previously discussed. In addition, cold diminishes local blood flow and helps constrict capillaries in the area of injury. The local application of cold also decreases clotting time because it increases the viscosity of the fluids and decreases the rate of flow in the injured area. This quicker clotting reduces hemorrhaging in the area of injury. Another important effect of cold is to lower tissue temperature, thus decreasing the metabolic demands and slowing the chemical actions in cells surrounding the injured area. This reduces the build up of waste products in the area and allows more tissue cells to survive the period of temporary hypoxia. To summarize, applying cold to an injured area reduces tissue damage and results in a smaller hematoma to be resolved. Cold applications are also beneficial in reducing the amount of muscle spasms that usually accompany athletic injuries. Therefore there is less discomfort associated with the pain-spasm cycle.

Compression

The purpose of compression on an acute injury is to help control or reduce the amount of edema and provide mild support. Compression about an injured area is normally accomplished by the use of an elastic wrap or appropriate taping. Compression acts as a physical deterrent to swelling by preventing fluids from accumulating in the injured area. Compression also increases the tissue pressure outside the blood vessels, thus helping to prevent edema caused by plasma seepage or extravasation. Normally, compression will also make an injured area feel more comfortable. Although an elastic wrap offers only mild support, the pressure does appear to provide some relief of pain.

Elevation

Elevation of an injured area limits fluid pooling and encourages venous return. Elevating an injured area also decreases the hydrostatic pressure within the blood vessels, which helps decrease the amount of edema by decreasing the volume of fluid filtered out of the blood vessels

and into the tissue spaces. Controlling the edema associated with an injured area decreases tissue damage and results in a smaller area to be repaired.

Rest

Resting an injured area is necessary to allow the body time to get the effects of the trauma under control and to avoid additional stress and damage to injured tissue. The period of rest required will vary, depending on the athletic trainer's and physician's philosophy and on the severity of the injury. The length of rest may range from a 10-minute break in a practice to many months of postoperative recovery. Athletes who continue to participate with an acutely injured area may increase hemorrhage and the amount of initial tissue damage as well as the amount and severity of secondary injury response, such as edema formation and the accumulation of tissue debris from hypoxic damage. All of this can result in a larger hematoma, slower healing, and a longer recovery period.

The purpose of the initial treatment procedures of ice, compression, elevation, and rest is to minimize the effects of an injury at its onset and to create an optimal environment for healing, thereby reducing the loss of function and length of the recovery period. Normally these procedures are used for at least 2 to 3 days after a significant injury. Although athletic trainers can do little to speed up the actual healing process, they can have a tremendous effect on the total recovery time and on the quality of the repair.

Follow-up treatment procedures

Treatment procedures used after the immediate postinjury period are designed to rehabilitate the athlete toward full functional use of the injured area and return him or her to an optimal level of performance in a minimal period of time. Both heat and cold modalities are used after the initial treatment period; however, heat should not be

REHABILITA- TION
Exercise
Heat or cold applications

used until you are relatively sure no further bleeding or swelling will occur. Heat is used primarily to increase the circulation to an area. Cold is used primarily to relieve pain, thereby allowing early and more extensive range of motion. Both of these modalities should always be used in conjunction with some type of exercise. Exercise is the primary modality used to rehabilitate an injured area and is the most effective method of increasing blood flow to an area. The increased blood flow helps resolve the hematoma and deliver oxygen and nutrients required in rebuilding injured tissues.

Athletic trainers must be familiar with rehabilitation procedures. He or she must assume a leadership role in convincing an injured athlete that the key to a good rehabilitation program is continued progressive exercise, not just an extension of passive treatment activity for a longer period of time. The type of exercises used to restore normal function depend on the nature and severity of the injury as well as the athletic trainer's philosophy. Basically, exercises should be performed essentially pain free and progress as fast as possible from active range of motion to full participation. This may be completed in days or may take 3 to 4 weeks or longer. Pain is the primary governing force for all treatment procedures. As long as the exercise is pain free, the athlete should be encouraged to increase the level of activity. If the exercise is painful or if residual swelling and pain are present following treatment, the activity is too strenuous and should be modified.

Chronic inflammation

Chronic is defined as long lasting. Although there is no sharp delineation of time between acute and chronic, *acute* generally refers to a matter of hours or days, whereas chronic refers to weeks, months, or years. Chronic inflammation may result from overuse, improper technique, continued stress, or repeated injury to a structure or area of the body. For whatever reason, the inflammatory response continues to repeat itself and can be detrimental to an athlete's performance. Such conditions as tennis elbow, jumper's knee, and shin splints are typical examples of chronic inflammations. They can progress to a point at which they disable an athlete. Although these seem to be different conditions, chronic inflammatory responses are basically alike and require the same treatment; rest, local heat, protection against reinjury, and often anti-inflammatory medications prescribed by a physician. In chronic conditions, identification of possible causes and preventive measures is more important than the cure. The purpose of any training program is to build up the body's structures gradually so they are able to withstand progressively heavier workloads, thus increasing their strength, endurance, and ability to avoid injury. Once a chronic inflammatory condition occurs, it is up to the athletic trainer or physician to attempt to identify and eliminate the possible causes. These problems can be magnified by the fact that in many cases relief will require a sharp reversal of activity. A period of complete rest may be required, which must then be followed by a gradual increase in workload. This can become very frustrating and burdensome to the athlete, athletic trainer, or coach, especially if the injury occurs during the athletic season. The athlete's impatience to resume activity too soon or at too great an intensity level often results in recurrence of the condition and an even more frustrating period of disability.

Summary

The body's response to trauma is generally well established and programmed. When some type of trauma occurs, there is a certain amount of damaged tissue and blood that accumulates as the result of the primary injury. In addition to hematoma formation, there is frequently a secondary response that causes the injury site to become even more extensive. This secondary response includes edema and hypoxia and may continue for 24 to 48 hours. The body responds to this trauma with an inflammatory reaction designed to localize the extent of the injured area, rid the body of waste products, and enhance healing. The processes of inflammation and healing form a continuum that can be subdivided into three phases; substrate (vascular changes and phagocytosis), fibroplastic (laying down of collagen fibers), and maturation (scar development). However, portions of these phases can occur simultaneously. For example, fibroplasia begins during the substrate phase, and scar maturation begins while collagen production continues. Possessing a fundamental knowledge of what happens to the body as a result of trauma provides the athletic trainer with a more rational basis for the management of various athletic injuries.

One of the primary responsibilities of an athletic trainer is to positively affect and influence the healing process to gain optimal treatment results with the injured athlete. This is initially accomplished through reducing the effects of the initial injury or trauma. Bleeding and swelling must be controlled as quickly as possible to minimize the magnitude of the hematoma. Limiting the hematoma allows the healing process to commence earlier, reducing the length of inactivity caused by the injury. Follow-up treatment procedures using exercise in conjunction with various methods of heat or cold applications are designed to optimally rehabilitate the injured athlete in a minimal period of time. It is not the intent of this text to discuss the various modalities and treatment procedures used by athletic trainers. We recommend that you aggressively seek out new information in this area and continue to improve and refine your treatment and rehabilitation techniques.

SHOCK

Another of the body's responses to trauma is shock. Shock is a state of collapse or depression of the cardiovascular system. It does not occur very often in athletics; however, any significant athletic injury can result in shock. The possibilities of shock developing are much greater with severe bleeding (external or internal), spinal injuries, major fractures, and significant intrathoracic or intra-abdominal injuries. There are three main causes of shock: (1) the heart is damaged so that it fails to pump properly, (2) blood is lost so that there is an insufficient volume of fluid in the circulatory system, and (3) blood vessels dilate so that blood "pools" in the larger vessels, resulting in a diminished amount of fluid available to provide efficient circulation. One of these last two causes are most often responsible for shock when it occurs because of athletic injuries.

The result of shock is the same no matter what the cause; that is, a diminished amount of fluid available in the circulatory system. This results in an insufficient perfusion of blood providing oxygen and nutrients through the tissues and organs of the body. All bodily processes are affected. Body systems are depressed, and vital functions slow down. Shock is always serious; if this condition is not treated properly and promptly, death can result.

Shock develops in distinct stages. It can progress quite rapidly or develop over a period of hours. Fig. 6-2 traces a continuous cycle of traumatic shock and outlines how each of the signs of shock develop. It is important for an athletic trainer to recognize these signs and to be prepared to properly care for an injured athlete. The important signs indicating possible shock are:

1. Rapid, weak pulse
2. Cool, clammy skin
3. Rapid, shallow breathing
4. Profuse sweating
5. Pale skin, and later, cyanotic mucous membranes
6. Nausea, possibly vomiting
7. Dull, lackluster eyes; pupils may dilate
8. Steadily falling blood pressure
9. Unconsciousness

As soon as the athletic trainer recognizes any of these signs, the athlete should be treated for shock. Shock is a serious condition, but if recognized quickly and treated effectively, it can be reversed. The general treatment for shock is as follows:

1. Keep the athlete lying down, and elevate the lower extremities if the injury will not

be aggravated. If there is a head, spinal, or abdominal injury or breathing difficulties, keep the athlete flat or in a comfortable position.

2. Establish and maintain a clear airway.
3. Control obvious bleeding.
4. Loosen or remove any pieces of uniform or equipment that may hinder breathing or circulation.
5. Maintain body temperature as near normal as possible. In cold temperatures, keep the athlete warm and reduce the loss of body heat.
6. Do not give anything to eat or drink.

7. Give oxygen if available.
8. Transport the athlete to medical facilities or summon medical assistance.

BODY'S RESPONSE TO THERMAL EXPOSURE

It is extremely important for the athletic trainer to understand the body's response to thermal exposure, especially any abnormal responses such as heat exhaustion or heat stroke. Athletes participating in activities such as running, tennis, cycling, baseball, and softball regularly engage in vigorous exertion during hot and humid weather. Early season practices in fall sports

Fig. 6-2. Continuous cycle of traumatic shock.
(From Brennan, W.T. and Ludwig, D.J., Guide to problems and practices in first aid and emergency care, ed. 3, Dubuque, Iowa, 1976, William C. Brown Co.)

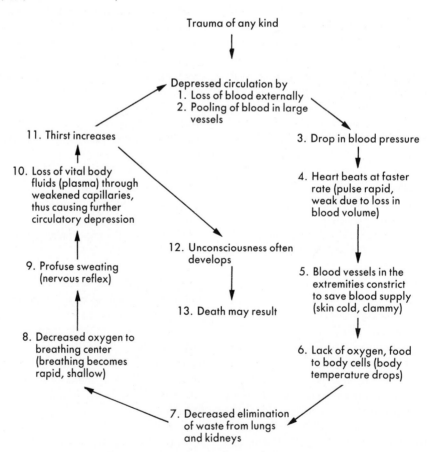

such as football, cross country, soccer, or field hockey frequently necessitate participation in a hot, humid environment. It is possible to find these same environmental conditions indoors, such as in wrestling rooms and gymnasiums. The recent popularity of distance running and marathons has also increased problems related to heat stress. Heat-related problems vary in severity from temporary heat cramps to fatal heat strokes. Life-threatening situations in athletics are rare; however, they occasionally occur as the result of heat stress. The devastating effects of heat illness are needless and preventable. The athletic trainer can have a tremendous impact on prevention of heat-related illnesses by intelligently counseling coaches and athletes about the variables concerning activity in hot weather. Therefore it is extremely important for athletic trainers to understand the physiologic mechanisms active in thermoregulatory responses and how environmental conditions can significantly

contribute to heat illness. The athletic trainer must also know how to acclimate athletes, initiate preventive measures to avoid potentially fatal heat-related incidents, recognize associated signs and symptoms indicating the development of heat-related conditions, and be proficient in the use of emergency procedures required to care for athletes suffering from heat-stress conditions.

Physiologic basis of heat exposure

The human body is continually attempting to maintain a constant internal (core) temperature of 98.6° F (37° C). The brain and the thoracic and abdominal visceral structures are considered core organs. To maintain constant temperature to these organs, heat lost must equal heat gained. If heat gain exceeds heat loss, the core temperature will rise; conversely, core temperature falls when heat loss exceeds heat production. The body has various mechanisms to gain as well as lose heat (Fig. 6-3), and it is extremely important

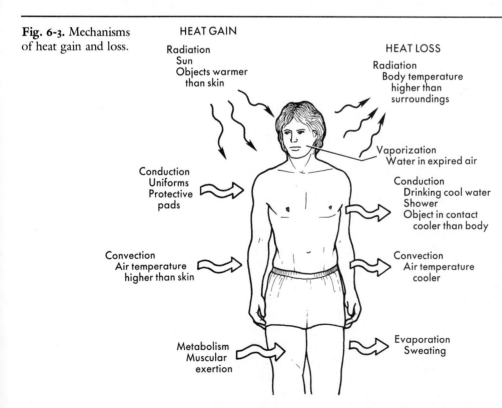

Fig. 6-3. Mechanisms of heat gain and loss.

HEAT GAIN

Radiation
Sun
Objects warmer
than skin

HEAT LOSS

Radiation
Body temperature
higher than
surroundings

Conduction
Uniforms
Protective
pads

Vaporization
Water in expired air

Conduction
Drinking cool water
Shower
Object in contact
cooler than body

Convection
Air temperature
higher than skin

Convection
Air temperature
cooler

Metabolism
Muscular
exertion

Evaporation
Sweating

to maintain a balance between these mechanisms during athletic activity.

Heat production

The body produces both heat and energy during *metabolism.* During exercise and muscular exertion accompanying athletic activity, the metabolic rate increases, as does the heat production. The greater the energy expenditure, the greater the heat production. This heat diffuses from the muscle cells to capillary blood, which passes through the lungs. A relatively small amount of heat is lost through *vaporization* of water in the air expired during respiration. However, most of the heat is carried by the blood into the circulatory system.

Heat gain

Heat can be gained by the body from the environment through radiation, conduction, and convection (Fig. 6-3). We gain heat by *radiation* from the sun and surrounding objects. On an athletic field, a considerable amount of heat can be gained from the sun in this way. This is especially true when there is little or no cloud cover, or during the middle portion of the day when the sun is directly overhead and the radiation is more concentrated. Remember, the heat radiating from an artificial turf is usually higher than that radiating from a natural or grass playing field. We also gain heat by radiation from objects surrounding the body when they are warmer than the skin's temperature.

Convection is the transfer of heat from one place to another by motion or circulation. If the temperature of the air surrounding the athlete is higher than the athlete's temperature, he or she may gain heat through convection. An increase in the athlete's core temperature may also occur through *conduction* or contact with protective equipment and uniforms. This is especially true in football, in which much of the body's surface is covered with pads or a full uniform.

Heat dissipation and loss

As excess heat is produced or gained by the body, it must be eliminated or dissipated in order to keep the body temperature from reaching detrimental extremes. Heat loss is accomplished by radiation, conduction, convection, and evaporation (Fig. 6-3). There are a number of strategies and preventive measures athletic trainers employ to encourage or promote the dissipation of heat from the body and minimize the risk of heat-related illness during athletic activity; these are discussed on pp. 110 to 113.

The body eliminates heat primarily by cutaneous vasodilation and sweating. When the core temperature rises, for whatever reason, the body responds by increasing the peripheral blood flow in an attempt to transfer the heat from the core to the periphery. This brings an increase of body heat to the skin's surface, where it can be dissipated to the outside environment. When the body temperature is warmer than surrounding objects, we lose heat through radiation. When the air temperature is cooler than the body's, we can lose heat by convection. Athletes who are running can lose heat in this manner, as can those standing in a breeze. The amount of heat lost by convection depends on the temperature and speed of the air flow over the body. The body can also lose heat by conduction, providing the object in contact with the body is cooler. Examples of this are drinking cold water, wiping off with a cool, wet towel, or taking a cool shower.

The major portion of heat loss during athletics is through *evaporation* of sweat from the surface of the body. This is the body's major defense mechanism against overheating and serious heat illness. The body produces sweat that accumulates on the surface of the skin and cools the body as it evaporates. Our bodies are cooled only if the sweat evaporates. The effectiveness of this sweating and evaporation mechanism is strongly influenced by the relative humidity or the moisture in the air. That is, the lower the humidity, the faster the evaporation rate. As the relative humidity rises, the rate of the evaporation diminishes, until between 70% and 80% humidity, effective evaporation may cease. Therefore the combination of high temperature and high humidity decreases the body's ability to cool down, and increases the possibilities of heat-related conditions. The rate of sweating also depends on the intensity of the activity, the physical condition of the athlete, how acclimated the athlete is, and the amount and type of clothing and equipment worn.

Temperature regulation

The function of the thermoregulatory system is to maintain a relatively constant internal body temperature, whether the body is at rest or participating in strenuous activity. This system is controlled by the temperature regulatory center in the hypothalmus, which receives its information from various thermal receptors located throughout the body. The role of this center in the brain is analogous to that of the thermostat in a house. As information comes in that heat is being gained, the thermoregulatory center automatically relays information to appropriate thermal effectors, and mechanisms of vasodilation or sweating, are initiated.

Cutaneous vasodilation brings warm blood to the body's surface, where excess heat can be dissipated. This mechanism functions well as long as heat levels are not excessively high and the outside temperature is lower than the skin's surface. It is possible for an athlete's rate of heat gain and storage to become excessive in a very short period of time. If this occurs, it may overwhelm the body's mechanisms of heat loss. Such a situation can quickly develop into a serious heat illness. In addition, as the external temperature approaches that of the skin's surface or actually becomes higher, the heat dissipated by cutaneous vasodilation diminishes and may eventually cease completely. Body heat must then be dissipated primarily by the evaporation of sweat. If peripheral vasodilation is quite marked, the effective volume of the vascular system is decreased, and the heart must increase its output to compensate and maintain adequate blood flow. This is accomplished by an increase in both heart rate and stroke volume. Unfortunately, at least some degree of vasomotor control of the cutaneous vessels may be lost during heat stress. The result is pooling of blood in the extremities. As

blood is progressively shunted into the periphery, less and less blood flows to the internal organs and central nervous system. These effects may combine to cause symptoms of headache, dizziness, exhaustion, restlessness, and impaired thinking.

Another important physiologic consideration is the volume of sweat lost from the body. Profuse sweating can cause excessive losses of body water, which can result in a decreased blood volume and dehydration and a decreased rate of sweating and cooling by evaporation. If this water is not replaced, circulatory collapse (shock) may result from the continuing decrease in blood volume. As sweating decreases there is also a decrease in evaporative cooling, which can cause an excessive rise in core temperature. As water loss becomes extremely excessive, the mechanism of sweating is shut off to maintain or conserve blood volume. When this happens, internal body temperature soars, giving way to a serious heat condition, heatstroke, which is discussed on p. 110.

Increased physical exertion during athletic activity, combined with varying degrees of increased air temperature and humidity, can place abnormal demands on the thermoregulatory system. When this system fails, or the heat gained exceeds that lost, athletes are subjected to the effects of heat-related conditions. This is especially prevalent during early season workouts. The athlete who is not acclimated to physical activity in hot, humid weather is particularly susceptible. Acclimation is an important preventive measure, as most serious heat-related problems occur in the first few days of practice.

Heat acclimation

Heat acclimation is the process of becoming accustomed to athletic activity in hot weather. It improves the circulatory and sweating responses, and facilitates the dissipation of heat. Heat acclimation helps minimize changes in body temperature. Acclimation renders the athlete more capable of adapting to or tolerating the stresses of heat and is the most efficient method of handling increased external temperatures. The acclimated athlete exhibits less heat stress during workouts in hot, humid weather than does the nonacclimated athlete. As an athlete becomes acclimated, several important body adjustments occur to allow the athlete to more effectively handle the stresses of heat. The body responds to heat acclimation by increasing cardiac output, circulating blood volume, and venous tone. The basal metabolic rate, core temperature, and pulse rate are reduced. In addition, the body is able to more precisely regulate sweat production, electrolyte concentrations, and peripheral blood flow and maintain a more stable blood pressure under varying conditions of stress.

For heat acclimation to occur, athletes must workout or exercise in hot weather. It is best for an athlete to acclimate gradually over a period of time before scheduled practices or an athletic season begins. Each athlete will acclimate at a different rate. Further, the athlete in good condition is capable of more work in the heat and will acclimate more rapidly than the nonconditioned athlete. It is believed that optimal acclimation requires an athlete to exercise with progressively increasing intensities between 1 to 2 hours daily. With this type of a schedule, acclimation is usually well developed in 5 to 7 days and complete in 12 to 14 days. In addition, athletes should have adequate access to water during the acclimation period, because withholding fluids significantly retards this process.

Heat-related conditions

Three specific heat illnesses or syndromes can result from thermal exposure; (1) heat cramps, (2) heat exhaustion, and (3) heatstroke. These three are listed in order from the least serious to the most serious. Each is normally caused by the same set of circumstances; that is, strenuous activity in a combination of hot and humid weather, resulting in a loss of body water and a derangement of the body's thermoregulatory system. Although the cause of these heat-related conditions is normally the same, each represents a different bodily reaction to excessive heat, with

their own set of signs and symptoms and treatment procedures. It is extremely important for athletic trainers to be familiar with signs and symptoms that indicate the development of heat illnesses, as well as emergency measures necessary to adequately care for athletes suffering from serious heat stress.

It is important to remember that heat cramps and heat exhaustion can lead to heatstroke. This is especially true when working with athletes. In most types of activity, a person will voluntarily stop working and seek relief from the heat when either heat cramps or heat exhaustion appear to be developing. Athletes, on the other hand, especially highly competitive or motivated athletes, are more likely to continue working out or exercising even though symptoms may be developing. Athletes in a sport such as football are required to wear heavy protective equipment and uniforms that cover much of the body and add to the problem of heat dissipation. Athletes are also engaged in strenuous activity under the influence of the coaches' or trainers' philosophies concerning the number of breaks, availability of water, and the intensity of the exercise sessions. All of these factors are pertinent to the development of heat-related conditions.

Heat cramps

Heat cramps are the least serious of the three heat illnesses. These cramps are painful spasms of skeletal muscles. Past training literature suggested that heat cramps are caused by salt or electrolyte loss. More recent literature, however, suggests that heat cramps result from a fluid volume problem and can normally be prevented by providing unlimited amounts of water to athletes throughout activity in hot weather.

When heat cramps do occur, they normally accompany strenuous physical activity and profuse sweating in hot weather. The most common muscles involved are the calf muscles or abdominals, but any of the voluntary muscles can be affected by a sudden and painful spasm or cramp. Heat cramps may be mild, with slight cramping, or they may be quite severe and incapacitating, with intense pain. Athletes suffering heat cramps are normally alert and oriented to their surroundings. The skin will be wet and warm as a result of excessive sweating. The body temperature, pulse, and respiratory rate should be normal or slightly elevated.

In most cases heat cramps are not a serious problem and can be relieved by slowly stretching the contracted muscle. The application of firm pressure or gentle massage may facilitate relief. The athlete should also be encouraged to drink liquids. Many times the athlete will resume activity after alleviation of the muscle spasms; however, a severe episode of heat cramps may require the athlete to avoid further exertion for a longer period of time, perhaps 12 to 24 hours. Should heat cramps frequently recur in the same athlete, additional assessment of specific causes is warranted, and medical referral may be necessary. Remember, athletes who suffer heat cramps should be closely observed, as this condition may precipitate heat exhaustion or heatstroke.

Heat exhaustion

Heat exhaustion is probably the most common condition caused by exertion in hot weather. The physiologic basis for heat exhaustion has been previously described; that is, peripheral vasodilation, loss of vasomotor control, and vascular pooling. Because of this peripheral vascular collapse, these athletes are suffering from an abnormally decreased volume of blood (hypovolemia) circulating in the body.

It is important for an athletic trainer to recognize the signs and symptoms associated with heat exhaustion and be able to differentiate them from those associated with heatstroke. Fig. 6-4 illustrates the main signs and symptoms associated with both conditions, with a (■) representing those most important.

Heat exhaustion is characterized by profuse

Fig. 6-4. Main signs and symptoms associated with heat exhaustion and heatstroke.

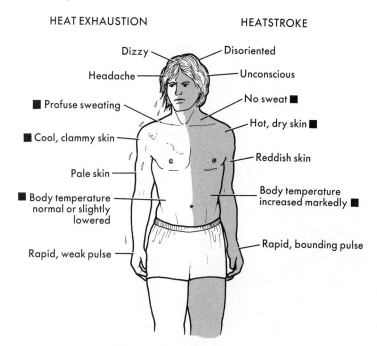

HEAT EXHAUSTION   HEATSTROKE

Dizzy — Disoriented

Headache — Unconscious

■ Profuse sweating — No sweat ■

■ Cool, clammy skin — Hot, dry skin ■

Pale skin — Reddish skin

■ Body temperature normal or slightly lowered — Body temperature increased markedly ■

Rapid, weak pulse — Rapid, bounding pulse

sweating, which makes the skin wet, cool, and clammy. The skin may also appear pale or gray. The decrease in blood volume normally results in headache, weakness, dizziness, fatigue, nausea, and occasionally unconsciousness. The athlete may be disoriented, and heat cramps may accompany this condition. The body temperature is usually normal or slightly below normal, and the respiration usually fast and shallow. Heat exhaustion may lead to complete collapse of the thermoregulatory system if not properly identified and treated.

Heat exhaustion is normally not life threatening, but proper medical care is required. The athlete should be treated as if in shock; that is, taken out of the hot environment and placed supine with the feet elevated. Remove as much equipment and uniform as possible. The cooling process can be assisted by sponging or toweling the athlete with cool water (Fig. 6-5). If the athlete is conscious, allow him or her to drink cool fluids. The athlete will normally feel better in a short period of time; however, should symptoms persist, the athlete should be transported to a medical facility. Athletes suffering heat exhaustion should be withdrawn from further activity for the remainder of that day and closely observed.

Heatstroke

Heatstroke (sunstroke) is the least common of the heat-related conditions but certainly the most serious. Heatstroke occurs when the thermoregulatory system of the body is completely overwhelmed or the volume of circulating blood becomes so low that the sweating mechanism is shut off to conserve depleted fluid levels. When either of these occur, the body temperature rises rapidly to dangerous and ultimately fatal levels. The body temperature may go over 106° F (41.1° C).

Heatstroke is a severe medical emergency and must be recognized and treated immediately. This condition is characterized by hot, dry skin and a rising temperature. The athlete's skin is normally reddened or flushed. As the temperature rises, the pulse becomes very rapid and strong. Initially the athlete may experience headache, dizziness, and weakness, which are often followed by convulsions and unconsciousness.

The immediate emergency care for an athlete exhibiting signs of heatstroke is to reduce the body temperature as quickly as possible by any means available. This may include cooling the body by placing ice or cold towels around the body, immersing the athlete in cold water, directing a fan at the athlete, or sponging the body with cool water or alcohol. Remove clothing and equipment to prevent the retention of body heat. If the athlete is conscious, allow him or her to drink cool water. Athletes suffering from heatstroke are critically ill and must be taken to a medical facility as soon as possible. Aggressive efforts to lower the body temperature should continue during the referral and transfer process.

Preventive measures

Although acclimation is probably the most important method of preventing problems re-

Fig. 6-5. Assisting the cooling process.

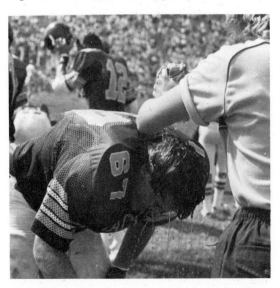

lated to heat stress, there are other measures an athletic trainer can take to prevent or reduce the impact of heat stress on the body.

Medical history. Obtain a complete medical history, including any previous heat illnesses or problems caused by the heat. Has the athlete ever fainted from excessive heat? Has the athlete ever had any sweating problems? Athletes who have suffered previous heat-related problems may have some permanent damage to the thermoregulatory center and are more prone to future heat disorders.

Physical condition. Evaluate the general physical condition of the athlete. Has he or she been working out in the heat? Inquire about the duration and intensity of work and training activities. In some sports, athletes may be required to com-

plete a physical fitness test, such as 12-minute run, before hot weather practice. Athletes in poor physical condition are candidates for heat illness. In addition, athletes who are overfat have an appreciably decreased ability to dissipate heat.

Recording temperature and humidity. It is important for the athletic trainer to measure the temperature and humidity during hot weather activity. The information an athletic trainer must have to make reasonable estimates of the severity of climatic conditions as they may affect athletes is minimal. Effective environmental guidelines can be constructed from easy-to-obtain temperature and humidity measurements taken on the practice or playing fields. These measurements should be made before and during training ses-

Fig. 6-6. Weather guide for the prevention of heat stress.
(From Fox, E.L., and Matthews, D.K.: The physiological basis of physical education and athletics, ed. 3, Copyright (c) 1981 by CBS College Publishing. Copyright 1971 and 1976 by W.B. Saunders Company. Reprinted by permission of Holt, Rinehard and Winston, CBS College Publishing.)

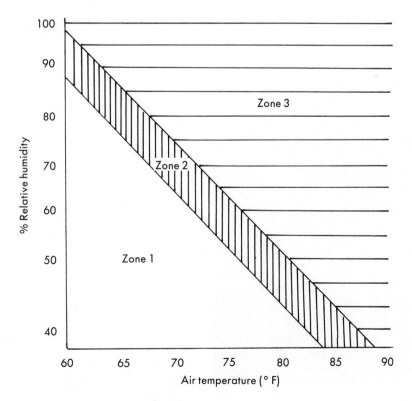

sions, and adjustments or modifications in activity made if so indicated. These adjustments include decreasing intensity levels of activity, providing more breaks and fluids, eliminating unnecessary clothing, or delaying or postponing practices until conditions improve.

There are several methods of monitoring the temperature and humidity. These readings can be obtained from the local weather bureau and then charted on a graph such as Fig. 6-6. This type of guide was developed from weather data gathered at the time of heatstroke fatalities occurring in football. Any combination of environmental conditions in zone 1 would be considered safe. Conditions in zone 2 would be a warn-

Fig. 6-7. Using a sling psychrometer to monitor environmental conditions.

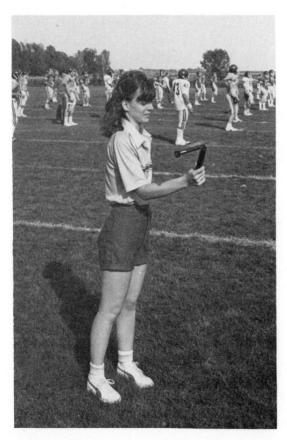

ing area, and athletes would need to be carefully observed for signs and symptoms of heat illness. Zone 3 would be the danger area. If conditions in this zone were present, practices would have to be modified or postponed, and athletes closely observed. Note that humidity is a significant factor, even in the presence of moderate temperatures.

Readings can also be taken on the athletic field using various devices developed to measure environmental conditions, such as a wet-bulb thermometer or sling psychrometer (Fig. 6-7). These are more accurate methods because deviations of several critical degrees often exist between onsite recordings and those from the weather bureau. This is especially true with artificial surfaces, as they tend to be several degrees hotter than grass fields.

Fluid replacement. Water is one of the major necessities of life. As previously discussed, decreased body fluid associated with profuse sweating diminishes the available blood volume and sweating necessary for body cooling. *Fluids must be provided.* Athletes should have unlimited and easy access to water during all athletic activity in hot weather (Fig. 6-8). It is better for athletes to drink small amounts frequently than to schedule a break every hour or so, when they may gulp large amounts of water. Deliberately withholding water from athletes for purposes of weight loss may be extremely hazardous in hot weather.

Clothing and uniforms. In hot or humid weather, clothing and uniforms should be lightweight, loose fitting, and light colored to reflect the sun. Porous or net shirts expose more of the body surface for evaporation of sweat and dissipation of body heat. Avoid the use of long stockings, long sleeves, excess clothing, and sweat suits during hot weather activity. This type of clothing can seriously limit heat loss by reducing evaporative cooling. Rubberized clothing should never be used in hot weather, as it does not allow the evaporation of sweat and dissipation of body heat.

Rest periods. Provide rest periods during hot

weather activities to dissipate accumulated body heat. If possible, athletes should rest in cool, shaded areas with some air movement. Loosen or remove heavy or tight-fitting jerseys to expose more skin surface. Allow football players to remove their helmets. In areas where hot weather conditions are especially severe, unique arrangements for moving air, such as placement of large fans, may be required.

Weight charts. Weight charts can facilitate the detection of an athlete who may be more susceptible to heat stress. Daily measurements of weight loss, which mainly reflects water loss, should be taken and recorded. Athletes losing excessive amounts of weight each day, in excess of 3% of their body weight, which is not made up in a 24-hour period, should be observed carefully; they may be candidates for heat illnesses.

Diet. A well-balanced diet is essential to athletic activity and will normally replenish any electrolytes or body minerals lost during hot weather. For example, sufficient salt replacement will normally occur with a balanced diet. It is not usually recommended that athletes ingest salt tablets.

Summary

The body's response to thermal exposure is basically one of maintaining heat balance; that is, the same amount of heat must be lost as produced or gained by the body during activity in hot weather. Heat is gained by the body mainly through metabolism but may also be gained through radiation, convection, and conduction. Heat is lost from the body by radiation, convection, conduction, and evaporation. The body functions to maintain a relatively constant temperature throughout the thermoregulatory system.

Our body eliminates heat gained during activity in hot weather, primarily by cutaneous vasodilation and sweating. Peripheral blood flow is increased to transfer heat from the core of the body to the periphery, where it can be dissipat-

Fig. 6-8. Athletes enjoying free access to water during practice.

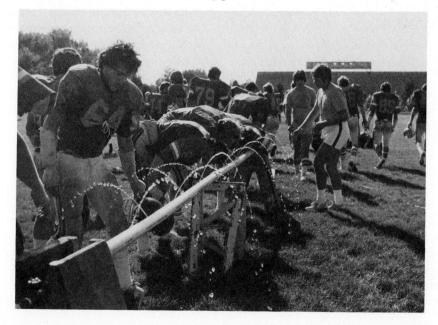

ed. The evaporation of sweat from the skin's surface is the body's major defense mechanism against overheating. There are many factors, both internal and external, that influence or affect these two important heat-dissipating mechanisms. Whenever abnormal demands are placed on the thermoregulatory system and the heat gained exceeds that lost, athletes are subjected to the effects of heat-related conditions. These conditions can be significantly reduced through heat acclimation, adequate water replacement, and the awareness of various factors imposed on the athlete by the combinations of exercise, environment, and clothing.

Heat-related conditions include heat cramps, heat exhaustion, and heatstroke. Heat cramps are the least serious, heat exhaustion the most common, and heatstroke the most serious. Each of these is caused by basically the same set of circumstances, but each represents a different bodily reaction to excessive heat. It is extremely important for the athletic trainer to be familiar with signs and symptoms that indicate the development of these heat conditions, as well as emergency measures that should be immediately initiated should they occur.

BODY'S RESPONSE TO COLD EXPOSURE

Unlike heat-related conditions, injuries resulting from exposure to cold are seldom a problem in athletics. Activities such as ice-skating and skiing are normally performed in cold weather. Athletes running or jogging outside during the winter months are subjected to cold environmental conditions. Occasionally other sports, due to a change in the weather, must be performed in a cold environment. Exposure to cold under these circumstances normally does not present a significant problem for two reasons: (1) exercise, as previously discussed, increases the heat production of the body, and (2) adequate clothing is usually worn by the athlete. Even though exposure to cold is seldom a problem, athletic trainers should possess a basic knowledge of how the body responds to cold, as well

as the associated signs and symptoms and emergency measures necessary to care for athletes suffering from cold-related injuries.

Physiologic basis of cold exposure

The physiologic basis required for regulation of a constant core temperature has been discussed. Just as the body has mechanisms to guard against overheating, there are thermoregulatory mechanisms designed to prevent abnormal cooling (hypothermia).

Heat production

As previously described, metabolism is the body's main source of heat. During cold weather, an athlete will normally increase his or her muscular activity in an effort to increase metabolism, thus producing more heat to stay warm. If the voluntary increase in muscular activity is not sufficient, the athlete normally begins to shiver, which also increases metabolism. If the core temperature continues to drop, the basal metabolic rate will accelerate in an effort to increase heat production.

Heat preservation

During cold weather, the body attempts to conserve heat and maintain its core temperature. The skin and subcutaneous tissue, especially fat, form a natural insulation. As the body temperature decreases, cutaneous vasoconstriction occurs, shunting blood away from the skin and the cold environment to which it is exposed. This prevents excessive transfer of heat from warmer parts of the body to those areas being cooled by significantly reducing the amount of blood circulating in the extremities. This does not include the head, from which, on a cold day, a large amount of heat can be lost if it is uncovered. This vasconstriction decreases surface temperature of the extremities, making them more susceptible to the injurious affects of exposure to cold. This is especially true of the fingers or toes, as they provide a large surface area that is often poorly protected.

Athletes provide additional insulation to the

cold weather by the clothing worn. The effectiveness of this insulation is more dependent on thickness and layering than the type or style of clothing.

Heat transmission

Heat is transmitted, or lost, from the body primarily by the mechanisms described earlier; that is, radiation, conduction, convection, and evaporation. Depending on the severity of exposure, athletes must attempt to reduce the transmission of heat from the body in order to prevent cold-related injuries. The amount of heat lost through radiation can be reduced by covering the exposed surface areas of the body, especially the head. Other body areas with a large surface/volume ratio, such as the ears, hands, and feet, are also particularly likely to lose heat by radiation. Reducing heat loss by conduction is accomplished mainly by avoiding contact with objects colder than the body. When the object is large and a good conductor of heat, such as water or metal, the heat loss can be considerable. Decreasing heat loss by convection can be achieved primarily by avoiding the cold wind and dressing appropriately. Persons exposed to a cold environment are normally not sweating. However, athletes who exercise or perform in cold weather usually sweat. Sweating dampens the clothing, which aids in the conduction of heat away from the body. Therefore, during cold weather, athletes should wear several layers of light, loose clothing that will trap air, a very effective insulator, and provide adequate ventilation to allow moisture to escape. Athletes should also change clothing, especially socks and gloves, when they become damp with perspiration. Clothing that becomes wet loses its ability to trap air and increases conductive heat loss by up to 20 times over dry clothes.

Cold-related conditions

When heat regulating mechanisms fail or are insufficient to maintain the temperature of the core (brain, lungs, heart and abdominal organs) or shell (skin, muscles and extremities), injury

from cold can occur. There are two specific cold-related conditions that may result from cold exposure: (1) *frostbite* and (2) *hypothermia.* Although these conditions are seldom a problem in athletics, athletic trainers should be familiar with signs and symptoms that indicate their development, as well as emergency procedures necessary to adequately care for athletes suffering from exposure to cold. It is important to recognize the early stages of cold-related conditions and take preventive measures to avoid serious consequences.

Frostbite

Frostbite is freezing of a part of the body and occurs when the heat supply to that part is insufficient to counteract the heat loss, causing the intracellular and interstitial water to crystallize. The resulting mechanical damage caused by formation of ice particles can result in tissue injury or death. The frozen area is normally small and most commonly occurs on exposed body areas such as the nose, ears, cheeks, or fingers. However, unexposed body areas, such as the toes, may also be affected. The penis is another commonly affected area of the body, especially in the northern climates. This condition occurs when an inadequately clothed but perspiring male athlete is running in extremely cold temperatures. With growing numbers of year-round runners and the common use of nylon shorts, the incidence of this condition is increasing. The extent of the injury from frostbite depends on such factors as temperature, wind velocity, duration of exposure, humidity, lack of protective clothing, or the presence of wet clothing.

There are various degrees of frostbite. A minor case, or first-degree frostbite, often called *frostnip,* involves the skin's surface. The affected skin may at first become flushed or reddened, and burning and tingling sensations are common. With continued exposure, the skin may suddenly turn white and become painless. Because of this loss of sensation, the athlete may be unaware of the danger. This is the most common type of frostbite affecting athletes and, if identified early, can be reversed without any tissue damage. The treatment consists of rewarming by some means, such as covering the area, holding a warm hand over the area, blowing hot breath against the area, or holding the frost-nipped portion against the body. Rewarming usually produces burning and itching sensations accompanied by local redness and swelling.

Superficial frostbite involves the skin and subcutaneous tissue. The skin becomes firm, white, and waxy although the tissue beneath it remains soft. Athletes with superficial frostbite should be removed from the cold, and the affected area should be carefully rewarmed as described for frostnip or in a warm water bath (100° to 105° F). The area should not be rubbed. As the area is warmed, it may turn purple and swell. If superficial capillaries are damaged, edemic fluid will leak out into the tissue, causing superficial blisters to appear. Stinging, burning, or aching pain may follow and last several days to weeks. This area of the body is often extremely sensitive to further cold exposure and should be protected during additional activity in cold weather.

Deep frostbite involves freezing of the entire tissue depth, including muscles and bone. This type of frostbite occurs when someone is exposed to freezing weather for a prolonged period of time. This is a serious injury, and these persons should be transported to a medical facility immediately. There is often permanent damage associated with this type of injury.

Hypothermia

Hypothermia is a condition in which the core temperature falls below 95° F (35° C). At temperatures below 95° F the body's thermoregulatory mechanism is overwhelmed, and the body is unable to rewarm itself without outside assistance. If the body temperature drops below 86° F (30° C), a life-threatening medical emergency exists. This condition will seldom affect an athlete, but if present, can result in a serious and potentially fatal injury. Participation in winter sports, such as cross-country skiing, can present opportunities that may result in a general cooling of the body to dangerous levels. In most cases of athletic-related hypothermia, exhaustion is a predisposing problem. In addition to cold temperatures, wind and wetness are the major contributing environmental factors.

The degree of hypothermia present determines the signs and symptoms manifested. As can be seen in Table 6-1, as the core body temperature falls, drastic changes in respiration and cellular metabolism occur, and the associated signs and symptoms become progressively more severe. Early signs of hypothermia include shivering, depressed respiration, and a slow irregular pulse. The skin is cold and pale. As body temperature decreases, a person may show signs of an altered mental state, such as irritability, incoordination, stumbling, clumsiness, weakness, and difficulty in speaking. Continued temperature depression leads to muscular rigidity, collapse, coma, and failure of the respiratory and cardiovascular systems. The treatment of hypothermia is basically to prevent further heat loss, rewarming by any means possible, and prompt transportation to a medical facility.

Table 6-1. Signs and symptoms of hypothermia

Core body temperature		Signs and symptoms
°C	°F	
37	98.6	Peripheral vasoconstriction $\uparrow$Heart rate, $\uparrow$Respiratory rate
35	95	$\uparrow$Muscle tone, $\rightarrow$Shivering
32	89.6	$\downarrow$Heart rate, $\downarrow$Respiratory rate Muscular rigidity Altered mental status
30	86	Basal metabolic rate Dilated pupils
28	82.4	Cardiac arrhythmias
27	80.6	Coma
25	77	Hypotension and shock
24	75.2	Respiratory arrest
15	59	Cardiac standstill

From Parcel, G.S.: Basic emergency care of the sick and injured, ed. 2, St. Louis, 1981, The C.V. Mosby Co.

Summary

The body's response to cold exposure is primarily one of maintaining a constant core temperature. Just as the body has mechanisms to guard against overheating, there are thermoregulatory mechanisms designed to prevent abnormal cooling. Metabolism is the body's main source of heat. During cold weather, athletes normally increase muscular activity, which increases metabolism, producing more heat. If muscular activity is not sufficient, the athlete will begin to shiver, which also increases metabolism. The body also prevents an excessive transfer of heat from warmer parts of the body to those areas being cooled by cutaneous vasoconstriction, which reduces the amount of blood circulating in the extremities. Athletes can reduce the transmission of heat from the body by covering exposed surfaces, avoiding contact with colder objects or wind, and wearing several layers of light, dry, loose-fitting clothing.

Cold-related conditions include frostbite and hypothermia. Frostbite is freezing of a part of the body and can result in tissue damage or death. There are three degrees of frostbite. Frostnip involves only the skin's surface and can usually be easily reversed without any tissue damage by various means of rewarming. Superficial frostbite involves the skin and subcutaneous tissue, whereas deep frostbite involves the entire tissue depth, including muscles and bones. Superficial frostbite will often leave surface blisters after rewarming. There is often permanent damage associated with a deep frostbite.

Hypothermia is a condition in which the body temperature falls below 95° F (35° C), and the body is unable to warm itself without outside assistance. This condition seldom affects an athlete but can be a life-threatening emergency. The early signs of hypothermia include shivering, depressed respiration, and a slow, irregular pulse. The skin is cold and pale. As body temperature decreases, an athlete may show signs of an altered mental state and failure of the respiratory and cardiovascular systems. The treatment of hypothermia is to prevent further heat loss, rewarm the athlete by any means, and transport to a medical facility.

KEY TERMS

acute Of short duration

adhesions Fibrous bands that may connect or unite two adjacent surfaces of parts

atrophy Wasting away or deterioration of a tissue, organ, or part

chronic Of long duration

collagen Main supportive protein in skin, tendon, bone, cartilage, and connective tissue

conduction Process of transfer by direct contact

convection Transfer of heat from one place to another by motion or circulation

deep frostbite Freezing of the entire tissue depth, including muscles and bone

diapedesis Movement or migration of blood or its elements through the intact vessel wall

edema Accumulation of excessive amounts of blood fluids in the tissue spaces

evaporation Dissipation in the form of vapor

extravasation Process of escaping or passing out of a vessel into the tissues

exudate Fluid that has escaped from a tissue or its vessels

fibroblasts Connective tissue cells that form collagen fibers

fibroplasia Production of fibrous tissue

fibroplastic phase Initial phase of the healing process in which fibrous tissue is produced

frostbite Localized freezing of a part of the body

frostnip Initial stage of frostbite involving only the surface of the skin

healing by first intention Primary union by fibrous adhesions without formation of infection and pus

healing by second intention Secondary union accompanied by infection and delayed healing

heat acclimation Process of becoming accustomed to athletic activity in hot weather

heat cramps Painful muscle spasms resulting from a fluid volume problem

heat exhaustion Heat stress condition characterized by profuse sweating, which makes the skin cool and clammy

heatstroke (sunstroke) Heat stress condition characterized by lack of sweating and resulting in hot dry skin and a rising body temperature

hematoma Accumulation of extravasated blood that becomes organized into a localized mass

hypothermia Systemic condition in which the body temperature falls below 95° F (35° C)

hypoxia Inadequate or reduced oxygen content

inflammation Basic response of vascularized tissues to an injurious agent, whether the source is physical, bacterial, thermal, or chemical

margination Accumulation of white blood cells on the inner surface of blood vessels near the site of an injury

maturation phase Final stage of the repair process, in which the newly formed fibrous connective tissue matures and becomes stronger

metabolism Chemical process by which energy is produced

necrosis Death of one or more cells, or of a portion of tissue or organ

phagocytosis Ingesting and disposing of unwanted substances such as elements of the hematoma

primary injury Initial insult or injury resulting directly from the trauma

radiation Process of emitting radiant energy in the form of waves

secondary injury Additional responses or damages that occur after the primary injury

shock State of collapse or depression of the cardiovascular system

substrate phase Initial phase of the acute inflammatory response, characterized by localized vascular changes

superficial frostbite Freezing of the skin and subcutaneous tissue

vaporization Conversion of a liquid or solid into a vapor

SUGGESTED READINGS

American Academy of Pediatrics: Climatic heat stress and the exercising child, Physician Sportsmedicine 11:155-159, 1983.

Appenzeller, O., and Atkinson, R.: Sports medicine, Baltimore, 1981, Urban & Schwarzenberg, Inc.

Brennan, W.T., and Crone, W.J.: Guide to problems and practices in first aid and emergency care, ed. 4, Dubuque, Iowa, 1981, Wm. C. Brown Co., Publishers.

Bryant, J.C.: Psychology in contemporary sport, ed. 2, Englewood Cliffs, N.J., 1983, Prentice-Hall, Inc.

Bryant, W.M.: Wound healing, CIBA Clinical Symposia 29: 3, 1977.

Dunn, R.: Psychological factors in sports medicine, Athletic Training 18:34-35, 1983.

Fox, E.L., and Mathews, D.K.: The physiological basis of physical education and athletics, ed. 3, Philadelphia, 1981, W.B. Saunders Co.

Hafen, B.Q., and Peterson, B.: First aid for health emergencies, St. Paul, 1980, West Publishing Co.

Knight, K.L.: Cryotherapy in sports medicine. In Scriber, K., and Burke, E.J., editors: Relevant topics in athletic training, Ithaca, N.Y., 1978, Movement Publications.

Nelson, W.E., and others: Treatment and prevention of hypothermia and frostbite, Athletic Training 18:330-332, 1983.

Ryan, A.J., and Allman, F.L.: Sports medicine, New York, 1974, Academic Press, Inc.

Ryan, G.B., and Majno, G.: Inflammation: a scope publication, Kalamazoo, 1977, The Upjohn Co.

Strauss, R.H.: Sports medicine and physiology, Philadelphia, 1979, W.B. Saunders Co.

Vinger, P.F., and Hoerner, E.F.: Sports injuries, the unthwarted epidemic, Boston, 1982, John Wright—PSG Inc.

Williams, J.G.P., and Sperryn, P.N.: Sports medicine, ed. 2, 1976, Baltimore, The Williams & Wilkins Co.

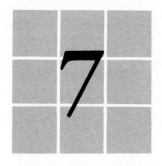

7

Athletic injuries and related skin conditions

An *athletic injury* is defined as a disruption in tissue continuity that results from athletic or sports-related activity, causing a cessation of participation or restriction of usual activity. This definition implies that an athletic injury is more than the aches and pains that may accompany but not interfere with athletic participation. There is an almost infinite array of possibilities in the spectrum of athletic injuries, ranging from minor problems to severe and potentially lethal types of trauma. The care of athletic injuries also involves a wide range of treatment possibilities,

from as little as the application of a Band-aid to multiple operations and months of rehabilitation. Athletic injuries or illnesses that athletic trainers must often assess and manage are discussed in this chapter.

Athletic injuries result from the application of forces or stresses in excess of the body's or body part's ability to adapt. The manner and location by which these excess forces or stresses are applied to the body, better known as the *mechanism of injury,* determines the exact nature and extent of the injury and the tissues involved.

These forces or stresses may be applied (1) instantaneously, resulting in an *acute traumatic injury,* or (2) over a considerable period of time, resulting in a *chronic overuse syndrome.* Traumatic injuries such as sprains, strains, and contusions are common to athletic activity, particularly during contact sports. Overuse syndromes such as tendinites, bursites, stress fractures, and shin splints are becoming much more common in athletic activity because of the increasing intensity of training and conditioning programs. As a group, the overuse injuries occur more often in athletic activity requiring specific repetitive movements.

Athletic injuries are grouped into two main classifications, depending on the integrity of the skin: (1) the *exposed* injuries, and (2) the *unexposed* injuries. Exposed, or open, injuries are those that disrupt the continuity of the skin. Unexposed, or closed, injuries are those that are internal and do not break the skin. An athlete can suffer an injury in both classifications simultaneously; for example, an external blow resulting in a laceration as well as a contusion. This chapter deals with the skin and with athletic injuries in both classifications, and with the associated signs and symptoms that indicate their presence. Guidelines for determining the severity of injury and when medical assistance should be sought are also presented.

SKIN

The skin is the largest and one of the most important organs of the body, and when intact, it serves as a barrier to protect us from many types of physical, chemical, and even biologic attacks. In terms of surface area, the skin is as large as the body itself—probably 1.6 to 2.0 square meters (m^2) in most adults. For the athletic trainer, the skin is often the window through which the physical assessment is performed. A large portion of the athletic injury assessment process takes place at the skin surface. Careful visual inspection of the skin, followed by palpation of structures beneath its surface, can provide valuable information when assessing athletic injuries. To gain this useful information, athletic trainers must possess an understanding of the anatomy, structure, and functions of the skin.

Visual inspection

Unless a specific lesion is the chief complaint of the athlete, the initial visual examination of the skin during the secondary survey can be completed quickly. Look at the exposed skin surface in its entirety. Include in your examination the mucous membranes of the lips, mouth, and nasal openings. Assessment of specific skin lesions is covered later in this chapter.

Color, temperature, and texture

Skin color is influenced by a number of factors in addition to pigment distribution. For example, a bluish tint to the skin (cyanosis) may occur as a result of inadequate oxygenation of the blood, whereas a flushed or ruddy appearance may accompany fever or sunburn. Shock or exposure to cold temperatures will decrease blood flow to the skin and result in generalized pallor. Small, nonelevated patches of purplish or red discoloration may be the result of blood vessel trauma and localized hemorrhage into the layer of skin or mucous membranes. If very small or almost pinpoint in size, such localized lesions are called *petechiae* or petechial hemorrhages. Hemorrhagic spots larger than petechiae are called *ecchymoses.* Special attention should always be given to areas of increased or decreased pigmentation in skin that is otherwise normally pigmented.

In palpating the site of an injury, any detection of a localized increase in skin temperature would suggest the presence of an inflammatory process or an increase in localized blood flow. A decrease in skin temperature is often noted in areas of inadequate circulation. In areas of swelling, the skin becomes stretched, and the texture feels tight and smooth. A highly skilled athletic trainer can detect edema in a body part by changes in skin texture long before obvious swelling occurs. Good assessment techniques and keen observational skills are especially important if the symptoms of a particular injury are insidious and gradual in their appearance. Remember, when involved in assessment of an injured extremity, always compare the skin and characteristics of the contralateral limb.

Anatomy and structure

Two main layers compose the skin: an outer thinner layer, the **epidermis,** and an inner thicker layer, the **dermis** (Fig. 7-1). The epidermis consists of stratified squamous epithelial tissue, the dermis of fibrous connective tissue. Underlying the dermis is subcutaneous tissue, or superficial fascia, made of areolar and, in many areas, adipose tissue. The epidermis has four layers in all parts of the body except the palms of the hands and soles of the feet. In the skin of the palms and soles, there are five layers of epidermis. From the surface in, they are as follows:

1. *Stratum corneum* (horny layer): Dead cells converted to a water-repellant protein,

Fig. 7-1. Microscopic view of the skin. The epidermis is shown raised at one corner to reveal the underlying dermis.

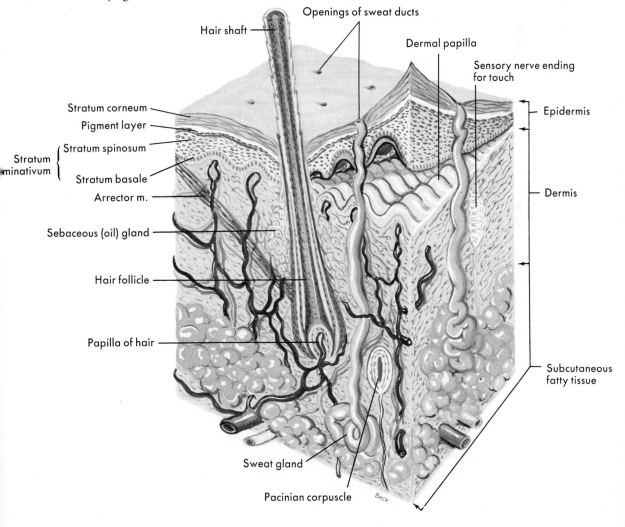

called keratin, that continually flakes off (desquamates).

2. *Stratum lucidum:* So named because of the presence of a translucent compound (eleidin) from which keratin forms; present only in thick skin of palms and soles.

3. *Stratum granulosum:* So named because of granules visible in the cytoplasm of cells (cells die in this layer).

4. *Stratum spinosum* (prickle-cell layer): Several layers of irregularly shaped cells.

5. *Stratum germinativum* (basal layer): Columnar-shaped cells, the only cells in the epidermis that undergo mitosis; new cells are produced in this deepest stratum at the rate old keratinized cells are lost from the stratum corneum; new cells continually push surfaceward from the stratum germinativum into each successive layer, only to die, become keratinized, and eventually flake off, as did their predecessors. Incidentally, this fact illustrates nicely the physiologic principle that while life continues the body's work is never done; even at rest it is producing new cells to replace millions of old ones.

An interesting characteristic of the dermis is its parallel ridges, suggestive on a miniature scale of the ridges of a contour-plowed field. Epidermal ridges, the ones made famous by the art of fingerprinting, exist because the epidermis conforms to the underlying dermal ridges.

Accessory organs

The accessory organs of the skin consist of hair, nails, and microscopic glands.

Hair. Hair is distributed over the entire body except the palms and soles. The structure of a hair has several points of similarity to that of the epidermis. Just as the epidermis is formed by the cells of its deepest layer reproducing and forcing upward the daughter cells, which become horny in character, so a hair is formed by a group of cells at its base multiplying and pushing upward and in so doing becoming keratinized. The part of the hair that is visible is the shaft, whereas that which is embedded in the dermis is the root. The root, together with its coverings (an outer connective tissue sheath and an inner epithelial coating that is a continuation of the stratum germinativum), forms the hair follicle. At the bottom of the follicle is a loop of capillaries enclosed in a connective tissue covering called the hair papilla. The clusters of epithelial cells lying over the papilla are the ones that reproduce and eventually form the hair shaft. As long as these cells remain alive, hair will regenerate even though cut, plucked, or otherwise removed.

Each hair is kept soft and pliable by two or more sebaceous glands, which secrete varying amounts of oily sebum into the follicle near the surface of the skin. Attached to the follicle, too, are small bundles of involuntary muscle known as the arrector pili muscles. These muscles are of interest because when they contract, the hair stands on end, as it does in extreme fright or cold, for example. This mechanism is also responsible for gooseflesh. As the hair is pulled into an upright position, it raises the skin around it into the familiar little goose pimples.

Hair color results from different amounts of melanin pigments in the outer layer (cortex) of the hair. White hair contains little or no melanin.

Some hair, notably that around the eyes and in the nose and ears, performs a protective function in that it keeps out some dust, other types of particulate matter, and insects. For the hair on the bulk of the skin, however, no function seems apparent.

Nails. The nails are epidermal cells that have been converted to keratin. They grow from epithelial cells lying under the white crescent (lunula) at the proximal end of each nail.

Glands. The skin glands include three kinds of microscopic glands, namely, sebaceous, sweat, and ceruminous.

Sebaceous glands secrete oil for the hair. Wherever hairs grow from the skin, there are sebaceous glands, at least two for each hair. The oil, or sebum, secreted by these tiny glands has value not only because it keeps the hair supple but also because it keeps the skin soft and pliable. Moreover, it prevents excessive water evaporation from the skin and water absorption through the skin. And because fat is a poor conductor of heat, the sebum secreted into the skin lessens the amount of heat lost from this large surface.

Sweat glands, although very small structures, are important and numerous—especially on the palms, soles, forehead, and axillae (armpits). Histologists estimate that a single square inch of skin on the palms of the hands contains about 3000 sweat glands.

Ceruminous glands are thought to be modified sweat glands. They are located in the external ear canal. Instead of watery sweat, they secrete a waxy, pigmented substance, the cerumen.

Functions

Vital, diverse, complex, extensive—these adjectives describe in part the function of the skin, its accessory organs, and related structures. Skin functions are crucial to survival and include protection from trauma (physical, chemical, biologic, and thermal), excretion, and sensation. In addition, the skin plays an extremely important role in maintaining fluid and electrolyte balance and normal body temperature. Sweat, in evaporating, cools the body surface. It also contains some nitrogenous wastes and therefore serves as a vehicle for both excretion and water loss.

In athletics, the function of the skin in temperature regulation is particularly important. The skin is very vascular and contains a large number of uniquely arranged blood vessels. The number of capillaries in the skin far exceeds what is required. Therefore, under resting conditions, a large quantity of blood is normally shunted around the excess capillary beds through direct connections (anastomoses) between small arteries and veins. These arteriovenous anastomoses can be closed if the internal body temperature increases, such as occurs in strenuous exercise. If these shunt vessels are closed, blood is forced into the many extra capillary beds near the skin surface, and excessive heat can be radiated into the environment.

EXPOSED ATHLETIC INJURIES

Exposed athletic injuries are those in which there is a disruption in the continuity of the skin. These injuries are common in athletics and include open wounds as well as various skin lesions that may or may not break the skin.

Open wounds

Open wounds are normally caused by physical trauma and may range from a simple scratch to a large, deep, freely bleeding laceration. Table 7-1 outlines the five common types of open wounds. It is important for the athletic trainer to remember that an open wound may only be surface evidence of a more severe and often "hidden" athletic injury. Most open or exposed athletic injuries are minor in severity and do not result in significant hemorrhaging or loss of tissue. However, any bleeding must be controlled before a complete evaluation of the wound itself or of the possible involvement of deeper anatomic structures. The application of direct pressure over the site of bleeding, preferably with a sterile dressing (Fig. 7-2), should be sufficient to control the hemorrhaging of most open wounds. The risk of infection is usually a greater concern for the athletic trainer treating an exposed wound than the amount of bleeding. Any open wound is susceptible to contamination with pathogenic bacteria or other harmful microorganisms. They may enter the body through even the smallest break in the skin. Contaminants may also be carried into the body by the object causing the wound. Although not all open wounds bleed freely, the flow of blood can aid in flushing out contaminants. Therefore minor wounds can be cleaned while they are bleeding in an attempt to clean out all dirty material and contaminants. The signs and symptoms of a wound infection generally appear 8 to 48 hours after the injury occurs. The typical signs and symptoms of a wound infection can be readily remembered by the acronym SHARP, which stands for *S*welling, *H*eat,

Table 7-1. Types of open wounds

Type	Cause	Characteristics	Care
Abrasion	Fall Scraping or rubbing portion of skin away	Superficial Little bleeding, oozing, or weeping	Clean Remove debris Apply antiseptic treatment Apply sterile dressing Change dressing daily
Laceration	Wound made by tearing	Jagged edges May bleed freely Contusion and tearing Often leaves scar	Control bleeding Clean Suture if necessary Inspect daily
Incision	Cut by sharp object	Smooth edges Freely bleeding	Control bleeding Clean Suture if necessary Inspect daily
Puncture	Penetration by sharp object	Small opening Minimal bleeding	Clean Refer to medical assistance Inspect daily
Avulsion	Tearing loose flap of skin	Completely loose Hanging as a flap May bleed freely	Control bleeding Clean Save avulsed tissue Refer

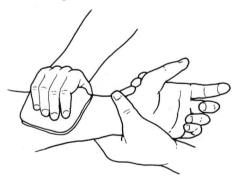

Fig. 7-2. The application of direct pressure to control bleeding.

*A*ching, *R*eddness, and *P*us. Wound infections should be recognized and promptly managed or referred to a physician for definitive treatment.

Abrasions

Abrasions occur when the epidermis and a portion of the dermis is scraped or rubbed away (Fig. 7-3). This type of injury is very common in athletic activity and is usually caused by falling on a firm or rough surface. Athletes commonly refer to abrasions as "mat burns," "floor burns," or "cinder burns," depending on the surface that caused them. A reddish, irregular surface appearance gives rise to the descriptive name "strawberry." The bleeding associated with abrasions is usually limited to blood oozing from underlying injured capillaries. Although these injuries may be painful, the primary concern is that of infection. The abrased area will often contain contaminants such as bits of dirt, debris, or bacteria embedded in the injured tissue.

An abrasion must be cleaned thoroughly. Soap and water will work quite well, as will a

Fig. 7-3. Abrasion. **A,** Schematic of typical abrasion injury. Note that tissue damage is confined to epidermis. **B,** Posterior forearm abrasion.

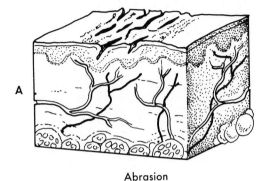

Abrasion

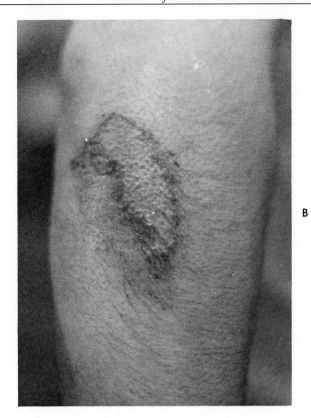

B

number of appropriate commercial preparations. Care must be taken to remove all foreign material from the wound. Any dirt or debris left in an abrased area may cause infection or become incorporated into the healing tissue and leave an unsightly "traumatic tattoo." Depending on the circumstances of injury, you may have to use a soft brush to clean the area thoroughly. Once the wound is cleaned, an antiseptic should be applied and the wound covered with a sterile nonadhesive dressing. Abrasions occurring in the vicinity of a joint may respond better to an ointment dressing so that a scab does not form and be continually reopened during activity. The wound should be cared for daily with these routines.

An abrasion should be referred to a physician for any of the following reasons:

1. It is impossible to remove all the foreign material by washing the wound.

2. The area surrounding the abrasion becomes inflamed and infected a few days after the injury.

3. There is doubt about the status of the abrasion.

Lacerations

Lacerations are wounds or cuts made by tearing and are common in athletics (Fig. 7-4). These injuries are usually the result of some type of direct blow to the skin and are especially common over bony prominences. The skin may be stretched and actually torn apart. Lacerations are often described as a combination of contusion and tear. They generally lack the clean appearance of a typical incised wound. The edges of a laceration are usually jagged or irregular and at least some surrounding tissue damage occurs in most laceration injuries. The severity of lacerations can range from a very small crack in the skin to a large, deep wound with associated damage to surrounding and deeper structures. The nature and severity of bleeding associated with lacerations is quite variable.

Incisions

Incisions are wounds caused by cutting with some type of sharp object, such as a knife (Fig. 7-5). The edges of an incision are smooth and cleanly cut, with little damage to surrounding tissue. Occasionally, an incised wound will be deep and damage blood vessels, muscles, tendons, or nerves well below the skin surface. Fortunately, severe incision wounds rarely occur as a result of athletic activity.

The initial care for incisions is essentially the same as for lacerations. Once bleeding has been controlled, carefully clean and inspect the

Fig. 7-4. Laceration. **A,** Schematic of typical laceration injury. Note that injury extends into the dermis. **B,** Facial laceration.

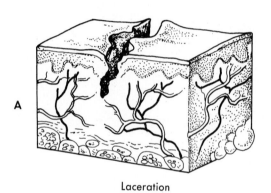

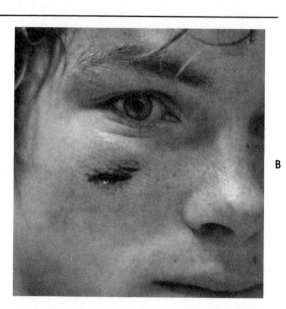

Laceration

Fig. 7-5. Incision. **A,** Schematic of incision injury. **B,** Incision caused by glass fragment.

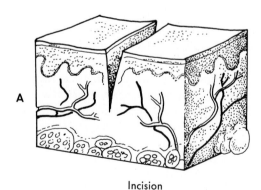

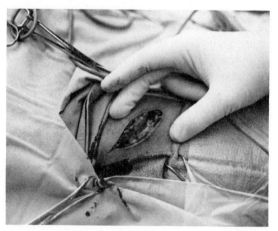

Incision

wound. Is there any foreign material embedded in the wound? How deep is the wound? Was the mechanism of injury sufficient to cause other injuries in addition to the open wound? Remember, a laceration is caused by a crushing type of force, and there is probably an associated bruise. Close the edges of the cut or tear with adhesive strips such as butterfly closures or Steri-Strips and apply a sterile dressing. Occasionally this is all that will be necessary. In many cases, however, sutures are indicated. Because of activity required during athletics, sutures are more frequently recommended for athletes than nonathletes. Lacerations and incisions also need to be protected against additional trauma and stretching when the athlete returns to participation. The wound should be inspected daily for any signs of infection or further trauma. The athlete should be referred to a physician for any of the following reasons:

1. The wound may need sutures for adequate closure
2. There is foreign material embedded in the wound which cannot be removed

3. Bleeding persists despite all efforts to control it
4. The wound is on the face or another part of the body where scar tissue will be noticeable after healing
5. The surrounding area becomes inflamed or infected
6. There is doubt about how the laceration or incision should be treated

Puncture wounds

Puncture wounds occur as a result of direct penetration of the skin by a pointed object (Fig. 7-6). The opening may be quite small, with little or no bleeding. The penetrating object may, however, damage underlying structures and carry contaminants into the body. One of the first considerations in caring for a puncture is to determine the depth of penetration and the possibility of underlying damage. Only if the puncture is very minor and the penetrating object small, with little depth of penetration, is the athletic trainer justified in simply cleaning the wound and observing for signs of infection. The

Fig. 7-6. Puncture. **A,** Schematic of puncture injury. **B,** Puncture injury resulting from archery range accident.

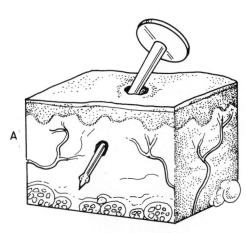

Puncture wound

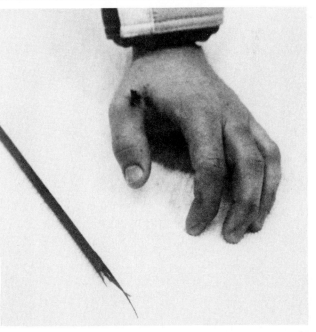

B

A

majority of puncture wounds should be cleansed and promptly referred to a physician. Large items that remain imbedded should be left in place until a physician can remove them. A tetanus toxoid booster is often indicated with puncture wounds. Punctures are not common in athletics but should be properly cared for when they occur. These wounds should be inspected frequently for signs of infection.

Avulsions

An avulsion is the tearing away of part of a structure. When referring to an open wound, an avulsion is the tearing loose of a piece of skin, which may be torn completely free or remain partially attached, hanging as a flap (Fig. 7-7). There may or may not be much bleeding. If an avulsed piece of skin or tissue of significant size is torn completely free of the athlete, it should be saved and transported with the athlete to a medical facility. The avulsed portion should be wrapped in sterile gauze and kept moist and cool. Occasionally, significant portions of avulsed tissue may be successfully reattached. When the avulsed part remains attached, the flap of skin should be placed back in its normal position before bandaging and referral. Small flaps of skin, especially in highly vascular body areas such as the scalp and face, may remain viable and heal if replaced.

Fig. 7-7. Avulsions. **A,** Schematic of avulsion injury. **B,** Avulsion injury to tibial area. Note avulsed skin flap.

(Courtesy Dr. James Garrick, Center for Sports Medicine, St. Francis Memorial Hospital, San Francisco.)

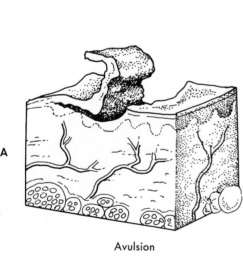

A

Avulsion

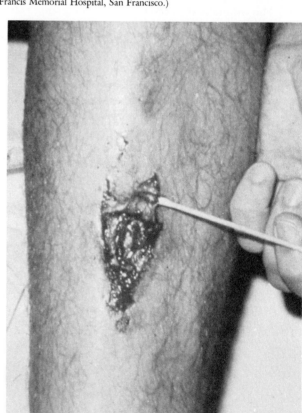

B

Common skin lesions

There are a variety of skin lesions or disorders that can cause disability or impair athletic performance. These conditions may or may not break the surface of the skin, but they are discussed along with exposed athletic injuries because they do involve the integrity of the skin. The integrity of the skin can be altered in many ways. Examples include physical trauma, infectious agents, and exposure to irritants in the environment, plant or insect poisons, and caustic chemicals. The skin problems and symptoms arising from these varied insults differ greatly between athletes. Prevention of skin problems, as well as the correct assessment and treatment of skin disorders when they do occur, should be a major concern of the athletic trainer.

The assessment of any skin lesion should begin with a determination of the general characteristics of the eruption. This information is valuable in attempting to determine the nature and cause of the skin lesion and in describing the skin disorder when consulting a physician or dermatologist. The general characteristics of skin lesions include the (1) location, (2) configuration, and (3) structure of the eruptions. Location refers to the body areas affected. For example, contact dermatitis is sharply limited to the area of the body in contact with the causative agent. Configuration refers to the arrangement or position of several lesions in relation to each other (Fig. 7-8). For example, ringworm is characterized by reddened circular areas. Structure refers to the physical signs used to classify skin lesions. It is important for the athletic trainer to recognize the structure of individual lesions in order to identify the specific problem.

Lesions are classified as primary and secondary. *Primary lesions* are those that appear initially in response to some change in the internal or external environment of the skin. *Secondary lesions* do not appear initially but result from the primary lesions. For example, a blister (primary lesion) may break and leave a small, moist area of skin called an erosion (secondary lesion). Some of the more common skin lesions are classified by structure in Fig. 7-9 and described in the following section.

Fig. 7-8. Configurations of skin lesions. **A,** Grouped (cluster); **B,** girdle (encircling pattern); **C,** ring-shaped (cyclic); **D,** linear.

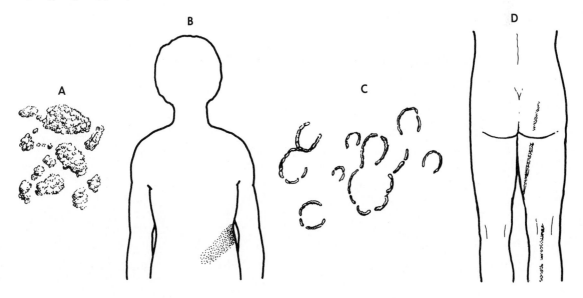

Fig. 7-9. Common skin lesions classified by structure. **A,** Macule, a small (less than 1 cm) circular discoloration of the skin without elevation or depression. (A lesion larger than 1 cm is called a patch.) **B,** Papule, a small (less than 1 cm) solid elevated area of the skin, usually involving the epidermal structures. A lesion larger than 1 cm is called a plaque. **C,** Nodule, a small, solid mass in dermal or subcutaneous tissue; deeper than a papule. **D,** Vesicle, a circumscribed, elevated lesion containing serous fluid and usually less than 1 cm in diameter. These may form within the epidermis or between the epidermis and dermis. **E,** Bulla, a vesicle larger than 1 cm in diameter. **F,** Pustule, a vesicle containing purulent exudate or pus.

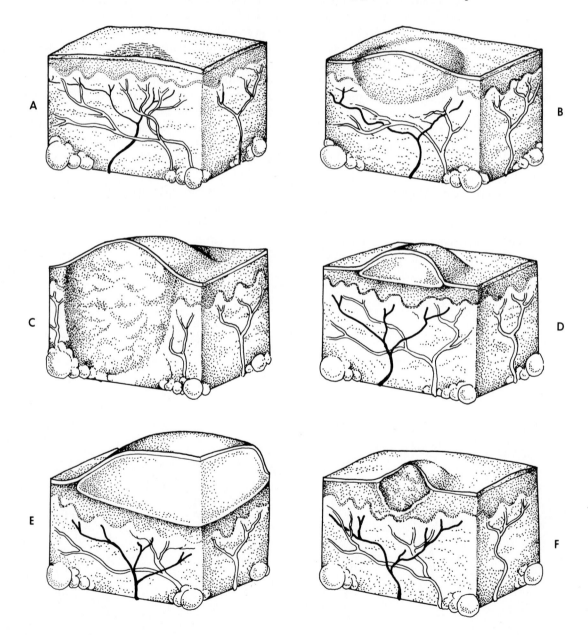

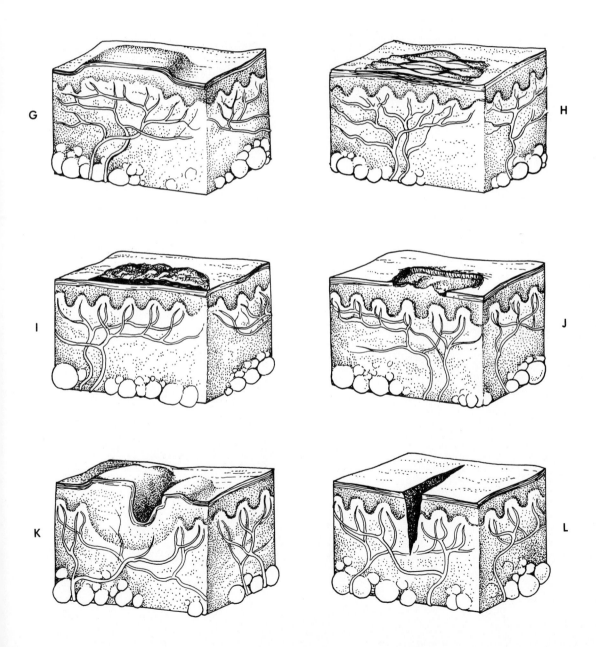

Fig. 7-9, cont'd. G, Wheal, a circumscribed flat-topped, firm elevation of the skin with a palpable margin, resulting from edema in the skin. **H,** Crust, dried exudate of serum, blood, or purulent material on the surface of the skin. **I,** Scale, dried thin plates of epithelial cells. **J,** Erosion, a moist, circumscribed and often depressed area that reflects loss of partial or full-thickness epidermis. **K,** Scar, an area of replacement fibrosis of the dermis or subcutaneous tissues resulting from destruction of these layers. May be depressed or raised. **L,** Fissure, a deep linear split in the skin extending into the dermis.

Fig. 7-10. Examples of friction blisters.
(Courtesy A.G. Edwards, A.T.,C., University of Nevada–Las Vegas.)

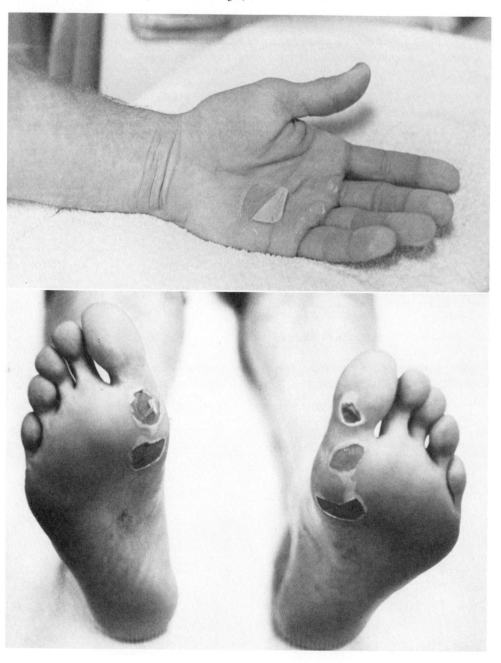

Mechanically produced lesions

Blisters. Blisters are normally caused by some type of skin friction or irritation. Many friction or shearing forces will cause the epidermis to separate from the dermis; the area between these layers then fills with fluid (Fig. 7-10). This fluid is normally a clear exudate that has escaped from tiny blood vessels in the area. If the shearing force actually ruptures a blood vessel, such as might occur with a sharp pinching action, the blister may be filled with blood. Occasionally, a blister will become infected and the area between the two layers of skin will become purulent, that is, filled with pus.

Friction blisters can occur anywhere on the body, but are most common on the feet and hands. This is especially true early in an athletic season, when the skin of the feet and hands is soft and not accustomed to athletic activity. Over a period of time the skin will be able to accommodate the friction, becoming tougher and much less likely to blister. The friction or shearing forces that cause blisters are enhanced by such things as poor-fitting or faulty equipment (especially shoes), participating on extremely hard surfaces, continued repetitive activity, or activity requiring frequent starting, stopping, and changing of direction. Athletes will normally feel a blister developing by detecting a "hot spot." This is an ideal time to care for the blister if at all possible.

Blisters can be very handicapping to an athlete. Evaluating the severity of the blister and determining proper care will depend on the cause, location, size, depth, and affect on performance. Identifying the cause, such as poor-fitting shoes or a spike or cleat coming through the sole of a shoe, can help alleviate further complications. Many blisters can be drained and the skin protected, thus permitting the athlete to continue normal activity. In some cases the activity level will have to be modified for a few days so that the athlete does not continue to aggravate the blistered area. Infected blisters may require medical assistance.

Calluses. Calluses are a thickening of the outer layer of skin (epidermis) normally present on the hands and feet. An excessive accumulation of callous tissue is usually found over a bony prominence and can develop from constant friction, pressure, or irritation (Fig. 7-11). This excess callus can become disabling and painful to an athlete as the mass becomes hard and inelastic. The most frequent sites for excessive callus formations are under the metatarsal bones at the ball of the foot, outer edge of the heel, inner edge of the big toe, or on the palm of the hand over the metacarpal heads. If left untreated, these hard masses are vulnerable to tearing and cracking

Fig. 7-11. Calluses. Note placement of calluses over the heads of the metatarsals.
(Courtesy Steve Yoneda, California Polytechnic State University.)

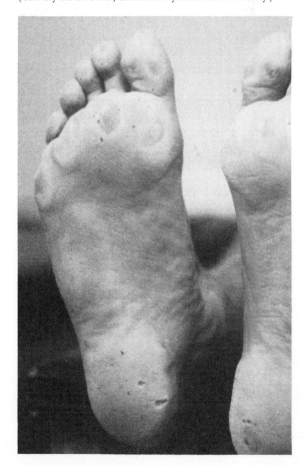

and may cause painful bruising of the underlying tissues. Blisters may also develop under calluses.

Calluses can be differentiated from similar skin lesions, such as warts, by the skin lines, which will continue through to the surface. Treatment consists of preventing the excess callus accumulation and protecting the involved area. This may include redistribution of weight bearing in the shoe, proper foot hygiene, or the application of some type of pad or glove to reduce constant irritation. Once excess callous tissue has formed, it should be softened and trimmed periodically to prevent further problems and reduce the severity of symptoms.

Contact dermatitis. Contact dermatitis is an acute inflammatory reaction of the skin resulting from direct contact with a substance to which the skin is sensitive. The first apparent change in the skin is a redness (erythema) that is sharply limited to the area of contact with the causative agent (Fig. 7-12). Depending on the duration of contact and the intensity of the reaction, this initial irritation may develop quite rapidly into an intense inflammatory response. Along with the erythema, small itching papules (bumps)

may form, and blisterlike elevations (vesicles) may develop. These vesicles may rupture, causing a crusty appearance.

Some of the possible causes of contact dermatitis in athletes are adhesive tape, dyes in leather or uniforms, elastic wraps, locally applied ointments, chemical powders, soaps, detergents, perfumes, deodorants, plants, such as poison ivy, and certain topical medications. When an athlete exhibits signs of contact dermatitis, the athletic trainer must attempt to identify the causative agent. This will require a complete and careful history. Investigate recent exposures to all possible causes, such as those listed previously. It may be possible to determine the cause and decrease the athlete's exposure to or remove the suspected irritants. If the problem persists or the inflammation becomes severe, oozing and spreading, the athlete should be referred to a physician specializing in skin care.

Bacterial lesions

The normal bacterial flora of the skin includes both pathogenic and nonpathogenic organisms, the major pathogenic type being the staphylo-

Fig. 7-12. Contact dermatitis.

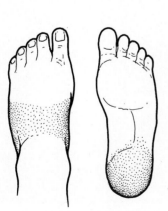
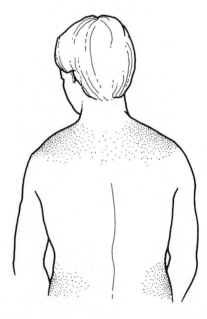

coccus, followed closely by the streptococcus. The normal integrity of the skin, and the immune and cellular defenses, act as barriers to most bacterial organisms. Whenever the integrity of the skin is altered by any means, the potential for infection is increased. Skin trauma, friction, sweating, bruises, and warm, moist areas under equipment and protective pads, which are common in athletics, predispose to bacterial infections. Oily skin, exposure to another infected person, and poor hygiene can also facilitate or spread infections.

When dealing with bacterial infections, it is extremely important for the athletic trainer to prevent the infection from spreading over the body or to other athletes. Thorough cleansing of the area with soap and water will help prevent many bacterial infections, including impetigo, from spreading. An antibacterial ointment should be applied and covered with a thin dressing, which should be changed frequently. The athlete's towel, uniform and clothing, should be isolated until thoroughly laundered. The skin should be kept dry, with special attention given to the affected area because dryness inhibits the growth of bacteria. The affected athlete may have to be isolated from close contact with others and under a physician's care and taking antibiotic medication.

To prevent bacterial infection from spreading, it is important for the athletic trainer to aggressively care for *all* cutaneous lesions, no matter how small. This consists of cleansing the lesion and applying an antiseptic, and perhaps an antibacterial ointment dressing if the lesions are draining or moist. It is also important that the athlete carry out a sound personal hygiene program. The athletic trainer must constantly watch for bacterial infections to treat them effectively and prevent them from spreading. It is also important that facilities and equipment used by athletes, such as wrestling mats and shower rooms, be well cleaned each day. Bacterial infections are a constant area of concern for athletic trainers. A bacterial infection allowed to spread can sideline numerous athletes or an entire team

in a short period of time and disrupt an entire athletic season.

Boils and impetigo. Two of the more common bacterial skin infections are boils (furuncles) and impetigo.

Boils are formed by staphylococci invading the skin through sebaceous glands or hair follicles. These follicles become inflamed, and the bacterial infection is localized in a painful red nodule and eventually a pustule. As a boil matures it becomes enlarged, hard, and tender. Most boils will eventually rupture spontaneously, releasing the contained pus. Occasionally, boils are lanced by a physician. The most frequent sites for boils are the upper extremities, buttocks, thighs, neck, and chest.

Impetigo is a highly contagious bacterial (streptococcal) inflammation of the skin. It is characterized by the appearance of small vesicles, which form pustules and eventually honey-colored, weeping crustations. Impetigo can be transmitted by direct contact with an infected athlete or contact with infected equipment or towels. Persons with impetigo should not engage in contact sports during the contagious period and should practice careful hygiene to protect other athletes. Treatment includes both topical and systemic antibiotics.

Fungal lesions

Fungal infections of skin, hair, and nails are common among athletes. Fungi are microscopic plants related to mushrooms and propagated by seeds called spores. Most fungal spores are highly resistant to drying or freezing and can survive for many years. These organisms thrive in dark, warm, and moist places, conditions often found in dressing rooms and lockers. There are many different fungi that grow in or on the human skin and can be transmitted from one athlete to another without bodily contact. This makes fungal infections an occupational hazard among athletes. Some athletes have a greater susceptibility to fungal infections than others.

The more common athletic fungal infections appear as an itching red rash consisting of small bumps or blisters and scales on the skin. Generally, a fungal infection tends to create more tissue reaction at the advancing borders of the infection than in the older center. This accounts for the ring-shaped lesions frequently seen, although not all fungal infections react in this manner. Sweating, heat, and physical activity contribute to the growth of fungi, commonly called ringworm (tinea) and classified according to the area of the body affected. The most common fungal infections among athletes are athlete's foot, jock itch, and ringworm.

Athlete's foot (tinea pedis) is a troublesome infection, causing redness, scaling, cracking, and itching on the skin surface of the feet. This condition is most common between the toes. *Jock itch* (tinea cruris) is a fungal infection that affects the groin, causing blistering, itching, swelling, and occasionally severe discomfort (Fig. 7-13). Jock itch can accompany athlete's foot, which is

frequently spread by wiping the feet before drying the rest of the body. *Ringworm* (tinea corporis) generally involves the upper extremities and trunk. These lesions are characterized by reddened, ringlike areas that may be scaly or crusted.

The best management of fungal infections is, of course, prevention. Athletes must establish good daily personal hygiene habits, such as washing and drying well, especially between the toes and in the groin and wearing clean clothes. Natural material, such as cotton, is best. Synthetic materials, such as nylon, trap moisture and may cause additional irritation. It is also important to keep the shower and locker rooms clean. In treating mild cases of fungal infections, it is important to minimize heat and moisture in the affected areas. The athlete can accomplish this by drying thoroughly after a shower, applying a fungicide, and wearing clean white clothing. Fungal infections will generally respond well to these routines. In moderate to severe cases of fungal infections, the athlete may also be under a physician's care and possibly removed from activity until the condition improves. Remember, individual susceptibility varies from person to person.

Viral lesions

Herpesvirus. The most common viral infection seen in athletics is *herpes simplex* (type 1) virus. This is commonly called a fever blister or cold sore and is an acute infection of the mucous membranes and skin by this form of herpesvirus. The herpes simplex (type 1) virus is carried inactively by the majority of the population and does not erupt until a person's resistance is lowered by another condition, such as sunburn, fever, stress, irritation, fatigue, or a dietary problem. The lesion is the result of recurrent infections that commonly affect the border of the lips, cheeks, mouth, and conjunctiva; however, it can occur on any skin surface. (Most genital lesions are caused by herpesvirus type 2 and are beyond the scope of discussion for this text. Athletes with genital herpes should always be re-

Fig. 7-13. Tinea cruris (jock itch).
(Courtesy A.G. Edwards, A.T.,C., University of Nevada–Las Vegas.)

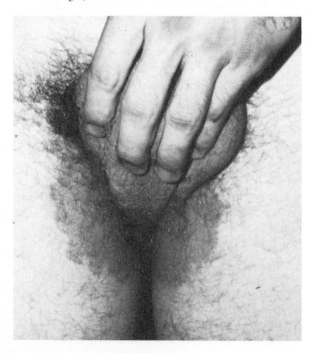

ferred to a physician for treatment.) Initially, groups of herpesvirus lesions appear as blisters, which rupture and form a crusted surface. The appearance of the vesicles is preceded by a burning and itching sensation. The condition is normally self-limiting and will disappear in 1 to 2 weeks. Some athletes are more susceptible to this condition, and lesions frequently recur at the same site. If an athlete develops this condition frequently, there may be an underlying causative factor that demands medical attention. The herpes simplex virus can be transferred from one person to another by direct contact during the vesicular phase, so contact with the infected area should be avoided until the crusted area is gone.

There is no cure presently available for herpes simplex. Treatment consists of keeping the area dry and clean to promote healing and prevent secondary infections. The athlete may have to be held out of competition to avoid contaminating other athletes. A detailed history of foods, medications, and activities of the athlete may help in finding and eliminating the initiating trigger or stimulus, thus preventing recurrence.

Warts. Warts are also caused by a virus. True warts are small tumors that may appear anywhere on the skin surface. They are characterized by small dark spots in their center. The black central spot is actually a capillary or vascular bud in the center of the wart. Warts also have a distinct border at which all skin lines end. Normally, warts are treated only if they interfere with athletic activity. They frequently disappear with no treatment.

Plantar warts develop on the sole of the foot. They may cause pain and disability, especially if they are located on a weight-bearing surface. During competition, plantar warts are protected with a donut-shaped pad to relieve pressure over the lesion. After the athletic season, the plantar wart can be removed by a physician or podiatrist.

Environmentally produced lesions

Sunburn. Sunburn is an injury to the skin caused by overexposure to ultraviolet rays of the sun or sunlamps. These lesions will vary in intensity from a first-degree burn characterized by a mild erythema (pink color) to a second-degree burn marked by the formation of large blisters. In addition to the reddening of the skin, pain is normally present, and in severe cases the athlete may complain of headaches and even exhibit a fever. Persons with very light complexions are more susceptible to sunburn than are those with darker complexions. Athletes not accustomed to being in the sun are also more vulnerable to the effects of the sun's rays. Sunburns and their associated signs and symptoms occur between 4 and 12 hours after exposure to the ultraviolet rays, which makes it difficult to judge the optimum time necessary to prevent overexposure. The effects of a sunburn usually dissipate in 2 to 4 days.

Prevention of sunburn can be accomplished by asking athletes to follow several guidelines. Athletes should acclimate themselves to the sun's rays. The initial exposure should be brief and gradually increased each day until the athlete can tolerate being in the sun without ill effects. Avoiding exposure during midday, when the ultraviolet rays are at their peak, will help reduce burning of the skin. The use of some type of sunscreen designed to filter out the shorter ultraviolet rays, which are the burning rays, is also very helpful in avoiding a sunburn. Absorbent sunscreens containing paraaminobenzoic acid (PABA) affords the most effective protection against the harmful ultraviolet rays of the sun. Many sunscreens are labeled with a number between 1 and 15. This number is a sun protective factor and helps indicate how long a person can remain in the sun. For example, a sunscreen with a number 4, indicates you can stay in the sun four times as long as you could without any protection. Sunscreen must be applied frequently to ensure adequate protection if the person perspires heavily or goes swimming.

The treatment of sunburns is the same as for any thermal burn and depends on the degree of severity and extent of body area involved. Cool water immersion, cool compresses, or soothing

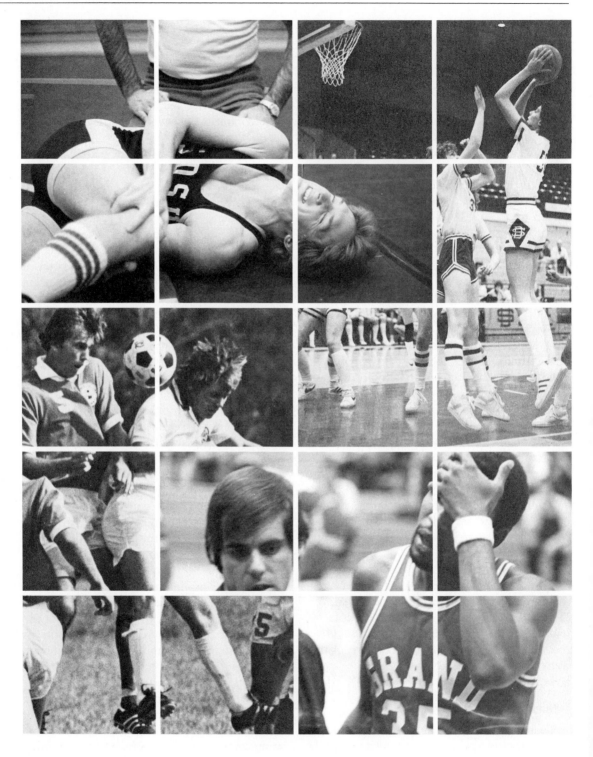

lotions are helpful in milder cases. Aspirin is often administered to relieve pain and some of the inflammatory effects. In severe cases in which blistering and fluid loss is evident, a physician should be consulted for appropriate treatment.

Frostbite. Frostbite occurs when isolated areas of the body are exposed to severe cold. The ears, nose, cheeks, fingers, and toes are the body areas most frequently involved. As a result of exposure to cold, the superficial blood vessels constrict, decreasing the blood supply to the exposed areas. The extent of the injury depends on such factors as temperature, duration of exposure, wind velocity, humidity, and lack of protective clothing. The exposed area initially becomes red and inflamed, then, if allowed to continue, progressively turns grey. If freezing occurs, the affected area takes on a waxy white appearance. As these changes occur, the athlete will normally experience burning or stinging of the affected area, followed by pins-and-needles sensations and finally numbness. An athlete may be unaware of the development of severe frostbite because of loss of sensations.

Frostbitten areas should be gently handled and rapidly rewarmed. In mild frostbite, rewarming will usually produce mild itching and burning sensations and some local redness and swelling. In severe frostbite there may be some blister formation and possible tissue death and permanent damage to the area. Athletes with severe frostbite should be referred to a physician.

UNEXPOSED ATHLETIC INJURIES

Unexposed, or closed, athletic injuries are said to be internal, with no associated disruption or break in the continuity of the skin. Unexposed injuries can result in massive bleeding and significant damage to underlying structures, with little or no visible signs at the skin surface. Structures commonly involved in athletic injuries of this type include soft tissues such as muscles, tendons, blood vessels, and ligaments. Bones are also subject to unexposed injuries. Unexposed athletic injuries also involve such structures as

nerves and internal (visceral) organs and their linings. The common unexposed athletic injuries are classified into contusions, strains, sprains, dislocations, and simple fractures (Table 7-2).

Contusions

A contusion is a bruise and is among the most common type of injury occurring in athletic activity. Contusions usually result from a direct blow or impact being delivered to some part of the body, which causes damage to underlying blood vessels. The resulting bleeding into the skin or subcutaneous tissues may produce symptoms that range from very minor areas of discoloration to extremely large, debilitating masses (Fig. 7-14). The collection of blood that forms at the site of a contusion is called a *hematoma*. As the blood leaks into the subcutaneous tissues, it will often cause a black and blue discoloration known as *ecchymosis*. In addition to the swelling, a bruise usually results in an area of local tenderness.

The tissues involved in a contusion, as well as the amount of damage and bleeding, will depend on the force of the impact, the size and shape of the object causing the bruise, and the part of the body receiving the blow. For example, a blow to a large muscular area such as the thigh will result in damage or bruising to the muscles. The involved muscles respond by protective muscle spasms, causing a decreased excursion of the muscle fibers and a reduced range of motion at the associated joints.

The objective of the initial treatment of contusions is to control the bleeding by means of ice, compression, and elevation. Heat and activity during this initial period may encourage or promote bleeding and should be avoided. Once bleeding has stopped and the athlete exhibits a near normal range of motion without a significant increase in pain, activity may be resumed. The level of activity is increased according to the athlete's tolerance until participation is at the level demanded by the sport. During recovery the athlete should be protected from reinjury by padding the bruised area and by avoiding

Table 7-2. Types of closed wounds

Type	Cause	Characteristics	Care
Contusion (bruise)	Direct blow	Hematoma Ecchymosis Local tenderness	ICE Symptomatic care Protect
Strain	Overstretching Overstressing Violent contraction Strength imbalance to muscle tendon units	1°—Stretching Some discomfort No disability	ICER Symptomatic care Minimal support
		2°—Tearing of fibers Pain Disability	ICER Symptomatic care Support during activity
		3°—Complete rupture Disability Deficit	ICER Referral
Sprain	Joint forced in abnormal direction	1°—Stretching Some discomfort No instability	Symptomatic care Support during activity
		2°—Tearing of ligament Pain Swelling Instability	ICER Protection Support during activity
		3°—Rupture of ligament Instability Swelling	ICE Referral
Dislocations	Joint forced beyond anatomic limits	Deformity Pain Loss of function	Cold Immobilization Referral
Fractures	Direct blow Indirect blow Twisting force Repetitive stress	Pain Crepitation Deformity Loss of function Guarding	Cold Immobilization Referral

Fig. 7-14. Schematic and examples of contusion injuries.

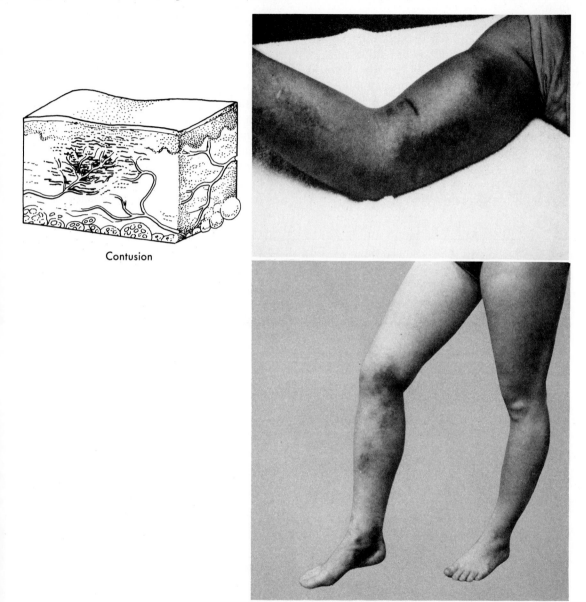

Contusion

excessive activity, which may aggravate injured tissues.

A complication to be aware of when dealing with contusions is *myositis ossificans,* the formation of bone within or around a muscle, commonly called a calcium deposit. Myositis ossificans can result from a contusion injury and occurs when part of the hematoma is replaced with bone (Fig. 7-15). It is believed that the bony deposits are caused by periosteal cells invading the hematoma following the injury. The invasion of the hematoma by periosteal cells can occur when a severe bruise involves the bone as well as the muscle, causing a subperiosteal hema-toma, or when the trauma causes a partial avulsion of muscle fibers from the periosteum. The bony deposit may be a separate piece of bone lying entirely within the muscle, or it may be attached to a bone. This complication seldom occurs as a result of a single injury. It is more likely to occur after chronic irritation, such as continued use of an injured part or repeated trauma to a body area. Whatever the reason, if the hematoma fails to resolve normally, myositis ossificans may result. The formation of myositis ossificans can be recognized by normal plain film radiographs about 3 to 4 weeks after periosteal cell activity begins. It is important for the ath-

Fig. 7-15. Myositis ossificans resulting from contusion injury to right biceps brachii.

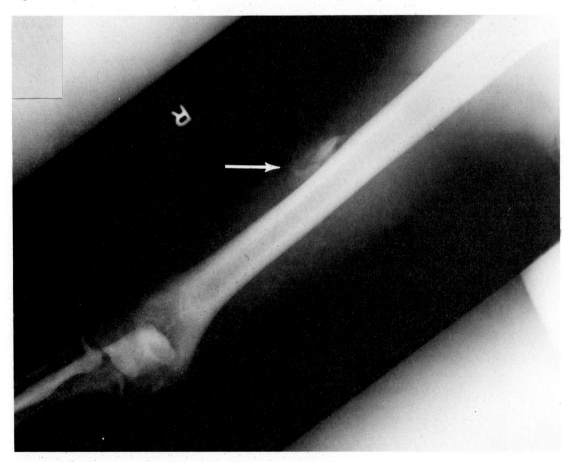

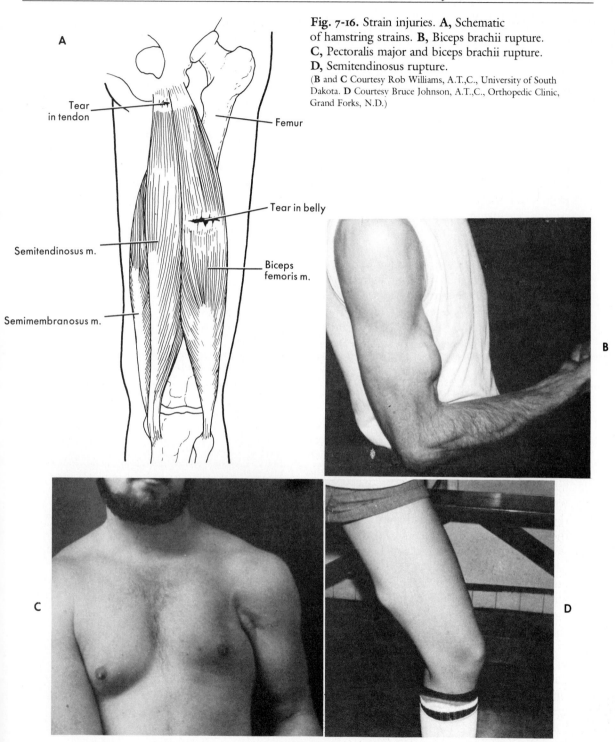

A

Tear
in tendon

Femur

Tear in belly

Semitendinosus m.

Biceps
femoris m.

Semimembranosus m.

B

C

D

Fig. 7-16. Strain injuries. **A,** Schematic
of hamstring strains. **B,** Biceps brachii rupture.
C, Pectoralis major and biceps brachii rupture.
D, Semitendinosus rupture.
(**B** and **C** Courtesy Rob Williams, A.T.,C., University of South
Dakota. **D** Courtesy Bruce Johnson, A.T.,C., Orthopedic Clinic,
Grand Forks, N.D.)

letic trainer to recognize the possibility of myositis ossificans after a severe contusion or repeated bruising. Myositis ossificans can occur anywhere in the body but most frequently involves the quadriceps. This condition should always be suspected if hematoma formation does not promptly resolve and pain, a palpable mass within the muscle, and loss of motion persist for 2 to 3 weeks. In this type of case the athlete should be withheld from activity until severe symptoms subside. It is important that athletes suffering from severe contusions should undergo frequent periodic evaluations.

Strains

Strains are injuries involving the musculotendinous unit and may involve the muscle, tendon, and the junction between the two as well as their attachments to bone (Fig. 7-16). Strains or pulls can be caused by a variety of mechanisms, such as overstretching, overstressing, a violent contraction against heavy resistance, a strength imbalance between agonists and antagonists, or an abnormal muscular contraction. These injuries are generally dynamic; that is, there is no outside intervention and the athlete injures himself or herself. The portion of the musculotendinous unit that is damaged depends on which component is the weakest link in the chain at the moment of injury. Generally, in younger athletes whose growth centers have not closed (ossified), the muscles and tendons are stronger. With these athletes, the attachments to the bone may fail and actually avulse a piece of bone with the tendon or separate at the epiphyseal, or growth, line (epiphyseal fracture) (Fig. 7-17). In older athletes, the tendons and musculotendinous junctions become the weaker links and are more susceptible to injury.

Strains are graded into three groups by level of severity. Each is determined by the amount of damage to the fibers of the musculotendinous unit. The definitions, and the signs and symptoms delineating each grade of severity, are as follows.

A *mild strain (first degree)* involves stretching and a minimal amount of tearing of the involved tissues. Although there is some discomfort during function after a mild strain, there is generally little or no disability. An athlete has normal or near-normal range of motion and experiences only insignificant loss in strength. Athletes with these injuries require only minimal protection and support, such as an elastic wrap, to continue participation. Many times an athlete will continue activity and not report mild strains unless symptoms become more severe.

A *moderate strain (second degree)* involves a significant tearing of fibers, although at least some continuity of the musculotendinous unit

Fig. 7-17. Epiphyseal fracture of the femur in a young athlete.
(Courtesy Bruce Johnson, A.T.,C., Orthopedic Clinic, Grand Forks, N.D.)

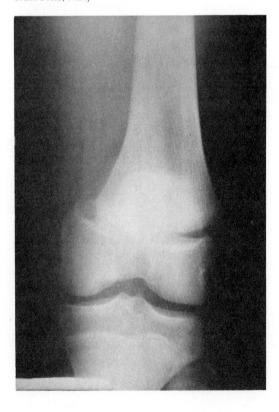

remains. A few fibers may be torn, or the majority of the fibers in a given unit may be damaged. An athlete may complete a workout or activity in pain after suffering a moderate strain and then experience disability later that day or the next morning. The second-degree strain is the most common types of strain cared for by the athletic trainer. Signs and symptoms accompanying moderate strains include varying degrees of pain, swelling, loss of strength, and loss of flexibility. The athlete may hear or feel a snap at the time the tissue tears. An area of point tenderness is evident on palpation, as is local pain expressed during active, resistive, or stretching movements. Occasionally a palpable gap, or deficit, is evident immediately after the injury. The athlete should be treated symptomatically and returned to activity as tolerated. The time required for return to complete activity varies from a few days to several weeks after a moderate strain. Athletes normally require protection and support for the injured area when they return to activity.

A *severe strain (third degree)* involves complete destruction of the continuity of the musculotendinous unit, thus causing instant disability. The rupture may occur anywhere along the musculotendinous unit or may involve an avulsion of a piece of bone at its attachment. Frequently the athlete will hear or feel a snap as the tissue ruptures. Usually there will be an associated palpable, and many times visible, gap at the site of injury. The muscle may bunch up because of spasmodic contractions. The athlete will experience a significant weakness and loss of function as a result of the injury. Severe strains should be treated initially with cold, compression, and elevation and then be referred to a physician for further diagnosis and treatment.

Strains should be referred to a physician for any of the following reasons:

1. A visible or palpable gap is noted.
2. Muscle fibers bunch as the result of spasmodic contractions and lack attachment of one extremity to a fixed point.

3. The athlete demonstrates a significant weakness and loss of function.
4. There is doubt about the status of the strain.

Acute musculotendinous strains resulting from athletic activity occur most frequently in the lower extremities. Treatment is aimed at restoring flexibility and strength. A period of complete inactivity will often result in a shortened, atrophied muscle that must be gradually stretched and strengthened to its normal state before full activity can be resumed. Severe strains therefore require repeated evaluations by the athletic trainer in order to return the athlete to full activity as quickly as possible.

Chronic strains can result from abuse or overuse of the musculotendinous unit. The most frequent mechanisms of injury involve workloads that are too stressful for the musculotendinous unit to withstand. Training and conditioning programs are designed to strengthen this contractile unit gradually, so that it is able to withstand progressively heavier work loads and thereby avoid strains. Chronic inflammation of a muscle may result if an athlete trains too intensely, performs specific repetitive movements over a considerable period of time, or continues to use an injured area. Any area of the musculotendinous unit can become irritated and inflamed, such as the muscle *(myositis)*, the tendon *(tendinitis)*, the musculotendinous junction, the tendon and its protective synovial sheath *(tenosynovitis)*, or the tendinous attachment to bone. Although each of these chronic overuse syndromes involves a different area of the contractile unit, they require basically the same treatment. Treatment procedures normally include rest, local heat, anti-inflammatory medication, and protection against continued aggravation. Most treatment programs require a modification of activity, or perhaps complete rest, which may be difficult and frustrating for both the athlete and the coach. After the cessation of symptoms, the athlete must resume activity gradually and progress within tolerable limits to avoid recurrence of the injury.

Sprains

A sprain is an injury involving a ligament. Ligaments are basically inelastic and designed to prevent abnormal motion at a joint. Whenever a joint is forced to move in an abnormal direction, ligaments are stressed (Fig. 7-18). If the ligament is forced beyond its limit, damage will occur at the weakest link in the ligament. The damage may be within the ligament itself or at one of its attachments. The severity of damage depends on the amount and duration of the abnormal force. Hinge joints, those designed to function in only one direction or plane, are the most frequently sprained. Sprains may occur dynamically; for example, the injury may be self-inflicted during twisting or turning activity. Most sprains, however, involve some outside intervention, such as getting hit on the side of the leg or landing on someone or something in the wrong way.

Ligament sprains are among the more common injuries in athletics. They also are graded into three levels of severity, determined by the amount of ligament damaged.

A *mild sprain (first degree)* involves minor stretching or tearing, with minimal disruption in the continuity of the ligament. Although there may be some discomfort during function, there is little or no disability. The athlete will have no instability or abnormal motion of the joint during passive stress tests. The ligament is not weakened significantly, and the treatment is symptomatic. An athlete may continue activity and not even report a mild sprain.

A *moderate sprain (second degree)* involves a tearing of ligament fibers and a partial break in the continuity of this noncontractile structure. Like second-degree strains, moderate sprains include the widest range of severity and are the type most commonly reported to the athletic trainer. Moderate sprains are the most difficult to assess. Long experience and refined assessment skills are needed to determine with accuracy the amount of damage sustained by a ligament in a second-degree sprain.

Moderate sprains include varying degrees of pain, swelling, and instability. The athlete may

---

Fig. 7-18. Sprain injuries. **A,** Ligament sprain resulting from inversion of the ankle during weight bearing. **B,** Second-degree sprain of anterior talofibular ligament 5 days after injury.
(Courtesy Neal Dutton, A.T.,C., Bethel College, St. Paul, Minn.)

A

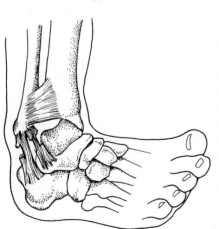

B

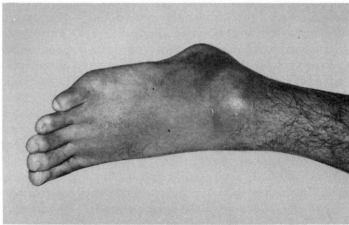

hear or feel a snapping sensation as well as sense something giving way at the time of the injury. The torn fibers of the injured ligament will produce local pain and instability. The amount of instability will depend on the number of ligament fibers torn or ruptured. As long as some of the ligament remains intact, the passive stress test will normally have an end point, or a perceived limit to abnormal motion.

The goal when caring for moderate sprains is primarily to protect the injured ligament during the healing process. Protection is mandatory to keep the damaged fibers immobile and close together in order to promote efficient repair. If injured ligaments are subjected to repeated stresses and reinjury during this healing process, they may heal in a lengthened and weakened state, resulting in an unstable joint. In most cases protection must be provided by external means, such as a cast, brace, splint, or tape. Once the healing ligament is moderately strong, the surrounding muscles can be rehabilitated to assist in support and to provide protection. Remember, ligaments heal by developing scar tissue, which takes a minimum of 6 weeks to develop and may take 6 months or longer to mature and provide maximum strength. Assessment, treatment, and rehabilitation of second-degree sprains provide the athletic trainer with a considerable challenge.

A *severe sprain (third degree)* involves a complete rupture and break in the continuity of the ligament. This may involve the ligament pulling loose a piece of bone at its point of attachment, causing an avulsion fracture. The athlete frequently hears or feels the ligament snap and has the sensation of the joint giving way in this type of injury. The athlete may or may not have pain initially with a completely torn or severed ligament. Passive stressing will produce significant instability and no endpoint of motion. Chapter 9 discusses some factors that may interfere with passive evaluation procedures.

Athletes suspected of having severe sprains should be treated with routine initial proce-dures, splinted, and referred to a physician for further diagnosis and surgical repair if necessary. Frequently surgical repair is required to reposition the ligament ends to ensure healing at or near normal length.

Sprains should be referred to a physician for any of the following reasons:

1. Significant instability is demonstrated by passive stress tests.
2. Significant joint effusion occurs within a few hours after the injury.
3. There is doubt about the status of the sprain.

Dislocations

A dislocation is the displacement of contiguous surfaces of bones composing a joint (Figs. 7-19 to 7-21). This type of injury results from forces, usually external, that cause the joint to go beyond its normal anatomic limits. This may occur as a result of excessive force or from force in an abnormal direction. When there is an incomplete displacement of the bone ends, the injury is called an incomplete dislocation or *subluxation.* Because ligaments function to prevent displacement or abnormal motion at joints, all sprains result in some degree of subluxation. A complete dislocation, or *luxation,* occurs when there is a complete separation of the bone ends. A dislocation will either remain displaced after injury or reduce spontaneously and move back into place. It may be difficult to evaluate exactly what happened unless the athlete can document the dislocation. Many times the athlete is aware that the bones are out of place, and can relate the position of the joint when it was dislocated. Dislocations may be accompanied by avulsion fractures, which can be verified by radiographs, and by torn ligaments, resulting in moderate to severe sprains.

Joints that are designed to function in one direction or plane, such as hinge joints, are those more severely injured when dislocated. For example, when the ankle, knee, or elbow are dislocated, there is normally a significant amount of

Fig. 7-19. Elbow dislocation. **A,** Schematic of posterior displacement. **B,** Actual posterior displacement injury.
(Courtesy A.G. Edwards, A.T.,C., University of Nevada–Las Vegas)

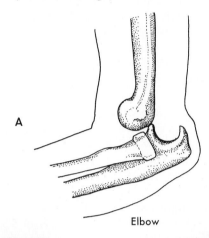

Elbow

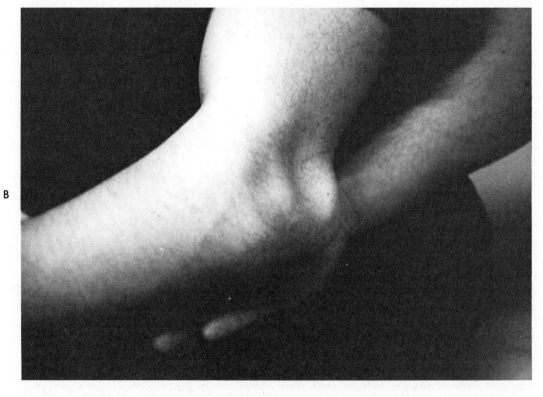

Fig. 7-20. Shoulder dislocation. **A,** Schematic of anterior displacement. **B,** Actual anterior displacement injury.
(Courtesy Steve Yoneda, A.T.,C., California Polytechnic State University, San Luis Obispo, Calif.)

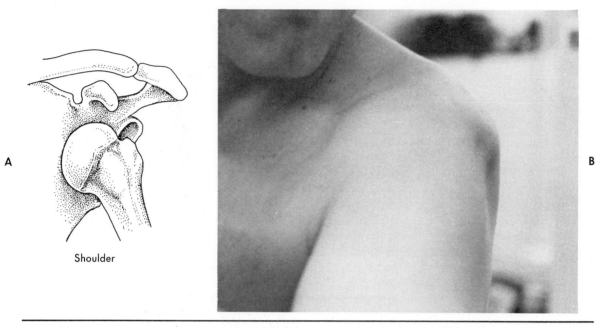

A

Shoulder

B

Fig. 7-21. Finger dislocation. **A,** Schematic of proximal interphalangeal joint dislocation.
B, Actual interphalangeal joint dislocation.
(Courtesy A.G. Edwards, A.T.,C., University of
Nevada–Las Vegas.)

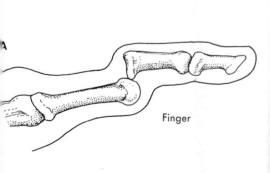

Finger

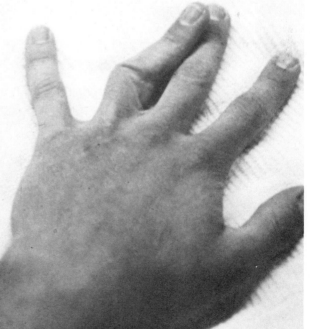

B

damage to surrounding structures. Damage to nerves and blood vessels is also more likely. On the other hand, when the shoulder, which has a great range of motion and few restrictions, is dislocated, long-term complications and damage to nerves and blood vessels are not as common.

Dislocations that remain displaced are generally easy to recognize. Deformity is almost always apparent. Occasionally the athletic trainer may have to palpate and compare body contours with the uninjured extremity to reveal minimal deformity. Dislocations also cause a significant amount of pain as well as loss of limb function. The objective of treatment is reduction of the dislocation by a physician. Initially, the athletic trainer should splint or support the injured joint to prevent any further damage. All dislocations and suspected dislocations should be referred to a physician for radiographs and further evaluation.

Treatment for dislocations, once they are reduced, depends on the joint involved, but essentially is the same as that for severe sprains. Surgical intervention is sometimes required, and the injured ligaments must be supported and protected throughout the healing process. Unprotected joints may heal with increased laxity in the ligaments, making the joints more vulnerable to subsequent subluxations and total dislocations.

Fractures

A fracture is a disruption in the continuity of bone and can range in severity from a simple crack to the severe shattering of a bone with multiple fragments. Fractures are unique injuries in that they heal with the same type of tissue (bone) that was injured and can thus regain their preinjured strength. Bones can be fractured in several ways. A direct blow may cause a break at the point of impact, such as an athlete getting kicked in the lateral aspect of the leg, resulting in a fractured fibula. An indirect blow may cause a fracture away from the point of impact, such as an athlete landing on his or her hand and breaking one of the bones of the upper extremity. Severe twisting forces, such as turning and cutting maneuvers, may also cause a fracture. As

previously described, severe sprains or strains may result in avulsion fractures.

Prolonged repetitive activity or chronic overuse can lead to another type of fracture, *stress fracture,* sometimes called fatigue fracture. These types of fractures occur over a considerable period of time and without history of an acute traumatic episode. Stress fractures are generally incomplete fractures and seldom result in separation of bone fragments. Many times the initial plain-film radiographs will be negative, and the stress fracture will not be confirmed until the appearance of new periosteal bone formation is recognized on follow-up radiographs 2 or 3 weeks later. The actual fracture line may never appear on radiographs. The athletic trainer should suspect a stress fracture when an athlete reports painful stress and tenderness over a bony area without any specific trauma but is involved in an activity with repetitive stress. If symptoms persist, repeated radiographs or a bone scan may be required to obtain a definitive diagnosis.

Fractures are divided into two major classifications according to involvement of the overlying skin. Fractures that do not break the skin are called *closed (simple) fractures,* whereas fractures that are associated with a tear of the skin are *open (compound) fractures* (Fig. 7-22). Compound fractures may be caused by a broken bone end tearing the skin, or by a direct blow that lacerates the skin at the time of fracture (Fig. 7-23). These are generally the more serious type of fractures because of the additional possibilities of infection and external bleeding.

Fractures are also described by the manner in which the bone is broken. This classification is determined and confirmed only by radiographs. Although the athletic trainer is obviously not responsible for classifying fractures according to radiographic appearance, he or she should be familiar with the terminology. Various types of fractures are illustrated in Fig. 7-24. Other terms an athletic trainer should be familiar with concerning fractures include:

Contrecoup: A fracture occurring at a distance away from the point of impact, such as a skull fracture caused by a blow to the opposite side.

Fig. 7-22. Two major classifications of fractures; closed and open.

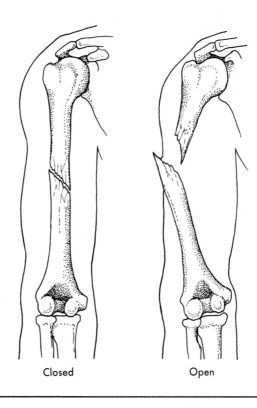

Closed   Open

Fig. 7-23. Compound fracture of the ulna.

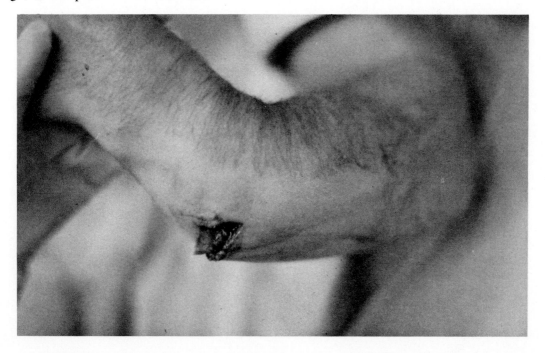

Fig. 7-24. Various types of fractures. **A,** Avulsion, a fracture in which a piece of bone is pulled loose at the attachment of a tendon, ligament or muscle, normally occurring with a sudden violent contraction or stress. **B,** Chrondral, a fracture involving the articular cartilage. **C,** Communited, a fracture in which three or more fragments are produced. **D,** Compression, an impacted fracture characterized by crushed bone tissue, such as the body of a vertebra. **E,** Depressed, in which part of a flat bone is depressed inward or below the surface, such as the skull or cheek bone. **F,** Epiphyseal, a fracture at the growth plate of long bones. Occurs in growing children, as this is the weakest link along the bone.

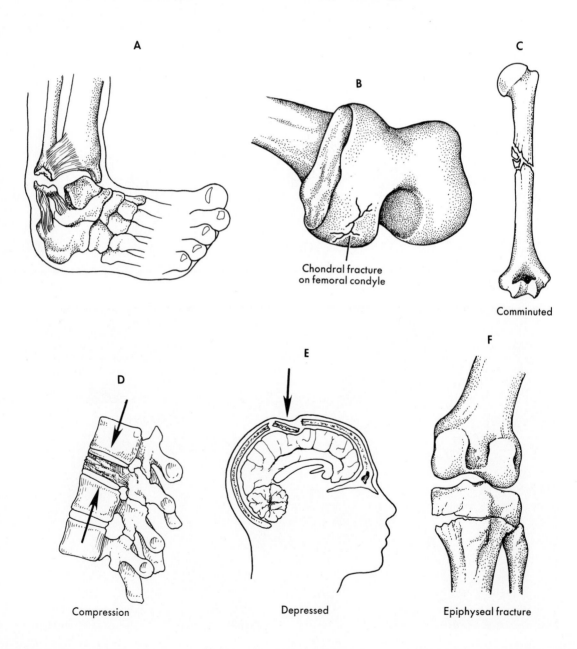

A

B

Chondral fracture
on femoral condyle

C

Comminuted

D

Compression

E

Depressed

F

Epiphyseal fracture

Fig. 7-24, cont'd. G, Greenstick, an incomplete fracture of a long bone that occurs in adolescent athletes whose bones are still pliable. A common example would be a greenstick fracture of the clavicle in children. **H,** Impacted, a fracture in which one fragment has been driven into and imbedded in another fragment. **I,** Oblique, a fracture that crosses the bone at an oblique angle to its long axis. **J,** Osteochondral, a fracture involving the articular cartilage and underlying bone. **K,** Spiral, a break that twists around and through the bone and is usually caused by a twisting injury. **L,** Stress (fatigue), a fracture occurring after prolonged repetitive activity. **M,** Transverse, a break across the bone at a right angle to its long axis, often caused by a direct blow.

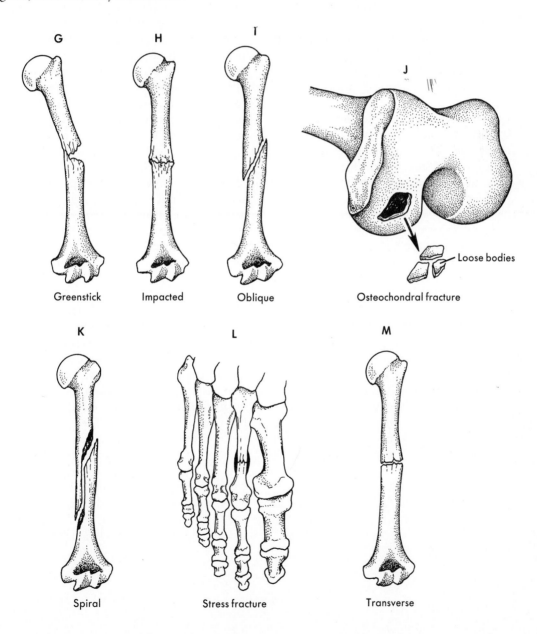

G

H

I

J

Greenstick   Impacted   Oblique   Osteochondral fracture

Loose bodies

K   L   M

Spiral   Stress fracture   Transverse

Delayed union: A fracture that has not united successfully within expected period of time although the healing process continues.

Nonunion: Failure of the ends of a fracture to unite.

Malunion: A fracture that has united with faulty alignment of fragments.

Overriding: A fracture in which the fragments overlap, resulting in shortening of the bone.

Rotated: A fracture in which one of the fragments has rotated in relation to the other.

Fracture-dislocation: A fracture near a joint that occurs simultaneously with a dislocation.

Displaced: A fracture in which bone fragment is out of normal alignment.

Nondisplaced: The pieces of bone lie in relatively normal alignment. Occasionally this type of break may be difficult to see on a radiograph.

There are many signs and symptoms that may assist the athletic trainer in recognizing a fracture. The primary symptom is pain localized at the fracture site that remains consistent with motion, palpation, or stress maneuvers. The athlete may report the sound or sensation of something breaking or snapping. The athlete may also experience a grating or grinding sound (crepitation), which is caused by the bone ends rubbing against each other during any type of movement. There may be an obvious deformity or irregularity of the involved area such as swelling, protrusion, or shortening of a limb. With a compound fracture, a broken bone end may or may not be protruding through the open wound. There may be a loss of function or disability associated with a fracture. However, a loss of function does not always accompany a fracture and it is a myth to believe, "If the injured part can be moved, it's not broken." The detection of any of these signs and symptoms deserves additional assessment procedures and referral to medical assistance for further diagnosis and radiographs. Forceful manipulation or stress procedures to evaluate bone integrity should be reserved as a final check of structural continuity, not as further proof of that which already clearly requires further diagnosis and radiographs. Athletes may demonstrate false motion or abnormal movement in an area, which is commonly called a false joint. However, in the presence of the above signs and symptoms there is little need to demonstrate false motion. In the absence of signs and symptoms indicating a fracture, more vigorous procedures should be applied to evaluate the bony integrity. A forceful levering both longitudinally and cross-wise to the bone should be performed before pronouncing any such injury free of fracture. Athletic trainers must maintain a high index of suspicion and never allow an athlete to return to activity with an injury that suggests a fracture. Similarly, athletic trainers must not decide any suspected fracture is safe from aggravation by continued athletic activity without further diagnosis.

The treatment for suspected fractures is that of protection for the injured area so that no further damage occurs because of improper handling or movement. This is normally accomplished by splinting the injured area. Remember to immobilize the joint above and below a fracture site to avoid movement to the bone fragments. If there is an open wound associated with the fracture, control the bleeding and apply a sterile dressing before splinting the area. Treat for shock if necessary. The athletic trainer should also feel for a pulse distal to major fractures to ensure circulation is adequate. Whenever circulation is jeopardized, a medical emergency exists and the injured athlete must be transported to a medical facility immediately.

KEY TERMS

abrasion Break in skin continuity occurring when the epidermis and a portion of the dermis is scrapped or rubbed away

acute traumatic injury Athletic injury occurring instantaneously as a result of some type of trauma

athletic injury Disruption in tissue continuity that results from athletic activity, causing a cessation of participation or restriction of usual activity

avulsion Tearing away of part of a structure, which may be torn completely free or remain partially attached, hanging as a flap

chronic overuse syndrome Athletic injury resulting from forces or stresses applied to a structure or tissues over a considerable period of time

closed (simple) fracture Fracture that does not break the skin

contusion (bruise) Skin or soft tissue injury that usually results from a direct blow or impact delivered to some area of the body

dermis Inner and thicker layer of the skin

dislocation Luxation or displacement of contiguous surfaces of bones comprising a joint

ecchymoses Extravasations of blood generally caused by trauma to skin or muscle

epidermis Outer and thinner layer of the skin

exposed injury Athletic injuries or conditions that disrupt the continuity of the skin

fracture Disruption in the continuity of bone

incision Open wound caused by cutting the skin with a sharp object such as a knife

laceration Open wound or cut made by tearing the skin, which usually results from some type of direct blow to the skin and is especially common over bony prominences

luxation Complete dislocation

mechanism of injury Manner and location by which excess forces or stresses are applied to the body, resulting in athletic injuries

myositis ossificans Formation of bone within or around a muscle, commonly called calcium deposits

open (compound) fracture Fracture associated with break in the skin

petechiae Small, nonelevated, pinpoint purplish or red discolorations resulting from localized hemorrhage into the skin or mucous membranes

primary lesion Lesion that appears initially in response to some changes in the internal or external environment of the skin

puncture wound Open lesion occurring as a result of direct penetration of the skin by a pointed object

secondary lesion Lesions that do not appear initially but result from a primary lesion

sprain Athletic injury involving a ligament

strain Athletic injury involving the musculotendinous unit

stress fracture Incomplete break in a bone, occuring after prolonged, repetitive activity

subluxation Incomplete dislocation

unexposed injury Internal athletic injuries with no associated disruption or break in the continuity of the skin

SUGGESTED READINGS

American Academy of Orthopaedic Surgeons: Emergency care and transportation of the sick and injured, ed. 3, Chicago, 1981, The Academy.

Arnheim, D.D.: Modern principles of athletic training, ed. 6, St. Louis, 1985, Times Mirror/Mosby College Publishing.

Grant, H.D., and others: Emergency care, ed. 3, Bowie, Md., 1982, Robert J. Brady Co.

Hafen, B.Q., and Karren, K.J.: First aid and emergency care, skills manual, Englewood, Colo., 1982, Morton Publishing Co.

Malasanos, L., and others: Health assessment, ed. 3, St. Louis, 1985, Times Mirror/Mosby College Publishing.

O'Donoghue, D.H.: Treatment of injuries to athletes, ed. 4, Philadelphia, 1984, W.B. Saunders Co.

Stauffer, L.W.: Skin disorders in athletes: identification and management, Physician Sportsmedicine **11**:101-121, 1983.

Strauss, R.H.: Sports medicine and physiology, Philadelphia, 1979, W.B. Saunders Co.

The Nurse's Reference Library: Assessment, Springhouse, Pa., 1982, Intermed Communications, Inc.

Warner, C.G.: Emergency care, assessment and intervention, ed. 3, St. Louis, 1982, The C.V. Mosby Co.

White, W.B., and Grant-Wels, J.M.: Transmission of herpes simplex type I infection in rugby players, J.A.M.A. **252**(4): 533-535, 1984.

U N I T

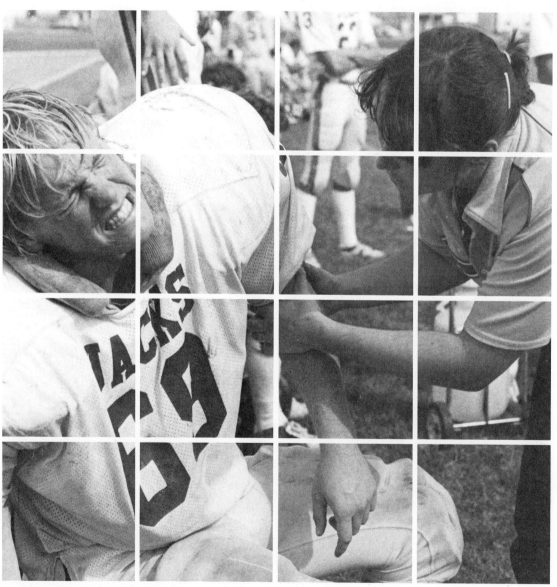

Injured athlete undergoing assessment.

T H R E E

Athletic injury assessment process

The athletic injury assessment process is a necessary and extremely important skill for anyone who shares the responsibility for the medical care of athletes. One of the primary factors in the successful management of athletic injuries is the earliest possible determination of the type and extent of injury. To ensure a complete and effective evaluation, the athletic trainer must have meaningful and well-established assessment procedures to follow with every injury. In addition to the skilled execution of carefully organized steps in an assessment sequence, the athletic trainer must constantly sharpen and refine basic observation and communication skills essential for effective information gathering. This unit is designed to assist the athletic trainer in preparing his or her assessment techniques. The remainder of this text is concerned with evaluative techniques for injuries to specific areas of the body.

8   Factors related to athletic injury assessment

9   Assessment procedures

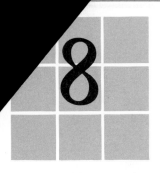

Factors relating to athletic injury assessment

Athletic injury assessment is defined as the comprehensive evaluation of an athletic injury beginning when the injury occurs and continuing through the healing process until the injured area has been rehabilitated to its fullest extent. The initial evaluation involves accurately recognizing the nature, site, and severity of the athletic injury. This is the first step in properly caring for an injury and is accomplished by talking with and listening to the athlete and observing, touching (palpating), and perhaps stressing or manipulating the injured area. The knowledge gained during this initial evaluation will assist the athletic trainer in formulating the most effective and appropriate follow-up care and treatment procedures. This information will also provide the basis for decisions that may be required concerning referral to medical assistance. Without this knowledge, an injured area may not be cared for properly, which can result in further injury or delay recovery. Thus effective treatment and recovery programs depend on the accuracy of the initial assessment of athletic injuries.

The athletic injury assessment process involves more than just the initial evaluation of an injury. Periodic reevaluations after the injury are necessary to give the physician, athletic trainer, coach, and athlete information about the current status of the injured area. The knowledge gained during these repeated evaluations is used to determine such things as how the injured athlete is progressing, whether or not the treatment or rehabilitation programs should be changed, and when the athlete can return safely to activity. The entire process of assessing an injured area ends only after the part has healed and been rehabilitated to its fullest.

Athletic injury assessment is not an easy task. The recognition and accurate identification of an injured area is often difficult and challenging.

Knowledge, experience, practice, and acquired skills are all necessary prerequisites for competence in the assessment of athletic injuries. Of course, there is no substitute for experience and practice. The knowledge surrounding the athletic injury assessment process can be categorized into five main areas (Fig. 8-1). Each of these areas is interrelated and important to the total process.

ANATOMY

To accurately evaluate an injured area, the athletic trainer must understand the anatomy of the involved body part. A total assessment involves isolating and evaluating each anatomic structure suspected of being injured. This isolation process should be performed systematically to permit identification of the involved structures as well as to assess the severity of involvement. Athletic trainers should be able to visualize the actual structures being evaluated (Fig. 8-2). Without a good understanding of the underlying anatomic structures, it will be difficult or

Fig. 8-1. The five major areas of an athletic injury assessment process.

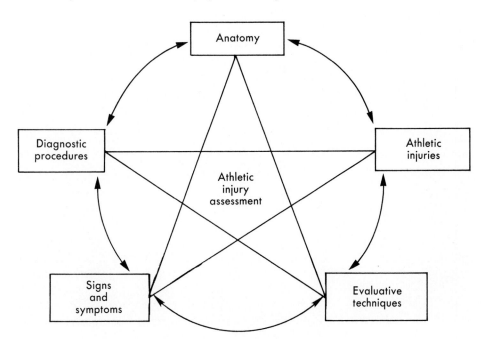

impossible to accurately evaluate the injury. A review of basic bone, joint, and muscle anatomy was presented in Unit One; more detailed regional anatomy is presented with each body area discussed throughout the remainder of this text. However, it is strongly recommended that courses in anatomy and kinesiology be taken by athletic trainers to strengthen their knowledge in these areas. Frequent review of this important information is encouraged.

ATHLETIC INJURIES

An overview of the body's response to trauma and the common athletic injuries was presented in Unit Two. Everyone who has the responsibility for the medical care of athletes should be familiar with these processes and the various injuries that may result from athletic activities. To accurately assess these injuries, it is extremely important to understand how the body responds to trauma and how the associated signs and symptoms develop. Furthermore, it is important

to have a general understanding of the mechanisms causing common injuries. All of this information can greatly assist the athletic trainer in the assessment process.

EVALUATIVE TECHNIQUES

An important aspect of the athletic injury assessment process is the use of an organized examination sequence. Although each injury is unique, an evaluation of the injured area is easier to perform by using a systematic approach. Each athletic trainer must develop his or her own evaluative techniques within the limits of individual abilities and training. This text is intended to offer guidelines for development of athletic injury assessment skills, not to make medical diagnosticians out of athletic trainers. A properly trained person present at the time an injury occurs has the best opportunity to make an accurate initial evaluation, and most of the time this responsibility will fall on the athletic trainer. In the absence of trained personnel, the initial eval-

Fig. 8-2. Reviewing anatomy of the knee.

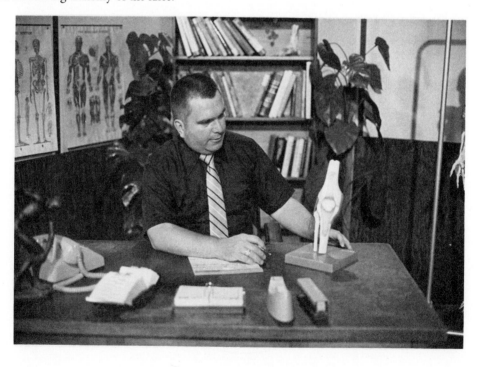

uation may be neglected and the injured athlete told to "wait and see" or "walk it off." In many cases an injured athlete is simply referred to a physician, and by the time the evaluation is performed, pain, swelling, and spasm make the assessment more difficult. Further, initial evaluations performed by an athletic trainer immediately after a serious injury can be of great importance to the physician in establishing early treatment and planning of follow-up care.

SIGNS AND SYMPTOMS

Signs and symptoms exhibited by an injured athlete yield valuable information needed to make an accurate assessment (Fig. 8-3). A *symptom* is subjective evidence of the injury, or something the athlete tells us. For example, pain that is associated with an injury is felt and can only be described by the athlete. A *sign* is objective evidence of the injury, or something you as the examiner can see, hear, or feel. An example of a sign is swelling associated with an injury, which can be observed and felt by the athletic trainer. Interpretation of the signs and symptoms recognized during the assessment process provides information for the type of care the athlete should receive.

DIAGNOSTIC PROCEDURES

Diagnostic procedures include all of the techniques a physician may employ to assist in the diagnosis of an athletic injury. Several tests or procedures are often required to pinpoint the location, extent, and seriousness of some injuries. An increase in the number, availability, and sophistication of these diagnostic procedures has made them extremely valuable tools in sports medicine. In many cases complex laboratory tests or radiographic studies are required for a physician to complete the diagnosis of some athletic injuries. Because of their importance and frequency of use, several of these procedures will be discussed. It is the responsibility of the athletic trainer to refer the injured athlete for addi-

Fig. 8-3. Signs and symptoms of athletic injuries.

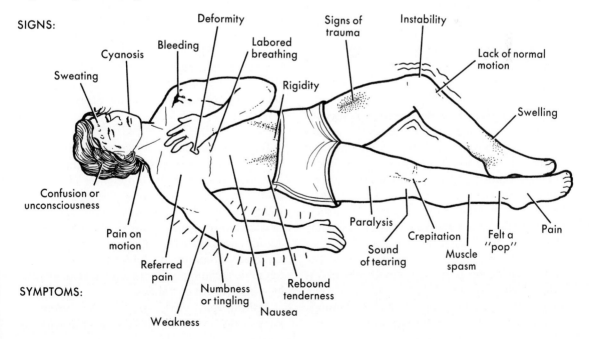

SIGNS:

Deformity

Signs of trauma

Instability

Bleeding

Cyanosis

Labored breathing

Lack of normal motion

Sweating

Rigidity

Swelling

Confusion or unconsciousness

Paralysis

Pain

Pain on motion

Crepitation

Felt a "pop"

Referred pain

Sound of tearing

Muscle spasm

SYMPTOMS:

Numbness or tingling

Rebound tenderness

Weakness

Nausea

tional diagnostic procedures when indicated by the information gained during the assessment process.

It is not the intent of this text to discuss in any great depth the additional procedures a physician may use in diagnosing an injury. However, because they are important to the total assessment process, athletic trainers should possess some knowledge of these procedures. Such information is frequently useful in helping to prepare an athlete for referral or in explaining the rationale for specific procedures before or after they are performed. Following is a brief description of the more common diagnostic procedures a physician may use to assist in diagnosing an athletic injury.

Radiology

Radiologic studies are very important and useful in diagnosing many athletic injuries or related conditions. Radiologic images or tests include a wide variety of techniques or procedures used individually or in combination to provide the physician with information necessary to assist in making a diagnosis. Radiologic techniques or procedures used most often in the diagnosis of athletic injuries are (1) plain film radiography, (2) contrast-enhanced radiography, (3) computed tomography, and (4) nuclear imaging.

Plain film radiography

The term *plain film radiography* is used to describe those radiologic procedures that use no special techniques or material to enhance the contrast of the various structures of the body. These procedures are adequate when natural radiographic contrast exists between body structures, such as bone and adjacent soft tissues. These are the most common types of radiologic procedures used in sports medicine. Plain film radiographs are used to clarify or confirm the clinical assessment in many types of athletic injuries. Plain film examinations are commonly used for bone and joint injuries, and the findings include information concerning bone integrity,

atrophy, hypertrophy, erosion, contours, and density, as well as the relationships between articulating bones (Fig. 8-4).

Stress radiographs. A stress radiograph is a procedure using radiographs taken while stress is being applied to the joint. These types of radiographs are normally performed with the athlete under anesthesia to eliminate pain and accompanying muscular contractions. An unstable joint or one showing abnormal motion will be demonstrated on a stress film by a widening of the joint space as the stress is applied (Fig. 8-5). This finding generally confirms a clinical impression of ligament instability. It is also possible to show the disruption of the growth plate in younger athletes by the use of stress radiographs.

Tomography. Tomography is a technique using radiographs taken with a specialized computer to give a two-dimensional view of one particular area of tissue at any depth (Fig. 8-6). This is like taking a radiograph of one slice or section at any level of the extremity. As the x-ray is focused on a particular area, the x-ray tube and film are synchronized and move in opposite directions. This opposing movement blurs out unwanted structures while keeping the focal area in sharp contrast. Tomograms are helpful in delineating specific areas and are frequently used to evaluate bony structures. Tomography has been shown to significantly improve the diagnostic success in injuries involving the cervical spine.

Contrast-enhanced radiography

Contrast-enhanced radiographic procedures are those used to examine structures that do not have inherent contrast differences from surrounding tissues. With this type of radiologic technique, it is necessary to use one of a variety of contrasting agents. These preparations can be administered orally, rectally, or by injection into the body. Some of the contrast-enhanced radiographic techniques that may be used with athletic injuries are as follows.

Arthrography. Arthrography is the study of joints using a contrast medium, with or without

Fig. 8-4. Plain film radiography. **A,** Procedure for taking sunrise view of patellae; **B,** the resulting radiograph.

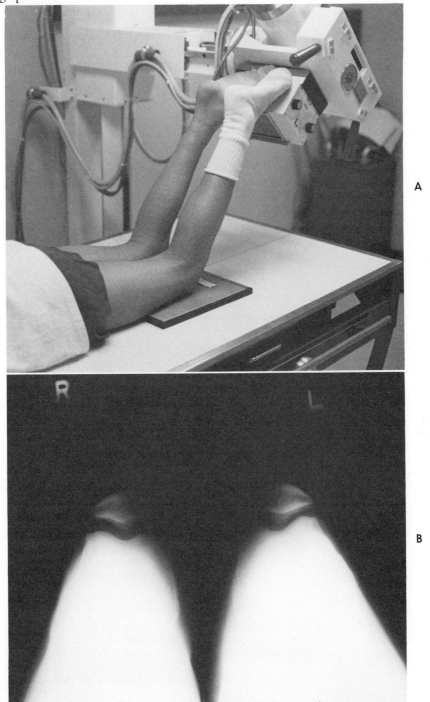

Fig. 8-5. Stress radiograph. **A,** procedure for taking a stress radiograph of an ankle. **B,** An ankle stress film.

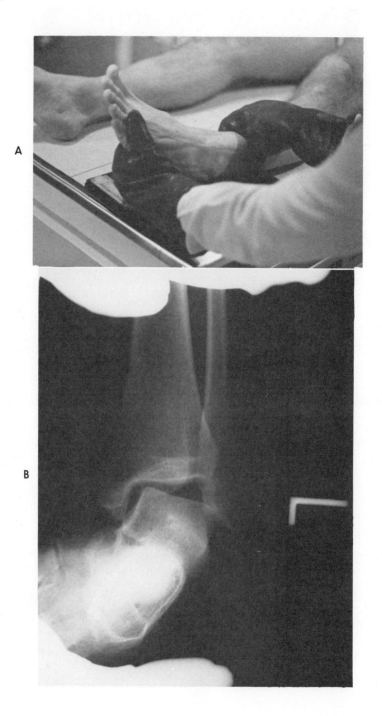

Fig. 8-6. Tomograms of a fractured right proximal tibia, showing successive sections or slices of the fracture site from superficial (**A**) to deep (**F**).

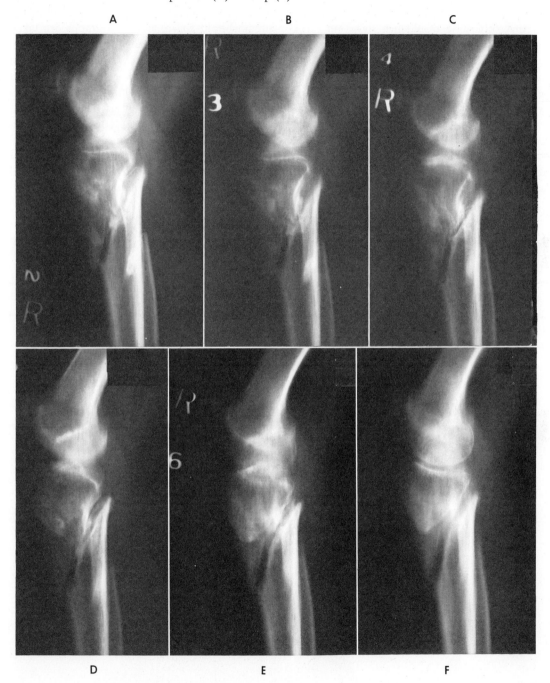

air, which is injected into the joint space. A radiograph is then taken, called an *arthrogram,* which outlines the soft tissue structures of a joint that otherwise would not show up on a plain film radiograph (Fig. 8-7). the radiopaque dye will outline any irregularities in the soft tissue structures of the joint. After injection, the dye is generally absorbed by the body within a few hours. This procedure is frequently performed on athletic injuries involving the knee, especially those in which cartilage damage is suspected. As arthroscopy techniques improve, less arthrography is being done, but it still has its place in the diagnosis of certain conditions.

Myelography. Myelography is the radiographic study of the spinal cord and canal. A contrast medium is injected into the spinal canal in the subarachnoid space, and radiographs are taken (Fig. 8-8). Cerebrospinal fluid may also be removed for laboratory studies at this time. An abnormality present on the resulting *myelogram* will show up in the dye column. The most common lesion evaluated by myelography is an intervertebral disc herniation with evidence of spinal cord or nerve root compression. The material normally injected is either an oil-type agent that must be withdrawn from the spinal canal later, or a water-soluble agent that is absorbed by the body.

Fig. 8-7. Arthrography of the knee joint. **A,** Procedure for injecting radiopaque dye into the joint. **B,** An arthrogram showing vertical tear in the posterior portion of the medial meniscus.

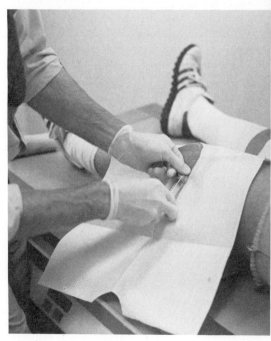

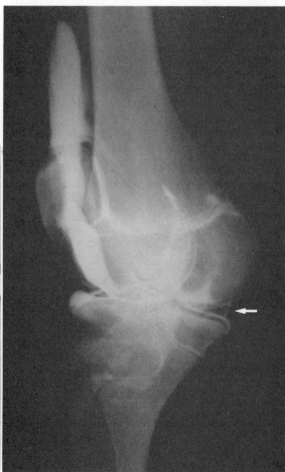

Discography. Discography is the radiographic study of the spine for visualization of an intervertebral disc. Radiopaque dye is introduced into the disc space between two vertebrae, and a radiograph, called a *discogram,* is taken (Fig. 8-9). Ruptures of the intervertebral disc will be indicated by an abnormal dye pattern between the vertebrae.

Angiography. Angiography is the radiographic study of the vascular system. A water-soluble radiopaque dye is injected either intra-arterially *(arteriogram)* or intravenously *(venogram),* and a rapid sequence of radiographs are taken to follow the course of the contrast material through the blood vessels (Fig. 8-10). These tests are useful in diagnosing injury to or partial blockage of blood vessels.

Urography. Urography is the radiographic study of the urinary tract. A contrast medium is injected into the athlete intravenously and

Fig. 8-8. Myelography. **A,** Injecting contrast medium into the spinal canal. **B,** A myelogram.

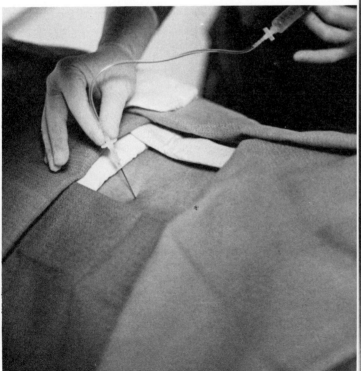

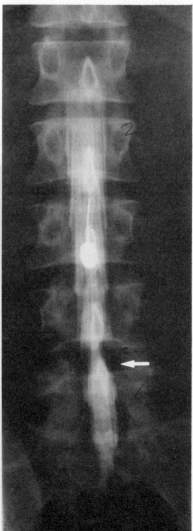

A

B

Fig. 8-9. Discography. **A,** Injecting radiopaque dye into the disc space between vertebrae. **B,** Normal discogram (L$_4$-L$_5$) showing needle in place. Note that dye remains encapsulated at point of injection. **C,** Abnormal discogram (L$_5$-S$_1$). Note that dye has extravasated beyond injection site because of herniation.

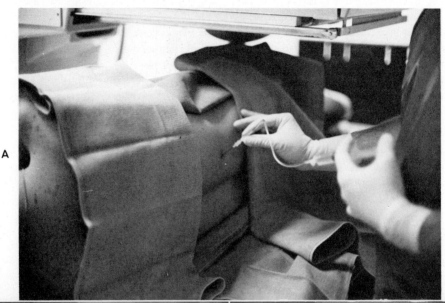

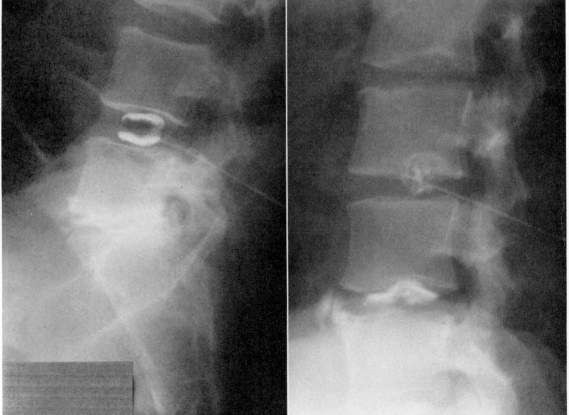

Fig. 8-10. Angiography. **A,** Injecting radiopaque dye into the right femoral artery. **B,** Arteriogram. Arrow points to right common iliac artery. Note absence of this artery on the left side.

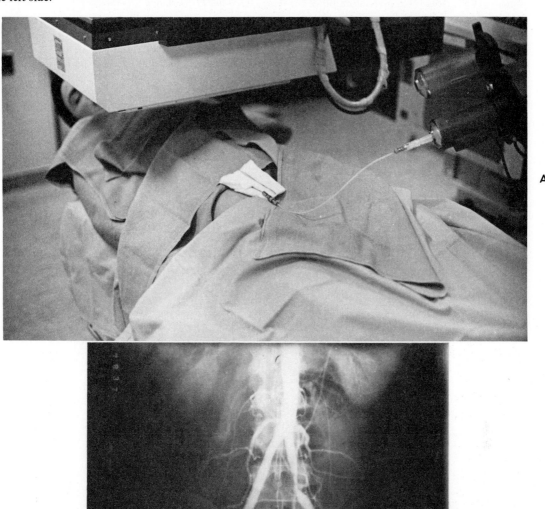

Fig. 8-11. Urography. **A,** Injecting a contrast medium intravenously, and **B,** an intravenous pyelogram (IVP). Note the nonvisualization of the left ureter *(arrow)* following a contusion to the left kidney.

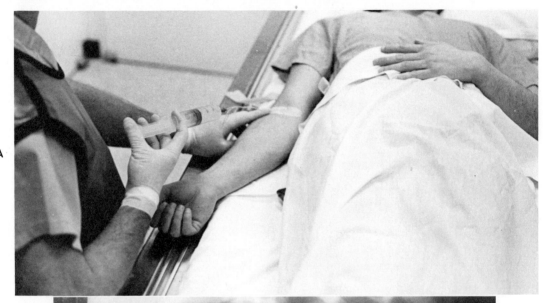

A

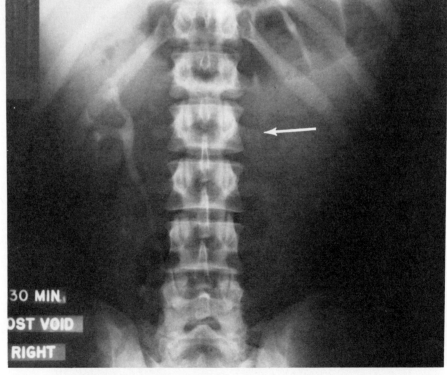

B

30 MIN.

OST VOID

RIGHT

quickly passes into the urine. Radiographs are then taken of the kidneys, ureters, and urinary bladder (Fig. 8-11). This is called an *intravenous pyelogram* (IVP) and is a common procedure when urinary tract injuries are suspected.

Computed tomography

Computed tomography (CT scan) is a sophisticated test that is performed with computerized radiographic equipment. The images obtained give almost a three-dimensional view of the affected area. Images are displayed on a television monitor during the procedure, and permanent films are recorded at various levels or slices during the examination sequence (Fig. 8-12). This is a representation of what would be seen with the athlete cut open on a transverse plane. The normal examination of the head uses 8 to 10 slices and of the body, 12 to 15 slices. CT scanning is the primary imaging procedure used in trauma involving the head, as it shows both the contents of the skull and any injury that may have occurred. Small hematomas, localized swelling, and cerebral atrophy can be picked up by the CT scan almost unfailingly. This diagnostic procedure can also be used effectively on the trunk and extremities. In these cases, a contrasting agent is frequently injected intravenously to enhance the appearance of certain visceral structures.

Nuclear imaging

Nuclear imaging depends on the selective and unique absorption characteristics of certain radioactive compounds by different organs of the body. Typically, a radioactive isotope with a very short half-life is injected into the body, and the resultant radioactivity in a given area, organ, or tissue is calculated on a counter and recorded on a scanner. The most common nu-

Fig. 8-12. Computed tomography (CT scan). **A,** taking a CT scan.

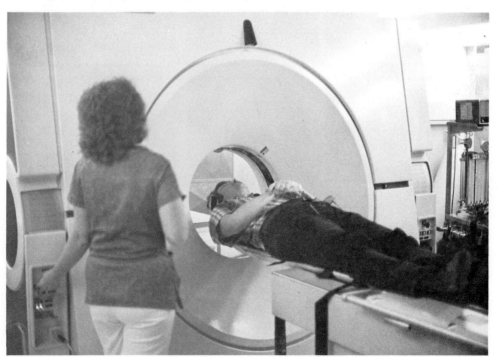

A

Continued.

Fig. 8-12, cont'd. B, the resulting CT scan film series.

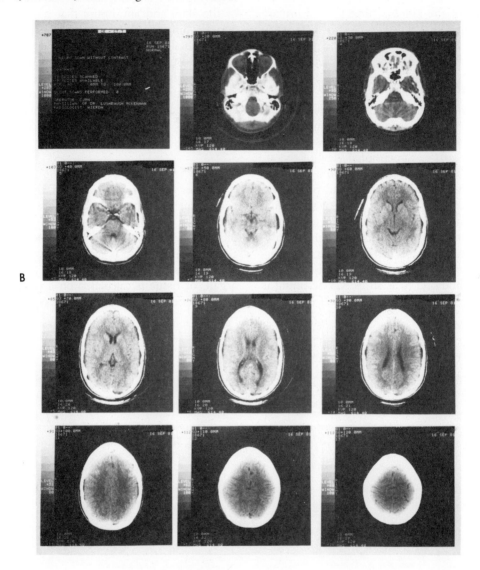

B

Fig. 8-12, cont'd. C, one of the individual sections.

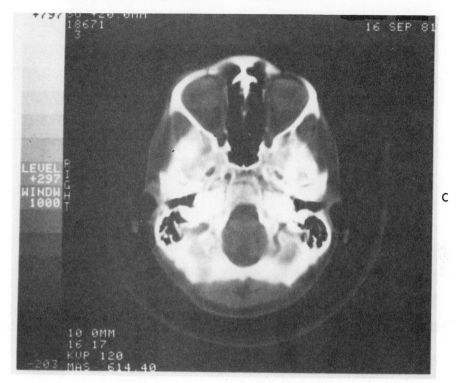

Fig. 8-13. Nuclear imaging. **A,** Procedure for taking a bone scan; **B,** a total body view bone scan. Note increased activity *(arrows)* in the midshaft of the left tibia, indicating a stress fracture.

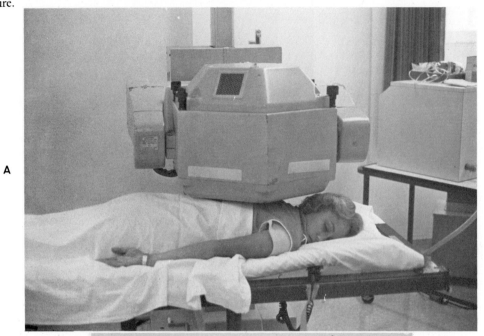

A

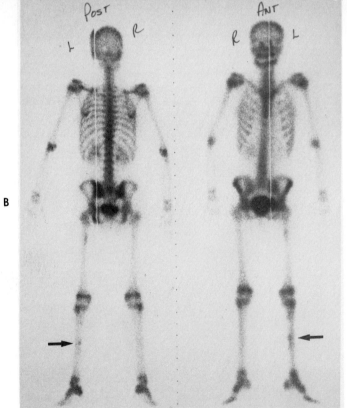

B

clear imaging technique associated with athletic injuries is the **bone scan** (Fig. 8-13). This test will detect particular areas of abnormal metabolic activity within a bone, which may indicate a tumor, infection, or recent fracture. Bone scans can detect sites of stress in a bone before a conventional radiograph shows any abnormality. Bone scans will often detect stress fractures before they are symptomatic. This can lead to an earlier diagnosis, earlier and more effective treatment, and less disability for the athlete. Bone scans can also be useful in determining if myositis ossificans or spondylolysis are still active or if they have matured. Nuclear imaging can also be used for examination of soft tissue areas. Examples include scans of the brain (largely replaced by CT scans), liver, lung, heart, or thyroid.

Laboratory evaluations

There is a large and ever-increasing variety of laboratory evaluations or procedures that can be performed to supplement the assessment of athletic injuries. Laboratory tests make the basic sciences available to those who participate in the diagnosis and treatment of an injured athlete. In many cases, the professional athletic trainer needs to know, at least in general terms, the purpose of a particular test, how it is performed, and the significance of its results in order to serve effectively as a member of the sports medicine team. Biochemical data gained from laboratory studies of blood, urine, synovial fluid, cerebrospinal fluid, aspirates, or other materials can reveal information essential to diagnosis and treatment. For example, analysis of synovial fluid aspirated or removed from a joint (Fig. 8-14) will distinguish certain characteristics between infections, arthritides, acute injuries, and occasionally tumors or other unusual diseases. In acute injuries, blood is frequently present in the synovial fluid, which indicates that damage has occurred to a structure located within the joint capsule or to the joint capsule itself. An associated benefit of joint aspiration is the frequent relief of pain and an increased range of motion.

Fig. 8-14. Aspirating a knee joint.

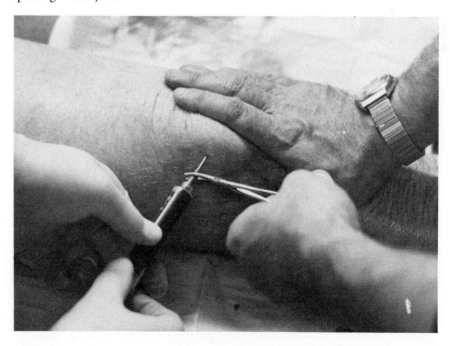

Fig. 8-15. Electroencephalography. **A,** electrodes are applied to the scalp. **B,** The resulting electroencephalogram.

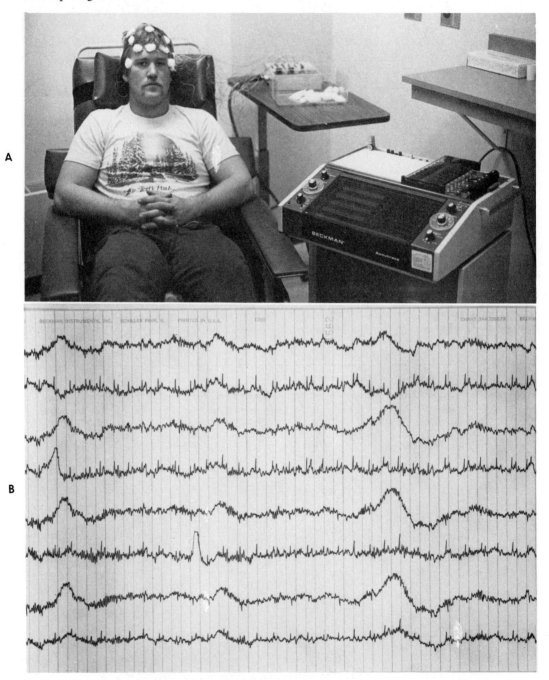

Electroencephalography

Electroencephalography is the study of electrical currents emitted by the brain. This electrical activity is picked up by electrodes applied to the scalp and displayed on a monitor or printed on readout paper (Fig. 8-15). The graphic recordings are called an *electroencephalogram* (EEG). The patterns and changes in electrical activity allows the neurosurgeon or neurologist to base a diagnosis on the activity of the brain rather than relying solely on neurologic assessments.

Electrocardiography

Electrocardiography is the study of electrical activity of the heart. This measure of electrical activity is picked up by electrodes placed on the chest and extremities and displayed on a monitor or recorded on paper (Fig. 8-16). The graphic recordings are called an *electrocardiogram* (ECG) or EKG) and are valuable in suspected heart lesions.

Echocardiography

Echocardiography is a technique that uses echoes or reflected high-frequency sound waves to locate and observe the activity and integrity of cardiac structures. The images are recorded on videotape and are often processed by computer for quantitation and enhancement of detail (Fig. 8-17). During the test, sound waves are generated by a transducer placed over the chest wall. The technique is said to be noninvasive because it does not break the skin or interfere in any way with the events that are being observed. Echocardiography is often used to measure the size of the cardiac chambers in order to detect filling defects after injury. It is the most frequently used test in the area of clinical cardiology after the electrocardiogram.

Electromyography

Electromyography is the study of the electrical potentials generated in muscles. Electrodes placed on the surface of a muscle, or sterile needle–type electrodes inserted into the muscle itself, pick up the electrical potentials that are generated when the muscle contracts. These electrical signals are then displayed on an oscilloscope or printed on a paper strip recording (Fig. 8-18). The graphic recordings are called an *electromyogram* (EMG). Interpretation of the electrical activity generated with slight and maximal-effort contractions is helpful in diagnosis of peripheral nerve injuries, muscle denervation, and intrinsic muscle disease.

Arthroscopy

Arthroscopy allows a surgeon to actually view the interior of a joint through a series of very small lenses with a fiberoptic light source. This diagnostic procedure is performed under sterile technique and either local or general anesthesia. After the joint is distended with saline solution, a small incision (2 to 3 mm) is made, and the arthroscope is inserted into the joint space. A fiber bundle transmits light into the joint, and the surgeon, peering through an eyepiece, inspects the interior of the joint (Fig. 8-19). The image can also be displayed simultaneously on a television screen.

The knee, because of its structure, easily lends itself to arthroscopy, although this procedure is now used to examine many joints of the body. Arthroscopy can contribute significantly to the preoperative diagnosis and has almost eliminated unnecessary exploratory surgery. This procedure frequently precedes more major and "open" surgical procedures. In certain conditions, such as loose bodies or a torn cartilage in the knee, the necessary surgery can be performed through or in conjunction with the arthroscope. This greatly reduces an athlete's recovery time and results in improved medical care for athletes.

Pulmonary function tests

A large number of pulmonary function tests are available to measure the functioning of the respiratory system as a whole and the relationships of its various parts. As a group these tests are used to determine the presence of disease or injury, the type of disease or lesion that might be present and the extent of disability, and the

Fig. 8-16. Electrocardiography. **A,** Placement of electrodes, and **B,** the resulting electrocardiogram.

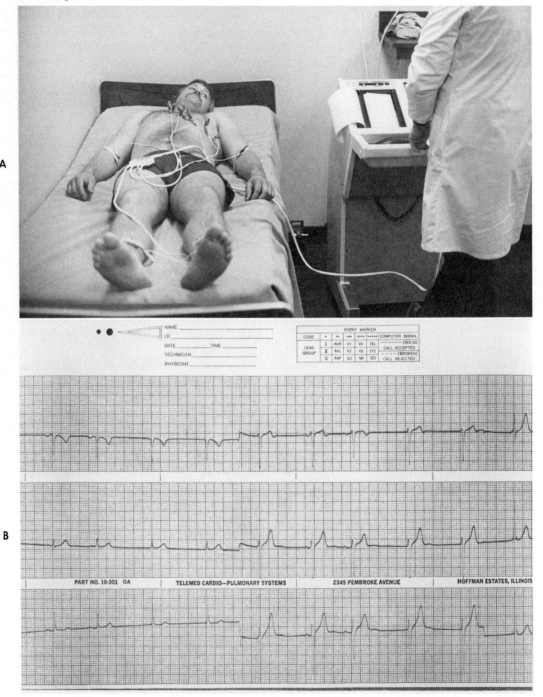

Fig. 8-17. Echocardiography. **A,** placement of electrodes and sound head on athlete's chest, and **B,** portion of the resulting echocardigram.

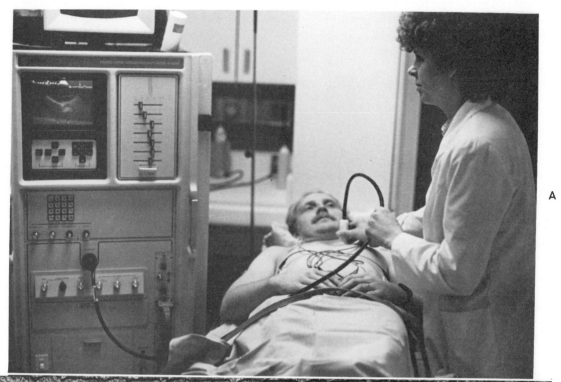

A

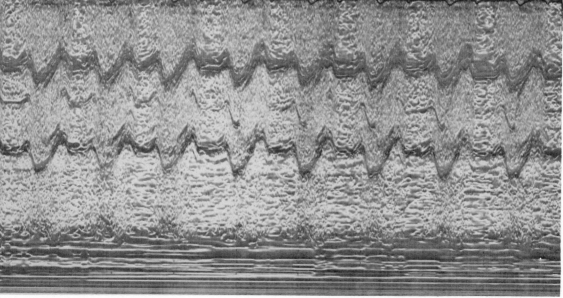

B

Fig. 8-18. Electromyography. **A,** Surface electrodes pick up electrical potentials and display them on an oscilloscope. **B,** Picture of oscilloscope display.

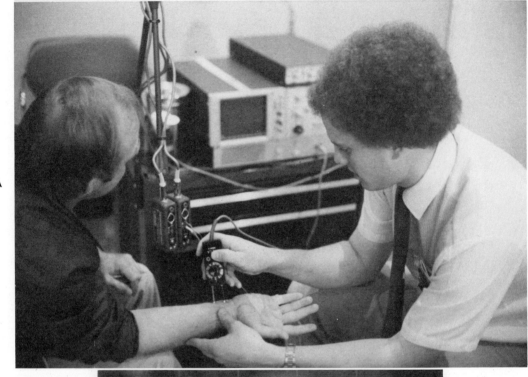

A

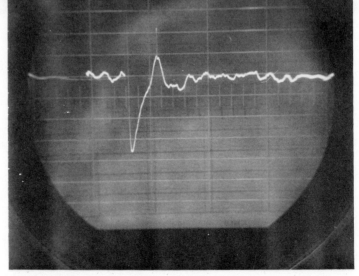

B

Fig. 8-19. Arthroscopy of a knee joint. The arthroscope is inserted into the knee joint and hooked up to a television monitor. Note on the television screen the probe inside the joint cavity.

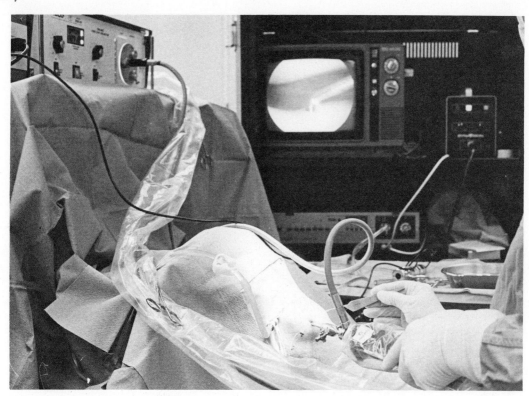

Fig. 8-20. Pulmonary function test. **A,** Athlete performing a forced vital capacity test. **B,** The resulting graph.

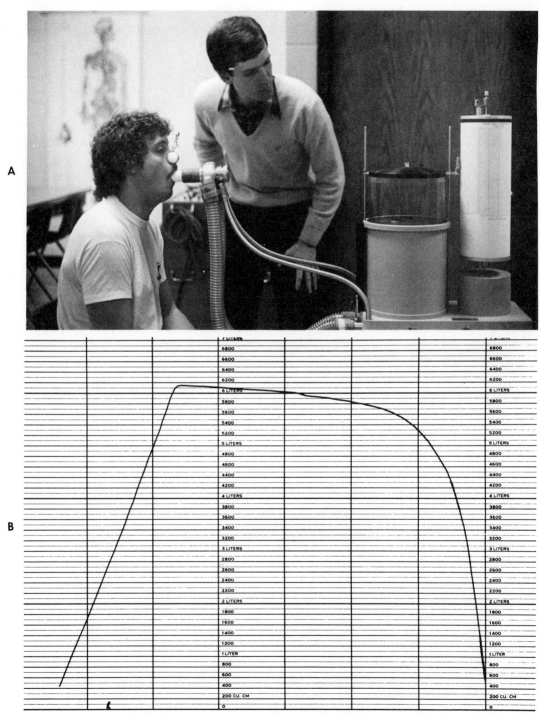

proper course of treatment or therapy. Examples of pulmonary function tests include: (1) determination of lung volumes, such as vital capacity, (2) ventilation measurements, such as tidal volume and respiratory rate, and (3) pulmonary mechanics tests, such as forced expiratory volume and airway resistance (Fig. 8-20).

Summary

The preceding five areas, anatomy, athletic injuries, evaluative techniques, signs and symptoms, and diagnostic procedures, are each important to the total athletic injury assessment process and are interrelated. Neglecting any of these areas can result in decreased effectiveness when evaluating an athletic injury. Accurate evaluations require that you possess knowledge in each of these areas and are able to apply that knowledge to specific injuries.

ASSESSMENT CONSIDERATIONS

There are many considerations related to the total picture of athletic injury assessment. In addition to signs, symptoms, and diagnostic procedures, other factors are important and must be considered by the athletic trainer. The remainder of this chapter discusses important considerations you should be aware of as you prepare to evaluate athletic injuries.

When to assess

The optimal time to begin assessing an athletic injury is as quickly as possible after it has occurred. As time passes, some of the signs and symptoms necessary for an accurate evaluation may be masked by pain, swelling, inflammation, and muscle spasms. If the evaluation is delayed for a period of time until the athlete is referred to medical assistance, an accurate diagnosis may be hindered by conditions that have developed since the onset of injury. In addition, the period of least discomfort for the athlete is usually right after the injury occurs. Hours or days later the injured area may be very painful and swollen, making an accurate evaluation very difficult. Of course, not all injuries are reported when they occur. There will be times when an athlete will

not report an injury for days or even weeks. Such a delay in reporting an injury will make the evaluation more difficult and may require that you wait for the pain and swelling to subside in order to gain an accurate assessment.

Where to assess

Athletic injuries occur almost anywhere and at any time during athletic activity. Whenever possible, the ideal place to evaluate an injured athlete is right where the injury has occurred. If an injury occurs during a scheduled contest or game, the initial assessment may be limited to a cursory evaluation as to the nature and severity of the injury. After this evaluation, if indicated, the injured athlete can then be removed from the contest to a place where clothing and equipment can be removed and a more thorough examination conducted. If any serious injury is suspected, a thorough examination should be conducted on the playing field without moving the injured athlete and using all the time necessary.

Athletic injuries during practices should also be assessed where they occur if at all possible. It is easier to evaluate an injury without a cluster of players or fans around. If spectators are present, ask them to move elsewhere or complete a limited examination to determine the nature and severity of the injury and then move the athlete to an area more suitable for a thorough assessment.

Personal assessment skills

Athletic injury assessment is not an easy task. The ability of one person to accurately interpret what is felt by another can be difficult. Signs and symptoms may be masked and misleading, or there may be some abnormal preexisting conditions present that complicate the evaluation. The athlete may feel excitement, panic, or concern about the injury, and facts may be distorted. Many factors may contribute to making the assessment difficult. However, if you are responsible for the injury evaluation, there are some personal skills you should be aware of and practice to help you make the injury assessment procedures less difficult and more informative.

Know the athletes. Knowing the athletes can

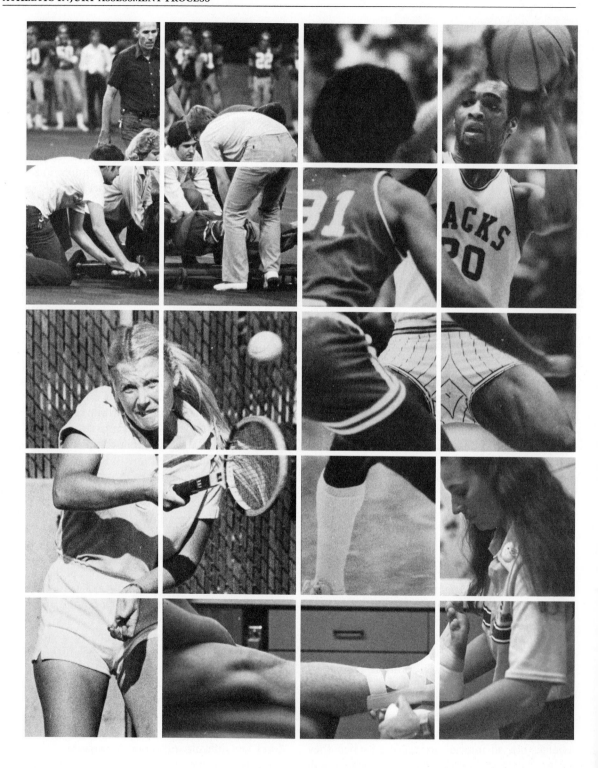

be quite an asset when they become injured. All coaches and athletic trainers should make an attempt to get acquainted with each athlete. The more you know about an athlete, the better prepared you are to assess athletic injuries occurring to that person. This knowledge includes the medical history as well as the current medical status of the athlete. Does the athlete have any current injuries, diseases, allergies or other medical problems? Is the athlete on any medications or under psychologic stress? Does the athlete wear contact lenses or have dental appliances?

It is also important to know something about the athlete's personality. How do they react to emergencies or stressful situations? How do they react to pain? Some athletes complain about every little pain, whereas others never complain of pain even though it can be seen he or she is hurting. It is important to know and understand psychologic and personality traits for effective athletic injury care. You should observe each of the athletes, trying to ascertain more about his or her personality.

Know the sport. Unlike a coach, who may work with only one sport, an athletic trainer works with all athletes in all sports. Therefore athletic trainers must understand the basic fundamentals and physical demands of each sport with which they may be working. This information can be an asset when deciding whether or not an athlete can return to activity after an injury. The physical skills demanded in one sport may prevent an injured athlete from participating, whereas an athlete with a similar injury may be able to safely participate in another sport.

Remain calm. Try to remain calm. Do not get excited. In many situations the first task is to calm the injured athlete. It is difficult to evaluate an injured area when the athlete is excited, scared, or anxious. If the athletic trainer is equally excited, the athlete may become more anxious about the severity of the injury than warranted by the circumstances. Action and words should not reflect panic. Do not hurry the assessment. Make it as thorough as possible under the circumstances.

Be alert. Be alert during athletic activity. Watch more than just the play or performance. Attempt to observe all the athletes. Is anyone not getting up? Is anyone staggering, limping, or acting unusual? Observing an injury as it occurs allows the athletic trainer to have a better idea of the cause of the injury and what to expect when performing evaluation procedures.

Use good judgment. There are many outside influences surrounding athletic injuries, thus making it important to always use good sound judgment and common sense. Athletic trainers frequently work under a certain amount of pressure to quickly return the athlete to activity. The athlete is usually in good physical condition at the time of injury and strongly motivated to return to activity. The athlete expects the evaluation to be carried out quickly and accurately and wants to know exactly what is wrong as well as when a return to action can be expected. Athletic trainers may have additional pressure from the coach, parents, fans, or other athletes. Because of the nature of the sport, athletic trainers may even be under time restraints to hurry the evaluation. Remember, everyone makes mistakes, but it is better to error on the conservative side by being cautious, especially when you are unsure of the nature and severity of the injury. In athletic injury assessment, trainers must make rapid and accurate judgments. Use sound judgment based on knowledge and experience.

Experience. There is no substitute for experience in assessing athletic injuries. Athletic trainers can gain the anatomic background, a knowledge of the specific signs and symptoms associated with various injuries, and the specific assessment techniques through study. However, the confidence developed in assessment skills will only increase through practice. It takes experience to refine assessment skills.

Patience. To become proficient at athletic injury assessment, athletic trainers must develop patience. There is an extremely wide range in the type and severity of athletic injuries. Some injuries may constitute an obvious evaluation and solution. Other injuries will constitute a grey area and will be very difficult to accurately assess. The injury may be masked by pain, swelling, or muscle spasm. The signs and symptoms may be insidious. These types of athletic injuries may require a long, meticulous evaluation to recognize the nature of the injury. A hurried evaluation may result in an inaccurate assessment.

Referral skills

An area often neglected by those assessing athletic injuries is that of referral. Contacting a physician and scheduling the athlete to be examined is not all there is to referring. Information gained at the initial evaluation must also be conveyed to the next link in the injury management chain. As has been previously discussed, by the time the physician evaluates the athlete, pain, swelling, muscle spasms, and inflammation may have developed, making the assessment more difficult. Therefore the information gained on the initial assessment should be recorded and passed along whenever an injured athlete is referred. This information can assist in the overall assessment of the injury.

Do not hesitate to refer an athlete to a physician or other professional person if you feel uncomfortable or have questions about the assessment. It is better to be cautious initially than sorry later that you did not refer the athlete. There will be some athletic injuries that will also require consultation with a specialist. Again, these injuries should be referred at the earliest possible time so the specialist can take advantage of the optimal time for treatment.

Plan of action

The coach or athletic trainer who has the responsibility for the medical care of athletes should have a plan of action worked out ahead of time should an injury occur. Plan emergency procedures as well as routine assessment techniques in advance so that these procedures may be carried out as easily and efficiently as possible. Any moving, lifting, or transporting should be thought out and practiced in advance so that these maneuvers will go smoothly. A well-practiced plan of action can reassure athletes that they are and will be handled in the best possible manner. Maintain a calm environment and initiate the preplanned steps of the emergency network. Plan for the worst and hope for the best. If you have not planned for a severe emergency and it occurs, there is a good chance it will be poorly handled.

Know how to obtain professional assistance. The ambulance, hospital, and physician's phone numbers should be readily accessible, as should a telephone with an outside line. Emergency equipment must be readily available and not locked up some distance away. This emergency equipment must also be operable, and the people handling it should be trained in its use.

Summary

As athletic training students develop procedures for assessing athletic injuries, many factors must be considered. These factors directly influence the effectiveness of the athletic injury assessment process and include knowledge and proficiency in those topics discussed in this chapter. In addition, athletic trainers must continue to refine and improve these assessment skills in an attempt to provide their athletes with optimal medical care.

KEY TERMS

angiography Radiographic study of the vascular system, using a contrast medium injected either intra-arterially (arteriogram) or intravenously (venogram)

arthrography Radiographic study of joints, using a contrast medium to outline the soft tissue structures; the resulting radiograph is called an arthrogram

arthroscopy Surgical procedure that allows the surgeon to actually view the interior of a joint through a series of small lenses with a fiberoptic light source

athletic injury assessment Comprehensive evaluation of an athletic injury beginning when the injury occurs and continuing through the healing process until the injured area has been rehabilitated to its fullest extent

bone scan Nuclear imaging technique used to detect particular areas of abnormal metabolic activity within a bone

computed tomography (CT scan) Sophisticated procedure using computerized radiographic equipment to get a three-dimensional image of the area

discography Radiographic study of the spine, using a contrast medium injected into an intervertebral disc; the resulting radiograph is called a discogram

echocardiography Technique that uses echoes or reflected high-frequency sound waves to visualize the heart

electrocardiography Study of electrical activity of the heart; the graphic recordings are called an electrocardiogram (ECG or EKG)

electromyography Study of electrical potentials generated in muscles; the graphic recordings are called an electromyogram (EMG)

electroencephalography Study of electrical currents developed by the brain; the graphic recordings are called an electroencephalogram (EEG)

myelography Radiographic study of the spinal cord and canal, using a contrast medium injected into the spinal canal; the resulting radiograph is called a myelogram

nuclear imaging Radiographic study using short-term radioactive substances injected into the body and recorded on a scanner

plain film radiography Procedure that uses no contrast material to enhance the various structures of the body; the most common types of radiographic procedures used in sports medicine

sign Objective evidence of an injury, or something the athletic trainer can see, hear, or feel

stress radiograph Radiograph taken while stress is being applied to the joint; normally performed with the athlete under an anesthesia

symptom Subjective evidence of an injury, or something the athlete relates

tomography Radiographic technique using a specialized computer to give a view of one particular area of tissue at any depth; resulting radiograph is called a tomogram

urography Radiographic study of the urinary tract using a contrast medium injected intravenously; resulting radiograph is called an intravenous pyelogram (IVP)

SUGGESTED READINGS

Allman, F.L.: What a trainer ought to be, Athletic Training, **5**:3-7, 1970.

Arger, P.H., and others: Computed tomography in orthopedics, Orthop. Clin. North Am. **14**:217-231, 1983.

Daffner, R.H.: Introduction to clinical radiology, a correlative approach to diagnostic imaging, St. Louis, 1978, The C.V. Mosby Co.

Hair, J.E.: Intangibles in evaluating athletic injuries, J. Am. Coll. Health Assoc. **25**:228-230, 1977.

Lee, B.C.: CT scans of the head: basic interpretation, Hosp. Med. **18**:21-42, 1982.

Radiology in sportsmedicine—a round table, Physician Sportsmedicine, **9**:61-80, May, 1981.

Zarins, B: Arthroscopic surgery in a sports medicine practice, Orthop. Clin. North Am. **13**:415-421, 1982.

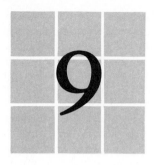

9 Assessment procedures

A comprehensive and accurate evaluation of athletic injuries or related conditions often requires a detailed and systematic assessment process. This chapter presents an approach to athletic injury assessment. It will discuss, in orderly sequence, those assessment procedures that should be performed by an athletic trainer when an athlete is injured. Everyone responsible for the medical care of athletes should develop an organized sequence of assessment procedures to perform a more accurate evaluation of athletic injuries. Mastery of complex assessment techniques requires a substantial personal commitment on the part of the athletic trainer in terms of the time and effort expended. In addition, it is essential that the student in an athletic training program have individualized professional super-vision, guidance, and support. We hope the procedures presented in this chapter will aid in the development of those skills essential to the successful assessment of athletic injuries.

A thorough athletic injury assessment can be broken down into two major parts: (1) the primary survey and (2) the secondary survey. Each survey is important and should be considered with each injury.

PRIMARY SURVEY

The *primary survey* is that portion of the assessment concerned with evaluation of the basic life support mechanisms: Airway, Breathing, and

> **THE PRIMARY SURVEY**
> Airway
> Breathing
> Circulation

Circulation. These are usually referred to as the ABCs of life support. The probability that life-threatening situations will arise as a result of athletic injuries is minimal; however, everyone involved in athletics must be aware that the potential for serious injury does exist. Critical injuries do occur, and death can result from an athletic injury. Life-threatening conditions must be recognized immediately and dealt with effectively to prevent needless loss of life. Persons responsible for the medical care of athletes must be trained to recognize and react appropriately to various life-threatening situations.

With most athletic injuries, the primary survey is completed easily and quickly. The experienced and observant athletic trainer will initiate a part of the primary survey even before reaching the injured player. Although a serious injury may exist that will only be revealed through a thorough examination, the critical life-support mechanisms (ABCs) can be evaluated almost immediately. For example, if an injured athlete is conscious and talking, one can assume that he or she is breathing and has a pulse. This type of basic observation is often completed while approaching the injured player. With this initial observation, the primary survey is begun.

Success in athletic injury assessment depends on the development of observational skills and the ability to remain calm and objective in times of stress and confusion. As you approach an injured athlete, be very observant. Survey the situ-

Fig. 9-1. Implementing athletic training skills. Note position of athlete's left foot and ankle. (Courtesy Rochester Post-Bulletin, Rochester, Minn.)

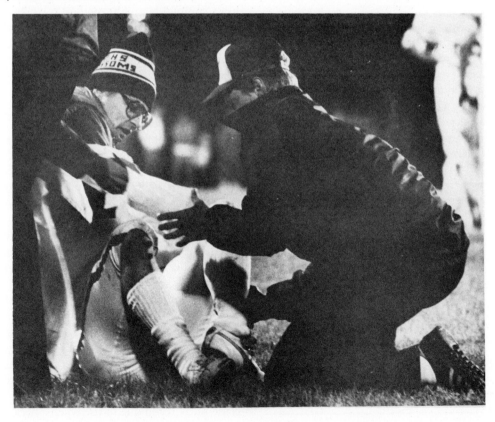

ation quickly and completely. As you conduct the primary survey, you should also note important details such as severe bleeding, level of consciousness, and body position. Completion of the primary survey can be accomplished quickly if you are disciplined in the use of an appropriate mental checklist.

Although athletic injuries are seldom life threatening, it is important to consider and understand the aspects of basic life support. This section presents assessment techniques used to recognize possible life-threatening conditions. The purpose is not to present a discussion of specialized techniques, such as cardiopulmonary resuscitation (CPR), that are used to manage specific emergency situations. It should be emphasized, however, that a thorough understanding of basic life-support procedures is a necessary prerequisite to the study of assessment techniques.

Airway

Anything that blocks the passage of air through the trachea or windpipe into the lungs causes an airway obstruction. The most common cause of airway obstruction is blockage of the windpipe opening by the tongue. This may occur when an athlete is unconscious. In these cases the tongue may fall toward the back of the throat (pharnyx) and block the airway opening

Fig. 9-2. Tongue blocking the airway.

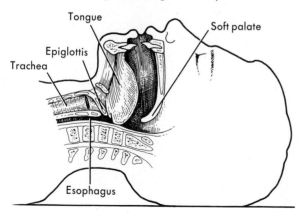

into the trachea (Fig. 9-2). This situation is life threatening and requires immediate action. Because the tongue is attached to the lower jaw, moving the lower jaw forward will usually lift the tongue away from the back of the pharnyx and open the airway. This may be all that is required for breathing to resume spontaneously. There are several methods of opening the airway.

Head tilt is the most important step in opening the airway. Tilting the head backward as far as possible will cause the lower jaw to move forward if there is sufficient tone in the muscles of the jaw. With the athlete on his or her back, place the hand closest to the athlete's head on the forehead and apply firm backward pressure (Fig. 9-3). This will tip the athlete's head backward. The head tilt may be augmented by either the neck lift or chin lift maneuvers (Fig. 9-4).

Head tilt–neck lift. Head tilt–neck lift is the most commonly taught method for opening an airway. In addition to performing the head tilt maneuver, place your other hand under the neck to lift and support it upward (Fig. 9-4, *A*). The hand lifting the neck should be placed close to the back of the head to minimize movement of the cervical spine.

Head tilt–chin lift. Another method of assisting the head tilt maneuver for opening an airway is the chin lift. To augment the head tilt, place the tips of your fingers under the lower jaw on the bony rim and lift the chin forward (Fig. 9-4, *B*). You must be careful when compressing the soft tissues under the chin, because this could obstruct the airway. The chin should be lifted so that the teeth are almost brought together.

Jaw thrust without head tilt. When a neck injury is suspected, movement of the cervical spine must be avoided. The jaw thrust method should then be used to open the airway. This can be accomplished by grasping the angles of the athlete's lower jaw and lifting with both hands to move the jaw forward (Fig. 9-5). Your elbows should be on either side of the head and resting on the surface on which the athlete is lying. This is the safest technique to use when a neck injury

Fig. 9-3. Opening the airway using the head tilt.

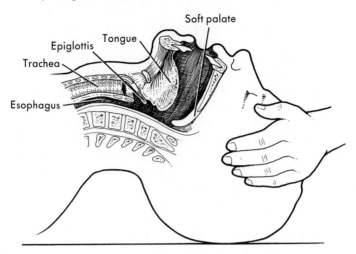

Fig. 9-4. Opening the airway and assessing breathlessness using **A,** head tilt-neck lift and **B,** head tilt-chin lift procedures.

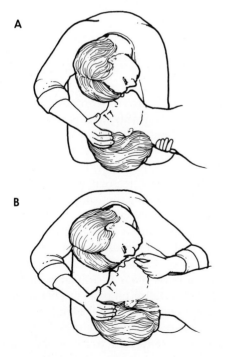

Fig. 9-5. Jaw thrust procedure without head tilt. This is the safest technique to use to open an airway when a neck injury is suspected.

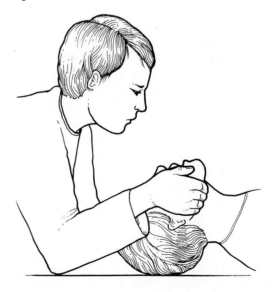

is suspected because it can be accomplished in most cases without movement of the neck.

The airway can also become obstructed by various foreign objects, such as dental appliances, chewing tobacco, chewing gum, or a mouth guard. Athletes should be advised not to compete with substances other than a mouthpiece in their mouth. Take the time to explain the mechanism of airway obstruction. If an athlete understands how foreign objects in the mouth can easily block the trachea, such advice will more likely be followed. Any foreign object in the mouth should be removed immediately when assessing airway and breathing. If an object becomes lodged and occludes the airway, an effective method for removing it is the Heimlich maneuver. Although serious complications following use of the Heimlich maneuver are rare, the procedure does involve some risk. Proper instruction in executing this emergency care procedure is essential.

Breathing

The term *apnea* refers to any temporary cessation of breathing. An athlete may stop breathing or be in respiratory arrest for a variety of reasons, the most common being an obstructed airway. The airway may be obstructed by the tongue or foreign object, as previously discussed, swelling in the throat caused by allergic reactions, or tissue damage caused by a severe blow to the neck. Respiratory arrest may also result from cardiac arrest, poisons, drugs, drowning, and intrathoracic injuries. Regardless of cause, it is extremely important that the person in charge recognize the condition immediately and initiate appropriate emergency care procedures. Assessment of breathing and adequacy of airway are closely coupled. The first priority in assessment and care of injuries involving an athlete's breathing is to establish an open airway. Remember, when the airway is opened, an athlete suffering from apnea may begin to breathe spontaneously. If it does not appear that the athlete is breathing, put your ear close to the athlete's mouth and nose as shown in Fig. 9-4. Listen for an exchange of air. Feel for any breath

against your cheek or ear and watch the chest for any breathing movements. If the athlete is not breathing after opening the airway, appropriate techniques of artificial ventilation must be initiated immediately.

A more common respiratory problem observed in athletes is difficult or labored breathing, called *dyspnea*. This can be a terrifying and serious condition for the athlete. In the absence of chest or lung injuries, dyspnea is often the result of *hyperventilation* by the athlete. This is described as over-breathing to the extent that the carbon dioxide level in the blood is abnormally lowered. Hyperventilation can be a psychologic response to pain and trauma caused by an athlete breathing very rapidly and deeply. The athlete may be terrified that he or she cannot get enough air into the lungs. Athletes suffering from dyspnea may experience dizziness, faint feelings, chest pains, and sensations of numbness or tingling of the hands and feet. You should treat the athlete in a calm and reassuring manner. Talk to the athlete and encourage slow, relaxed breathing. A procedure used to build up the blood carbon dioxide level is to ask the athlete to breathe into a paper bag. In this way the athlete will rebreathe exhaled air and raise the carbon dioxide level in the blood to a normal or near-normal level. It is important to explain this technique to the athlete to gain his or her confidence. Once the athlete is calmed down and breathing more normally, it is possible to continue the assessment of any associated injuries.

Circulation

There are several reasons why an athlete's heart may stop beating, but should it occur, the exact cause is immaterial to the athletic trainer. Of utmost importance is the recognition of cardiac arrest and the immediate initiation of emergency measures. Circulation is assessed by palpating for a pulse. *Pulse* is defined as the alternate expansion and recoil of an artery caused by the intermittent ejection of blood from the heart. The carotid artery in the neck (Fig. 9-6) is the most commonly used artery to check for a pulse during an emergency situation. This is the main artery in the neck, and lies superficially in a groove between the sternocleidomastoid muscle and the trachea, or windpipe. The carotid artery is normally not obstructed by clothing or equipment and is easily accessible. Position yourself on one side of the athlete, place your index and middle fingers on the windpipe, and slide them toward you as shown in Fig. 9-7. Press gently into the soft part of the neck next to the wind-pipe. The carotid pulse can be felt in the groove formed by the sternocleidomastoid muscle and the trachea. Always feel for the carotid pulse on the side of the neck closest to you.

If the athlete does not exhibit a pulse, appropriate emergency techniques of artificial circulation must be initiated immediately. Every athletic trainer must have a working knowledge of current cardiopulmonary resuscitation tech-

Fig. 9-6. Anatomic illustration of neck showing the carotid artery.

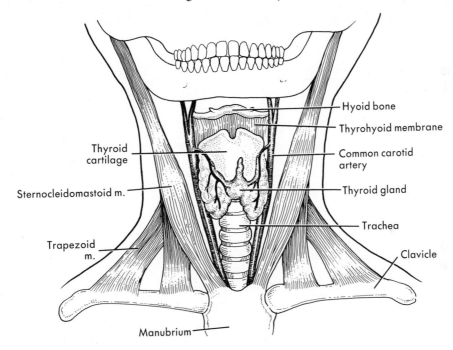

Fig. 9-7. Assessing pulselessness by **A,** placing your index and middle finger on the windpipe and **B,** sliding them downward into the groove formed by the sternocleidomastoid muscle and the trachea.

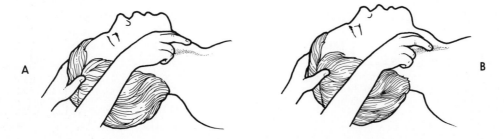

niques. This knowledge can be gained only through supervised training and practice and should be reviewed at least annually.

Fig. 9-8 is a flow chart illustrating the basic steps of the primary survey in sequential order. Once the primary survey concerning the ABCs of life support has been completed and all life-threatening conditions have been brought under control, the secondary survey begins.

SECONDARY SURVEY

The *secondary survey* is that portion of the assessment that examines the athlete in an attempt to recognize and evaluate all injuries. In sports medicine, it is the secondary survey that usually comprises the largest portion of the total athletic injury assessment procedure. It consists of an ordered sequence of procedures used to assess the nature, site, and severity of an athletic injury. When injury occurs, early, accurate assessment is essential in developing an effective treatment and rehabilitation program. In addition, the assessment can provide the athletic trainer with useful information for the development of programs to prevent similar injuries.

The importance of using a detailed and properly sequenced checklist in the assessment procedure cannot be overemphasized. By following

Fig. 9-8. Basic steps of the primary survey.

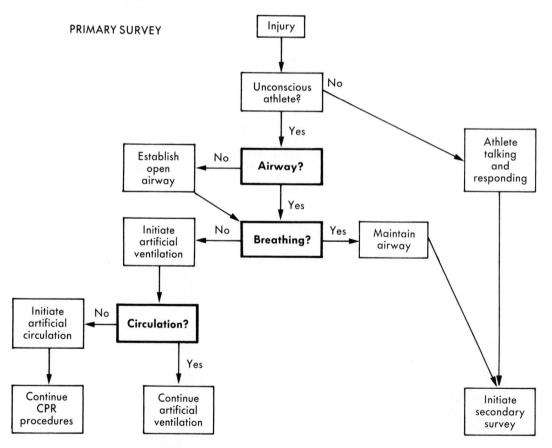

a consistent pattern in your evaluation procedures, you are less likely to forget a procedure or miss an important detail. Pilots, for example, learn early in their flight training about the importance of using checklists. Sample checklists are provided for each body area discussed throughout the remainder of the text.

The secondary survey can be divided into four basic steps. These can be easily remembered by the acronym HOPS, which stands for *History*, *Observation*, *Palpation*, and *Stress*. Each step is important and should be carried out thoroughly and efficiently to accurately assess an athletic injury. Of course, not all the procedures discussed under each step of the secondary survey will be carried out with each athletic injury. The nature, type, and severity of the injury will determine the evaluative techniques used. Every athletic trainer will at some time be faced with an athletic injury requiring very few assessment skills; for example, a fractured arm with the bone protruding through the skin. With this type of an injury, immediate first aid and referral skills are the primary concern of the athletic trainer. Except in these types of obvious injuries, the athletic trainer should always initiate and conduct some type of a sequential assessment process. Short cuts in evaluating athletic injuries should be avoided, as they increase the risk of overlooking or missing important information. Athletic trainers must continue to improve and refine their assessment skills.

> **THE SECONDARY SURVEY**
> *History*
> *Observation*
> *Palpation*
> *Stress*

History

Obtaining an accurate history of an injury is one of the most important steps in the secondary survey portion of the total athletic injury assessment process (Fig. 9-9). Taking a history in-

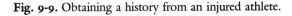

Fig. 9-9. Obtaining a history from an injured athlete.

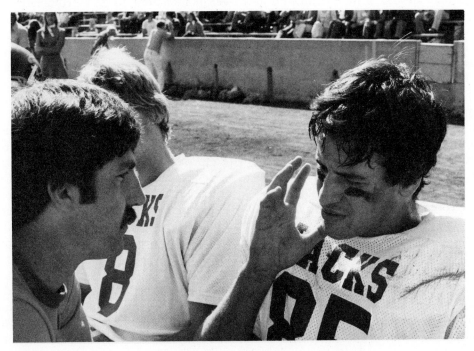

volves finding out as much information as possible about the actual injury and the circumstances surrounding its occurrence. This is accomplished by talking with the injured athlete or others who have either witnessed or observed the injury. Information gained in a thorough history can provide important clues in determining which structures may be injured and which assessment techniques will be appropriate as you continue the examination.

Athletic injuries can happen almost anywhere and anytime during activity. They basically appear in two ways; (1) suddenly, such as those caused by trauma, and (2) gradually, such as the overuse syndromes that develop over a period of time. The direction taken when obtaining the history depends on the nature of the injury and how it occurred.

Injuries that appear suddenly. The history of a sudden traumatic injury is usually easy to obtain. This type of an athletic injury is frequently witnessed by persons who can provide useful information to help in completing the history. In many cases the athletic trainer will witness the injury and have an idea of the mechanisms involved before formal questioning begins. Sometimes, however, the athletic trainer does not witness the injury and must question the athlete and others who were present in an attempt to establish the facts. In some cases an athlete may not report the injury at the time it occurs or when the symptoms initially appear. Then, in addition to the history of the injury, you must find out what, if anything, has occurred since the injury happened. Specific questions required to elicit necessary information will vary, depending on the nature of the injury in question. Piecing together the complete history requires time, skill, patience, and thoroughness.

Injuries that appear gradually. Accurate assessment of athletic injuries that develop over a period of time, such as chronic injuries and overuse syndromes, requires a very detailed history. If the athlete understands the importance of the history in assessing the extent of injury, he or she will be more likely to be patient and cooperative in answering questions. Sometimes the onset of the symptoms may be insidious, and the athlete will have few recollections of any injury or stress. The symptoms usually begin as a mild and sporadic ache and gradually become more painful and continuous. You must attempt to gain as much information as possible related to the injury. Did the symptoms appear suddenly or did they come on gradually? What has the athlete been able to do since the symptoms first appeared? Inquire about functional capabilities such as the ability to walk, climb stairs, twist, throw, or whatever activity is involved with the body area injured. What aggravates the injured area? Is it relieved by rest? Injuries that appear gradually may be caused by any of a number of factors, such as errors in training, inappropriate or improperly fitted equipment, playing surfaces, structural abnormalities, poor flexibility, or poor conditioning. The history must take into consideration all of these factors. A meticulous history is required when attempting to assess injuries of this type.

There are several important factors to remember in attempting to gain a comprehensive history (Fig. 9-10). Each of these factors has to do with the development and use of communication skills.

To gain an accurate history of the injury, you must communicate with the injured athlete if at all possible. The athlete is the only person who has experienced the injury and knows exactly how it feels. Of course, there will be times when it will be impossible to talk to the injured athlete; for example, if he or she is unconscious or unresponsive for any reason. When this occurs, you must question other athletes or persons who might have witnessed the injury. Attempt to gain as much information as possible from whomever observed the injury or has knowledge of important factors associated with its occurrence.

There are other factors to keep in mind as you attempt to talk with an injured athlete. Immediately after an injury, the athlete may not feel like talking. He or she may be in pain and frightened or panicky. Perhaps the last thing the athlete wants to do at that time is carry on a conversation about the injury. You should appreciate that every athlete responds differently to an injury. Some explain their injury in great detail, whereas others volunteer little if any information. Some athletes try to minimize their injury, whereas others try to maximize it. In addition, some persons become very emotional when in pain or under stress. These circumstances often complicate the assessment process and underscore the need to communicate with an injured athlete in a calm and reassuring manner. Make every attempt to relax the athlete so that he or she will be able to discuss the injury and respond to questions.

When speaking with the athlete, keep the questions simple. Most athletes are not interested in carrying on lengthy conversations after sustaining an injury. Ask only one question at a time, and get the answer before proceeding on to the next. Attempt to follow an orderly format in taking an athlete's history, but allow for modifications on the basis of his or her responses. A format often used by nurses in eliciting information during a history is to divide the information into five groups remembered by the acronym PQRST: (1) *Provocative-palliative*, (2) *Quality*, (3) *Region-radiation*, (4) *Scale of severity*, and (5) *Timing*.

In asking provocative or palliative questions, an attempt is made to determine: What caused it? What makes it better? Or worse? Quality questions include, How does it feel, sound, and look? Region-radiation questions determine where the injury is located and if the resulting pain or abnormal sensations are localized or radiating. Asking "How does it feel on a scale of 1 to 10?" can often reveal a great deal about how the athlete views the severity of his or her injury.

Fig. 9-10. Factors related to obtaining an accurate and thorough history of an athletic injury.

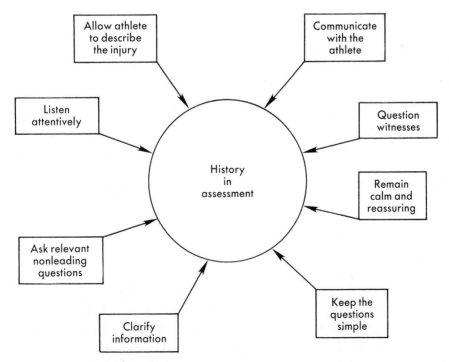

Timing questions are questions such as: When did it begin? How often does it occur? Was the onset sudden or gradual?

So called standard or canned questions are seldom useful. Each injury and each injured athlete is unique. The athletic trainer must develop interview or questioning skills that can be applied in a wide variety of situations. Clarify the information being gathered and ask questions that will elicit further essential information. Ask relevant, nonleading questions of an injured athlete. Examples of leading questions are "Did you turn your ankle under?" and "Does it hurt right here?" It is much easier for an athlete in pain to answer "yes" to such questions than to describe the injury in detail. If you lead the athlete with your questions, you may actually develop a false impression of the injury. Let the athlete describe the injury and tell you what happened.

As the athlete explains how the injury occurred, it is important to listen attentively to what he or she is saying. Many clues as to the structures injured, as well as severity of injury, can be gained by listening to the athlete's description of the injury. It is easy to make assumptions about an injury, especially if the injury was witnessed. If the athlete says he or she heard and felt a popping or cracking sensation and believes something is broken, it must be assumed correct until proved otherwise. Give the athlete the benefit of the doubt, even if it appears that he or she is overreacting to the injury. Do not start the assessment with your mind made up about the injury. Each new injury must be evaluated separately. Begin with a complete history, and allow the athlete to describe the injury and spell out in detail exactly what happened. The importance of being a good

Fig. 9-11. Information gained by taking the history of an athletic injury.

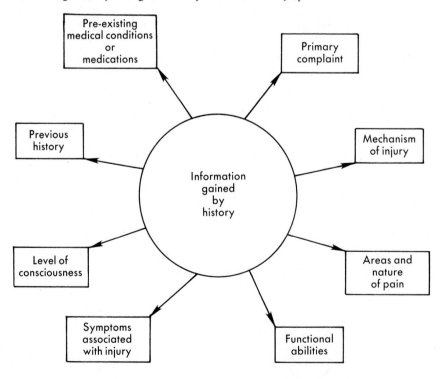

listener cannot be overemphasized. Obtaining a good history requires a high degree of proficiency in listening skills.

The importance of the history-taking process cannot be overemphasized; a vast amount of information can be gained by conducting an accurate and thorough history of all athletic injuries and related conditions (Fig. 9-11). The history is of special significance because the physical findings associated with athletic injuries are often minimal.

In communicating with an injured athlete, determine the primary complaint early in the assessment process. Where does it hurt? What type of injury has the athlete suffered? Attempt to find out the exact *mechanism of injury*. How and when did the injury occur? Did the athlete fall or was there a twist? Did the athlete receive a blow, and if so, from what direction? Did the athlete hear or feel anything? Attempt to recreate in your mind the mechanism of injury and visualize the position of the body when the injury occurred. It is important to have a clear conception of the mechanism of injury.

Attempt to locate the areas of pain. It is helpful if the athlete can point to where the pain is. Notice how he or she points to the painful area. Is the pain localized or is it spread over a large body area? Be as exact as possible in determining anatomic location. Is the pain around a joint, along a bone, or in a muscular area?

Inquire about the functional abilities of the injured athlete. Athletes may be able to perform with minimal amounts of pain or only occasional pain. Is there pain only during function or movement? Is the pain intensified by movement or activity? Is the pain constant or intermittent? Seek specific information concerning the nature of pain associated with athletic injuries.

In addition to the pain, ask the athlete to describe any other symptoms associated with the injury in as much detail as possible. Is the athlete experiencing any numbness, tingling, weakness, or burning sensations? Is reference made to any type of grinding or grating sensations (crepitation). Did the athlete experience any abnormal sounds or sensations at the time of the injury? Does the athlete feel any tightness, tension, or swelling associated with the injury?

Talking with an athlete will also assist in assessing his or her level of consciousness. For example, is the athlete alert and responsive or confused and disoriented? It is important to evaluate the athlete's level of consciousness and establish a neurologic baseline early in the assessment process, especially when the injury involves the head. The importance of level(s) of consciousness will be discussed in greater detail in Chapter 11.

Knowledge of past injuries or problems can greatly help in assessing the nature of current injuries. Inquire about any previous injuries to the affected part or surrounding body area. If there was a previous injury, probe for additional details. What type of injury? How long was the recovery period? Was the recovery complete? What kind of treatment and rehabilitation programs were followed? All this information can be helpful in assessing current injuries. Also attempt to find out about any other pre-existing medical conditions that may have a relationship to the injury, or any medications the athlete may be taking.

The more relevant information that can be gained from a history, the more accurately the injury can be evaluated. Do not overlook the importance of obtaining the history even though you witnessed the injury and believe you know exactly what is injured and how it occurred.

Observation

The next step of the secondary survey, observation, begins when you first see the injured athlete and continues until the assessment process is completed (Fig. 9-12). Much information can be gained through observation skills. Several important points should be remembered in observing an injured athlete (Fig. 9-13). Begin by quickly surveying the entire scene. Notice the position of the athlete. Did you observe the mechanism of injury? Was there any apparatus or equipment associated with the injury? Look

Fig. 9-12. Observing and inspecting an injured area.

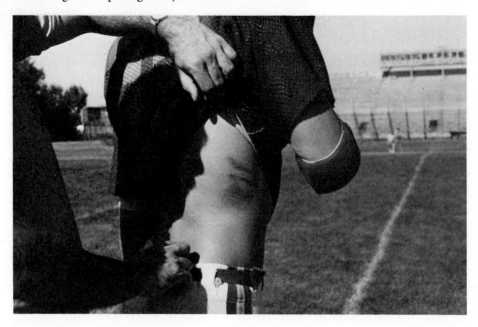

Fig. 9-13. Factors related to observing an injured athlete.

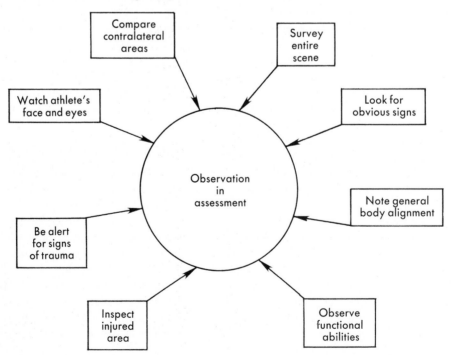

for any obvious bleeding, deformity, swelling, discoloration, or any other signs of injury. Note general body alignment and posture of the athlete. Is the athlete holding a body part or grasping some body area? If the athlete is moving around, observe his or her functional abilities. Is the athlete using the injured part or protecting it? Is he or she limping?

After a general survey of the injury scene, carefully inspect the injured area and assess the results of the athletic injury. This is often accomplished in conjunction with the history-taking process. Watch closely as the athlete describes the injury. What is the position of the injured part? Be alert for any signs of trauma, such as abrasions or contusions, that may indicate the mechanism of injury. Some athletes try to disguise or minimize the extent of their injury. Observing the athlete's face and eyes as he or she describes the injury may give further clues

as to the extent of pain. More pain may be reflected in the athlete's face than he or she is willing to admit.

When inspecting an injury, clothing and equipment that may obscure the area should be removed. Consider the athletes modesty in removing clothing and equipment. If possible, adequate exposure should permit visualization of the area above and below the injury. Do not limit your examination solely to the area of injury. You should always compare the injured body part to the contralateral uninjured part and note any obvious differences. However, you must be aware of any abnormalities in the uninjured body part caused by such things as congenital conditions or previous injuries. If the athletic trainer has been involved with a preseason screening program of the uninjured athlete, this information will be readily available. Attempt to gain as much information as possible by observation (Fig. 9-14).

Fig. 9-14. Information that can be gained during observation of an injured athlete.

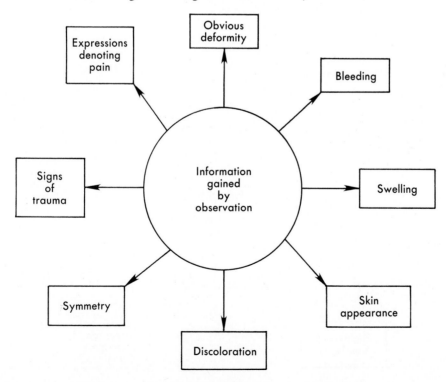

Fig. 9-15. Palpating an injured area.

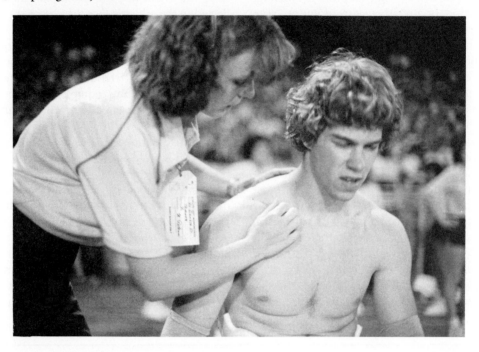

Fig. 9-16. Factors associated with palpating an injured area.

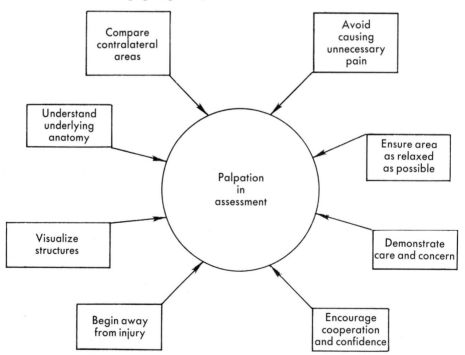

Palpation

Palpation means to touch and feel the injured area. After the history and observation steps, you can gain additional physical information concerning the injury by carefully palpating the affected body area (Fig. 9-15). There are several important points to remember as you prepare to palpate an injured athlete (Fig. 9-16). Palpation procedures should begin in a tender manner to avoid unnecessary pain. If you cause the athlete unnecessary pain, he or she may become tense and uncooperative, making palpation assessment of the injury more difficult, if not impossible. To accurately palpate an injured area it should be as relaxed as possible. Treating the athlete gently helps demonstrate your concern and helps establish confidence and cooperation. The intensity or pressure used with each palpation maneuver can then be increased, depending upon the athlete's tolerance and the severity of the injury. It is also a good practice to begin palpating away from the injury site to encourage the athlete's cooperation and confidence. In addition, by doing this you are not as likely to become so involved with the obvious injury that you overlook another, less apparent injury.

It is important that you visualize what structures are under your fingers. Are you feeling approximately where ligaments should be? Are you feeling an isolated tendon or a musculotendinous junction? Are you palpating predominately muscular tissue or bone? To visualize the structures that are being palpated, you must have an understanding of the underlying anatomy. It may be helpful to look at anatomic charts or drawings to verify underlying anatomy and show them to the injured athlete to help him or her understand the injury. Remember to also compare contralateral areas.

Important information can be gained by care-

Fig. 9-17. Information that can be gained during palpation of an injured athlete.

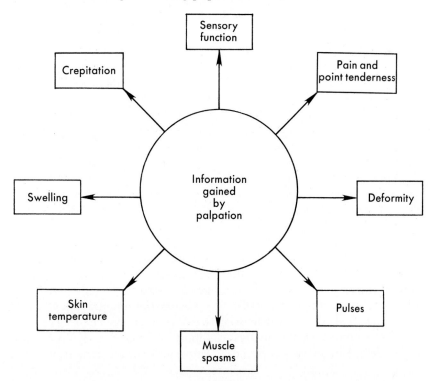

ful palpation procedures (Fig. 9-17). Pain is one of the most obvious and consistent symptoms of injury. Use of palpation techniques to localize pain is extremely useful in assessing athletic injuries. It is especially important to locate areas that are most painful to touch. These are called areas of point tenderness. Regardless of the anatomic structures involved, point tenderness is usually found at the site of injury. This location of *point tenderness,* along with knowledge of underlying anatomic structures, can provide important clues in evaluating the site and nature of an injury. It may be necessary to observe the athlete's face for wincing or grimacing if he or she cannot provide reliable verbal responses.

Another physical sign that can be recognized by palpation is swelling. Swelling or edema may be localized at the injury site or diffused over a larger area. Swelling may result from bleeding caused by trauma or by accumulation of pus or tissue fluid as a result of some inflammatory process (described in Chapter 6). As a rule of thumb, the amount of swelling is generally related to the severity of injury. There are cases, however, in which serious injuries produce very limited swelling, and minor injuries cause severe and extensive swelling or edema. In areas of extensive swelling, the skin becomes stretched and feels tight and smooth.

Additional information gained during palpation may be related to the temperature and surface moisture of the skin. Normal skin is moderately warm and dry. In palpating the site of an injury, any indication of an increase in skin temperature would suggest the occurrence of an inflammatory process. A decrease in skin temperature may be felt in areas of inadequate circulation. In addition, various combinations of skin color, temperature, texture, and moisture can assist in identification of generalized conditions such as shock and problems associated with body temperature regulation.

Muscle spasm may also be recognized while palpating an injured area. This is a body defense mechanism designed to protect an injured area from further trauma. When an injury occurs, the surrounding muscles often involuntarily contract or become tight as the body attempts to splint or brace the injured area. The area surrounding an injury may then feel tense or tight as you palpate the area. Remember to instruct the athlete to relax the injured area as much as possible before beginning palpation procedures.

Deformity is another physical sign that may be discovered during palpation. The cause may be a fracture, dislocation, or the tearing of soft tissue such as ligament, muscle or tendon. Deformity may be quite obvious and easily seen on observation, or it may be very discreet and only recognized after careful palpation of the injured area. If there is any question regarding what the normal contour of the area should be, the corresponding uninjured side should be palpated as a basis for comparison.

Circulation in an extremity can also be evaluated by palpation. After a severe fracture or dislocation it is especially important to palpate for a pulse distal to the injury to determine if the extremity has sufficient circulation. If no pulses are found distal to a severe injury, a medical emergency exists, and appropriate care and referral measures must be initiated immediately.

Additional assessment of the neurologic status, that is, sensory function, can also be evaluated by palpation procedures. This is accomplished by applying stimuli to test the dermatomes of major peripheral nerves. The stimulus can be lightly touching, pinching, or pricking the area with a sharp object. Note any increase or decrease in sensations. This is especially important in assessing head and spinal injuries but should also be used after significant injuries involving the extremities. Check sensations distal to the injury to determine neurologic involvement. If necessary, check the same area on the uninjured side to compare sensations. If distal sensations are normal, it may be assumed the nerve is intact.

Crepitation is a grating, grinding, or sticking sensation that may be produced by various conditions. When crepitation is associated with athletic injuries, it is commonly caused by the broken ends of a bone rubbing together or the thickening of synovial or bursal fluid and membranes. An athlete may describe a grinding sensation on movement of an injured part, and you may feel crepitus as you palpate the injured area.

Up to this point in the assessment process, the injured athlete does not have to move or be moved. If necessary, history, observation, and palpation can be completed with the athlete remaining in the original position he or she is in immediately after injury. The next step of the assessment does involve some movement of the athlete. However, should a serious injury be suspected, it is not necessary to continue on to the next assessment step. Instead, appropriate emergency measures should be initiated.

Stress

The final step of the secondary survey involves selective use of stress tests, or manipulation of the injured body area (Fig. 9-18). Stress tests are employed in an attempt to further locate and define the structures involved in the injury as well as to evaluate the integrity of affected tissues. Information gained in this way is extremely valuable and usually cannot be obtained in any

Fig. 9-18. Applying stress procedures to an injured area. **A,** Active range of motion. **B,** Manual resistance applied against an injured body part. **C,** Passive stress applied to a joint. **D,** Functional activities performed by an athlete.

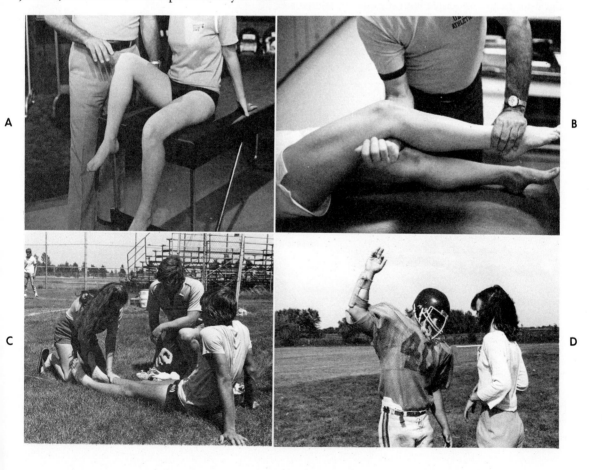

other manner. Invaluable information can be obtained about an athletic injury through the history, observation, and palpation steps of the secondary survey. It is important to realize, however, that a complete and detailed evaluation is not possible unless the injury is subjected to some stress. Unfortunately, this important step in athletic injury assessment is often neglected or even omitted completely. There are several important factors to remember as you prepare to stress an injured area (Fig. 9-19).

Stress procedures should not be applied to an injured area until the history, observation, and palpation steps have been completed. You must have an idea as to the nature of the injury before you attempt to move the affected body part. For example, you would not attempt to stress an injured area when you suspect a dislocation or fracture. In addition to the information gained, completion of the first three steps in the secondary survey serves another useful purpose. It provides the time necessary to calm and relax the athlete before manipulation and stress testing begins.

It is essential that you explain what you are going to do and elicit the athlete's cooperation before stress testing begins. It is extremely difficult to use stress tests effectively in assessment procedures if the injured athlete is tense and unable to relax. A mutual sense of trust between the athlete and the athletic trainer is essential to gain accurate information from the assessment.

Fig. 9-19. Factors associated with stressing an injured area.

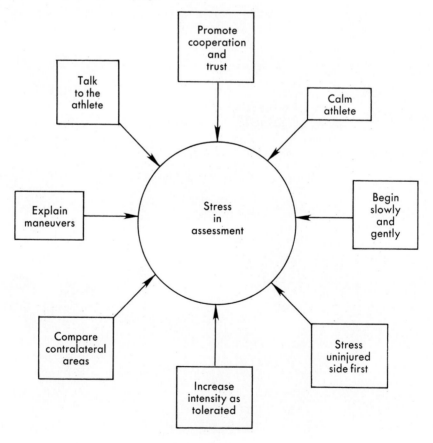

In addition to development of trust, the ability to communicate effectively is especially important during this step of the evaluation process.

Applying stress to an injured area will undoubtedly cause some additional pain. However, these procedures should not cause unnecessary pain, or you will most likely lose the cooperation of the injured player. Any stress applied to the athlete should begin slowly and gently to minimize pain and protective muscle spasms. In a painful injury, it is a good practice to begin stress maneuvers on the uninjured side. This will help lessen apprehensions and prepare the player for procedures that will be carried out on the injured side. This can also give you information necessary to compare the injured to the uninjured side.

Although there are many procedures for applying stress to an injured area, they can be divided into four basic types of maneuvers, called (1) active, (2) resistive, (3) passive, and (4) functional movements. Seldom is it necessary to subject an injury to tests from all four groups. Information gained during the first three steps in the assessment process will enable you to select the most appropriate procedure. Information that can be gained by careful stress procedures is outlined in Fig. 9-20.

Active movements

Active movements are those that can be initiated and completed by the athlete without assistance of any kind. Such movements are usually the least stressful. To initiate this type of maneuver the athlete is asked to move the injured part as directed by the athletic trainer. Active motion is used to evaluate the ability to move and the integrity of contractile and related tissues such as

Fig. 9-20. Information that can be gained by using stress procedures on an injured athlete.

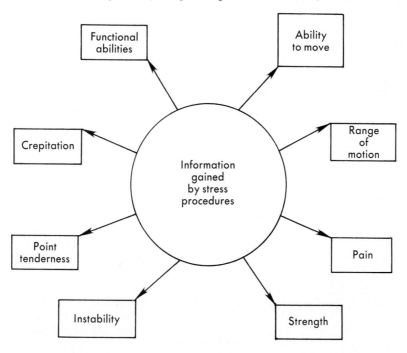

muscles and tendons and their junctions, attachments, integration, and control by the nervous system.

Another important factor that can be evaluated with active motion is the range of motion (ROM) of surrounding joints. For example, an athlete may be asked to actively move an injured extremity through the pain-free ROM. Active motion will indicate the athlete's ability and willingness to perform the movements requested as well as the range of motion possible. Pain will normally limit active motion so that additional injury to damaged structures does not occur as a result of the assessment process. Note the limits of active motion and if necessary compare it to the ROM of the uninjured side.

Resistive movements

Resistance may be applied against active motion to further evaluate the integrity of the contractile tissues. Whenever a muscle or tendon injury is suspected or indicated, resistive movements can assist in identifying specific tender areas. Usually resistance is applied manually by the athletic trainer. Manual resistance can be applied throughout the range of motion or iso-

metrically in various positions in the range. Low initial resistance against movement is gradually increased, depending on the athlete's tolerance. The ability of the athlete to tolerate increasing resistance loads can reveal a great deal about the extent of injury involving the contractile tissues. Note the site of pain at any specific point throughout the resisted range of motion.

Resistive movements are also used to evaluate the strength of a body part. During the acute stages of an athletic injury, pain will normally limit an accurate evaluation of muscular strength. However, on repeated assessments used to determine when an injured athlete is ready to return to activity, manual muscle tests can be very beneficial in evaluating muscular strength. In recent years numerous mechanical and electronic devices have been developed to test muscular strength. Depending upon their availability and applicability, these devices can provide valuable information concerning muscle function. However, manual muscle testing remains a readily available and inexpensive tool for the athletic trainer.

Manual muscle testing is normally performed throughout a full range of motion for each mus-

Table 9-1. Grading for manual muscle testing

Numeric grade	Percentage of normal	Muscular contraction	Functional level
5	100%	Normal	Complete range of motion against gravity, with *full* manual resistance appropriate for age and sex
4	75%	Good	Complete range of motion against gravity, with *some* manual resistance appropriate for age and sex
3	50%	Fair	Complete range of motion against gravity and *no* manual resistance
2	25%	Poor	Complete range of motion with gravity eliminated
1	10%	Trace	Evidence of slight contractility; no joint motion produced
0	0%	Zero	No evidence of muscular contraction by either palpated or visible means

cle or group of muscles. The athlete is positioned in such a way that isolates the muscle or group of muscles being tested and allows movement through the full range of motion. Substitution by muscles other than those being tested can usually be eliminated by careful positioning. Manual resistance is then applied throughout the movement by the athlete or the athlete offers resistance to the movement performed by the athletic trainer. Those same resistive movements are usually performed by the contralateral or uninjured side for a comparison of strength. It is often necessary to carefully repeat manual muscle tests, comparing the strength to the normal side, because weaknesses can be subtle. Note weaknesses and differences in strength.

Manual muscle testing is graded subjectively; that is, according to the athletic trainer's judgment of the athlete's responses. Various grading criteria and classifications have been used to record manual muscular strength. Table 9-1 indicates traditional systems frequently used. Other evaluators prefer descriptive words, such as severe weakness, moderate weakness, minimal weakness, and normal. Whatever grading system is used, manual muscle tests should always be performed consistently, and movements should be coordinated and painless.

Passive movements

Passive movements are procedures performed completely by the athletic trainer and are the most difficult stress procedures to perform and evaluate. The athlete is asked to relax the injured area so that the effects of conscious control and muscular effort can be eliminated. Great care must be exercised in performing passive movements, as the potential to cause additional pain or injury is much greater than during active and resistive movements. Initially, these stress procedures must be performed very gently and slowly to avoid causing unnecessary pain and muscle spasms. The intensity of the procedures can then be increased, depending on the athlete's tolerance and the severity of injury.

Passive movements are used to evaluate the integrity of noncontractile tissues such as bones, joint capsules, ligaments, and bursae. There are numerous passive tests designed to analyze and locate any instability, pain, or crepitation present as the result of an injury. For example, each ligament about an injured joint should be stressed to check for pain and instability. The extent of instability or laxity must be recognized and noted to properly determine the severity of injury. These passive tests are often designed to reproduce the mechanism of injury. Specific passive procedures used to locate pain and instability in athletic injuries are described and illustrated throughout the remainder of this text.

Functional movements

Functional movements are a series of active movements or activities the athlete performs that simulate the type of activity required in a particular sport. These tests can be used during the initial assessment of an athletic injury, but are most often used to determine if recovery is complete and if the athlete is ready to return to full participation or activity. The athlete is asked to perform specific movements necessary or required in his or her sport. In most cases the first functional movements are designed to generate relatively little stress. Stress intensity is then increased for subsequent movements until the extent of injury is determined or full recovery is apparent. For example, the athlete with an injured leg may be asked to begin jogging; if that does not cause any pain or problems, the athlete may progress on to running and then jumping or cutting activities, depending on the sport.

Functional testing should always precede the return of the athlete to full activity. An athlete who has full strength and no pain or instability on active or passive stress tests must also demonstrate the ability to perform any activities required of his or her sport before returning to full participation.

ATHLETIC INJURY ASSESSMENT CHECKLIST

Primary survey

———— Airway
———— Breathing
———— Circulation

Secondary survey

———— History
    ———— Primary complaint
    ———— Mechanism of injury
    ———— Areas of pain
    ———— Functional abilities
    ———— Other associated symptoms
    ———— Level of consciousness
    ———— Previous injuries
    ———— Pre-existing conditions and medications
———— Observation
    ———— Bleeding
    ———— Deformity
    ———— Swelling
    ———— Discoloration
    ———— Signs of trauma
    ———— Skin appearance
    ———— Expressions denoting pain
    ———— Symmetry
———— Palpation
    ———— Point tenderness
    ———— Pain
    ———— Swelling
    ———— Deformity
    ———— Crepitation
    ———— Muscle spasms
    ———— Skin temperature
    ———— Pulses
———— Stress
    ———— Range of motion
    ———— Pain
    ———— Instability
    ———— Point tenderness
    ———— Crepitation
    ———— Functional abilities
    ———— Ability to move
    ———— Weakness

EVALUATIONS OF FINDINGS

The remainder of this text includes a variety of evaluative maneuvers and stress procedures that can be used to assist in the evaluation of athletic injuries. Obviously, not all athletic injuries require as complete and systematic a survey as outlined in this chapter. Athletic trainers must learn to select the appropriate evaluation procedures based on the injured body part and the findings obtained throughout the assessment process. To become skilled in athletic injury assessment, a person must be well versed in both functional anatomy and the procedures used during the evaluation process.

KEY TERMS

apnea Temporary cessation of breathing

crepitation Grating, grinding, or sticking sensation, produced by a variety of conditions

dyspnea Difficult or labored breathing

history procedures Gathering as much information as possible about the injury itself and the circumstances surrounding its occurrence

hyperventilation Over-breathing or very rapid deep breathing, resulting in abnormally lowered carbon dioxide levels in the blood

mechanism of injury Manner and location by which excess stresses are applied to the body, resulting in injury

observation procedures Recognizing, noticing, and inspecting an injured area and the circumstances associated with its occurrence

palpation procedures Examination by touch

primary survey Portion of the athletic injury assessment process concerned with evaluation of the basic life-support mechanisms of airway, breathing, and circulation

secondary survey Portion of the athletic injury assessment process that examines the athlete in an attempt to recognize and evaluate all athletic injuries and related conditions; it consists of an ordered sequence of procedures used to assess the nature, site, and severity of an athletic injury

stress procedures Manipulative techniques used to locate and define the structures are involved in the injury and to evaluate the integrity of affected tissues

SUGGESTED READINGS

Arnheim, D.D.: Modern principles of athletic training, ed. 6, St. Louis, 1985, Times Mirror/Mosby College Publishing.

Bowers, A.C., and Thompson, J.M.: Clinical manual of health assessment, ed. 2, St. Louis, 1985, The C.V. Mosby Co.

Cyriax, J.: Textbook of orthopaedic medicine, vol. 1, Diagnosis of soft tissue lesions, ed. 7, London, 1981, Macmillan Publishing Co., Ltd.

Daniels, L., and Worthingham, C.: Muscle testing, ed. 4, Philadelphia, 1980, W.B. Saunders Co.

Kessler, R.M., and Hertling, D.: Management of common musculoskeletal disorders, Philadelphia, 1983, Harper & Row, Publishers, Inc.

Malasanos, L., and others: Health assessment, ed. 3, St. Louis, 1985, Times Mirror/Mosby College Publishing.

O'Donoghue, D.H.: Treatment of injuries to athletes, ed. 4, Philadelphia, 1984, W.B. Saunders Co.

The Nurse's Reference Library: Assessment, Springhouse, Pa., 1982, Intermed Communications Inc.

Warner, C.G.: Emergency care: assessment and intervention, ed. 3, St. Louis, 1982, The C.V. Mosby Co.

U N I T

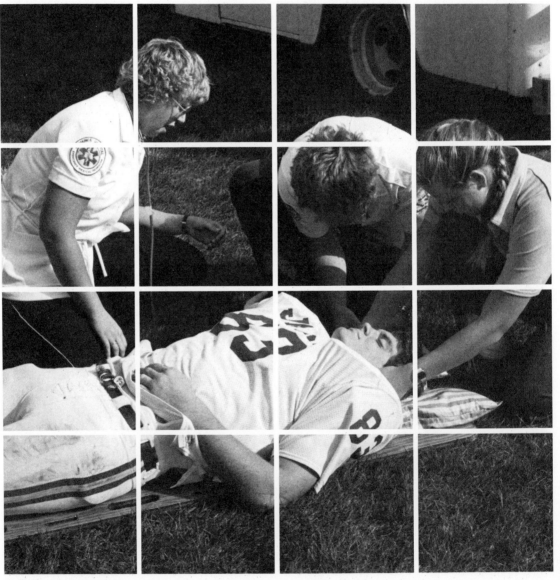

Cervical spine injury.

F O U R
Athletic injuries of the axial region

Athletic injuries to the axial region of the body are discussed first because of the vital organs within this region and the possibility that injuries involving these organs can be life threatening. The axial division of the body includes not only the head and spine but also the trunk, or torso, with its thoracic and abdominal subdivisions.

10   The unconscious athlete

11   Head and face injuries

12   Spine injuries

13   Throat, chest, abdomen, and pelvis injuries

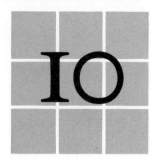

IO The unconscious athlete

One of the most difficult situations an athletic trainer may face is the assessment of an unconscious athlete. In most athletic injuries, the advantage of eliciting responses from the injured athlete greatly assists in making an accurate assessment. The unconscious athlete offers an unusual challenge in assessment, which again emphasizes the importance of having a prearranged sequence of evaluative techniques and a plan of action in the event you must care for an unconscious athlete.

UNCONSCIOUSNESS

Unconsciousness is defined as the inability to respond to any sensory stimuli, with the possible exception of those causing deep pain. The un-conscious athlete is unaware of his or her surroundings and is unable to make purposeful voluntary movements. Consciousness is one of the highest functions of the brain, and evaluating the level of consciousness is one of the most reliable mechanisms for determining the neurologic status of an athlete. An athlete is normally alert, oriented, and awake. Several terms are used to describe the various levels of consciousness. An athlete may be called *lethargic* when he or she seems drowsy but can be awakened easily by sound or a nudge, and when awake will answer questions. *Stuporous* is used to describe an athlete who is partially or nearly unconscious. This condition is marked by reduced responsiveness. The stuporous athlete will fall asleep easily but can be awakened for short periods of time by verbal or physical stimuli. He or she may be able to answer questions but rapidly falls asleep repeatedly. An *unconscious* athlete cannot be aroused to answer questions, but may pull away from or attempt to push away painful stimuli. *Coma* is a state of unconsciousness from which the athlete cannot be aroused, even by powerful stimuli. For the athletic trainer it is much more practical to describe behavior than to label and define various levels of consciousness.

In most instances the unconscious athlete will regain consciousness in a short period of time. Should this occur, the assessment process takes on a different focus, which is discussed in Chapters 11 and 12. This chapter is concerned only with assessment of the unconscious and unresponsive athlete. It is extremely important that athletic trainers evaluate and monitor the level of consciousness of each injured athlete throughout the assessment process.

Causes of unconsciousness in athletic activity

There are various reasons why an athlete may be rendered unconscious. Unconsciousness may result from derangement of the brain itself or from a problem in the body that interferes with the supply of oxygen and nutrients to the brain. The most common cause of unconsciousness in athletics is traumatic head injury. Injuries of this type are discussed in more detail in Chapter 11. An athlete may also become unconscious from conditions such as heatstroke, diabetes, epilepsy, and cerebral or cardiac malfunctions. The fact that it may be difficult to determine the exact cause of unconsciousness underscores the importance of developing a systematic approach to managing an unconscious athlete.

Seizures

Seizures, or convulsions, are discussed at this time because they are periods of unconsciousness that must be managed before the assessment process can continue. Seizures occur suddenly and result from abnormal electrical discharges within the brain. The most common cause of seizures during athletics is trauma to the head. However, any condition that irritates or damages brain cells may produce seizures or convulsions. A disorder of the brain that is characterized by a tendency for recurrent seizures is called *epilepsy*. There are several types of seizures, each characterized by disturbances of movement, unconsciousness, and altered sensations, behavior, mood, or perceptions. In a common type of seizure the person will fall down and display uncontrollable jerking or shaking movements of the extremities. This is known as a *grand mal seizure*. The teeth are often clenched, and there may be excessive salivation and loss of bowel or bladder control. Breathing may be irregular because of spastic contractions of the diaphragm; as a result, a bluish color (cyanosis) is often noted in the lips and under the fingernails. Most seizures are self-limiting and cease after a few minutes. After a grand mal seizure, the person is usually tired and will want to rest. Caring for an athlete who is having a seizure is primarily protective in nature. Protect the athlete's head, arms, and legs as they flail about so the athlete is not injured. The athlete must be protected but not restrained. If it can be inserted easily, a bite stick (padded tongue blade) or other soft object may be placed between the teeth to prevent the athlete from biting the tongue. Do not attempt to pry the athlete's mouth open to force anything into the mouth. Never place your fingers into the mouth of an athlete during a seizure. A return to normal respiration almost always follows a single convulsion or seizure, and breathing is not a problem unless successive seizures occur in a short period of time *(status epilepticus)*. Should this ever occur, medical attention must be obtained immediately. An athlete who has experienced a seizure should also be referred to medical assistance. It is important to provide a careful description of the seizure on referral. This information can greatly assist in diagnosis and treatment by the physician.

ATHLETIC INJURY ASSESSMENT PROCESS
Primary survey

When approaching an injured athlete, always note if the person is alert and responsive. If the athlete appears unresponsive, try to communicate with him or her in order to evaluate level of consciousness. Call the athlete by name. It may be necessary to use loud and repeated verbal stimulation to evoke a response. An unconscious athlete will not respond to verbal or visual commands, and the status of the athlete's airway, breathing, and circulation require immediate attention. Emergency care procedures of artificial respiration and circulation may have to be initiated before further assessment techniques can be considered. Remember, whenever an athlete is unconscious there is always the possibility that a severe injury has occurred, and utmost care and caution should be used. Assume the unconscious athlete has a neck injury as well as a head injury, and treat accordingly. Whenever an unconscious athlete must be moved, extreme care must be taken to avoid causing additional injury.

Fig. 10-1. Positioning the airway in an unconscious athlete who is not breathing.

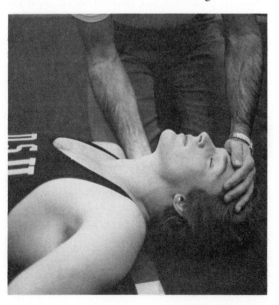

Airway

Immediate attention must be given to the airway of any unresponsive athlete. As previously discussed, the parapharyngeal muscles may relax, allowing the tongue to fall backward and block the airway, especially if the athlete is lying on his or her back (Fig. 10-1). In addition, the unconscious athlete may have lost the normal protective reflex of coughing, which increases the danger of aspiration should blood or vomitus be present. Therefore an adequate airway must be maintained and constantly monitored in the unconscious athlete.

Breathing

In the majority of instances, the unconscious athlete will be breathing. However, always make sure before continuing the assessment process. Assessing breathlessness was discussed in Chapter 9. If an unconscious athlete is wearing protective headgear, such as a football helmet with a face guard, assessing breathlessness and initiating cardiopulmonary resuscitation (CPR) techniques may be difficult or impossible. If the protective headgear of an unconscious athlete must be removed, extreme caution must be used, as there may be an associated cervical spine injury. Removing the headgear can cause dangerous motion of the cervical spine and produce additional trauma, which may result in spinal cord transection, paralysis, and even death. Therefore your plan of action in this situation must include procedures for removing the headgear or cutting the face guard away from the helmet without putting additional stress on the cervical spine. If the athlete is breathing sufficiently, leave the headgear in place, as it can assist in stabilizing the head and neck.

Face guards can be removed by cutting them away from the headgear. If the face guard is attached by the type of supports that allow it to swing upward, cutting the side supports with a sharp knife will allow it to swing up and away from the face during removal (Fig. 10-2). Large bolt cutters can also be used to cut the face guard at each point of attachment to the headgear. The face guard can then be lifted away from the face without moving the head and cervical spine. You should be prepared to carry out one of these procedures, depending on the style of face guards and supports used and removal equipment available.

If a football helmet must be removed from an unconscious athlete, the easiest and safest method is shown in Fig. 10-3. While one person holds the helmet firmly so there is no unnecessary movement, a second person removes the chinstrap and cheek pads. The cheek pads are removed with the help of a slender, flat object, such as a butter knife, spatula, tongue blade, screwdriver, or bandage scissors. It is a good practice to keep one of these objects (a butter knife is one of the best for this maneuver) readily available among your emergency supplies. The object is placed between the helmet and the cheek pad and twisted slightly to loosen the snaps holding the cheek pads in place. The cheek pads can then be carefully lifted out. The person holding the helmet then prepares to slide it off the athlete's head while the second person sup-

ports the head and neck. Putting the thumbs in the earholes of the helmet will assist in spreading the helmet to clear the ears as it is slid off. Throughout the removal process, the second person applies longitudinal traction to prevent movement of the head and maintain cervical alignment. After the helmet is removed the first person resumes responsibility for inline traction of the head and neck. This simple but critically important procedure should be practiced by anyone who has the responsibility of caring for injuries occurring in football. It should only be used when it is decided the helmet must be removed.

Circulation

In the majority of instances, the unconscious athlete will have a pulse. Assessing pulselessness is discussed in Chapter 9. If the unconscious athlete does not have a pulse and requires artificial circulation, uniforms and protective equipment may have to be removed. Removing a jersey or uniform top can be accomplished by cutting up the middle using bandage scissors (Fig. 10-4).

Fig. 10-2. Removing the face guard by: **A,** cutting the side supports with a sharp knife and **B,** swinging the face guard away from the face.

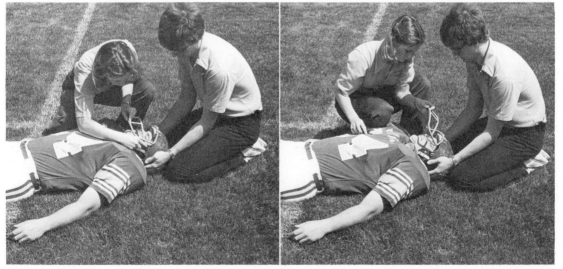

A   B

Fig. 10-3. Removing a football helmet from an unconscious player: **A,** supporting helmet so there is no unnecessary movement of neck, **B,** remove chin strap and loosen cheek pads with a slender flat object, **C,** lift cheek pads out and **D,** slide helmet carefully off while head supported.

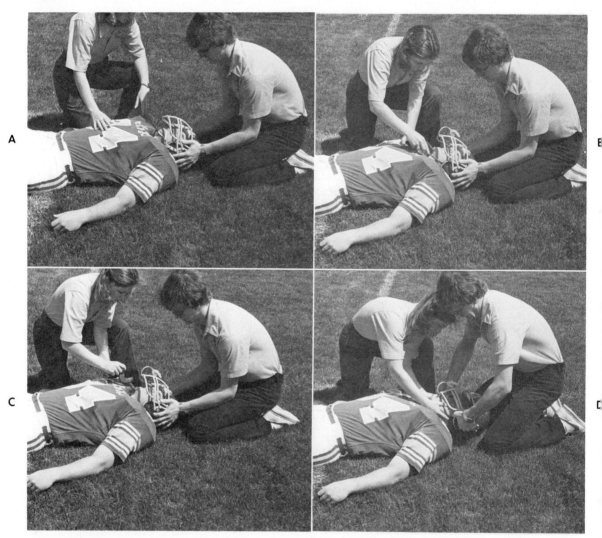

Fig. 10-4. Cutting football jersey off using bandage scissors.

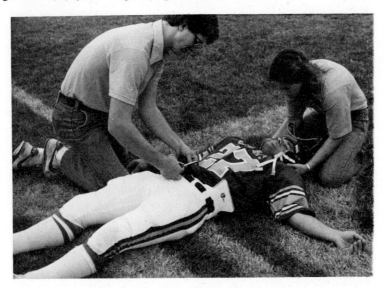

Fig. 10-5. Removing shoulder pads from the chest area by **A,** cutting laces in front and **B,** pulling halves laterally exposing the chest.

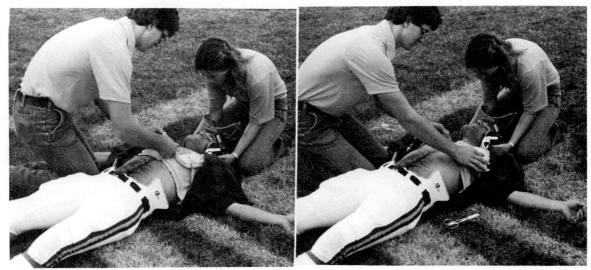

To remove shoulder pads from the chest area, cut the laces in the front and pull laterally so as to expose the sternum enough to permit chest compressions (Fig. 10-5).

In those instances in which an unconscious athlete is not breathing and does not have a pulse, emergency cardiopulmonary resuscitation (CPR) techniques must be initiated. However, most of the time the unconscious athlete will be breathing, have a pulse, and recover consciousness rather quickly. For these persons, the secondary survey remains the largest portion of the assessment process.

Secondary survey

The secondary survey is extremely important and at the same time more difficult to complete on the unconscious athlete. You must proceed, in sequence, to reconstruct the events and circumstances surrounding the injury, assess the extent of actual injury to the athlete in quesiton, and then initiate appropriate treatment, care, and transportation or referral procedures. Information gained during the secondary survey of an unconscious athlete is very important and can be useful to the physician who will diagnose the extent of the injury after referral. The information gained should be written down and passed along to the physician whenever an athlete who was or is unconscious is referred. It may be a helpless feeling to care for an unconscious athlete who is breathing normally and has a good pulse. However, continue the assessment process to gain as much information as possible.

Vital signs are important indicators of the health status of the injured athlete, and they may change. Monitor them throughout the assessment process. This is especially important for an unconscious athlete, because the extent of injury is seldom known. The vital signs will be discussed in more detail throughout the remainder of this chapter.

History

When the athlete is unconscious, the most important step in the athletic injury assessment process, the history, is not available from the usual source, the athlete. Nothing can narrow down the assessment more quickly than a good history. Even though the unconscious athlete is unable to communicate directly, proceed to obtain a complete and accurate history.

Find out as much as possible from whomever is available. Question athletes, officials, or others who observed what happened. Perhaps you witnessed the injury. If so, immediately complete a mental list of possible causes. Did the athlete suffer some sort of a blow to the head, or did he or she collapse unexpectedly in the absence of apparent trauma or injury? Remain constantly alert on the bench or sideline to witness any injury that may occur. Personal observation of circumstances surrounding an injury will make reliance on second-hand reports unnecessary and save considerable time. In addition, if you have a good working knowledge of the medical history of your athletes, you will be aware of possible conditions that may predispose them to unconsciousness, such as diabetes or epilepsy.

Level of consciousness. Evaluating the level of consciousness is a very important sign in assessing the status of the nervous system. Attempt to determine the level of consciousness of the injured athlete, and then ascertain whether it is stable, improving, or deteriorating. All subsequent changes must be recognized and recorded. Your observations and documentation of the level of consciousness can play a major role in assisting physicians in determining the proper care for the athlete. The physician must know if the loss of consciousness was immediate or developed over a period of time. The athlete who loses consciousness rapidly or shows a lack of improvement with time suggests that medical care is needed. The athlete who progressively develops into a very deep state of unconsciousness or coma also requires immediate medical attention.

Questions that should be answered include: How long was the athlete unconscious? Could the athlete be aroused? Was there a response to pain? What was the depth of unconsciousness?

Was the athlete aware of the correct time and oriented to the surroundings? Can he or she respond accurately to questions that require long- and short-term memory? The level of consciousness has a direct relationship to intracranial involvement. The deeper the unconsciousness, the more intensive the possible damage. Remember, this information is important in establishing a neurologic baseline and should be reported to the physician whenever the athlete is referred.

Observation

The unconscious athlete requires careful observation throughout the assessment process. Begin by observing the entire situation quickly. Note the alignment and position of the athlete. Look for any abnormal positions of the head or neck and unusual positions of any parts of the body. Note any apparatus or equipment that was in use at the time of injury. Look for any hemorrhaging and, if needed, initiate steps to control it. Measures to prevent or treat shock should also be initiated. Following are other vital signs that must be observed.

Respirations. Determine the number of respirations per minute of an unconscious athlete. This can be accomplished by watching for movement of the chest and by listening and feeling for air exchange at the mouth and nose. Another method would be to place a hand on the chest or upper abdomen and count the number of breaths per minute (Fig. 10-6). The normal adult respiratory rate will vary but is usually between 12 and 18 breaths per minute. In well-conditioned athletes the rate may be lower, and in younger athletes the rate may be slightly higher.

The character and pattern of the respirations should also be noted. Normal rate and rhythm of respirations in an unconscious athlete suggest that no severe brain damage has occurred up to that point. Abnormal breathing patterns suggest severe brain dysfunction and the need for immediate medical assistance. Table 10-1 briefly describes various abnormal breathing patterns that may indicate brain dysfunction. Any of these abnormal breathing patterns observed in an unconscious athlete, or in an athlete suffering from some sort of head injury, may indicate brain damage. The athletic trainer should be alert to recognize these patterns.

Fig. 10-6. Counting respirations by placing hand on upper abdomen of unconscious athlete.

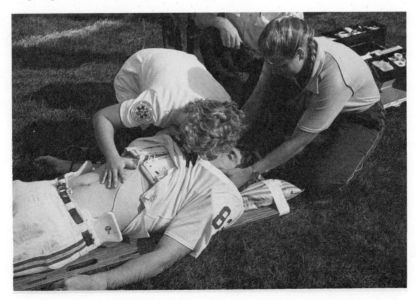

Table 10-1. Abnormal breathing patterns

Term	Description
Hyperpnea	Abnormal increase in the depth and rate of the respiratory movements
Apnea	Periods of nonbreathing
Ataxic breathing	Irregular breathing pattern, with deep and shallow breaths occurring randomly
Hyperventilation	Prolonged, rapid hyperpnea, resulting in decreased carbon dioxide blood levels
Cheyne-Stokes respirations	Periods of hyperpnea regularly alternating with periods of apnea, characterized by regular acceleration and deceleration in depth
Biot's respirations	Regular periods of hyperpnea and irregular periods of apnea
Cluster breathing	Breaths follow each other in disorderly sequence, with irregular pauses between them

Pupils. The pupils should be examined for size, equality, and reactions in any unconscious athlete. Pupils are normally round, equal in size, and react to light very quickly. Changes in pupil size or their reaction to light can give important information and must be noted. Check the size of the pupils of an unconscious athlete by gently raising the eyelids (Fig. 10-7). Are both the pupils the same size? Is one larger than the other? Pupils of unequal size may indicate an expanding lesion within the skull. The larger, or dilated, pupil will usually be on the side of the lesion and is caused by pressure on the third cranial or oculomotor nerve. However, both pupils may be dilated slightly in an unconscious athlete. If the pupils appear to be dilated, check their response to light. Normally the pupils constrict promptly when light is directed at them. The rapidity with which the pupils respond to light can vary somewhat between persons. It is the presence of the constricting response, or *pupillary reflex,* and the equality of the response between the right

Fig. 10-7. Checking size of pupils in an unconscious athlete.

Fig. 10-8. Using a flashlight to evaluate pupil response.

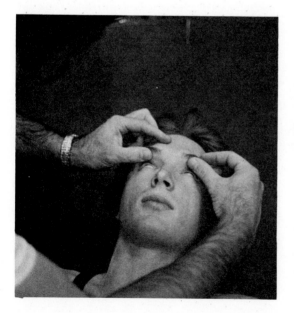

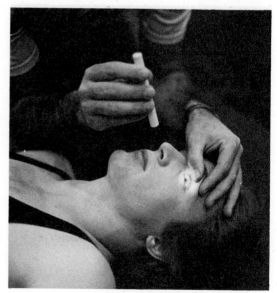

and left eye that is important to note. Pupillary response can be observed in two ways. You can use a flashlight to shine at the pupils to note the reaction (Fig. 10-8). If you do not have a flashlight, shade the athlete's eyes with your hand (Fig. 10-9) and then quickly take your hand away. When the sun or light hits the eyes, the reaction should be the same as using the flashlight. Failure of the pupils to react to light, or failure to react with equality, may indicate a serious situation. The athlete should be referred to medical assistance immediately.

Skin color. In assessing the unconscious athlete, changes in skin color can provide information useful in determining both adequacy of blood flow and blood oxygen concentration in a particular body part or area. In athletes with deeply pigmented skin, color changes related to blood flow or oxygenation are more apparent in the mucous membranes, the lips, the tongue, and the fingernail beds.

Those areas of the body that are particularly susceptible to color changes include the face (cheeks), the bridge of the nose, the neck and upper chest, and the midline of the abdomen. The flexor surfaces of the extremities and the backs of the hands are also said to be *pigment labile* and should be observed carefully for changes in skin color.

Color changes to be aware of are red, white, and blue. Reddening of the skin, *rubor,* indicates the capillary vessels are dilated, resulting in an increased blood flow. This may be present in an athlete suffering from heatstroke or high blood pressure. A pale or white skin color, *pallor,* is caused by constriction of blood vessels in the skin, which results in decreased circulation. This may indicate severe hemorrhaging or shock. A bluish color, *cyanosis,* results from poor oxygenation of the circulating blood and may be the result of heart failure or airway obstruction. Observation of changes in skin color can help determine immediate care for the injured athlete.

Signs of trauma. Look for any obvious signs of trauma, especially about the head and neck. Examine the scalp for lacerations, bumps, or deformities (Fig. 10-10). Is there blood in the hair? Check for any discharge coming from the ears *(otorrhea)* or nose *(rhinorrhea)* (Fig. 10-11). This discharge may be either blood or cerebrospinal fluid, or a combination of both. Cerebrospinal fluid is a clear fluid and indicates a probable skull fracture. Cerebrospinal fluid can be distinguished from blood when they are mixed together by collecting the discharge from the ears or nose on an absorbent pad, such as a gauze pad. The cerebrospinal fluid separates from the blood, forming a circle (halo) around the centrally located blood (Fig. 10-12). Blood draining from an ear, even in the absence of cerebrospinal fluid, may also be indicative of a skull fracture. Do not attempt to restrict the flow of cerebrospinal fluid or blood coming from the ear, because this may increase the intracranial pressure.

Look for discoloration or ecchymosis about the head and face. Discoloration over the mas-

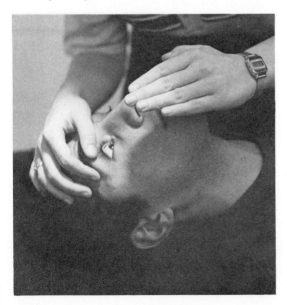

Fig. 10-9. Checking pupillary response by shading an athletes eye and quickly removing the hand allowing the light to reach the eye.

Fig. 10-10. Examining scalp for signs of trauma.

Fig. 10-11. Checking for discharge (otorrhea) coming from the ear.

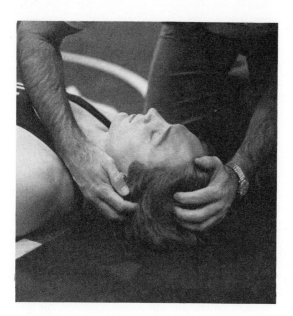

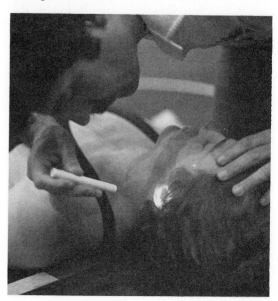

Fig. 10-12. An orange halo will form around the blood on a gauze pad if cerebrospinal fluid is present.
(From Judd, R.L., and Ponsell, D.D.: The first responder: the first critical minutes, St. Louis, 1981, The C.V. Mosby Co.)

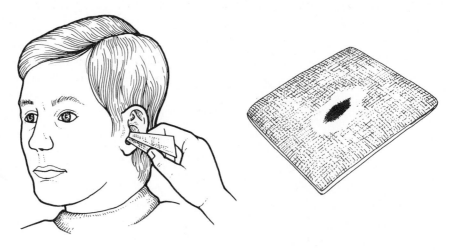

toid area just behind the ear may indicate a skull fracture and is called ***Battle's sign.*** Discoloration around the eyes, ***racoon eyes,*** may also indicate a skull fracture. However, either of these signs may not be present for 2 to 3 days after an injury.

Posturing. Neurologic signs called *posturing of the extremities* may occur as a result of severe brain injuries, which are seldom seen as a result of athletic activity. Although it occurs only rarely, persons who deal with athletic injuries should be aware of what posturing is and able to recognize it as a sign of severe brain malfunction. ***Decerebrate rigidity*** is a postural attitude that is characterized by extension of all four extremities (Fig. 10-13, *A*). ***Decorticate rigidity*** is a postural attitude that is characterized by extension of the legs and marked flexion of the elbows, wrists, and fingers (Fig. 10-13, *B*). Whenever posturing is noted in an unconscious athlete, an emergency exists and the athlete must be referred to medical assistance immediately.

Palpation

There are additional physical signs that may be evaluated by palpation. Remember, be gentle in palpating an unconscious athlete so as not to aggravate any existing injury or cause additional trauma.

Pulse. One of the first steps of the primary survey is to determine whether or not an unconscious athlete has a pulse. Continue to monitor the pulse to note any changes in rate or character, such as a change in rhythm or strength. The normal pulse rate for an athlete at rest will vary greatly but is usually between 50 and 80 beats per minute, depending on conditioning. Pulse readings can be taken at any area where an artery lies close to the surface of the skin. The most common pulse is taken at the wrist by palpating the superficial radial artery (Fig. 10-14). If circumstances make the radial pulse difficult to locate, the carotid pulse in the neck should be used. As intracranial pressure increases, an athlete's pulse rate slows down below normal.

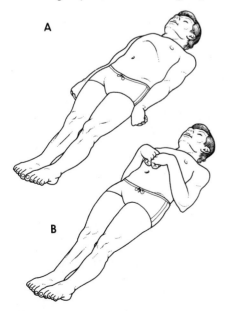

Fig. 10-13. Posturing of the extremities. **A,** Decerebrate rigidity. **B,** Decorticate rigidity.

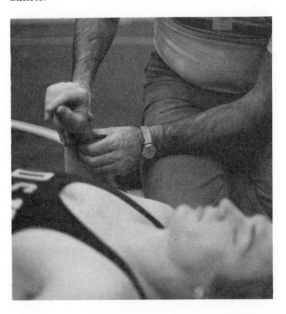

Fig. 10-14. Monitoring the pulse of an unconscious athlete.

Characteristics of the pulse indicate if the heartbeat is strong or weak, regular or irregular. These sensations are noted as you feel the pulse. Normally the pulse is strong and easily felt, indicating a full volume of circulating blood. Noting the rate, strength, and rhythm of the pulse can give important clues as to the health status of the athlete. A weak, rapid pulse is an indication of shock. A strong, rapid pulse may indicate fright or hypertension. The pulse rate and character should be noted immediately and then checked throughout the assessment process to detect any changes.

Remember, when evaluating an obvious deformity, such as a fracture or dislocation, you must also feel for a pulse distal to the injury. The absence of a pulse below an injury, when the athlete has a heartbeat, suggests severe arterial damage, such as transection or occlusion. The absence of a pulse distal to an injury should be regarded as an emergency requiring immediate referral to a physician for treatment.

Blood pressure. Another vital sign is blood pressure. Monitoring blood pressure in conjunction with pulse rates can be helpful in evaluating the status of an unconscious athlete. Blood pressure is the pressure that circulating blood exerts against the arterial walls. It is measured with a sphygmomanometer (blood pressure cuff) used in conjunction with a stethoscope. As the heart pumps blood into the closed circulatory system, a pressure wave is created, which keeps blood circulating throughout the body. The high and low points of this pressure wave are measured with the aid of the sphygmomanometer, which makes it possible to measure the amount of air pressure equal to the blood pressure in an artery. The blood pressure cuff is wrapped around the arm over the brachial artery, and air is pumped into the cuff by means of a compressible bulb. In this way, air pressure is exerted against the outside of the artery. Air is added until the air pressure exceeds the blood pressure within the artery or, in other words, until it compresses the artery. At this time no pulse can be heard through the stethoscope placed over the brachial artery at the

bend of the elbow along the inner margin of the biceps muscle. By slowly releasing the air in the cuff, the air pressure is decreased until it approximately equals the blood pressure within the artery. At this point the vessel opens slightly, and a small spurt of blood comes through, producing the first sound. This is followed by increasingly louder sounds that suddenly change as the air pressure decreases. They become more muffled, then disappear altogether. The first sound represents the *systolic blood pressure*. The lowest point at which the sounds can be heard, just before they disappear, is approximately equal to the *diastolic blood pressure*. Blood in the arteries of the average adult exerts a pressure equal to that required to raise a column of mercury about 120 mm high in a glass tube during systole, and 80 mm high during diastole. For sake of brevity, this is expressed as a blood pressure of 120 over 80 (120/80). Blood pressure readings can vary greatly among persons or in one person throughout the day. Differences in age, sex, and level of activity also contribute to variations in blood pressure from one person to the next.

Changes in blood pressure indicate changes in (1) blood volume, (2) integrity of the blood vessels, or (3) ability of the heart to pump blood. The loss of normal blood pressure indicates insufficient circulation. Whatever the cause of the decreased blood pressure in the cardiovascular system, the result will be insufficient perfusion of blood providing oxygen and nutrients to the tissues of the body. This is discussed in more detail under shock in Chapter 6. As shock develops, there is usually a reciprocal relationship between blood pressure and pulse; that is, blood pressure decreases and the heart pumps more rapidly to circulate the blood more efficiently.

Rising blood pressure in an unconscious athlete may indicate cerebral hemorrhage (see Chapter 11). This is especially true if the pulse rate is going down. Remember, athletes would have increased blood pressure and pulse rates during activity, which should return to normal as they rest. Blood pressure can change rapidly and should be monitored frequently in athletes remaining unconscious or suffering head trauma.

Skin temperature. Body temperature is normally taken with a thermometer. Because the skin is largely responsible for regulation of body temperature, you can evaluate gross changes in body temperature by feeling the skin. Feel the athlete's skin at several locations using the back of your hand (Fig. 10-15). The back of your hand is more sensitive to temperature change than the roughened fingers. The athlete in shock or suffering from heat exhaustion will have cool, clammy skin. Hot, dry skin is indicative of excessive body heat such as that associated with heatstroke or high fever.

Signs of trauma. Along with observing the head and neck for signs of trauma, you can also palpate the area. Run your fingers gently over the scalp, through the hair, and along the neck if this area is accessible and not covered by headgear (Fig. 10-16). Check for any depressions, lumps, or blood. You can also palpate for deformities and swelling in other areas of the body suspected of being injured.

Reaction to pain. Of course, the unconscious athlete is unable to respond and voluntarily move his or her extremities. However, it is normally possible to check the condition of the spinal cord of an unconscious athlete by providing a painful stimulus. A few methods of providing a painful stimulus include pricking the skin of the hands or feet lightly with a sharp object, pinching the skin, sternal compression, nipple pressure, calf pressure, and pinching the trapezius area (Fig. 10-17). If there is no spinal cord damage, the athlete may involuntarily pull away from the painful stimulus or attempt to push it away. If there is no reaction to the painful stimulus, it may indicate that the spinal cord is damaged or the athlete is in a coma. If the unconscious athlete responds to the painful stimulus by posturing of the extremities, severe brain malfunctioning is indicated.

Stress

As long as the injured athlete remains unconscious, manipulative or stress-type procedures are contraindicated. Because the athlete cannot respond, you are unable to assess the severity of associated injuries. The athlete may have a severe head or neck injury. Therefore the unconscious athlete should not be subjected to stress proce-

Fig. 10-15. Feeling the athletes skin for changes in skin temperature.

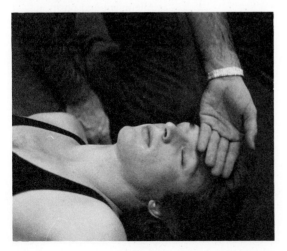

Fig. 10-16. Palpating cervical spine for any obvious signs of trauma.

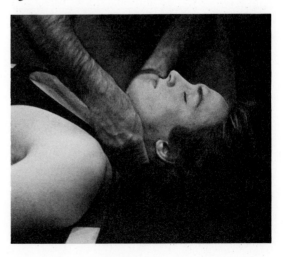

dures as previously described until he or she regains consciousness and is responsive.

Evaluation of findings

Fortunately, in most cases in which an athlete is rendered unconscious it is not a serious situation. Usually the athlete will be breathing normally, have a strong pulse, and regain consciousness in a short period of time. The assessment of the unconscious athlete may be limited to the primary survey and determination of the vital signs. In these persons the majority of the assessment process will take place after the athlete begins to regain consciousness. However, serious injuries resulting in extended unconsciousness can and do occur, and the athletic trainer must be prepared for these situations. Much important information can be gained during the evaluation of an unconscious athlete. This information will indicate what emergency care should be provided for the athlete and provide important clues to the nature and severity of the conditions surrounding the unconsciousness. It cannot be overemphasized that this information must be passed along whenever the athlete is referred to medical assistance. Observations can provide an important evaluative baseline for the physician's diagnosis and treatment.

When to refer the athlete

The unconscious athlete who regains consciousness in a matter of seconds and whose physical signs and symptoms appear normal may be treated by the athletic trainer. This is discussed further in Chapter 11. However, there are important physical signs which indicate that the unconscious athlete should be referred to a physician for additional assessment and treatment.

Fig. 10-17. Providing a painful stimulus to note reaction of unconscious athlete.

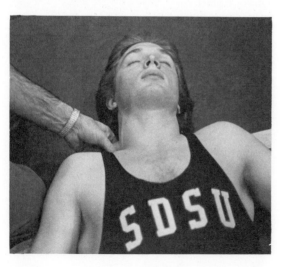

**ATHLETIC INJURY ASSESSMENT
CHECKLIST
UNCONSCIOUS ATHLETE**

Primary survey
———— Airway
———— Breathing
———— Circulation

Secondary survey
———— History
    ———— Question witnesses
    ———— Level of consciousness
———— Observation
    ———— Alignment and position
    ———— Bleeding
    ———— Respirations
    ———— Pupils
    ———— Skin color
    ———— Signs of trauma
    ———— Posturing
———— Palpation
    ———— Pulse
    ———— Skin temperature
    ———— Signs of trauma
    ———— Reaction to pain
———— Stress
No manipulative or stress procedures applied as long as the athlete remains unconscious

The athletic trainer should be able to recognize these signs. The following is a list of conditions that warrant referral to medical assistance:

1. Unconsciousness for an extended period of time (longer than 1 minute)
2. Unconsciousness that progressively develops into a coma
3. Rapid loss of consciousness
4. Dilated and unresponsive pupils
5. Pupils that are unequal in size
6. Signs about the head indicating possible skull fracture (clear fluid or blood coming from the ears, Battle's sign, racoon eyes, skull depressions)
7. Posturing of the extremities (decorticate and decerebrate rigidity)
8. Periodic or irregular breathing
9. Obvious deformities about the head and neck
10. No response to painful stimulus
11. Seizure following a head injury
12. Pulse that slows down below normal
13. Unconscious situation in which there is doubt about what should be done with the athlete

KEY TERMS

Battle's sign Discoloration appearing over the mastoid area

coma State of unconsciousness from which the athlete cannot be aroused, even by powerful stimulus

cyanosis Bluish discoloration of skin caused by poor oxygenation of the circulating blood

decerebrate rigidity Postural attitude characterized by extension of all four extremities

decorticate rigidity Postural attitude characterized by extension of the legs and marked flexion of the elbows, wrists, and fingers

diastolic blood pressure Force with which the blood pushes against the artery walls when the ventricles are relaxed

epilepsy Disorder of the brain characterized by a tendency for recurrent seizures

grand mal seizure Classic type of seizure in which the person will fall down and display uncontrollable jerking or shaking movements of the extremities

lethargy Condition of drowsiness

otorrhea Discharge from the ear

pallor Paleness or absence of skin coloration

pigment labile Area of the body that may show abnormal changes in skin color

pupillary reflex Contraction of the pupil on exposure of the retina to light

racoon eyes Discoloration around the eyes, indicative of a skull fracture

rubor Redness of the skin

rhinorrhea Discharge from the nose

status epilepticus Successive seizures occurring within a short period of time

stupor Partial or nearly complete unconsciousness

systolic blood pressure Force with which the blood pushes against the artery walls when the ventricles are contracting

unconsciousness Unresponsiveness to any sensory stimuli, with the possible exception of those causing pain

SUGGESTED READINGS

American Academy of Orthopaedic Surgeons: Emergency care and transportation of the sick and injured, ed. 3, Chicago, 1981, The Academy.

Grant, H.D., and others: Emergency care, ed. 3, Bowie, Md., 1982, Robert J. Brady Co.

Miller, R.H., and Cantrell, J.R.: Textbook of basic emergency medicine, ed. 2, St. Louis, 1980, The C.V. Mosby Co.

Parcel, G.S.: Basic emergency care of the sick and injured, ed. 2., St. Louis, 1982, The C.V. Mosby Co.

Rosen, P., and others: Emergency medicine: concepts and clinical practice, St. Louis, 1983, The C.V. Mosby Co.

Warner, C.G.: Emergency care, assessment, and intervention, ed. 3, St. Louis, 1982, The C.V. Mosby Co.

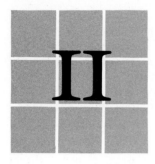

Head and face injuries

Injuries involving the head and cervical spine constitute the most potentially serious of all athletic injuries. Correct assessment procedures, followed by proper emergency treatment and timely referral, may mean the difference between rapid, complete recovery or paralysis or death. Because head and neck injuries can occur together and result from the same mechanisms of injury, it is important to always consider these areas together when assessing athletic injuries. This chapter is concerned with injuries occurring to the head and face and includes signs and symptoms that indicate the athlete should be referred for medical attention. Spinal injuries are discussed in Chapter 12.

HEAD INJURIES

The term "head injury" may be used to describe damage to the scalp, skull, or brain. It is important to realize, however, that all three of these structures may not be damaged in any one injury. For example, it is possible for a skull fracture to occur with little or no injury to either the scalp or the brain. As a matter of fact, most head injuries occurring in athletics are not associated with a skull fracture.

Head injuries can occur in any sport and in a variety of ways. However, most head injuries are caused by the application of some type of sudden force to the head. This sudden force is usually the result of a direct blow. Trauma of this type may be caused by the athlete colliding with another athlete or object such as a goalpost, wall, bleacher, or the floor or ground. It may also occur if the athlete is struck by some sort of athletic equipment, such as a baseball bat or hockey stick. In addition, the head may be injured by a blow from a projectile such as a baseball, golfball, discus, or hockey puck. The face or cervical spine may also be injured as a result of such sudden force.

Scalp

The scalp offers considerable protection for the skull. Without this protection, the skull could be fractured or the brain injured by much less force. It is important to understand the anatomy of the scalp because injury or infection to the scalp can also involve the skull or brain.

The scalp consists of five layers (Fig. 11-1):

S— Skin
C—Connective tissue (dense)
A—Aponeurosis of epicranius muscle
L—Loose connective tissue
P—Periosteum (pericranium)

The scalp is very vascular and has a profuse blood supply. Because of this, avulsed portions of the scalp can usually be saved and should never be cut away, even if points of attachment are minimal. In most instances, sufficient blood will reach the avulsed portion of the flap through remaining connections to permit healing if it can be sutured in place.

Skin. The skin of the scalp is denser than the skin anywhere else on the body and is similar in some ways to the thick skin of the soles of the feet and the palms of the hands. It is character-

Fig. 11-1. Layers of the scalp: skull, meninges, brain, and the connecting blood vessels.

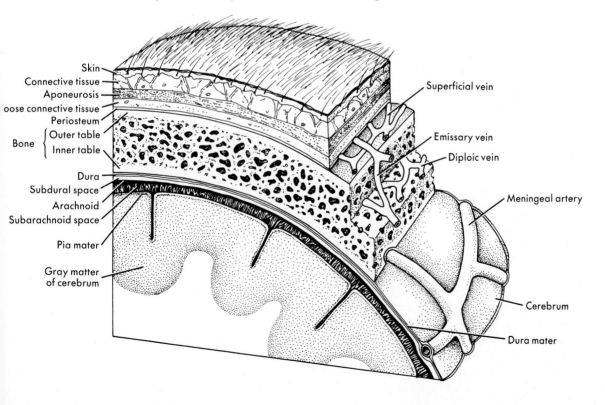

ized by great numbers of hairs and sebaceous glands. The sebaceous glands may become infected, making the scalp the most common site for sebaceous cysts, or *wens.*

Connective tissue (dense). The dense connective tissue layer acts to bind the skin above to the aponeurosis of the epicranius muscle below. This layer of the scalp, if cut, tends to bleed profusely because the blood vessels are firmly anchored by connective tissue and cannot retract. Because of the dense, unyielding nature of this layer of the scalp, inflammation here will generally result in only minimal swelling but much pain.

Aponeurosis. The aponeurosis (galea aponeurotica) is a very dense and strong membrane that becomes muscular over the frontal and occipital areas of the skull. It is this membrane that connects the muscular portions of the epicranius, or occipitofrontalis, muscle. This freely movable, dense fibrous tissue helps absorb the force of external trauma, particularly that of glancing blows. Scalp wounds do not gape unless this layer is cut or split.

Loose connective tissue. The loose connective tissue component of the scalp lies between the dense aponeurotic layer above and the pericranium, or periosteal covering, of the skull below. It forms a potential space called the *subaponeurotic space,* in which large quantities of blood or pus can accumulate under the scalp and extend over the whole dome of the skull without undue stretching.

Important emissary veins connect the large venous sinuses inside the skull with the superficial scalp veins that traverse this area. These veins may carry infections through the skull. Therefore whenever the galea has been lacerated and the wound is wide open, the athlete should be referred to a physician for careful debridement, irrigation, and closure of the wound. There is an old surgical axiom that states "if it were not for emissary veins, wounds and infections of the scalp would lose half their significance."

Periosteum (pericranium). This fifth and deepest layer of the scalp is only loosely attached to the surface of the skull except at the suture lines.

If this layer is torn as a result of a skull fracture, intracranial hemorrhage can leak into and collect in the subaponeurotic space of the scalp. Accumulation of blood in this space, instead of inside the skull, may for a time prevent compression of the brain and is aptly termed a "safety-valve" hematoma.

Scalp injuries

Injuries to the scalp may or may not involve the skull or brain. An athlete may suffer a severe brain injury without any observable trauma to the scalp; on the other hand, an athlete may have a dramatic-looking scalp injury with little or no brain damage. The true severity of head injuries may not be reflected by the appearance of scalp wounds. However, any scalp injury is indicative of forceful trauma to the head and suggests that further evaluation of the head should continue.

The most common athletic injuries to the scalp are contusions and lacerations. Because the scalp is highly vascularized and may bleed profusely if cut, scalp wounds many times appear worse than they actually are. Contusions about the scalp are marked by local tenderness and swelling. Bleeding between the skin and underlying tissue may result in a hematoma, which is commonly referred to as a "goose egg." If small blood vessels beneath the skin have been disrupted, there will be an ecchymosis in the area. Ecchymosis located in certain areas may indicate a possible skull fracture and is discussed on p. 225.

Lacerations of the scalp usually bleed quite freely and can give a rather frightening appearance initially. The source of bleeding should be located, and the bleeding controlled by direct pressure before continuing the evaluation of the head. Remember, scalp wounds are indicative of trauma to the head and are secondary considerations to neurologic assessment of the brain and spinal cord.

Skull

The skull consists of two major divisions: the cranium, or brain case, and the face. This section is concerned with the cranial portion of the

Fig. 11-2. Skull viewed **A,** anteriorly and **B,** laterally.

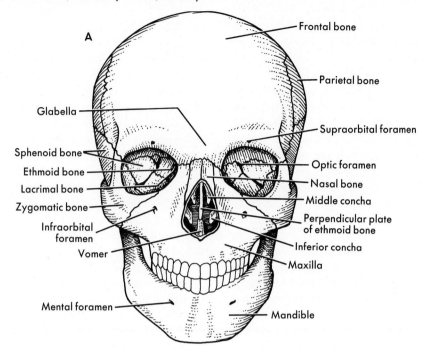

A

Frontal bone
Parietal bone
Glabella
Supraorbital foramen
Sphenoid bone
Optic foramen
Ethmoid bone
Nasal bone
Lacrimal bone
Middle concha
Zygomatic bone
Perpendicular plate of ethmoid bone
Infraorbital foramen
Inferior concha
Vomer
Maxilla
Mental foramen
Mandible

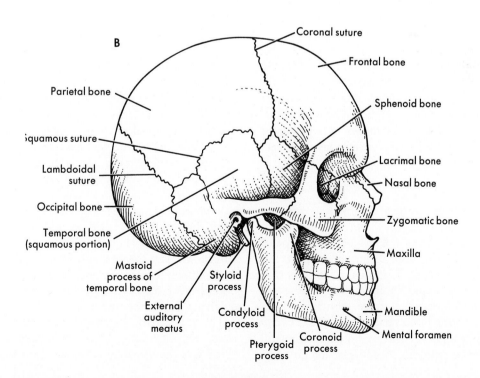

B

Coronal suture
Frontal bone
Parietal bone
Sphenoid bone
Squamous suture
Lambdoidal suture
Lacrimal bone
Nasal bone
Occipital bone
Temporal bone (squamous portion)
Zygomatic bone
Maxilla
Mastoid process of temporal bone
Styloid process
External auditory meatus
Condyloid process
Mandible
Mental foramen
Pterygoid process
Coronoid process

skull; injuries to the face are discussed on pp. 249 to 271. Review the anatomy of the cranial bones and landmarks in Fig. 11-2. Table 3-4 on p. 33, lists and gives a brief description of the eight bones of the cranium.

The cranium is a rigid, bony cavity encasing the brain. The rounded vault is composed of an inner table and an outer table of bone, between which lies cancellous bone (Fig. 11-1). Between these two layers of bone lie the *diploic venous system,* which is connected to the superficial venous system of the scalp by emissary veins. The inner table of the skull also contains grooves in which the meningeal arteries lie.

On your own head, palpate a few landmarks of the cranium. The *inion* is the apex, or most prominent portion, of the *external occipital protuberance.* You should be able to feel this structure on the occipital bone just above the base of the skull. The *mastoid process* of the temporal bone can be palpated just behind the ear. It serves as one of the most prominent landmarks on the lateral surface of the skull.

The average thickness of the skull is 2 to 6 mm. It is much thicker than this in the areas of the midfrontal and midoccipital bones, and much thinner than this in the temporal fossa.

The inner surface of the skull, which covers the hemispheres of the brain, is relatively smooth. In contrast, the base of the skull is irregular, containing many ridges and grooves, making this surface much rougher. These anatomic characteristics are important in understanding how the brain can be raked over bony irregularities during trauma.

Skull injuries

Skull fractures are not common in athletics but may occur when an athlete with an unprotected head receives a severe blow. This type of trauma would be more common in sports requiring a bat or club. Fractures of the skull may range from a simple linear fracture to a severe compound depressed fracture with bone fragments lacerating brain tissue. It may be very difficult to distinguish between a skull fracture and a subgaleal hematoma. Bleeding or the presence of cerebospinal fluid draining from the ear or nose may be the only indication of a skull fracture. The athletic trainer must be alert to recognize any signs of a possible skull fracture. As was described in Chapter 10, fractures to the bones at the base of the skull can cause discoloration over the mastoid area (Battle's sign) or around the eyes (racoon eyes) and may be accompanied by leakage of cerebrospinal fluid from the ear (ottorrhea) or nose (rhinorrhea).

It is possible for a fracture to involve only the inner or outer table of the skull. A fracture of the skull does not mean the brain has been injured; it simply indicates that the force was sufficient enough to crack the skull. Further neurologic tests should be carried out to assess the condition of the brain. However, a fracture line running through one of the grooves containing either the venous system or meningeal arteries may result in hemorrhage between the skull and the dura mater (epidural hemorrhage). This bleeding, especially if it is arterial hemorrhage, can produce serious results in a short period of time. Intracranial hemorrhaging is discussed in more detail on pp. 242 to 243.

Brain

The adult brain, one of our largest organs, generally weighs a little over 3 pounds. It consists of the following major divisions, named in ascending order beginning with the lowest part: brain stem (medulla, pons, and midbrain), cerebellum, diencephalon (hypothalamus and thalamus), and cerebrum. An understanding of the anatomy and generalized function of the brain stem, cerebellum, and cerebrum are of particular importance in initial assessment of head injury.

Brain stem. Three divisions of the brain make up the brain stem, so called because of its resemblance to a stem (Fig. 11-3). The medulla oblongata forms the lowest part of the brain stem, the midbrain forms the uppermost part, and the pons lies between them, that is, above the medulla and below the midbrain.

The brain stem is a fixed functional area between the more movable cerebral hemispheres above and the spinal cord below. If the brain is set in motion by a blow to the head, the neurologic symptoms that often result are caused by damage to the upper portions of the brain stem. The cerebral hemispheres move or rotate about the brain stem, which, because it is fixed and cannot move, tends to compress, or buckle, under the stress. The result is a brain stem concussion or the much more severe brain stem contusion.

The brain stem, like the spinal cord, performs sensory, motor, and reflex functions. Nuclei in the medulla contain a number of reflex centers. (The term "nucleus" used in reference to the nervous system means a cluster of neural cell bodies located in the gray matter of the central nervous system.) Of first importance among reflex centers in the medulla are the cardiac, vasomotor, and respiratory centers. Because their functioning is essential for survival, they are called the vital centers. They serve as the centers for various reflexes controling heart action, blood vessel diameter, and respiration. Because the medulla contains these centers, it is the most vital part of the entire brain—so vital, in fact, that severe contusions that result in actual tissue damage and hemorrhage in this area often prove fatal. Severe blows at the base of the skull will result in death if they interrupt impulse conduction by the vital respiratory centers. Other centers present in the medulla are those for various nonvital reflexes such as vomiting, coughing, sneezing, hiccuping, and swallowing.

Fig. 11-3. Sagittal section through midline of the brain. Note the components of the brain stem: medulla oblongata, pons, and midbrain.

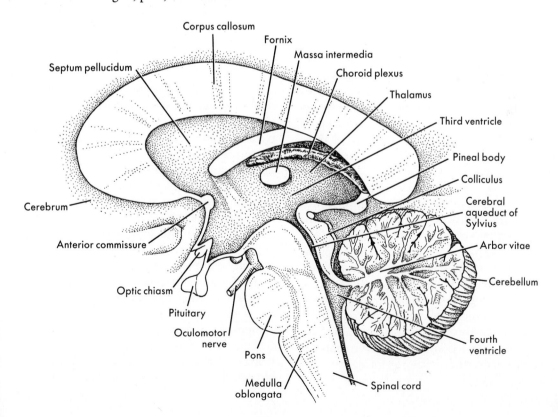

The pons contains centers for reflexes mediated by the fifth, sixth, seventh, and eighth cranial nerves. In addition, the pons contains the pneumotaxic centers that help regulate respiration.

The midbrain, like the pons, contains reflex centers for certain cranial nerve reflexes, for example, pupillary reflexes and eye movements, which are mediated by the third and fourth cranial nerves, respectively.

An important network of nerve fibers, called the *reticular activating system*, extends through the brain stem. This network serves as a control mechanism to regulate level of consciousness.

Cerebellum. The cerebellum, the second largest part of the brain, is located just below the posterior portion of the cerebrum and is partially covered by it. It occupies the most inferior and posterior aspects of the cranial cavity and is attached to the brain stem by three paired bundles of fibers.

The cerebellum performs three general functions, all of which have to do with the control of skeletal muscles. It acts with the cerebral cortex to produce skilled movements by coordinating the activities of groups of muscles. It controls skeletal muscles so as to maintain equilibrium and control posture. The cerebellum functions below the level of consciousness to make movements smooth instead of jerky, steady instead of trembling, and efficient and coordinated (synergic) instead of ineffective, awkward, and uncoordinated (asynergic).

Synergic control of muscle action is closely associated with cerebral motor activity. Normal muscle action involves groups of muscles, the various members of which function together as a unit. For example, in any given action the prime mover contracts and the antagonist relaxes, then contracts weakly at the proper moment to act as a brake, checking the action of the prime mover; the fixation muscles of the neighboring joint then contract. Through such harmonious, co-ordinated group action, normal movements are smooth, steady, and precise in force, rate, and extent.

Achievement of such movements results from cerebellar activity added to cerebral activity. Impulses from the cerebrum may start the action, but those from the cerebellum synergize, or coordinate, the contractions and relaxations of the various muscles once they have begun.

Injury to the cerebellum caused by hemorrhage or trauma produces certain characteristic symptoms, among which **ataxia** (muscle incoordination), **hypotonia,** tremors, and disturbances of gait and equilibrium predominate. One example of ataxia is overshooting a mark or stopping before reaching it when trying to touch a given point on the body (finger-to-nose test). Drawling and slurring of speech are also examples of ataxia. Tremors are particularly pronounced toward the end of movements and with the exertion of effort. Disturbances of gait and equilibrium vary, depending on the muscle groups involved, but the walk is often characterized by staggering or lurching and by a clumsy manner of raising the foot too high and bringing it down with a slap. Paralysis does not result from loss of cerebellar function.

Cerebrum. The cerebrum is the largest and most superiorly located division of the brain. A deep groove, the longitudinal fissure, divides the cerebrum into the right and left cerebral hemispheres. These halves, however, are not completely separate organs. A structure composed of white matter (tracts) and known as the corpus callosum joins them medially (Fig. 11-3). Prominent grooves, or fissures, subdivide each cerebral hemisphere into four lobes (Fig. 11-4). Each lobe bears the name of the bone that lies over it: frontal lobe, parietal lobe, temporal lobe, and occipital lobe.

Each hemisphere of the cerebrum consists of external gray matter, internal white matter, and islands of internal gray matter. The cerebral cortex is the thin surface layer of the cerebrum, composed of gray matter only 2 to 4 mm (roughly 1/12 to 1/6 inch) thick. Presumably, when early anatomists observed the outer darker layer of the cerebrum, it reminded them of tree bark—hence their choice of the name "cortex" (Latin for "bark").

The cerebrum performs three kinds of functions: sensory functions, motor functions, and a group of activities less easily named and even less easily defined or explained. "Intergrative functions" is one name for them. What most of us think of as mental activities are part, but not all, of the cerebrum's integrative functions. Consciousness, memory, use of language, and emotions are important integrative cerebral functions.

Very little is known about the neural mechanisms that produce consciousness. One known fact, however, is that consciousness depends on excitation of the cerebral cortex by impulses conducted to it through the brain stem reticular activating system. Without continual excitation of cortical neurons by reticular activating impulses, a person is unconscious and cannot be aroused (Fig. 11-5).

Meninges. Because the brain and spinal cord are both delicate and vital, nature has provided them with two protective coverings. The outer covering consists of bone: cranial bones encase the brain and vertebrae encase the spinal cord. The inner covering consists of membranes known as meninges. Three distinct layers compose the meninges: the dura mater, the arachnoid membrane, and the pia mater. Observe their respective locations in Fig. 11-6. The dura mater, made of strong white fibrous tissue, serves as the outer layer of the meninges and also as the inner periosteum of the cranial bones. The arachnoid membrane, a delicate, cobweblike layer, lies between the dura mater and the pia mater, or innermost layer of the meninges. The transparent pia mater adheres to the outer surface of the brain and contains blood vessels.

Between the dura mater and the arachnoid membrane is a small space called the subdural space, and between the arachoid and the pia mater is the subarachnoid space, which contains cerebrospinal fluid. This fluid serves as a protective cushion around and within the brain and spinal cord.

Fig. 11-4. Right hemisphere of cerebrum, lateral surface. Note the subdivision of the hemisphere into four lobes, each bearing the name of the bone that lies over it.

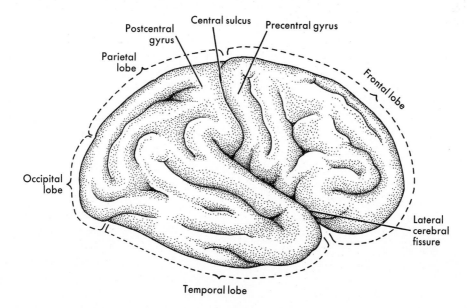

Fig. 11-5. Reticular activating system, consisting of centers in the brain stem reticular formation and fibers that conduct from the centers to widespread areas of the cerebral cortex. Functioning of the reticular activating system is essential for consciousness.

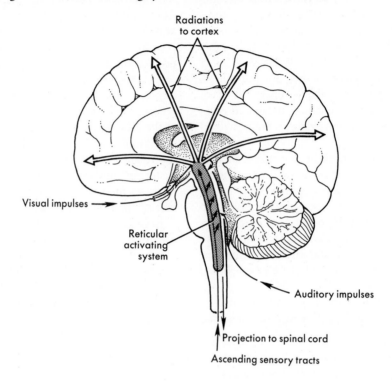

Fig. 11-6. Relationship of meninges to **A,** brain and **B,** spinal cord.
(From McClintic, J.R.: Human anatomy, St. Louis, 1983, The C.V. Mosby Co.)

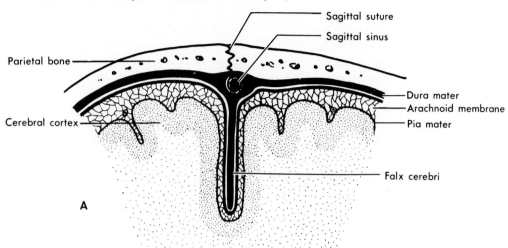

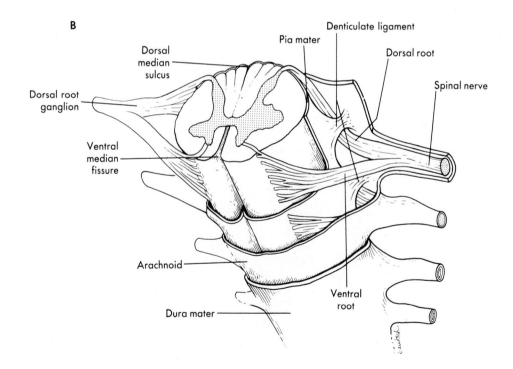

Brain injuries

Injuries to the brain constitute by far the most serious threat to an athlete. These injuries usually result from movement of the brain within the skull. The semisolid brain, surrounded by cerebrospinal fluid, has limited freedom to move about within the skull. Whenever a sudden force or impact is applied to the head, there can be an abrupt change of momentum for the brain, resulting in significant movement of the brain within the skull. This gives rise to the common mechanisms resulting in brain injury (Fig. 11-7).

A sudden forceful impact to the head can cause agitation of the brain, resulting in transient dysfunction (cerebral concussion). The brain may also be injured by direct transmission of force from the skull to the underlying brain tissue. This can result in the brain being contused (cerebral contusion) or lacerated as it impacts the skull. The brain can also be injured as it rebounds against the opposite side of the skull.

This mechanism is called a *contrecoup* injury and is possible due to the movement of the brain within the skull. The extent of the injury to the brain depends on the magnitude and direction of impact, the structural features of the inner skull, and the response of the brain to the force. Any blow to the head may be injurious to the brain. However, a brain injury is not necessarily the result of a single blow; it may be the cumulative effect of a series of blows.

In addition, injuries to the brain can occur as the result of a sudden force, causing tremendous twisting or swirling of the cerebral hemispheres within the skull. This can also result in cerebral contusions and lacerations as the moving hemispheres are raked over bony irregularities inside the skull. The twisting or swirling motion of the cerebral hemispheres can also cause a temporary malfunction of the brain stem. Consciousness depends on the interaction between the cerebral hemispheres and the upper brain stem. The

Fig. 11-7. Common mechanisms resulting in brain injury. A sudden impact to the head can cause *A,* shaking of the brain, *B,* direct transmission of force to the underlying brain tissue, *C,* contrecoup mechanism, or *D,* twisting or swirling of the cerebral hemispheres on the brain stem.

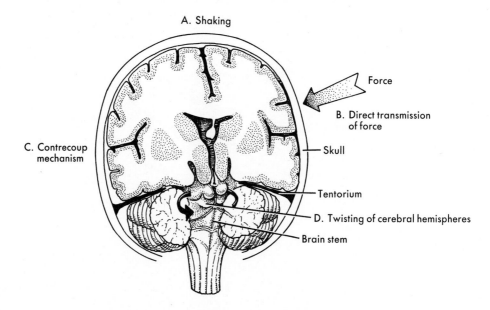

brain stem is not as free to move as the hemispheres, and the twisting motion can cause an interruption of neural functions of the reticular activating system (center of consciousness). This can result in a loss of consciousness for a brief moment to an extended period of time, depending on the severity of injury. Normally this does not result in permanent damage, and the brain stem recovers rapidly (brain stem concussion). However, a severe blow resulting in remarkable twisting of the brain stem may cause prolonged unconsciousness and tissue disruption (brain stem contusion) and hemorrhage from which the brain stem may not completely recover. The important signs to recognize during evaluation of injuries to the head will be discussed in more detail with each injury.

Concussion. There is no general agreement as to the exact definition of a concussion. A *concussion* appears to be a syndrome involving an immediate and transient impairment in the ability of the brain to function properly. It is usually caused by a direct blow to the head, as previously described. There have been various attempts to classify concussions by severity according to their accompanying signs and symptoms. A subcommittee of the American Medical Association Committee on the Medical Aspects of Sports classified concussions into the following three degrees of severity.

A *mild cerebral concussion* (first degree) is caused by a mild blow to the head, resulting in an agitation of the brain. The symptoms include no loss of consciousness. There may be momentary mental confusion, possible memory loss, a mild ringing in the ears *(tinnitus),* mild dizziness, and headache. There is usually no lack of coordination or unsteadiness. The athlete normally recovers quickly, with no residual symptoms. However, the athlete should be watched closely for any signs of changing orientation or additional postconcussion symptoms.

A *moderate cerebral concussion* (second degree) is caused by a blow of moderate intensity that results in a loss of consciousness lasting less than 5 minutes. This is usually followed by slight mental confusion and a temporary loss of memory (amnesia). Amnesia may take the form of *retrograde amnesia,* in which there is a loss of memory for events that occurred before the injury, or *anterograde amnesia,* in which there is a loss of memory for events occurring immediately after awakening. Dizziness, tinnitus, unsteadiness, blurred vision, double vision, nausea, and headache are also common symptoms and may be experienced in varying combinations.

The athlete usually recovers within 5 minutes but may have symptoms lasting several weeks. Athletes suffering moderate concussions should be referred to a physician for further evaluation and follow-up care. It is important that these athletes are closely observed for 24 hours for any changes or complications.

A *severe cerebral concussion* (third degree) is caused by a blow of severe intensity that results in a prolonged loss of consciousness (over 5 minutes). This is usually followed by prolonged retrograde amnesia, mental confusion, severe tinnitus, dizziness, headache, and marked unsteadiness. The recovery rate is slow and characterized by the presence of symptoms. This athlete must be referred to a physician.

Normally an athlete who has suffered a concussion will improve rapidly to an alert state of consciousness. The greatest concern for anyone who is responsible for caring for the athlete with a head injury is the possible development of an expanding intracranial lesion. The signs and symptoms of an athlete suffering from a concussion are reversible and will appear to be worse on the initial evaluation and then improve. If the signs and symptoms become progressively worse, it suggests that there is an expanding lesion within the cranium. For example, a neurologic assessment of an athlete who has a concussion should not reveal abnormalities in pupil size, movements, reflexes, sensations, strength, or respirations. Any deterioration in these neurologic signs indicate additional intracranial involvement, such as hemorrhaging or swelling. The neurologic evaluations are discussed in more detail later in this chapter as part of the assessment procedures.

Contusion. Contusions, or bruising of the brain, results when the brain impacts against the skull or is raked over bony irregularities, especially on the floor of the skull. Contusions to the hemispheres may result in a lack of nerve function of the bruised portion of the brain, but usually will not result in a loss of consciousness. Signs that suggest an athlete may have a cerebral contusion are any numbness, weakness, loss of memory, *aphasia* (loss of speech or comprehension), or general misbehavior when he or she is alert. An athlete with a cerebral contusion also remains stable or begins improving. Any deterioration suggests additional intracranial involvement.

Hemorrhage. Intracranial hemorrhaging is a potentially life-threatening consequence of a head injury. Hemorrhaging can lead to rapid deterioration of the athlete's condition and must be recognized if death or disability is to be averted. The same sudden forces that may result in concussion or contusion (to any area) of the brain may also cause blood vessel damage and hemorrhaging. The hemorrhaging forms a hematoma, which may continue to enlarge after the injury. Hematomas are classified as to their location within the skull.

A *subdural hematoma* develops when bridging cerebral vessels that travel from the brain to the overlying dura are torn. This condition is the most frequent cause of death from trauma in athletics. Rupturing of cerebral vessels can occur as a result of the twisting motion of the cerebral hemispheres or the stretching of these vessels on the side opposite the point of impact. Hemorrhaging can result in low-pressure venous bleeding or rapid arterial bleeding into the subdural space. The signs and symptoms of a subdural hematoma will vary, depending on the type of hemorrhaging. They may occur in rapid progression or may not be evident for hours or days following the injury.

An *epidural hematoma* develops when a dural artery is ruptured. Usually this hematoma is associated with a skull fracture, and it is commonly caused by a tear of the middle meningeal artery. The bleeding is between the dura mater and the skull. The clot formation is usually

Fig. 11-8. Hematoma causing increased intracranial pressure and shifting of the cerebral hemispheres away from the bleeding. Note the expanding pressure on the third cranial (occulomotor) nerve. This can result in a dilated pupil on that side of the head.

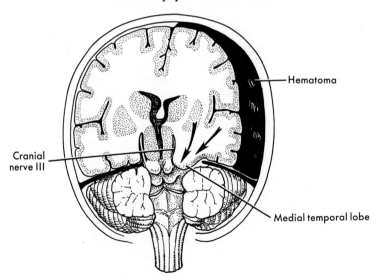

rapid, and signs and symptoms may occur in a matter of minutes to hours. An *intracerebral hematoma* develops when blood vessels within the brain are damaged. This may occur when a cerebral contusion is accompanied by significant bleeding.

Each of these hematomas can cause an increase in intracranial pressure and shifting of the hemispheres away from the hematoma (Fig. 11-8). This accounts for the deteriorating neurologic signs and symptoms, such as a decreasing level of consciousness, loss of movements, slowing of pupil reactions or a dilating pupil. It cannot be overemphasized how important it is for an athletic trainer to continue to evaluate an athlete suffering a head injury for neurologic signs that may indicate hemorrhaging and an expanding lesion within the cranium. Failure to do so can result in unnecessary death or disability for the athlete.

ATHLETIC INJURY ASSESSMENT PROCESS

As previously stated, head injuries are potentially the most serious athletic injuries. Although fatalities in sports are relatively rare, injuries to the head account for more fatalities than injuries to any other area of the body. Permanently disabling brain damage resulting from athletic activity is also rare. However, injuries to the brain do occur, and no head injury should be treated lightly. Anyone who has the responsibility of caring for athletic injuries should plan and prepare for devastating injuries. Head injuries can produce a wide array of complex symptoms, and correct assessment procedures by the athletic trainer are extremely important.

Primary survey

The importance of maintaining airway, breathing, and circulation has been discussed previously. These important steps of basic life support can never be neglected with any athletic injury. Always check and continue to monitor an athlete's airway, breathing, and circulation throughout the assessment process to recognize

and correct any life-threatening problems. Whenever an injured athlete is responsive, the primary survey can be completed quickly and with little difficulty.

Secondary survey

In evaluating an athlete with a head injury, it is extremely important to establish a neurologic baseline. This baseline gives the athletic trainer and the physician a point of reference. If the athlete improves from this baseline, there is a good chance that there is no additional intracranial involvement. Remember that intracranial involvement may take a period of time to develop. An athlete may appear to be doing fine immediately after an injury and then develop signs and symptoms hours later. An important aspect of the assessment of a head-injured athlete is the manner in which physical signs and symptoms progress. This is why it is important to do repeated evaluations over a period of time with an athlete who suffers an injury to the head. Physical changes are only appreciated if the athlete's initial status is evaluated and documented. When an athlete's condition deteriorates from the original neurologic baseline, it suggests additional intracranial involvement; he or she must be referred for medical assistance. This baseline information is extremely important to the physician who must diagnose the severity of injury after referral. It is, unfortunately, often neglected in the rush to get an injured athlete to medical assistance. Neurologic information should always be written down and reported to the physician. In reporting your evaluations, it is better to describe your findings in functional language. For example, to use a term such as "lethargic" is subject to misinterpretations. It is better to report the athlete's actions or behavior; for example, "the athlete responded accurately to verbal commands but would then fall asleep."

Whenever the trauma is sufficient enough to cause a head injury, remember that there may be an associated neck injury. Always handle the athlete with a head injury as though he or she has a cervical spine injury until proved otherwise. This includes protecting the injured athlete from any unnecessary movement during the assessment process. If movement of the athlete is necessary for any reason, absolute control of the head is essential.

Much information can be gained by performing a secondary survey on an athlete who has suffered an injury to the head. Throughout the evaluation process, look for signs and symptoms that may indicate the athlete has an expanding intracranial lesion or cervical spine involvement. Whenever any of these signs are recognized, it is not necessary to continue the assessment. It is time to seek medical assistance for the athlete. This point must be remembered and cannot be overemphasized.

History

It is vital to get a precise history for those injuries involving the head. Gain as much information surrounding the circumstances of the injury as possible. Attempt to determine the mechanism of injury and direction of force. Was there a loss of consciousness? Did the athlete have a seizure? Does the athlete have any medical problems that may be associated with the injury? Details of the injury, as well as specific time intervals between any changing clinical signs, should be recorded because this information is invaluable for diagnosis. Obtain as much information as possible from the injured athlete. Many symptoms may not be volunteered by the injured athlete but must be actively sought through questioning. If the athlete cannot remember or is stuporous or uncooperative, attempt to obtain information from anyone who witnessed the injury.

Level of consciousness. Establishing and monitoring the level of consciousness is the most important neurologic sign to be gained during the assessment of a head injury. Question the athlete in an attempt to evaluate the level of alertness, responsiveness, awareness, and orientation. Begin by checking the athlete's awareness to person, place, and time. Can the athlete answer simple questions such as "What is your name?"

"Where are you?" "How old are you?" "Do you know who I am?" Then ask the athlete questions that require more thought, such as "What do you do on a certain play?" Questioning along this line may require the assistance of a coach or another player who is aware of the correct answers. Also evaluate the athlete's memory. Can the athlete remember the events leading up to the injury? What was the first recollection following the injury? The severity of the injury is many times proportional to the lack of memory; that is, the longer the period of amnesia, the greater the injury to the brain.

Note the level of consciousness of the injured athlete and then ascertain any subsequent changes. In most instances the athlete's level of consciousness will improve in a short period of time. If the athlete regains consciousness quickly, the prognosis for a rapid and uneventful recovery is good. If the athlete regains consciousness slowly, the prognosis is more guarded. The athlete who shows minimal or very slow improvement should be referred to a physician or medical facility. A decrease in the level of consciousness is the most sensitive indicator of additional intracranial involvement; anytime the level of consciousness deteriorates, immediate medical attention is indicated.

Headache. Headache is another frequent symptom of a head injury, and an important consideration that should be discussed while talking with an injured athlete. A headache that becomes progressively more severe is an alarming symptom that may indicate additional intracranial involvement. The persistence of a headache indicates that whatever damage occurred to the brain has not subsided, and the athlete should not return to activity. The cessation of the headache is probably the most reliable indicator that adequate recovery has occurred and the athlete can return to activity, providing also that there are no other positive neurologic signs. As you periodically check on the health status of an athlete who has suffered an injury to the head, remember to question the athlete about his or her headache.

In addition to the mechanism of injury, level of consciousness, and headache, you should attempt to gain further information during the history portion of the assessment process. Question the athlete about his or her feelings concerning the head and neck. Is there any pain in the neck? Does the athlete feel any numbness, weakness, or tingling? Does the athlete complain of any ringing in the ears (tinnitus), dizziness, nausea, or blurred or double vision? All this information is important in establishing a neurologic baseline and should be obtained by talking with the injured athlete. In addition, question the athlete about any other painful or tender areas of the body that may require further evaluation.

Observation

An athlete suffering from a head injury requires close observation throughout the assess-

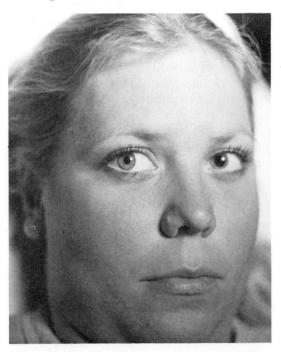

Fig. 11-9. Athlete exhibiting a dilated pupil following trauma to the head.

ment process. Watch the athlete carefully as you carry out the history-taking procedures. Notice if the athlete has any difficulty in finding or saying the right words or understanding commands *(aphasia)*. Check for any obvious deformities or abnormal positions of any body parts. Notice if the athlete attempts any movements of the head, neck, or extremities. Does the athlete demonstrate any weakness or paralysis? Watch for neurologic signs that may indicate the existence of expanding intracranial pressure, such as pupillary signs, irregular respirations, seizures, or a decreasing level of consciousness.

Pupils. It is important to check the quality and reaction of the pupils. Both pupils should be symmetric in size and react quickly and equally to light. When one pupil becomes larger and shows a decreased response to light, there is strong evidence for increased intracranial pressure. The athlete should be referred to a physician (Fig. 11-9). Also observe the eye movements. Normally the eyes gaze straight ahead, unless focused on something. The movement of the eyes should be coordinated; with a head injury, the gaze may be abnormal, or the eyes may turn in different directions. Any abnormal, uncoordinated, or involuntary movement of the eyes may indicate intracranial involvement. If the athlete is conscious, instruct him or her to follow your finger with the eyes and notice whether eye movement is paralyzed or decreased in any direction. For example, an athlete with a fracture of the orbit is usually not able to look upward as far on the fractured side. Involuntary rapid movement of the eyeballs in any direction *(nystagmus)* is another indication of intracranial involvement.

Respirations. Observe the respiratory rate and pattern. A normal respiratory pattern suggests that there is no apparent brain damage, at least at that time. Abnormal breathing patterns may indicate severe brain dysfunction and the need for medical assistance. These abnormal respiratory patterns are discussed in Chapter 10 and outlined in Table 10-1 on page 222.

Signs of trauma. Look for any signs of trauma,

which can give important clues as to the nature and severity of the injury. Examine the head, neck, and face for any deformities, lacerations, contusions, or hemorrhaging. Cuts and bruises are reliable signs that strong forces have been applied to the athlete's head. Watch for any discharge coming from the ears or nose. Look for any unusual or abnormal positions of any part of the body, which may indicate any additional injuries.

Palpation

Much of the information necessary to establish a neurologic baseline will be gained during the history and observation portion of the assessment process. However, once the injured athlete is stable, additional information can be gained through gentle palpation.

Pulse. It is important to evaluate the rate and nature of the pulse in an athlete who has suffered an injury to the head. The pulse should be felt periodically during the evaluation. Remember, the development of an unusually slow heart rate

after the athlete has calmed down may be another sign of increasing intracranial involvement.

Signs of trauma. Along with observing the head and neck for signs of trauma, you can also palpate these areas. Gently feel any painful areas indicated by the athlete for deformities, irregularities, tenderness, or swelling (Fig. 11-10). By carefully cupping your hand under the neck, the cervical spinous processes can be palpated with your fingertips to detect any localized deformity or pain. Tenderness or increased pain over these spinous processes is sufficient reason to suspect an associated cervical spine injury. The athlete should be handled appropriately.

Stress

Some stress movements by the injured athlete may be necessary to determine if there is associated spinal cord involvement. This is discussed further in the next chapter and should not be attempted until the steps of history, observation, and palpation have been carried out and you have some indication of the nature and severity of the injury. If the signs and symptoms already observed indicate a possible increasing intracranial lesion or spinal cord involvement, it is not necessary to subject the athlete to any movement or manipulation. Instead the athlete should be immediately protected from further trauma and referred to a physician or medical facility.

As an athlete recovers from a head injury, there are a few activities you can have the athlete perform to evaluate and monitor progress. One example would be coordination exercises. Have the athlete touch one knee with the opposite heel with the eyes closed (Fig. 11-11, *A*). Have the athlete touch the nose or ear with each index finger while the eyes are closed (Fig. 11-11, *B*). Repeat these maneuvers with increasing speed. Have the athlete touch each finger with the thumb of the same hand as rapidly as possible. Normally an athlete should be able to perform each of these maneuvers easily and quickly. Anything less than this indicates prolonged involve-

Fig. 11-10. Palpating the head and neck for signs of trauma.

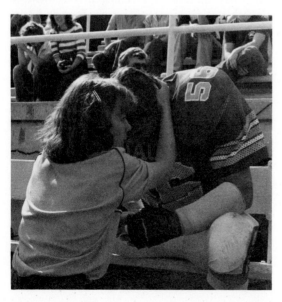

Fig. 11-11. Athlete performing coordination exercises: **A,** touching knee with opposite heel and **B,** touching nose with index finger while eyes are closed.

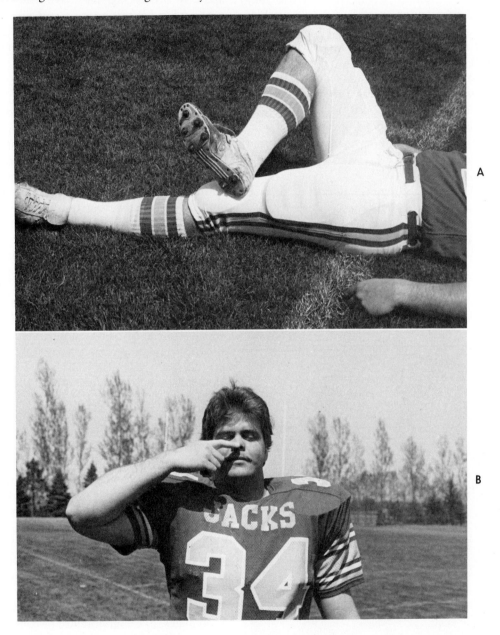

ment, and the athletic trainer should continue to monitor the athlete. Another activity that may be used to monitor an athlete is to have him or her stand with arms outstretched and eyes closed. If there is a tendency for one of the arms to drift outward and downward, it may indicate an expanding intracranial lesion on the side of the brain opposite the weak arm. An additional test often used on an athlete following a head injury is a check for a positive *Romberg's sign*. This is accomplished by having the athlete stand with his or her feet together, arms at the side, and eyes closed (Fig. 11-12). Normally a person can stand still in this position, but a tendency to sway or fall to one side is a positive Romberg's sign, which indicates continued intracranial involvement.

Fig. 11-12. Athlete performing Romberg's test. The ability to maintain correct posture while standing with feet together, arms at the side and eyes closed is interpreted as negative.

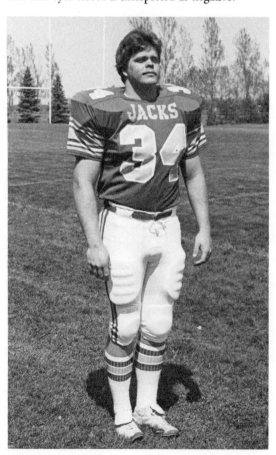

Evaluation of findings

Because of the potential seriousness of trauma to the head, athletic trainers must be able to recognize the signs and symptoms that may indicate severe injury. Failure to do so may result in permanent damage, paralysis, or even death to the athlete. Serious head injuries occur infrequently in athletics, but the mechanism for a catastrophic injury is present in most athletic activities.

The importance of the information gained during the assessment of a head injury cannot be overemphasized. This information indicates what emergency care should be provided for the athlete and provides clues to the nature and severity of the injury. This information also establishes the neurologic baseline for the physician's diagnosis and treatment plan and must be passed along whenever the injured athlete is referred to a physician.

When to refer the athlete

The athlete with an injury to the head, whose physical signs continue to improve or appear normal, may be handled by the athletic trainer. Remember that intracranial involvement may develop over a period of time. Repeated evaluations must be performed to note the progression of physical signs and symptoms associated with a head injury. If the athlete is not referred to a physician, it is important to inform someone who will be with the athlete for a period of time after the injury, such as the parents or roommates, of the importance of continued observation. It is a good idea to give this person a list of signs to watch for. This list should include information concerning the nature of the injury, the physical signs that may indicate an expanding intracranial lesion, and what to do or who to notify should these signs develop. A sample watch list is presented below.

Physical signs indicating that an athlete with a head injury should be referred to a physician for additional assessment and treatment are critically important. The list of conditions at right, should they appear, require that the athlete be referred to medical assistance.

FACE INJURIES

Although head and facial trauma may occur simultaneously, facial injuries are discussed separately because of the importance of recognizing trauma to the head. The remainder of this chapter discusses the anatomy for each area of the face, the common injuries or conditions that may result from athletic activity, and the associ-

1. Rapid loss of consciousness or progressive development of coma
2. Prolonged mental confusion
3. Prolonged amnesia
4. Increasing headache
5. Unequal size of pupils or their failure to react to light
6. Uncoordinated or involuntary movement of the eyes
7. Abnormal breathing patterns
8. Signs about the head indicating possible skull fracture (clear fluid or blood coming from the ears, Battle's sign, racoon eyes, skull depressions)
9. Unusual slowing of the heart rate
10. Doubt regarding the presence of an intracranial lesion

SOUTH DAKOTA STATE UNIVERSITY TRAINING ROOM

This is a medical follow-up sheet for your health and safety. Quite often signs of head injury do not appear immediately after trauma but hours after the injury itself. The purpose of this fact sheet is to alert you to the symptoms of significant head injuries, symptoms that may occur several hours after you leave the training room.

If you experience one or more of the following symptoms following a head injury, medical help should be sought.

1. Difficulty remembering recent events or meaningful facts.
2. Severe headache, particularly at a specific location.
3. Stiffening of the neck.
4. Bleeding or clear fluid dripping from the ears or nose.
5. Mental confusion or strangeness.
6. Nausea or vomiting.
7. Dizziness, poor balance or unsteadiness.
8. Weakness in either arm or leg.
9. Abnormal drowsiness or sleepiness.
10. Convulsions.
11. Unequal pupils.
12. Loss of appetite.
13. Persistent ringing of the ears.
14. Slurring of speech.

The appearance of any of the above symptoms tells you that you have had a significant head injury that *requires medical attention*. If any of the symptoms appear, contact J. Booher or B. Moran or Dr. B. Lushbough or report to the Brookings Hospital Emergency Room.

REMEMBER: Your health depends on how much you care about proper medical attention.

THE SDSU ATHLETIC TRAINING STAFF

ated signs and symptoms an athletic trainer should recognize during the assessment process.

Facial injuries are fairly common in athletic activity. However, their frequency and severity have declined in recent years, as more sports are requiring the use of protective devices such as mouth guards, eye guards, ear guards, and face masks. Athletes in many sports, however, have no protection for the face, and a variety of facial injuries can occur. The most common are contusions, abrasions, and lacerations of the skin.

These injuries are treated much as they would be if located anywhere else on the body; however, the need for optimal cosmetic results demands careful evaluation and care. Remember, any facial injury is indicative of trauma to the head, which can also result in injuries to the brain or spinal cord. Because of the great vascularity of the face, profuse bleeding can result in dramatic-appearing injuries (Fig. 11-13). Do not concentrate on facial trauma to the exclusion of possible associated injuries to the head or neck, which may be more serious.

ATHLETIC INJURY ASSESSMENT CHECKLIST
HEAD INJURIES

Primary survey

———— Responsiveness
———— Airway
———— Breathing
———— Circulation

Secondary survey

———— History
 ———— Mechanism of injury
 ———— Level of consciousness
 ———— Headache
 ———— Pain
 ———— Sensations (numbness, weakness, paralysis, tinnitus, dizziness, nausea, blurred or double vision)
———— Observation
 ———— Aphasia
 ———— Obvious deformities
 ———— Position and alignment
 ———— Movement in extremities
 ———— Pupil equality and symmetry
 ———— Eye movements
 ———— Respiratory rate and pattern
 ———— Signs of trauma
———— Palpation
 ———— Rate and character of pulse
 ———— Signs of trauma (deformities, irregularities, tenderness, or swelling)
———— Stress
 ———— Active motion in extremities
 ———— Coordination exercises
 ———— Romberg's sign

Fig. 11-13. Facial bleeding following forehead laceration.

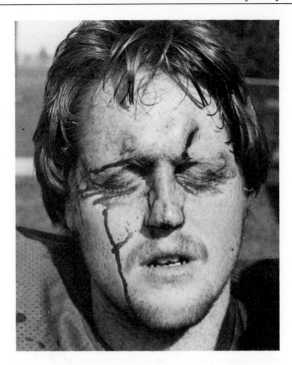

Fig. 11-14. Bony anatomy of the skull, face, and jaw.

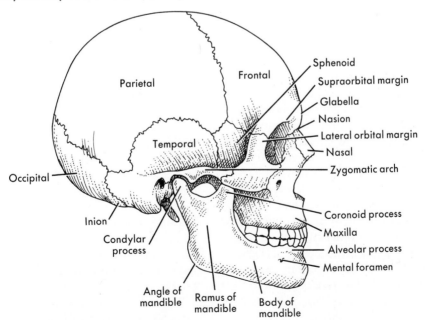

Facial bones

Review the anatomy of the facial bones as described in Chapter 3. Table 3-4 on p. 33 lists and gives a brief description of the 14 bones of the face. Refer to Fig. 11-14 to identify these bones. The facial bones are largely subcutaneous and readily palpable. Identify and note the position of the following bony structures or landmarks on your own face.

1. *Supraorbital margin:* This is the portion of the frontal bone that forms the upper margin, or ridge, over each eye orbit.
2. *Nasion:* This is a depression just above the nose, midway between the two supraorbital margins.
3. *Glabella:* This structure is felt as a prominent ridge of bone just above the nasion.
4. *Lateral orbital margins:* The sharp lateral (outer) margin of each eye orbit formed by the edge of the malar or zygomatic bone.
5. *Zygomatic arch:* This is the prominent portion of the cheek bone. The outline of the arch is easily traced by pressing gently along the undersurface of the orbit. The superficial temporal artery crosses the posterior extremity of this bony landmark. You should be able to feel the pulse at the point where the artery crosses the arch.

Jaw

The jaw is composed of an upper jaw, or maxilla, and a lower jaw, or mandible (Fig. 11-14). The mandible is the only movable bone in the skull and is the largest and strongest of the group. This bone has bony contact with the rest of the skull only at the *temporomandibular* joints and the teeth. The mandible consists of a curved, horseshoe-shaped body and two perpendicular rami that project upward at each end. Each flat ramus is joined to the body at the angle of the mandible. The upper border of the body bears the alveolar border, with 16 dental sockets for the teeth. Each ramus has two bony processes: (1) the posterior condyloid process, or head, that articulates with the undersurface of the skull in the temporomandibular joint, and (2) the ante-

rior coronoid process, which serves as an attachment for muscles. The coronoid process is thin and triangular. The mental foramen can be seen on the external surface of the body of the mandible just below the second premolar tooth on each side.

The temporomandibular joint is the only synovial, or diarthrotic, joint of the skull. The joint lies between the condyloid process of the mandible and the articular fossa on the undersurface of the temporal bone. The articular surfaces of both bones in the joint are covered by a unique type of fibrous (not hyaline) cartilage. A fibrocartilaginous articular disc divides the joint cavity into an upper and lower compartment. Each compartment is surrounded by a synovial membrane. You can palpate the joint by placing your finger just in front of the ear as you open and close the mouth.

The temporomandibular joint is enclosed in a thin, loose articular capsule that is weakly reinforced by support ligaments. The mandible can be elevated, depressed, protruded, retracted, and moved from side to side.

Jaw injuries

Injuries to the jaw normally occur as the result of a direct blow. Fractures to the mandible are more common than fractures to the maxilla or dislocations of the temporomandibular joint. The most common fracture of the mandible is near the angle of the lower jaw. Any contusion or suspected fracture of the mandible should be carefully palpated along the body to determine areas of point tenderness, swelling, or deformity. If there is no obvious deformity or abnormal movement observed, ask the athlete to open and close his or her mouth and appose the teeth. Does the jaw open and close normally on both sides? Do the teeth line up correctly? Palpate the temporomandibular joint as the athlete moves the jaw. If there is malocclusion of the teeth or increased pain on movement, the athlete should be referred to a physician for further assessment.

The most common fracture to the upper jaw involves the zygoma, or cheekbone. So-called tripod fractures of the cheekbone result from blunt trauma to the cheek or side of the face. If the zygomatic arch is fractured, the cheek will be depressed. In assessing potential facial injury, the athletic trainer should always look down over the forehead from behind the athlete (Fig. 11-15). Subtle differences in symmetry, indicating fracture, are often more apparent when the face is viewed from above and behind. Palpation of the involved bone can help supplement the overhead inspection, as tenderness and crepitus are common with zygomatic fractures.

A dislocation of the temporomandibular joint does not occur very often in athletic activity. However, when it does occur, it is normally the result of a blow to the side of the jaw with the mouth open. Uncomplicated dislocation of the jaw occurs only in a forward direction. Upward dislocation can only occur in association with

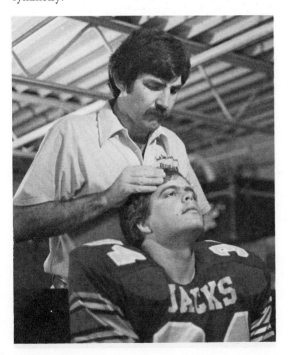

Fig. 11-15. Looking over the forehead of an athlete to note any subtle differences in symmetry.

extensive fracture of the base of the skull, and backward dislocation with smashing of the bony portion of the auditory canal, which lies immediately behind the joint. The major signs to recognize in a temporomandibular joint dislocation are loss of jaw movement and malocclusion of the teeth. These athletes should be referred to a physician for reduction.

Nose

The nose consists of an external and an internal portion. The external portion, the part that protrudes from the face, consists of a bony and cartilaginous framework overlaid by skin that contains many sebaceous glands. The two nasal bones meet at the nasion, where they are surrounded by the frontal bone to form the root of the nose. The nasal bones are surrounded by the maxilla laterally and inferiorly at the base of the nose. The flaring cartilaginous expansion forming the outer side of each nostril is called the *ala*.

The fact that the skin of the external nose contains many sebaceous glands has great clinical significance. If these glands become blocked, it is possible for infectious material to pass from facial veins in the area to the intracranial cavernous sinus. For this reason, the triangular zone surrounding the external nose is often known as the "danger area of the face."

The internal nose, or nasal cavity, lies over the roof of the mouth and is divided into right left cavities by a midline nasal septum. The nasal septum is made up of three structures: the perpendicular plate of the ethmoid bone above, the vomer bone, and the nasal cartilage below. The septum is frequently deviated to one side or the other, interfering with respiration and with drainage of the nose and sinuses.

Each nasal cavity communicates with the outside through the nostril, or anterior nares, and opens into the nasopharynx behind through the posterior nares. The nasal cavity also communicates with the middle ear through the eustachian tube and with the paranasal air sinuses—frontal, maxillary, sphenoid, and ethmoid—through their respective orifices. Communication with the conjunctiva of the eye exists through the nasolacrimal duct. These extensive relations of the nasal cavity are important in the spread of infection.

The roof of the nose is separated from the cranial cavity by a portion of the ethmoid bone called the *cribriform plate*. The cribriform plate is perforated by many small openings, which permit branches of the olfactory nerve responsible for the special sense of smell to enter the cranial cavity and reach the brain.

Separation of the nasal and cranial cavities by a thin, perforated plate of bone presents real hazards. If the cribriform plate is damaged as a result of trauma to the nose, it is possible for potentially infectious material to pass directly from the nasal cavity into the cranial fossa. If fragments of a fractured nasal bone are pushed through the cribriform plate and tear the dura, cerebrospinal rhinorrhea can result.

There are five paranasal air sinuses in the skull that communicate directly with the nose. The *frontal sinuses,* which are located inside the frontal bone, are perhaps the most important from the standpoint of potential for complications following a skull fracture. Note the close rela-

tionship of the frontal lobe of the brain to the wall of the frontal sinus (Fig. 11-16).

A skull fracture involving the sinus may tear the dura and injure the brain. If this should occur, a passageway is formed that will permit exchange of air and cerebrospinal fluid between the brain and nasal cavity. Air that enters and becomes trapped in the brain produces a condition called **pneumocephalus** (Fig. 11-16). As discussed previously, discharge of cerebrospinal fluid from the nose is called cerebrospinal rhinorrhea and is cause for immediate referral to a physician or medical facility.

Nose injuries

Nosebleeds (epistaxis). Hemorrhage from the nose is common in athletic facial injuries. Nosebleeds rarely become serious enough to jeopardize the life of the athlete. Because the nasal cavity is a bony space, even serious hemorrhage can usually be controlled by packing the cavity with gauze or cotton and applying pressure to the nostril of the bleeding side (Fig. 11-17). Cold compresses can also be applied to the nasal area in an attempt to constrict the blood vessels. Nosebleeds occur most often as a result of sep-

Fig. 11-16. Skull fracture involving the frontal sinus. Solid arrows indicate path of air, resulting in pneumocephalus; broken arrows indicate path of cerebrospinal fluid, resulting in cerebrospinal rhinorrhea.

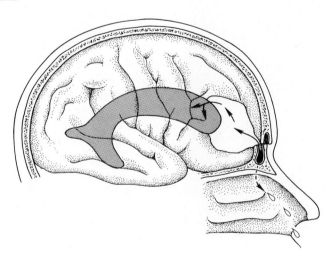

tal contusions caused by a direct blow to the nose.

Occasionally, the presence of insects or debris in the nose will produce inflammation or irritation and subsequent hemorrhage. If the presence of foreign bodies in the nose is suspected, the nasal interior should be examined and the athlete instructed to gently blow his or her nose while the unaffected nostril is pinched shut. If this does not rid the nostril of the foreign body, the athlete should be referred to a physician. Violently blowing the nose or probing for the foreign body may cause increased irritation.

Nasal fractures. The two nasal bones are the most frequently fractured bones in the face. Nasal fractures result from a blow to the nose; bleeding may be profuse and must be controlled. It is best to evaluate the nose as soon after injury as possible. Swelling is likely to occur, and once the area becomes swollen, important signs indicating a nasal fracture may be masked.

Fig. 11-17. Applying pressure to control a nosebleed.

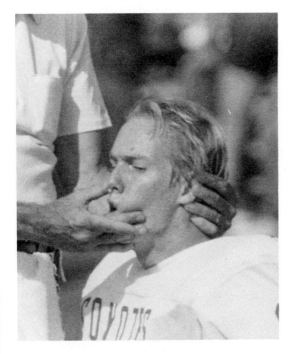

Begin the evaluation by carefully observing the nasal area for any deformity. A nasal fracture should be suspected with any abnormal deviation of the nose. Whenever there is a question about the abnormal deviation of an injured nose, it is a good practice to allow the athlete to view his or her nose in a mirror to evaluate the normal alignment and contour. Another method used to observe for any deviation is to view the injured nose by looking down the forehead and across the bridge of the nose when standing behind the athlete, as previously discussed.

If obvious abnormal deviation is not present, the injured area should be gently palpated. Carefully feel the two nasal bones between your thumb and forefingers to locate the areas of pain and tenderness. Palpation may also reveal deformity, increased mobility, or crepitation. All obvious and suspected nasal fractures should be referred to a physician promptly for further evaluation and reduction of the fracture.

Ear

As an organ of special sense the ear is both the organ of hearing and balance or equilibrium. It is divided into three parts (Fig. 11-18).

1. The external ear, consisting of (1) auricle, or pinna; (2) external auditory canal, or meatus, and (3) the tympanic membrane, or eardrum.
2. The middle ear cavity, containing (1) the ear ossicles and (2) the opening of the eustachian tube, which permits equalization of pressure on both sides of the eardrum.
3. The inner ear containing (1) the semicircular canals involved in maintenance of balance (equilibrium) and (2) the cochlea, which is the sensory organ for the perception of sound.

The visible part of the external ear is called the auricle, or pinna (Fig. 11-19). Except for the ear lobe, which is composed of connective tissue and fat, the auricle consists of fibroelastic cartilage with a very thin layer of tightly adhered and sensitive skin. It is important to realize that there is little or no subcutaneous tissue between the

Fig. 11-18. Components of the ear. Note in particular the external ear, consisting of the auricle (pinna), external auditory canal, and tympanic membrane (eardrum).

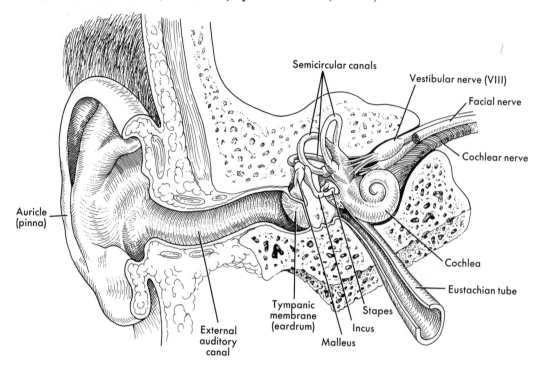

Fig. 11-19. The external ear, showing the component parts of the auricle (pinna).

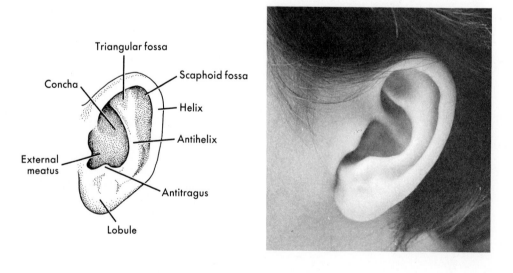

cartilaginous plates of the external ear and the overlying skin. As a result, there is no room between the skin and underlying cartilage to permit diffuse accumulation of tissue fluid or blood after an injury. Deformity occurs as blood or fluid accumulates in very localized areas.

The auditory canal, or meatus, is a tubelike structure about 1 1/4 inches long. It extends from the auricle into the temporal bone of the skull. The outer (lateral) third of the tube is cartilaginous, and the inner (medial) two thirds is bony. The canal terminates internally at the tympanic membrane, or eardrum. The skin that lines the canal is tightly adherent and very thin over the inner bony part, but is thicker over the outer cartilaginous portion, where it contains hair and sebaceous and ceruminous (wax) glands. It is in the outer portion of the tube that infections are most likely to occur, involving the sebaceous glands or hair cells.

The auditory canal is not a straight tube; the bony portion is directed downward and forward. This anatomic fact explains why it is necessary to draw the auricle upward and backward in order to align the cartilaginous portion with the nonmovable bony portion. When the canal

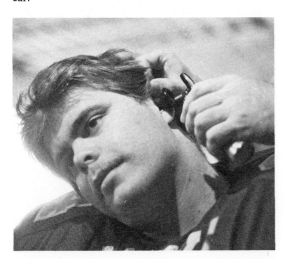

Fig. 11-20. Using an otoscope to examine an ear.

is straightened out it is possible to inspect its entire length for lacerations, foreign bodies such as insects, excess cerumen (wax), and infections. An otoscope is used to examine the auditory canal and eardrum (Fig. 11-20) and is used by some athletic trainers working under the supervision of a physician.

Ear injuries

Sports-related ear injuries are limited almost invariably to the components of the external ear. However, symptoms involving the middle and inner ear may be described by an athlete after an injury or sickness. These symptoms include defective hearing, tinnitus, *vertigo* (sensations of movement) or sensations of sudden fullness in the ear. Athletes expressing these symptoms should be referred to a physician or medical facility.

Assessment of the ear for potential injury after any type of head trauma should be a standard component of your examination sequence. You will need good illumination, proper positioning, and physical control of the athlete to complete a detailed assessment in this area. Always begin with palpation and examination of the surrounding mastoid and temporal areas of the skull. Look for ecchymosis, swelling, tenderness, and signs of localized trauma, such as lacerations or deformity.

As you focus your attention on the ear itself, look first for evidence of hemorrhage and carefully inspect the opening into the auditory canal for the presence of a foreign body (Fig. 11-21). If bleeding is noted after an injury, you should always consider the possibility of a basilar or temporal bone skull fracture. Leakage of cerebrospinal fluid (cerebrospinal otorrhea) from the ear following injury necessitates immediate referral. Most bleeding from the external ear is the result of simple canal lacerations. Although sometimes very painful, they are seldom serious.

Cauliflower ear (hematoma auris). Repeated contusions and twisting or friction-type injuries to the external ear, especially in the absence of protective ear guards, may result in a hematoma formation between the skin and underlying cartilage. If the hematoma remains untreated and is allowed to "organize," it becomes fibrotic and results in a *keloid*. A keloid is a raised nodular deformity that can only be removed by surgery. A cauliflower ear is the end result of keloid formation between the skin and underlying cartilage of an injured external ear, generally in the scaphoid fossa or concha areas (Fig. 11-22).

If assessment reveals continued swelling or hemorrhage after initial treatment of an ear injury with a cold pack and compression, the athlete should be referred to a physician. Ear deformity resulting from keloid formation can be avoided by timely aspiration of the hematoma and prompt initiation of compression therapy.

Swimmer's ear (external otitis). External otitis, or swimmer's ear, is a common infection of the external ear in athletes. It can be either bacterial or fungal in origin and is usually associated with prolonged exposure to water. The infection generally involves, at least to some extent, both the auditory canal and auricle. The ear as a whole is tender, and any pressure causes severe pain. The canal is red and swollen. Treatment of swimmer's ear often involves antibiotic therapy and prescription analgesics. Early referral to a physician is recommended.

Eardrum perforations. Traumatic rupture of the tympanic membrane can be caused by the penetration of a sharp object or a sudden blow across the ear. You should also suspect eardrum damage if hemorrhage is noted following a diving or altitude-related sports injury. Such injuries may be characterized by sharp pain, slight

Fig. 11-22. Hematoma auris (cauliflower ear), resulting in keloid formation in the scaphoid fossa (A). B, Onset of hematoma auris following acute trauma.

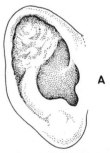

A

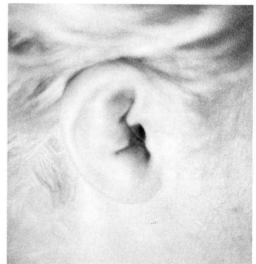

B

Fig. 11-21. Inspecting the external ear and auditory canal.

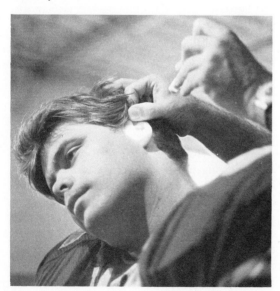

hearing impairment, tinnitus, and slight bleeding. Ruptured eardrums normally heal spontaneously but should be under a physician's care.

Frostbite. Athletes who participate in cold-weather sports are susceptible to frostbite. Superficial facial frostbite generally involves the ears, nose, and cheeks, the ears being particularly susceptible. Symptoms include burning, numbness, tingling, and blanching of the skin.

Teeth

There are 32 permanent teeth in the adult. Each tooth is composed of three main parts: crown, neck, and root (Fig. 11-23). The crown is the exposed portion of the tooth and is covered by enamel. The neck is that portion surrounded by the soft gingiva, or gum tissue. It is the root of each tooth that articulates with the jaw bone in the specialized gomphosis joint described in Chapter 4 (Fig. 4-1).

There are four types of teeth, which are easy to identify by direct inspection or by doing a little exploring with your tongue (Fig. 11-24):

1. *Incisors:* There are four chiseled, wedge-shaped incisors on top and four below.
2. *Canines:* The four canine, or eye teeth, are the longer, sharp teeth found on either side of the incisors; they are particularly prominent above but are found on both upper and lower jaws.
3. *Premolars (bicuspids):* Each premolar, or bicuspid tooth, has two points, or cusps, on the biting surface. There are two premolar teeth on each side, upper and lower, just behind the canines.
4. *Molars (tricuspids):* Each molar, or tricuspid tooth, has three major points (cusps) on the biting surface (Fig. 11-23). There are three molar teeth on each side, top and bottom. The third molars, or wisdom

Fig. 11-23. A molar (tricuspid) tooth sectioned to show its bony socket and details of its three main parts: crown, neck, and root.

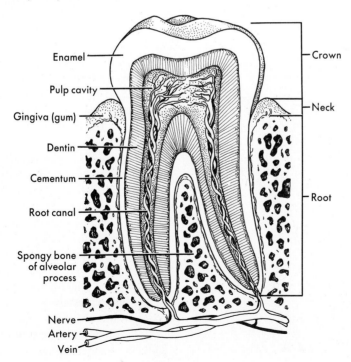

teeth, usually erupt between the ages of 16 and 23 and often come in twisted or misaligned.

Teeth injuries

Acquiring accurate and complete dental information should be an important goal of the preseason assessment process. Knowing about an athlete's dental crowns, bridges, and other appliances such as partial dentures before an injury occurs will greatly facilitate rapid assessment and treatment of an obstructed airway should these structures enter the respiratory passages following a facial injury.

Any tooth that is knocked out intact should be saved, cleaned, and either put back into the socket or transported with the athlete to a dentist as soon as possible. Many times the tooth can be saved by quick reimplantation. If a tooth has been chipped, cracked, or broken off, the athlete should be referred to a dentist. These conditions usually do not require a quick referral unless there is severe pain associated with them. Teeth that have been loosened but remain in place need no further treatment unless there is much discomfort in biting. The athlete may express a sensitivity to biting or to extremes of temperature for a short period of time after the injury. Encourage athletes to seek treatment of damaged teeth, as this may save teeth from being lost or subject to more extensive dental work.

Eye

The external structures visible in an anterior view of the eye are shown in Fig. 11-25. The structures of the eyelids and globe of the eye are illustrated in Figs. 11-26 and 11-27. As you view a person's eye from the front you see only a portion of the whole structure. Note in Fig. 11-25 that the upper lid will normally cover a small portion of the colored *iris* when the eyes are open. The space between the upper and lower lid margins is called the *palpebral fissure.* This distance should be equal in both eyes. The eyelids, or palpebrae, consist of voluntary muscle fibers and fat with a ridge of connective tissue, the *tarsal plate,* at the free edge. The overlying skin is very thin, with the eyelashes distributed evenly along the lid edges. A localized, painful infection of the small glands or hair follicles around the eyelashes at the lid margins is called a *sty* (Fig. 11-28).

A specialized membrane, the *conjuctiva,* lines the eyelids and covers the white (sclera) portion of the eyeball in front. Note in Fig. 11-27 that this membrane is divided into two portions: the shiny-pink *palpebral* portion that recesses into the superior and inferior fornix under the lids, and the *bulbar* portion over the eye itself. The bulbar portion is transparent but looks white because of the sclera below it.

Tiny blood vessels in the conjunctiva often become noticeable after periods of sleeplessness or stress. They often rupture in such situations, producing a small *subconjunctival hemorrhage.*

Fig. 11-24. The 32 permanent teeth.

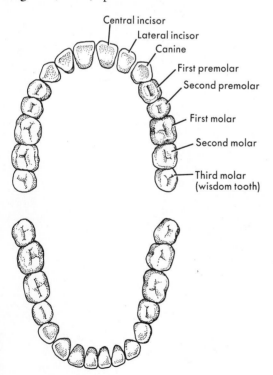

Central incisor
Lateral incisor
Canine
First premolar
Second premolar
First molar
Second molar
Third molar (wisdom tooth)

Fig. 11-25. Anterior view of the eye.

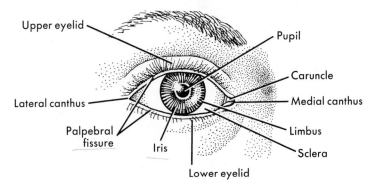

Upper eyelid

Pupil

Caruncle

Lateral canthus

Medial canthus

Palpebral fissure

Limbus

Iris

Sclera

Lower eyelid

Fig. 11-26. Horizontal section through left eyeball.

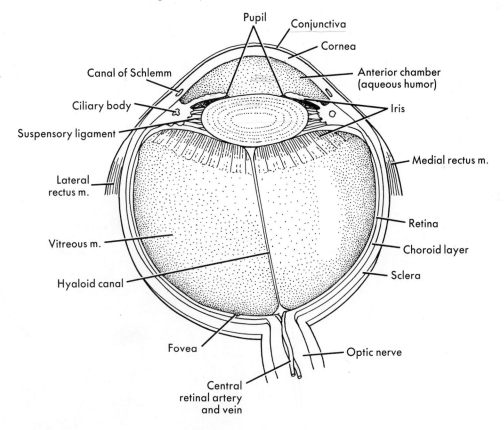

Pupil

Conjunctiva

Cornea

Canal of Schlemm

Anterior chamber (aqueous humor)

Ciliary body

Iris

Suspensory ligament

Medial rectus m.

Lateral rectus m.

Retina

Choroid layer

Vitreous m.

Sclera

Hyaloid canal

Fovea

Optic nerve

Central retinal artery and vein

Fig. 11-27. Longitudinal section through eyeball and eyelids, showing the conjunctiva, a lining of mucous membrane. Conjunctiva covering the cornea is called bulbar, and that lining the superior and inferior fornix is called the palpebral conjunctiva.

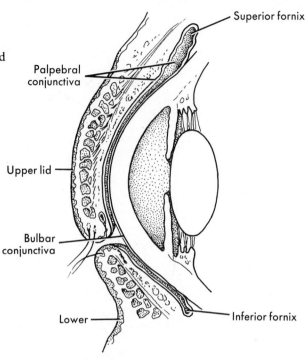

Superior fornix

Palpebral conjunctiva

Upper lid

Bulbar conjunctiva

Lower

Inferior fornix

Fig. 11-28. Lower lid sty.

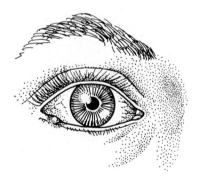

Fig. 11-29. Examining the inferior forni of the eye.

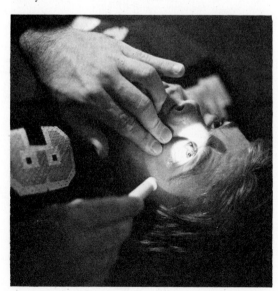

Such hemorrhages sometimes occur after such minimal stress as that produced by an episode of repeated sneezing or coughing. Subconjunctival hemorrhages can also result from trauma to the eye, such as that causing a contusion or abrasion. The red blood contrasted with the white sclera (called red eye), make these injuries appear to be more serious than they actually are. It is important to determine if red eye is associated with other, more serious eye injuries.

Eye injuries

Significant numbers of sports-related eye injuries occur as a result of head or facial trauma. Increased popularity and participation in tennis and racquetball, for example, have resulted in a dramatic increase in the number of eye contusion injuries. Such blunt blow injuries are often assessed initially by an athletic trainer. A knowledge of ocular assessment techniques permits rapid screening of eye injuries or related complaints and will facilitate rapid referral of the athlete to medical assistance when required.

Eye assessment is generally initiated as a result of complaints by an athlete of visual loss or ocular pain following head trauma or localized eye injury. The athlete's chief complaint and account of any injury will greatly assist in an accurate evaluation. In addition, the athletic trainer is often called on to assess ocular conditions that are not related to accident or injury. Examples of such noninjury problems include acute red eye and recentering of displaced contact lenses.

The conjunctiva lining the inferior fornix can be examined by moving the lower lid downward. The lid should be pressed and held gently against the lower ridge of the bony orbit without exerting pressure on the eyeball. After the lid is moved downward, ask the athlete to look up and to each side as you examine the inferior fornix (Fig. 11-29).

Fig. 11-30. Steps in everting the upper eyelid. **A,** Athlete looks downward. **B,** Grasp the eyelashes and tarsal plate and pull downward. **C,** Pull the lid over applicator. **D,** Hold the edge of the everted lid against the upper bony ridge of the orbit.

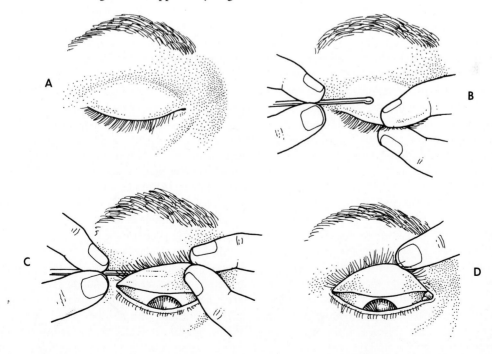

The conjunctiva lining the superior fornix is examined by eversion of the upper eyelid. The steps in everting the upper eyelid are illustrated in Fig. 11-30.

1. Ask the athlete to look downward but to keep the eyes open.
2. Grasp the eyelashes and the tarsal plate near the edge of the lid and pull gently downward. DO NOT pull the lid upward or outward.
3. Place a cotton-tipped applicator or lid evertor just above the tarsal plate of the lid and, while still holding the eyelashes, pull the lid over the applicator.
4. Hold the edge of the everted lid against the upper bony ridge of the orbit and examine the area for abrasions or the presence of a foreign body. DO NOT push against the eyeball.
5. The lid will return easily to its normal position when released if the athlete is asked to look upward and blink.

Foreign bodies and abrasions. Foreign bodies and abrasions are among the more common conditions of the eye to be managed during athletic activity. Athletes often express the feeling of having something in the eye. It is important to know that foreign bodies in the eye and abrasion injuries of the conjunctiva and cornea produce almost identical symptoms, that is, pain, increased tearing, and the sensation of something in the eye. To examine the eye for foreign bodies and abrasions, a penlight for illumination, a magnifying glass, cotton-tipped applicators or lid evertors, and an appropriate irrigating solution should be available.

Note in Fig. 11-26 that the cornea lies just below the bulbar conjunctiva and above the so-called anterior chamber of the eye. It covers the pupil and colored iris. Foreign bodies are often washed free from the cornea by the profuse tearing that occurs as a result of the initial irritation. Although a foreign body may not be present, the athlete who has suffered a corneal abrasion will continue to insist that something is in the eye. In these cases the abrasion and not the foreign body is responsible for the symptoms.

Examine the cornea by directing the penlight at it obliquely from several different positions. The iris should be fully visible, and the corneal surface should be smooth and free of irregularities. Superficial foreign bodies may be removed with a moistened cotton-tipped applicator or ophthalmic irrigating solution. If the foreign body cannot be removed or appears to be imbedded, the athlete should be referred to an ophthamologist or medical facility.

If no foreign bodies can be located on the corneal surface, the conjunctiva lining the inferior and especially the superior fornix should be examined carefully. If no foreign body can be located after the examination is completed, the presence of an abrasion should be suspected and, if symptoms continue, the athlete should be referred to a physician. It is also possible to check for a corneal abrasion by using a fluorescin dye strip (Fig. 11-31). The abrased area will be outlined by the dye when the lower fornix is touched by the moistened strip. Superficial abrasions normally heal without scarring or visual impairment.

Lacerations. The seriousness of lacerations involving the eye and surrounding tissues varies greatly. Any laceration of the eyeball itself is a serious injury with potentially grave consequences. The athlete will usually complain of pain in the eye and decreased vision. In looking at the eye, you may see the cut in the cornea, or the pupil may appear tear-shaped. If a laceration of the eyeball is noted, further examination in this area should stop. Reassure the athlete and refer him or her immediately to an ophthalmologist after placing a protective pad or shield over the eye. Often it is helpful to cover both eyes at the same time to reduce eye movement and lower the likelihood of further irritation. Do not exert any pressure on the eye.

Minor horizontal lacerations to the skin of the eyelid that do not involve the lid margin are generally not a serious problem. The cut edges are relatively easy to approximate, and after repair and healing the residual scar is minimal. If the margin of the eyelid is cut, the injury is much more serious. All lacerations that involve either the upper or lower lid margin should be referred to an ophthalmologist. Such lacerations may cut through the tarsal plate and lead to a "notched" lid, which can be disfiguring. In addition, persistent and troublesome tearing can also result from lacerations that cut the lower lid margin. In these cases the healed but notched tarsal plate interrupts the normal flow and direction of tears over the eye. Instead of flowing naturally toward the medial ducts which drain fluid into the nose, the tears escape from the eye. If the lower lid margin is cut near the nose (medial aspect) there is the added possibility that the duct, which drains tears into the nose, has also been cut. Such injuries require immediate referral so that the cut ends of the duct can be found and repaired. If the lower lid margin is lacerated near the nose, it should be assumed until proved otherwise that the tear duct has also been cut.

Blunt-blow injuries. The anatomy of the bony orbit makes the eye quite resistant to serious blunt-blow injuries. Contusion-type blunt-blow injuries can occur quite frequently, however, as a result of racquetball and handball injuries. It is fortunate indeed that in most cases damage is limited to subconjunctival hemorrhage (red eye) and periorbital contusion and ecchymosis (black eye) (Fig. 11-32).

Hemorrhage into the anterior chamber of the eye following a blunt blow is called *hyphema.* Assessment of this condition is usually no problem because the blood can be seen through the cornea as it collects in a pool in the lower portion of the anterior chamber of the eye (Fig.

Fig. 11-31. Use of fluorescein dye strip to detect corneal abrasions.
(From Barber, J.M., and Budassi, S.A.: Mosby's Manual of emergency care, St. Louis, 1979, The C.V. Mosby Co.)

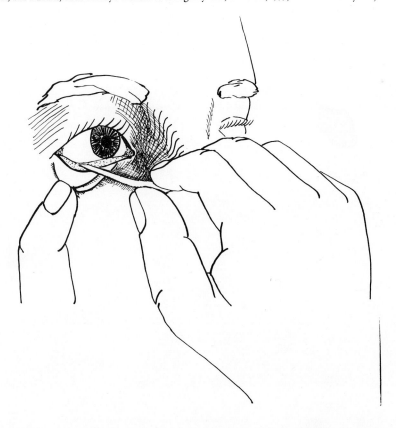

11-33). The athlete may also complain of pain in the eye and fuzzy vision. Although this condition clears spontaneously in almost all cases, referral to a physician is required because of the possibility of secondary hemorrhage.

A serious injury that can result from blunt-blow trauma to the eye is called a blow-out fracture. If the eye has been subjected to a severe blunt blow (such as a baseball or hockey puck injury), the possibility of a fractured orbit should always be considered. In blow-out fractures, the floor of the orbit is pushed into the maxillary sinus. As a result of the fracture, the mobility of the affected eye is restricted. This occurs because the ocular muscles are often trapped or pinched at the fracture site. If there is restriction of eye movement (especially an inability to look upward), or if the athlete complains of double vision *(diplopia)* following a severe blunt blow injury to the eye or face, an orbital fracture should be considered (Fig. 11-

34). In most cases of orbital fracture, multiple and potentially serious eye injuries occur. Referral to an ophthalmologist is essential.

Retinal detachment. Occasionally, athletes suffering trauma to the eye may suffer detachment of the retina. This may occur days, weeks, or even months after an injury. Athletes suffering a detached retina will normally complain of a "curtain" blocking his or her field of vision, together with light flashes or dark spots in front of the eyes. The athlete should be referred to an ophthalmologist immediately.

Displaced contact lenses. The use of contact lenses by athletes has greatly increased in recent years and presents some problems for the athletic trainer. Hard contact lenses are more likely than the newer soft lenses to cause eye abrasions, slip around, pop out, and become lost. The athletic trainer is often involved with locating and recentering displaced contact lenses (Fig. 11-35). To care for an athlete wearing contact lenses,

Fig. 11-32. Blunt blow injuries to the eye. **A,** Subconjunctival hemorrhage (red eye); **B,** periorbital contusion (black eye).

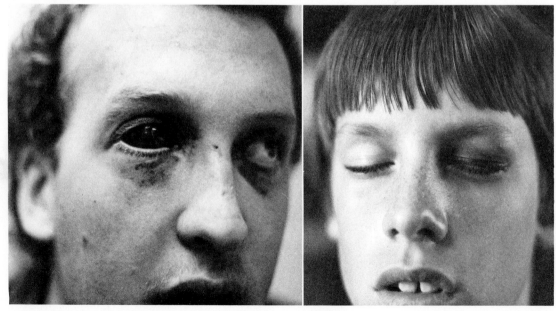

Fig. 11-33. Blood pooling in the lower portion of the anterior chamber of the eye following injury (hyphema).

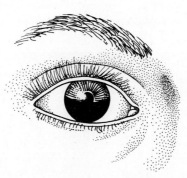

Fig. 11-34. A blow-out fracture of the left eye orbit. Inability to look upward on the injured side is the result of ocular muscles being trapped or pinched at the fracture site.

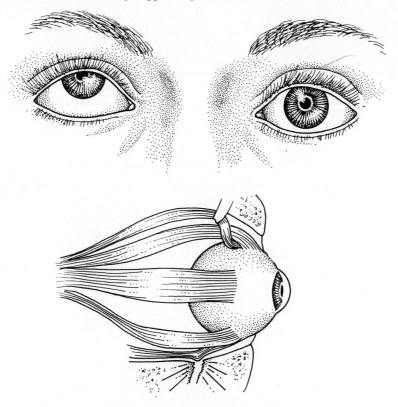

Fig. 11-35. Recentering of displaced contact lens. For purposes of illustration an opaque lens has been used. **A,** Lens is first located by pulling lids away from globe and looking in various directions. **B,** By pressing lens with lids, lens may be manipulated onto cornea. **C,** Lens displaced above. **D,** Lens recentered from displacement above.

(From Camp, R.H., et al.: In Girard, L.J., ed.: Corneal contact lenses, ed. 2, St. Louis, 1970, The C.V. Mosby Co.)

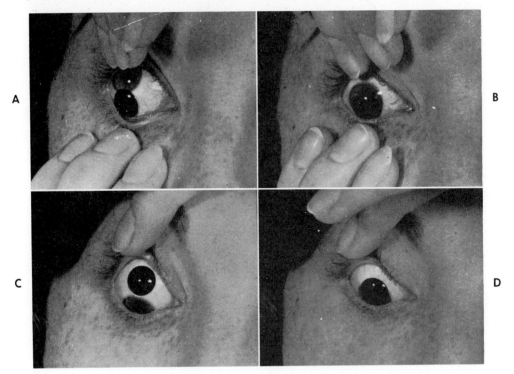

Fig. 11-35, cont'd. E, Lens displaced nasally. **F,** Eye is directed toward lens. **G,** Lens is recentered from nasal displacement. **H,** Lens displaced temporally. **I,** Lens recentered from temporal displacement.

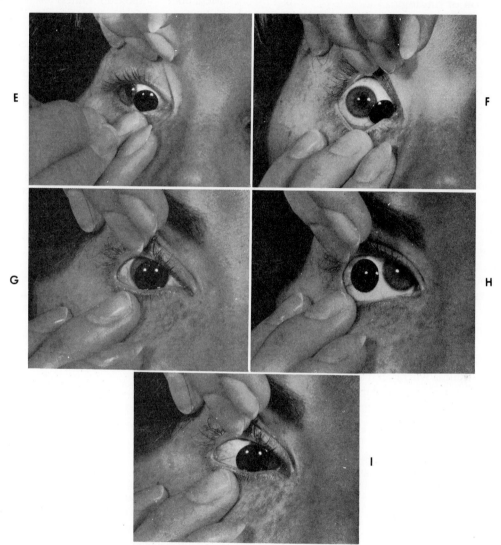

you should have wetting solution, lens cases, and a mirror available.

Evaluation of findings

The face is the most important cosmetic area of the body and the area involved with the senses of sight, smell, taste, and sound. A wide variety of athletic trauma can occur to the face. Facial trauma is an obvious area of concern and necessitates a careful, accurate assessment. Athletic trainers must remember that injuries to the face indicate trauma to the head, which can also result in injuries to the brain or spinal cord. Do not concentrate on facial trauma to the extent that associated injuries, which may be more serious, are overlooked.

When to refer the athlete

Because of the great vascularity of the face, injuries can appear very dramatic and sensational, although the underlying injuries may be minimal. Conversely, the appearance of facial trauma may not reflect the magnitude or seriousness of the injury. Therefore athletic trainers must carefully and accurately evaluate each facial injury. Medical assistance should be readily obtained for facial trauma whenever a significant injury is recognized or suspected. Athletic trainers who decide, incorrectly, that a facial injury is not serious enough to warrant medical referral place themselves and the athlete at risk. Following is a list of conditions that indicate an athlete should be referred to medical assistance.

Skin
  Lacerations requiring sutures
Facial bones (suspected fractures)
  Teeth do not fit together normally
  Deformity observed
  Pain at the site of injury, which is increased by palpation, forcefully biting down, or stress applied away from the site of trauma
  Crepitation
Temporomandibular joint (suspected dislocation)
  Loss of jaw movement
  Malocclusion of the teeth
Nose
  Discharge of cerebrospinal fluid
  Foreign body that cannot be easily removed
  Nasal deformity
  Crepitation or increased mobility on palpation
Ear
  Discharge of cerebrospinal fluid
  Foreign body that cannot be easily removed
  Athlete reports sensations of tinnitus, vertigo, or a sudden fullness in the ear that does not readily go away
  Hematoma formation
  Appearance of infection or inflammation
  Sudden hearing impairment
Teeth
  Chipped, cracked, broken or dislodged
  Athlete reporting continued sensitivity to biting down or extremes of temperature
Eye
  Loss of vision
  Ocular pain
  Imbedded foreign body
  Suspected abrasion on eyeball
  Laceration of eyeball or eyelid margin
  Irregularly shaped pupil
  Hemorrhage into anterior chamber
  Restricted eye movements
  Double vision
Doubt regarding facial injuries

ATHLETIC INJURY ASSESSMENT CHECKLIST
FACIAL INJURIES

Secondary survey

_____ History

    _____ Primary complaint

    _____ Mechanism of injury

    _____ Pain

    _____ Sensations (numbness, crepitation, dizziness, tinnitus, vertigo, loss of hearing, burning, tingling, loose teeth, visual loss, something in the eye)

_____ Observation

Jaw

    _____ Obvious deformity

    _____ Swelling

    _____ Signs of trauma

    _____ Malocclusion of teeth

    _____ Symmetry

    _____ Jaw movement

Nose

    _____ Epistaxis

    _____ Foreign body

    _____ Swelling

    _____ Deformity

    _____ Rhinorrhea

Ear

    _____ Hemorrhage

    _____ Foreign body

    _____ Otorrhea

    _____ Swelling

    _____ Infection or inflammation

    _____ Blanching of the skin

Teeth

    _____ Bleeding around teeth

    _____ Chipped, cracked, broken, or dislodged

    _____ Malocclusion

Eye

    _____ Foreign body

    _____ Abrasion

    _____ Increased tearing

    _____ Laceration

    _____ Pupil equality and symmetry

    _____ Red eye

    _____ Black eye

    _____ Hyphema

    _____ Diplopia

_____ Palpation

    _____ Tenderness

    _____ Swelling

    _____ Deformities

    _____ Crepitation

_____ Stress

    _____ Temporomandibular joint movement

KEY TERMS

anesthesia   Absence of touch sensations

anterograde amnesia   Loss of memory for events occurring immediately after awakening

aphasia   Loss of speech, writing ability, or comprehension of spoken or written language

ataxia   Failure of muscular coordination or irregularity of muscular action

concussion   Syndrome involving an immediate and transient impairment in the ability of the brain to function properly

contrecoup (counterblow)   Injury resulting from a blow on the opposite side, such as an intracranial injury

diplopia   Double vision

epidural hematoma   Hematoma outside the dura

epistaxis (nosebleed)   Hemorrhage from the nose

external otitis (swimmer's ear)   Common infection of the external ear in swimmers

hematoma auris (cauliflower ear)   End result of keloid formation between the skin and underlying cartilage of an injured external ear

hyphema   Hemorrhage into the anterior chamber of the eye

hypotonia   Condition of abnormally diminished tone, tension, or activity

intracerebral hematoma   Hematoma within the cerebrum

keloid   New growth or tumor of the skin, consisting of whitish ridges, nodules, and plates of dense tissue

nystagmus   Involuntary rapid movement of the eyeball

paresthesia   Abnormal sensation such as burning, itching, or prickling

pneumocephalus   Presence of air in the intracranial cavity

retrograde amnesia   Loss of memory for events leading up to the injury

Romberg's sign   Accomplished by having the athlete stand with his or her feet together, arms at the side, and eyes closed; normally a person can stand still in this position

sty   Localized, painful infection of the small glands or hair follicles around the eyelash

subconjunctival hemorrhage (red eye)   Rupture of the tiny blood vessels in the conjunctiva

subdural hematoma   Hematoma beneath the dura

tinnitus   Ringing in the ears

vertigo   Sensations of movements

wen   Sebaceous cyst

SUGGESTED READINGS

American Academy of Orthopaedic Surgeons: Emergency care and transportation of the sick and injured, ed. 3, Chicago, 1981, The Academy.

Arnheim, D.D.: Modern principles of athletic training, ed. 6, St. Louis, 1985, Times Mirror/Mosby College Publishing.

Budassi, S.A., and Barber, J.M.: Mosby's manual of emergency care: practices and procedures, ed. 2, St. Louis, 1984, Times Mirror/Mosby College Publishing.

Casson, I.R.: Brain damage in modern boxers, J.A.M.A. 251 (20):2663-2667, 1984.

Grant, H.D., and others: Emergency care, ed. 3, Bowie, Md., 1982, Robert J. Brady Co.

Miller, R.H., and Cantrell, J.R.: Textbook of basic emergency medicine, ed. 2, St. Louis, 1980, The C.V. Mosby Co.

O'Donoghue, D.H.: Treatment of injuries to athletes, ed. 4, Philadelphia, 1984, W.B. Saunders Co.

Parcel, G.S.: Basic emergency care of the sick and injured, ed. 2, St. Louis, 1982, The C.V. Mosby Co.

Rosen, P., and others: Emergency medicine, concepts and clinical practice, St. Louis, 1983, The C.V. Mosby Co.

Saunders, R.L., and Harbaugh, R.E.: The second impact in catastrophic contact-sports head trauma, J.A.M.A. 252(4): 538-539, 1984.

Subcommittee on Classification of Sports Injuries: Standard nomenclature of athletic injuries, Chicago, 1968, American Medical Association.

Torg, J.S.: Athletic injuries to the head, neck and face, Philadelphia, 1982, Lea & Febiger.

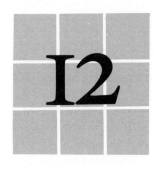

I2 Spine injuries

The human spine is a remarkable structure. During athletic activity the spine is able to withstand tremendous stresses and forces and at the same time remain quite flexible and mobile. The spine, or vertebral column, encases and provides protection for the spinal cord. Trauma to the spine can produce devastating athletic injuries. These injuries can be fatal or can cause irreversible damage to the spinal cord, resulting in permanent paralysis. To accurately assess and care for injuries to this area of the body, it is imperative that the athletic trainer possess a thorough understanding of the anatomic and mechanical characteristics of the spine.

ANATOMY OF THE SPINE

The spine consists of 33 vertebrae, which are subdivided into seven cervical, twelve thoracic, five lumbar, five sacral (fused), and four coccygeal (fused) vertebrae. The 24 nonfused vertebrae lying superior to the sacrum increase in size from the first cervical through the fifth lumbar. Between each of these vertebrae is an intervertebral disc. Discs act as shock absorbers and allow movement between adjacent vertebrae.

Intervertebral discs

Each intervertebral disc consists of two structures, the tough outer *annulus fibrosus* and the semisolid central **nucleus pulposus** (Fig. 12-1). The annulus fibrosus connects the bodies of adjacent vertebrae through obliquely arranged layers of fibrocartilage. Each layer of fibers is perpendicular to the adjacent layers. This arrangement gives the disc strength and elasticity. The annulus fibrosus is thicker anteriorly and laterally. This fact explains the larger number of posterior disc herniations. The nucleus pulposus is a gelatinous substance located in the center of the disc. It has a strong capacity to retain water.

Ligaments of the vertebral column

The bodies of adjacent vertebrae are connected by strong ligaments (Fig. 12-1). Two important longitudinal ligaments can be identified through the entire length of the spinal column. The *anterior longitudinal ligament* is a strong, bandlike structure composed of several layers of fibers that extends along and is firmly attached to the anterior surface of each vertebral body. It extends from the base of the skull to the sacrum. The *posterior longitudinal ligament* lies on the inside of the vertebral canal on the posterior surface of the bodies of the vertebrae. It is principally a structure that serves to connect the intervertebral discs. It consists of smooth, glistening fibers that commence on the body of the axis and continue downward to the sacrum.

In addition, the *ligamenta flava* bind the laminae of adjacent vertebrae firmly together. Spinous processes are connected by *interspinous ligaments*. The transverse processes of adjacent vertebrae are connected by *intertransverse ligaments*. The tips of the spinous processes of the cervical vertebrae are connected by the specialized *ligamentum nuchae*, which extends downward from the external occipital protuberance at the base of the skull to join the spinous processes of all seven cervical vertebrae. This strong and impor-

Fig. 12-1. Sagittal section of vertebral column.

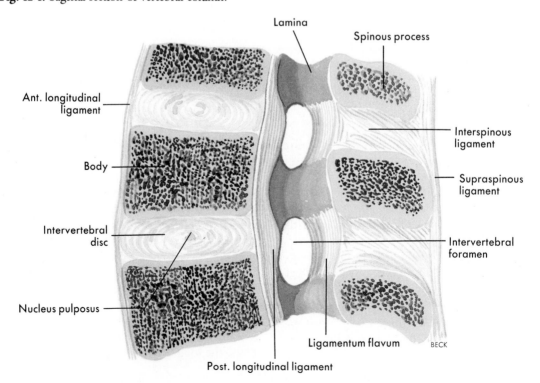

tant fan-shaped ligament lies in the midline and forms a septum between the neck muscles. The extension of this ligament, the *supraspinous ligament,* connects the tips of the rest of the vertebrae down to the sacrum.

Muscles acting on the vertebral column

The vertebral column, in part or as a whole, may be moved or acted upon by numerous muscles or muscle groups. Some muscles have both their origin and insertion on the spine and act directly on the column, whereas others act only indirectly on the spine and have their origin or insertion on some other bone or soft tissue component.

The superficial muscles of the back are, as a group, related to the upper limbs. The complex deep, or intrinsic, muscles of the back extend from the base of the skull to the pelvis on each side of the body. They control the movements of the vertebral column. The *short intrinsic muscles*

tend to steady adjoining vertebrae during movements of the column as a whole. The *long intrinsic muscles* or muscle groups are more involved in gross movements of the entire spine.

Muscles acting on the spine are extremely complex in morphologic detail and specific mechanisms of action. A brief functional grouping would include the following:

Flexion: Sternocleidomastoid, rectus abdominis, longus cervicis, and scaleni

Extension: Erector spinae, semispinalis, and splenius capitis

Lateral flexion: Iliocostocervicalis, longissimus, and the oblique muscles of the abdominal wall

Rotation: Rotatores, multifidus, and splenius cervicis

Spinal cord

The spinal cord (Fig. 12-2) is a continuation of the motor and sensory pathways from the brain

---

Fig. 12-2. Spinal cord surrounded by the three meningeal layers; dura mater, arachnoid, and pia mater.
(From McClintic, J.R.: Human anatomy, St. Louis, 1983, The C.V. Mosby Co.)

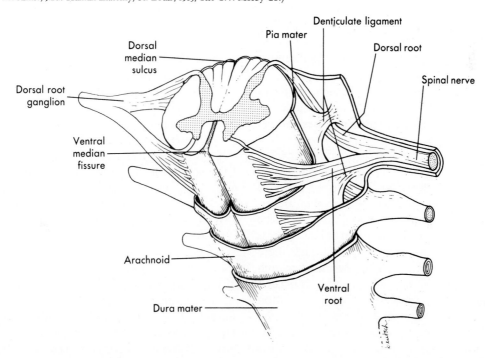

to the body and extremities. It is encased and protected within the bony spinal canal. The spinal cord is surrounded by the meninges, cerebrospinal fluid, a cushion of adipose tissue, and blood vessels. The cord extends from the foramen magnum to the lower border of the first lumbar vertebra, an average distance of 17 to 18 inches in the adult. Although the spinal cord terminates at the level of the first lumbar vertebrae, lumbar, sacral, and coccygeal nerve roots continue to descend in the canal. This gives the lower end of the spinal cord, with its attached spinal nerve roots, the appearance of a horse's tail, and prompted early anatomists to describe it as the *cauda equina.*

The spinal cord is oval and less than 1/2 inch in diameter. It tapers slightly from above downward and is extremely sensitive to injury. For example, it is said that if you were to drop a quarter on an exposed spinal cord from a height of 12 inches, neural function distal to the point of impact would be severely impaired. There are 31 pairs of spinal nerves connected to the spinal cord. They have no special names but are merely numbered according to the level of the spinal column at which they emerge. Thus, there are eight cervical, twelve thoracic, five lumbar, five sacral, and one coccygeal pair of spinal nerves. These spinal nerves leave the spinal cavity horizontally through the intervertebral foramina of their respective vertebrae and branch out to innervate the various parts of the body. Table 12-1 lists the spinal nerves and their plexuses and peripheral branches.

Dermatomes

Each spinal nerve supplies sensory fibers to areas of skin on the body surface that are arranged in a definite segmental pattern. Each strip of skin supplied by a given spinal nerve is called a *dermatome* (Fig. 12-3). Although there is considerable overlap in the innervation of each dermatome, sensation in each band is associated with a particular spinal nerve; loss of sensation in a dermatome segment suggests injury to the spinal nerve supplying that segment. If, for example, there is a loss of skin sensation in a band

that circles the trunk at the level of the umbilicus, a physician would assume injury to the spinal nerve root supplying that area (T_{10}).

Each segment of the spine is discussed separately in more detail along with the athletic injuries common to each area. Type and severity of athletic injuries varies, depending on which segment of the spine is involved. As a result, the evaluation and subsequent management must be specific to the area injured.

Cervical spine

The cervical spine is of paramount importance to the athletic trainer. This area of the spine has greater flexibility than any other vertebral segment. There are seven cervical (neck) vertebrae, which can be distinguished from other vertebrae by the presence of a foramen through their transverse processes. With the exception of the first cervical vertebrae, or atlas, each component of the cervical spine is characterized by the following component parts (Fig. 12-4):

1. The *body,* which is a flat mass located anteriorly and centrally. In the cervical vertebrae the body tends to be wider from side to side than in the anteroposterior diameter.
2. Two *transverse processes,* which project laterally from each vertebra.
3. The *spinous process,* a sharp palpable process that projects posteriorly and inferiorly from each vertebra.
4. Two *lamina,* which join the spinous process on either side with the body.
5. A central opening called the *vertebral foramen,* formed by the junction of the lamina with the body. This is the opening through which the spinal cord passes.
6. *Superior articular facets,* which are directed superiorly and posteriorly.
7. *Inferior articular facets,* which are directed anteriorly and inferiorly.

The bodies of adjacent vertebrae articulate with each other through the intervention of the intervertebral discs and through their articular facets or processes. The upper and lower pairs of articular processes between vertebrae are ar-

Fig. 12-3. Segmental distribution of spinal nerves (dermatomes). There is often considerable overlap between adjacent dermatomes. Injury to a single spinal nerve will seldom result in complete loss of sensation in a discrete dermatome area.

(From Judd, R.L., and Ponsell, D.D.: The first responder: the first critical minutes, St. Louis, 1981, The C.V. Mosby Co.)

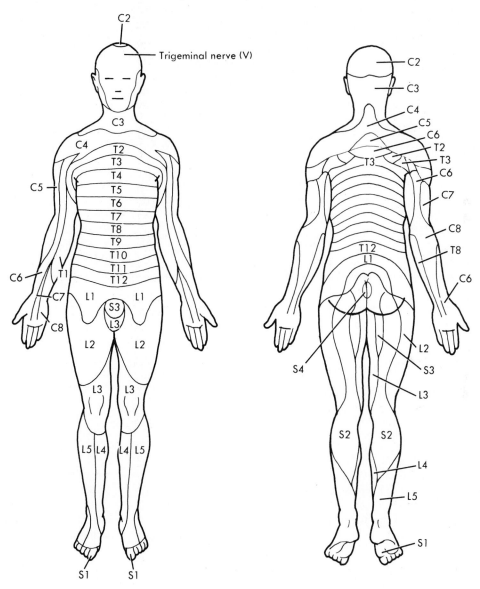

Table 12-1. Spinal nerves and peripheral branches

Spinal nerves	Plexuses formed from anterior rami	Spinal nerve branches from plexuses	Part supplied
Cervical 1 2 3 4	Cervical plexus	Lesser occipital Great auricular Cutaneous nerve of neck Anterior supraclavicular Middle supraclavicular Posterior supraclavicular Branches to muscles	Sensory to back of head, front of neck, and upper part of shoulder; motor to numerous neck muscles
Cervical 5 6 7 8 Thoracic (or dorsal) 1	Brachial plexus	Phrenic (branches from cervical nerves before formation of plexus; most of its fibers from fourth cervical nerve)	Diaphragm
		Suprascapular and dorsoscapular	Superficial muscles* of scapula
		Thoracic nerves, medial and lateral branches	Pectoralis major and minor
		Long thoracic nerve	Serratus anterior
		Thoracodorsal	Latissimus dorsi
		Subscapular	Subscapular and teres major muscles
		Axillary (circumflex)	Deltoid and teres minor muscles and skin over deltoid
		Musculocutaneous	Muscles of front of arm (biceps brachii, coracobrachialis, and brachialis) and skin on outer side of forearm
		Ulnar	Flexor carpi ulnaris and part of flexor digitorum profundus; some of muscles of hand; sensory to medial side of hand, little finger, and medial half of fourth finger
2 3 4 5 6 7 8 9 10 11 12	No plexus formed; branches run directly to intercostal muscles and skin of thorax	Median	Rest of muscles of front of forearm and hand; sensory to skin of palmar surface of thumb, index, and middle fingers
		Radial	Triceps muscle and muscles of back of forearm; sensory to skin of back of forearm and hand
		Medial cutaneous	Sensory to inner surface of arm and forearm

*Although nerves to muscle are considered motor, they do contain some sensory fibers that transmit proprioceptive impulses.

†Sensory fibers from the tibial and peroneal nerves unite to form the *medial cutaneous* (or sural) *nerve* that supplies the calf of the leg and the lateral surface of the foot. In the thigh the tibial and common peroneal nerves are usually enclosed in a single sheath to form the *sciatic nerve*, the largest nerve in the body with its width of approximately 3/4 of an inch. About two thirds of the way down the posterior part of the thigh, it divides into its component parts. Branches of the sciatic nerve extend into the hamstring muscles.

Table 12-1. Spinal nerves and peripheral branches—cont'd

Spinal nerves	Plexuses formed from anterior rami	Spinal nerve branches from plexuses	Parts supplied
Lumbar 1 2 3 4 5 Sacral 1 2 3 4 5 Coccygeal 1	Lumbosacral plexus	Iliohypogastric Ilioinguinal Sometimes fused	Sensory to anterior abdominal wall Sensory to anterior abdominal wall and external genitalia; motor to muscles of abdominal wall
		Genitofemoral	Sensory to skin of external genitalia and inguinal region
		Lateral cutaneous of thigh	Sensory to outer side of thigh
		Femoral	Motor to quadriceps, sartorius, and iliacus muscles; sensory to front of thigh and medial side of lower leg (saphenous nerve)
		Obturator	Motor to adductor muscles of thigh
		Tibial† (medial popliteal)	Motor to muscles of calf of leg; sensory to skin of calf of leg and sole of foot
		Common peroneal (lateral popliteal)	Motor to evertors and dorsiflexors of foot; sensory to lateral surface of leg and dorsal surface of foot
		Nerves to hamstring muscles	Motor to muscles of back of thigh
		Gluteal nerves, superior and inferior	Motor to buttock muscles and tensor fasciae latae
		Posterior cutaneous nerve	Sensory to skin of buttocks, posterior surface of thigh, and leg
		Pudendal nerve	Motor to perineal muscles; sensory to skin of perineum

ranged vertically, except in the cervical spine. In the cervical spine the more transverse arrangement of the articular facets between adjacent vertebrae makes dislocation possible without fracture. It is not possible for a simple dislocation to occur elsewhere in the spinal column because of the vertical direction of the articular processes. With the exception of the cervical spine, any dislocation injury must be a fracture dislocation, because the articular processes must break before the vertebral bodies can be separated.

The atlas (C_1) has large oval and concave facets that articulate with the occipital condyles of the skull. Nodding and lateral flexion movements occur at the atlantooccipital joint. The axis (C_2) is characterized by the dens (odontoid process) on the superior aspect of its body. Rotation of the skull occurs at the atlantoaxial joint, with the dens acting as a pivot. In addition to the longitudinal ligaments and articular capsules, a number of specialized ligaments help to stabilize the articulations between the skull and

Fig. 12-4. Component parts of a "typical" cervical vertebra. Note the almost transverse relationship between the articular processes between adjacent vertebrae.

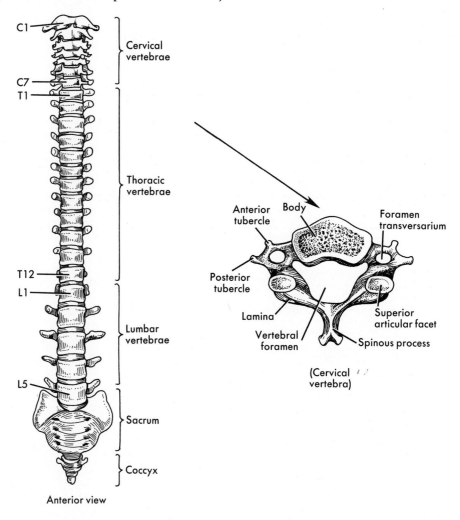

atlas and between the atlas and axis. The *transverse ligament of the atlas,* for example, protects the spinal cord in certain types of cervical fracture by limiting backward displacement of the dens into the vertebral canal. Rotation of the skull is limited by the lateral odontoid or "check" ligaments. These very strong fibrous bands extend from each occipital condyle at the base of the skull to the dens, or odontoid process, of the axis.

The seventh cervical vertebra (C_7) is called the *vertebra prominens* because of its relatively long and easily palpated spinous process. It is the first clearly palpable spine as you run your fingers downward along the vertebral crests, although the spine of the first thoracic vertebrae (T_1) immediately below it is in fact more prominent.

Cervical spine injuries

Injuries to the cervical spine can be the most serious of athletic injuries. These injuries range in severity from minor neck pain to complete paralysis or death. It is imperative that the athletic trainer protect the athlete from further injury whenever an injury to the cervical spine is suspected. Ill-advised assessment procedures and improper handling and transporting maneuvers may cause irreparable spinal cord damage to an athlete who has suffered a cervical spine fracture or dislocation. Therefore utmost caution must be used in evaluating, treating and handling the athlete who has suffered an injury to the neck region. This is one area of the body with which it is certainly better to be conservative and cautious in your assessment of injury rather than to risk a lifetime of paralysis, or possibly death, for the athlete.

Injuries to the cervical spine can involve the vertebrae, intervertebral discs, ligaments, muscles, nerve roots, or spinal cord. These structures can be injured by various mechanisms. The most common mechanism of injury to the neck is forced movements of the head on the cervical spine (Fig. 12-5). This can occur when the athlete receives a blow to the head that forces the neck beyond its normal limits of motion, resulting in forced hyperextension, flexion, lateral flexion, rotation, or a combination of these movements. The contractile tissue surrounding the cervical spine may be stretched or strained while attempting to resist this forced movement. If forced movement is severe or violent enough, serious injuries to the neck, such as fractures or dislocations, may occur. Injuries to the cervical spine may also be the result of cervical compression. When an athlete receives a head-on blow,

Fig. 12-5. Possible mechanism of neck injury. The cervical spine is forced beyond its normal limits of motion.

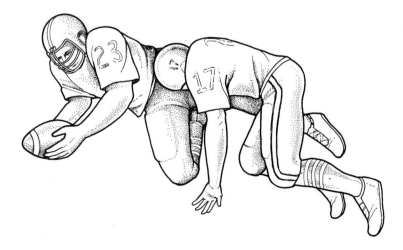

the force is transmitted through the cervical spine and may cause vertebral fracture or dislocation. The neck can also be injured by a direct blow. This mechanism usually results in contusions or bruising about the neck but can result in a serious spinal cord injury if the blow is violent enough.

The most common injuries to the neck are sprains and strains, which often occur simultaneously. These injuries vary in severity. Slight trauma may result in very mild injuries of little consequence. In these cases, the athlete will express no feelings of weakness or instability. Although there may be tenderness and pain at the site of the injury, the athlete can easily demonstrate a normal range of motion in the neck. In more severe injuries, the athlete will usually resist moving the neck through a full range of motion. With the more severe injuries there will be localized pain and muscle spasm, and the athlete may complain of an insecure feeling about the neck. Injuries resulting in moderate to severe neck sprains and strains should be referred to a physician for further evaluation.

Cervical nerve syndrome is an injury resulting from forced lateral flexion, causing the nerve roots to be either stretched or impinged. This is commonly known as a "pinched nerve," "burner," "stinger," or "hot shot" and is characterized by sharp, burning, radiating pain. When the cervical plexus is involved, the athlete may complain of pain shooting into the posterior scalp, behind the ear, around the neck, or down the top of the shoulder. If the brachial plexus is involved, the athlete may complain of radiating pain, numbness, and loss of function of the arm and possibly the hand. Symptoms usually subside in minutes, but such injuries may leave residual soreness and paresthetic areas. Severe or repeated cervical nerve syndrome episodes should be evaluated by a physician.

Serious injuries of the cervical spine, such as fractures or dislocations, are not common in athletics; however, they do occur. The potential for this type of an injury is inherent in almost any sport. Football, however, provides the greatest potential for serious cervical spine injuries, as the head is often used in blocking and tackling techniques. Diving and gymnastics also provide mechanisms for devastating neck injuries. Most fatal or paralyzing injuries occur when an athlete's neck is forced into hyperflexion, such as putting the head down and using the top of the head to make contact with an opponent. This type of mechanism can cause fractures or subluxations of the cervical vertebrae, which may produce lesions to the spinal cord. The major signs and symptoms that may indicate serious neck injuries include unremitting neck pain, muscle spasms, and evidence of spinal cord involvement such as numbness, loss of sensations, weakness, *paresthesia* (abnormal sensation such as burning or prickling), and partial or complete paralysis of the limbs. The athletic trainer must be aware of the significance of these important clues. They may indicate a serious spinal injury and require proper care and transportation of the injured athlete.

Because most mechanisms causing cervical spine injuries involve forces to the head, injuries to the head and neck must be considered together. In all cases, both areas should be evaluated following trauma to the head. As was discussed in Chapter 10, any head injury severe enough to render an athlete unconscious must be handled as if there is also associated cervical spine involvement. Whenever there is any question concerning a neck injury, treat the athlete as if he or she has a serious cervical spine injury until proved otherwise.

Thoracic spine

The basic anatomic characteristics typical of vertebrae in general are easily identified in the 12 components of the thoracic spine. The thoracic vertebrae show the least modification of the basic pattern. Fig. 12-6 shows the anatomic components of a typical thoracic vertebrae (T_8). Transitional changes in appearance occur in individual vertebra toward the cervical and lumbar ends of the thoracic region. The first and twelfth thoracic vertebrae are distinctly transitional.

Whereas T_1 has a long and almost horizontal spinous process, the spine on T_{12} is short and broadened. The remaining spinous processes of thoracic vertebrae are long and tend to slope sharply downward.

The heart-shaped body of a typical thoracic vertebra is intermediate in size between those of the cervical and lumbar segments. Unique *costal facets* are found on each side of thoracic vertebrae at the junction of the body and lamina. Adjacent facets of contiguous (touching) verte-

brae form an articular socket for the head of a rib. These facets are found only on thoracic vertebrae.

The thoracic spine is the most stable section of the vertebral column. Although a considerable range of motion is possible, including flexion, extension, rotation, and lateral bending movements, the actual displacement between vertebrae is limited. Stability of the thoracic spine results from the obliquely set articular facets, the thin intervertebral discs, the overlapping of the

Fig. 12-6. Typical thoracic vertebra, superior aspect.

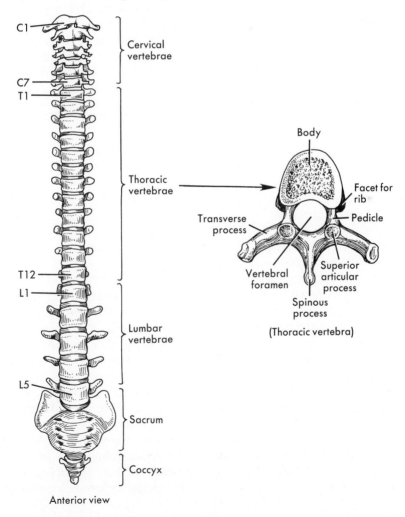

long spinous processes, and the attachment of the ribs. In addition, the well-developed anterior longitudinal and posterior longitudinal ligaments effectively limit motion. The functional price paid for stability in this region is restricted motion between individual vertebrae.

Thoracic spine injuries

The most common athletic injuries to the thoracic spine are contusions, sprains, and strains. Contusions caused by a blow to the thoracic area more commonly involve the paraspinal muscles, those muscles lateral to the spinous processes. Sprains and strains may be caused by overstretching of the soft tissue surrounding the thoracic vertebrae or by violent muscular contraction against resistance. On examination it may be difficult to distinguish between a sprain or strain. With either of these injuries there may be tenderness, spasm, and increased pain on active contraction or stretching. An athlete with a moderate to severe injury may exhibit a very stiff back and may resist any motion or movement of the thoracic spine.

Serious injuries to the thoracic spine are extremely rare in athletic activity. Fractures or dislocations are unusual because of the stable anatomy previously described. The most common serious injury is a compression fracture to the body of one of the thoracic vertebrae. The mechanism of injury is usually forced forward flexion of the thoracic spine, which compresses the anterior portion of adjacent vertebral bodies. Typically, the athlete will give a history of sharp forward flexion, resulting in a jackknifing effect. This can occur as an athlete falls violently on the buttocks or is forced into extreme flexion of the thoracic spine. An athlete with a compression fracture will usually have no neurologic complaints and will be able to move around and even walk. However, the athlete will complain of constant localized pain, which may be increased with any movement of this area of the spine. The athlete should be referred for further evaluation and radiographs.

Lumbar spine

The five lumbar vertebrae differ from the thoracic vertebrae in their larger size and absence of costal facets. A typical lumbar vertebra (L_3) is shown in Fig. 12-7. The massive bodies of these vertebrae are designed to stabilize and accommodate the increasing body weight that must be supported toward the lower end of the spinal column. The prominent lumbar curve, an anterior convexity somewhat deeper in women than men, helps to project the weight of the torso onto the lower limbs.

Progressive changes in appearance of specific vertebral components through the five lumbar vertebrae include a widening of the bodies from side to side and a marked separation between articular processes. The articular processes of lumbar vertebrae are oriented to facilitate a considerable range of movement, particularly in flexion, extension, and side-to-side bending. They do not, however, permit axial rotation.

The hatchet-shaped spinous processes of lumbar vertebrae are horizontal and extend posteriorly from a triangular vertebral foramen. The horizontal orientation of the spinous processes makes it possible to insert a needle between two adjacent vertebrae and enter the vertebral canal to sample cerebrospinal fluid. This process, usually accomplished between L_3 and L_4, is known as a *lumbar puncture.*

Lumbosacral joint

The body weight is supported by the opposing surfaces of the first sacral and fifth lumbar vertebra and by the two articulations between the superior sacral and inferior lumbar articular processes. Articulations between the last, or fifth lumbar vertebra and the sacrum are similar to the joints that exist between the movable vertebrae in the spine above. However, the intervertebral disc located between L_5 and the sacrum is very thick, especially along its anterior border. This articulation is the meeting place of the movable lumbar spine above with the fixed and rigid sacrum below. It is notorious as a frequent site of pain. The lumbosacral angle has a rather extensive normal range of variation but averages about 120° in most adults.

The anterior surface of the lumbosacral joint lies in a straight line directly below the occipital condyles when the body is erect and the posture normal. The joint also marks the termination of the lumbar convexity (which begins at T_{12}) and the commencement of the sacral concavity. The fifth lumbar vertebra may be joined in whole or in part to the sacrum. This is known as sacral-ization of the fifth lumbar vertebra. The condition is often devoid of symptoms but may be the cause of back pain in some athletes.

The two bones entering into the lumbosacral articulation are held together by a host of very strong ligaments. Sprains are common, however, if this body area is subjected to direct blows or sudden twisting movements. Lordosis increases the possibility of ligament sprains in this area. The major ligaments associated with the lumbosacral junction can be evaluated by

Fig. 12-7. Typical lumbar vertebra, superior aspect.

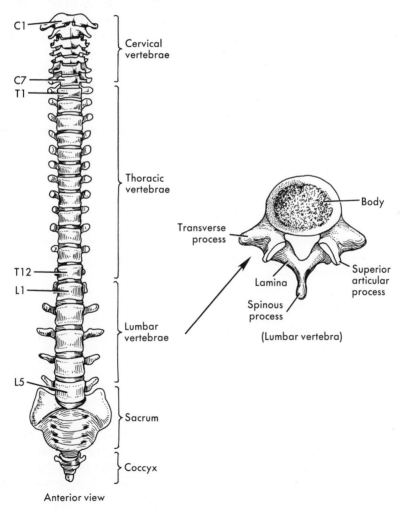

Cervical vertebrae

Thoracic vertebrae

Lumbar vertebrae

Sacrum

Coccyx

Anterior view

Transverse process

Body

Lamina

Spinous process

Superior articular process

(Lumbar vertebra)

asking the athlete to lie supine on a table and hyperflex both thighs on the abdomen. This position will stress the ligaments and elicit point tenderness and pain if ligament injuries are present.

The lumbosacral trunk (fourth and fifth lumbar nerves) is in close approximation to each side of the lumbosacral joint. Both the fourth and fifth lumbar nerves emerge from the spine through long bony canals, or tunnels, and are subject to compression injuries that may be caused by muscle spasms or direct trauma in the joint area. Because the fourth and fifth lumbar nerves are the principal constituents of the sciatic nerve (L_4, L_5; S_1, S_2, S_3), irritation to L_4 or L_5 can cause or contribute to the pain syndrome commonly called *sciatica*.

Lumbar spine injuries

The lumbar spine, or lower back, is an area that is subjected to many types of stresses and forces during athletic as well as nonathletic activity. The lower back is very susceptible to injury, and athletes frequently complain of pain in this area. The majority of low back pain in athletes is caused by either acute trauma or chronic stresses. Occasionally, low back pain is caused by structural defects in the vertebrae or intervertebral discs. All conditions affecting the lumbar spine can be aggravated by various contributing factors, such as inadequate or inappropriate conditioning, inflexibility, congenital anomalies, or poor postural habits. Each of these factors should be kept in mind when evaluating injuries to the lumbar spine area.

The most common athletic injuries to the lower back are contusions, sprains, and strains. Contusions are more common in the paraspinal muscles but may also occur over the subcutaneous spinous processes. The athlete will often have a history of a direct blow to the lumbar area, with localized tenderness and pain on movement. Sprains and strains are common in the multiplicity of muscles and ligaments in the lower back. Both of these injuries can be caused by the same types of mechanisms and may occur simultaneously. Violent muscle contractions against resistance, overuse, and overstretching are the most common mechanisms resulting in sprains or strains in the soft tissues along the spine. The complex anatomy of the lower back makes it very difficult to stress and evaluate specific muscles and ligaments. As a result, it is difficult to differentiate between a sprain and strain in this area. Fortunately, it is also usually unnecessary, as both of these injuries are treated symptomatically.

Severe injuries to the lumbar spine, such as fractures or dislocations, are extremely rare in athletic activity. Neurologic damage as a result of such an injury is also not as likely as in the cervical spine because the spinal cord ends at about the first lumbar vertebrae and the peripheral nerves in the cauda equina are more mobile and resistant to trauma. Compression fractures, as previously described in the thoracic spine, can also occur to the bodies of the lumbar vertebrae. However, the most common fractures in the lower back involve the spinous or transverse processes. These can occur as a result of a direct blow or violent muscle contraction. Fractures of this type are at times indistinguishable from severe strains or contusions without radiographs.

The most common structural defect of the lumbar spine in athletes is a condition called *spondylolysis,* which is a defect in the pars interarticularis of the vertebrae (Fig. 12-8). If this defect is bilateral, it may allow that vertebra to slip forward on the vertebra or sacrum below, a condition called *spondylolisthesis.* It may develop in athletes involved in strenuous exercise or competition. Many authorities consider this condition to be a stress fracture and the result of repeated trauma and stress rather than an acute fracture. It is also believed that spondylolysis and spondylolisthesis can be congenital. The athlete with spondylolisthesis will usually complain of low back pain associated with increased activity. With rest or inactivity the pain diminishes, only to return again once activity is resumed. In addition to the pain in the lower back, the athlete may complain of pain radiating into the buttocks and upper thighs. The appearance of radiating pain, as well as recurrent episodes of low back pain with activity, should alert the athletic trainer to refer this athlete for further diagnosis and radiographs. Occasionally the pain level remains tolerable and the athlete continues activity without ever knowing about the spondylolisthesis.

Another structural defect that may occur in the lumbar spine of an athlete is intervertebral disc herniation. In this condition the nucleus pulposus herniates through the annulus fibrosus and presses against the spinal cord or the spinal nerve roots. Although this condition is more common in people in their 30s and 40s, it can also occur in younger athletes. The athlete with a ruptured or herniated disc will normally have extreme pain and stiffness in the lower back, pain in the buttocks, and a unique type of radiating leg pain if the compression is severe. This leg pain is usually unilateral and follows the route of the sciatic nerve, which is formed by the fourth and fifth lumbar nerves and the first, second, and third sacral nerves. Pain may radiate down into

the thigh, calf, and foot, depending on the nerve roots involved. Sitting for prolonged periods of time, standing with both legs straight, or bending over will be especially uncomfortable for these athletes. Additional signs that may indicate a herniated disc include unilateral muscle weakness, sensory loss, or reflex loss in the leg. Athletes with signs and symptoms of this type must be referred for further evaluation.

Congenital anomalies are more common in the lumbar area than in any other segment of the spine. The most common of these is *spina bifida occulta,* which is a defect in the bony spinal canal without involvement of the spinal cord or meninges. This condition is usually noted only on a radiograph and, unless it is quite severe, causes only intermittent and moderate discomfort in the lower back. Athletes with spina bifida occulta have a higher incidence of low back pain and should be instructed in proper techniques to help protect this vulnerable area. Proper techniques include appropriate exercise and strength training, correct lifting procedures, and avoiding sudden stressful loads on the lumbar spine.

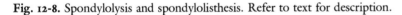

Fig. 12-8. Spondylolysis and spondylolisthesis. Refer to text for description.

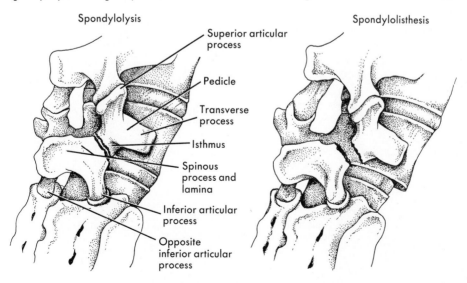

Spondylolysis

Spondylolisthesis

Superior articular process

Pedicle

Transverse process

Isthmus

Spinous process and lamina

Inferior articular process

Opposite inferior articular process

Sacrum and coccyx

The sacral and coccygeal portions of the spine are often referred to as the false, or fixed, vertebrae (Chapter 3). Together, the sacrum and coccyx form the terminal portion of the spinal column. In addition, they form the strong wedge-shaped posterior portion of the bony pelvis. Numerous ligaments of the sacrum and coccyx attach to portions of the lumbar vertebrae above and to points on the bony pelvis laterally and below.

The sacrum (Fig. 12-9) is a large wedge-shaped structure formed by the fusion of five vertebrae. The inner (pelvic) surface of the sacrum is smooth and concave, whereas the outer (posterior) surface is convex and rough. The upper portion (base) articulates with the body of the fifth lumbar vertebra, and the lower portion (apex) articulates with the coccyx below.

The concave inner surface is grooved by four

transverse ridges that show the points of separation between the original bodies of the five sacral vertebrae before fusion. At each end of the transverse ridges are large openings (sacral foramina), which accommodate the sacral nerves and arteries. The prominent *sacral promontory* is a bony prominence projecting from the anterior border of the base.

The coccyx forms the bony tip of the spine. It is generally a single, triangular bone fused from four rudimentary vertebrae. These vertebrae are very small and consist of only the fused body and poorly developed transverse processes. No laminae or spinous processes are present. Occasionally, the first element, or vertebrae, in the coccyx may be separate from the rest. The upper (superior) portion of the coccyx, called the base, articulates with the sacrum. The coccyx diminishes in size until it reaches the tip (apex). Athletic injuries to the coccyx are not common but

Fig. 12-9. Sacrum and coccyx. **A,** Anterior view; **B,** posterior view.

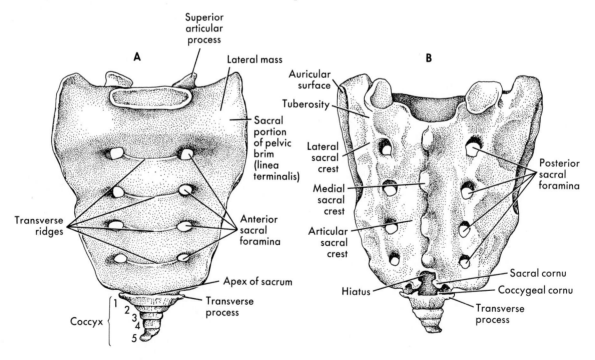

may occur from a direct blow to the area, such as a kick or a fall to a sitting position. Although these injuries may be painful, they generally are not disabling and require only routine treatment procedures.

Sacroiliac joints

The sacroiliac joint is formed by the articulation between the sacrum and the iliac portion of the hip bones (innominate bones) on each side of the pelvis. It is a true synovial joint (Chapter 4), but movement is limited by the presence of interlocking facets of bone and by extremely strong and dense ligaments. Any appreciable movement in either or both of the sacroiliac joints would lead to gross instability in the erect posture. In the sitting or standing position, the full weight of the body above the pelvis passes through these joints. Therefore freedom of motion must be sacrificed for stability.

The sacrum hangs from the sacroiliac joints and is kept from being pushed forward into the pelvis by the interlocking facets of bone and by the *posterior sacroiliac ligaments,* which are the strongest in the body. The dimple on each side immediately above the buttock is a useful external surface landmark that defines the center of the sacroiliac joint in most young adults. True sacroiliac sprains are extremely rare and almost never occur as a result of athletic activity.

ATHLETIC INJURY ASSESSMENT PROCESS

The potential for spinal injuries resulting in neurologic damage such as permanent paralysis or death is present in most athletic activities, especially contact sports. With any injury involving the spine, it is extremely important for the athletic trainer to recognize the possibilities for neurologic involvement as quickly as possible. Selection of appropriate assessment procedures, handling maneuvers, and transportation techniques depends on the possibility of involvement of the spinal cord. Added neurologic damage can occur during improper positioning or movement of an injured athlete. At no time in the assessment of athletic injuries is the principle "do no harm" more important than when evaluating and caring for injuries involving the spine.

Athletes suffering an injury to the spine generally present themselves in one of two modes. The athlete may suffer a traumatic injury and remain lying on the court or field. In these instances the injured athlete should be treated as though he or she has sustained a serious spinal cord injury until proved otherwise. This includes protecting the injured athlete from any unnecessary movement during the assessment process until you can be sure there is no spinal cord involvement. It is more common, however, for the athlete with an injury to the back or neck to be moving about. They often walk into the training room complaining of pain. In dealing with injuries of this type, it is relatively safe to assume there is no serious neurologic involvement. This large group of injuries include those caused by acute trauma and chronic stresses.

Primary survey

The primary survey is of utmost importance when an injured athlete remains down and appears to be unresponsive or unconscious. Maintenance of airway, breathing, and circulation must then be primary considerations. Remember, whenever a neck injury is suspected, movement of the cervical spine must not occur. If the athlete is unconscious and a neck injury is suspected, the jaw-thrust method of opening the airway is the safest technique to use. If the injured athlete must be moved to perform CPR techniques, it is extremely important that he or she be rolled or moved as a unit to avoid any unnecessary movements of the spine. After assurance that the respiratory and circulatory states of the injured athlete are adequate, proceed to the secondary survey and a more detailed neurologic evaluation.

Secondary survey

The evaluation procedures used during the secondary survey depend on the responsiveness and position of the injured athlete. A quick glance at the overall picture will generally determine the direction in which the athletic trainer will proceed with the secondary survey. It is important to maintain a high index of suspicion whenever assessing spine injuries, as there may be associated damage to the spinal cord or peripheral nerve roots. It can be very difficult for the athletic trainer to determine which spine injuries threaten nerve function and which do not. Therefore it is best to consider all spine injuries as potentially dangerous and handle them accordingly.

The athlete who remains unconscious must be managed as if a spinal injury has occurred, as discussed in Chapter 10. The athlete who is responsive but remains lying on the floor or ground following a traumatic injury must also be evaluated and handled with utmost caution. The athlete should be evaluated in the position he or she is found. If a spinal injury is unstable, the vertebral column is no longer able to protect the spinal cord and may actually cause added neurologic damage during any type of positioning or movement. If necessary, the entire secondary survey can be accomplished with the athlete remaining in the original position. Remember, whenever neurologic involvement is recognized or suspected, it is not necessary to continue the assessment process; it is time to seek medical assistance. It is of paramount importance to protect the injured athlete from further aggravation of any neurologic involvement. Examination of the neck and immobilization of the spine should precede all other maneuvers of the secondary survey in circumstances in which there is reason to believe that a spinal injury may have occurred.

Fortunately, the majority of athletic injuries involving the spine are not serious and consist of contusions, sprains, and strains. In these instances, the secondary survey can provide information necessary to recognize the structures involved and the extent of injury. In addition, the secondary survey can assist the athletic trainer in determining if referral and further evaluation is necessary, which treatment procedures to follow, and when the athlete can safely return to activity.

Always remember that a cervical spine injury can occur along with a head injury. Both areas should be evaluated simultaneously. As discussed in the previous chapter, it is important to establish and monitor an athlete's level of consciousness in order to recognize possible intracranical involvement associated with a head injury.

History

The history of an injury involving the spine is very important. If the athlete remains down after an injury, the initial questioning must be directed at determining the nature and site of the injury. If the head, neck, or back is involved in the injury, questioning must be directed at recognizing any possible neurologic involvement. Begin by asking the athlete to express his or her feelings and sensations.

Paralysis. Is there any paralysis? Paralysis is the most reliable sign of spinal cord injury. Spinal cord injuries in the neck may cause paralysis of all four extremities *(quadriplegia)* as well as breathing impairment. Spinal cord injuries below the neck may cause paralysis of the lower extremities *(paraplegia),* with no impairment of breathing functions. However, a spinal cord injury may not manifest itself with symptoms of complete paralysis. An athlete may demonstrate a partial, or incomplete, paralysis *(paresis)*.

Test muscle function by requesting very gentle active movements, such as asking the athlete to carefully move his or her fingers or toes. Then proceed to the larger joints such as the wrists, elbows, shoulders and ankles, knees, and hips. If the athlete has normal motion in the extremities, proceed to check the speed and strength of movements. The speed of movement can be evaluated by having the athlete open and close the fingers or move the toes quickly. Strength can be evaluated by putting resistance against the active motion or asking the injured athlete to grip your hand or fingers. Any demonstrable weakness or loss of function should be considered and managed as a spinal cord injury. Remember to always compare extremities on both sides of the body to note any difference in motion, speed, or strength. It is possible the spinal injury involved nerves on only one side of the body.

Sensations. The loss of voluntary movement in the extremities is usually accompanied by loss of sensations. Sensory function can be evaluated by stimulating the skin of the arms, trunk, and legs with a light touch or sharp object such as a safety pin. Does the athlete perceive the touch and/or pain stimulus appropriately and symmetrically? Are sensations absent *(anesthesia),* decreased, exaggerated, or delayed? Recalling the distribution of dermatomes allows you to locate those dermatomes where sensations are altered. Try to test as many dermatomes as possible by distributing the stimuli over the body. An athlete may also complain of abnormal sensations *(paresthesia)* such as burning, tingling, or prickling in the extremities. These paresthesias may follow a specific dermatome pattern. It is important that these be recognized as symptoms of possible spinal cord injury and appropriate emergency care measures initiated. It may take a detailed neurologic evaluation to detect minor neural problems, but if the injured athlete has normal sensations, motion, speed, and strength in the extremities, it can be assumed that no serious spinal cord injury has occurred.

Pain. Question the athlete about pain associated with the injury. Is there any pain in the neck or back? Where is the pain located? How severe is the pain? The athlete with unremitting neck or back pain should be handled as if there is spinal cord involvement. Occasionally, if the injured athlete is lying very still, he or she will not complain of much pain until movement of the injured area of the spine is attempted. If pain is increased significantly when an athlete attempts to move, he or she should be managed as if the spinal cord is involved. The athletic trainer should encourage an athlete with possible neck or back injuries to remain motionless.

At this time it may be necessary to palpate and localize the painful or tender areas. Avoid moving the injured athlete during this process. The spinous processes can be palpated by carefully placing your hand under the neck or back. Localized deformity, tenderness, or increased pain detected immediately over the spinous processes is sufficient reason to suspect an injury to the spinal column, and the athlete should be handled as if there is spinal cord involvement.

For the athlete who does not appear to have any spinal cord involvement, attempt to gain as much information surrounding the circumstances of the injury as possible. Continue to investigate the tender and painful areas. Are there muscle spasms or tightness associated with the pain? If possible, ask the athlete to point to the painful areas. Notice if the athlete can localize the pain or if it appears to cover a large area. Also notice if the athlete is complaining of pain in the soft tissues along either side of the spine or over the bony spinous processes. Does the athlete have a difficult time specifying where the pain is? Ask the athlete to describe the characteristics of the pain. For example, is the pain sharp, burning, or a dull ache? Is the pain constant or intermittent? Is there any radiating pain into the arms, shoulders, thighs, or legs? Are there certain types of movements or exercises that aggravate or increase the pain? Is the pain relieved by rest or certain positions?

Mechanism of injury. Attempt to determine the mechanism of injury, including the type of forces or stresses that occurred. Does the injury appear to be the result of an acute traumatic episode or the accumulation of chronic stresses that have developed over a period of time? Was the injury caused by a direct blow or was the spine stretched, strained, or twisted?

Previous history. Many injuries to the spine are chronic conditions that do not arise from a single acute injury. These chronic conditions represent an aggravation of previously existing circumstances, such as congenital abnormalities, structural deviations, postural habits, or previous injuries. Therefore a complete history of any previous neck or back complaints should be sought. The history should include information that might link previous injuries to the current problem. Ask how the symptoms began and what has occurred from the time of onset until the present. How did the pain first start? Was the athlete injured? Are the symptoms affected by posture, rest, or activity? What treatment procedures have been carried out on the injured athlete, and have they helped? Knowing the past history and behavior of symptoms gives the athletic trainer important information to assist in recognizing possible causes as well as determining treatment procedures.

Observation

Initial observations are extremely important in determining which assessment procedures to use and in what sequence. Watch very carefully as you approach an injured athlete. Is the athlete lying motionless? If so, you should expect and treat the athlete as if he or she has suffered a serious spinal injury until proved otherwise. Is the athlete attempting any movements of the neck or extremities? Remember, an athlete who has suffered a serious cervical spine injury will be very cautious and defensive of any movements of the neck.

Deformities. Watch very closely as you carry out the history process and talk with the injured athlete. Survey the athlete for obvious deformities or abnormal positions of any body parts. Observations may be difficult because of the position of the athlete. For example, if the athlete is lying on his or her back, it is extremely difficult to view the spine without some movement. Uniforms and equipment may also conceal the injured area. If the area can be viewed, look for any deformity of the spine. The spinous processes may appear crooked or out of place, which would be an extremely reliable sign. However, the spine rarely appears deformed, even with very severe injuries, and the absence of deformity in no way rules out the possibility of a fracture or dislocation.

Signs of trauma. Look for any signs of trauma that may give additional clues to the nature and severity of the injury. If the areas can be viewed, look for cuts and bruises about the head, face, shoulders, back, and abdomen. These physical signs can indicate what types of forces have been applied to the athlete's body and help establish the mechanism of injury. Also watch for any signs that may indicate neurologic involvement, such as paralysis or weakness.

Movements and positions. If the athlete is moving about and spinal cord involvement is not suspected, observe his or her movements and the positions preferred. Voluntary movements can be most revealing when the athlete is unaware you are examining his or her actions. During an obvious and intentional examination of gait or posture, an athlete may intentionally move or assume a position considered proper or one that depicts an extremely painful state. Either of these may not accurately reflect the symptoms associated with the injured neck or back. Every athletic trainer should develop a protocol for observing the main postures and positions of the body during all types of activity.

Watch the athlete's gait pattern and willingness to move about. Does the athlete appear to stand, walk, and move about normally and without pain? Does the athlete appear to move very cautiously as if in pain? Does the athlete avoid bending, twisting, or other motions that could be painful? Can the athlete relax, or does he or she seem to have a difficult time finding a comfortable position? Which standing, sitting, or lying positions does the injured athlete prefer or consciously avoid?

Alignment of the neck and back. Evaluating an athlete's postural alignment may reveal underlying causes of neck or back conditions. This is especially true of chronic or overuse conditions affecting the lower back. Athletic injuries and painful conditions can result from malalignments and poor postural habits, which are intensified by heavy or intense athletic activities. Therefore an athletic trainer should understand the fundamental concepts of body alignment and posture.

Posture is an individual matter. There is no

single best or most appropriate posture for all persons. For each athlete, the best posture is that in which the body segments are balanced in the position of least strain and most support. Posture and body mechanics must be considered from the standpoint of the athlete's body build and the activities in which the athlete is involved. Minor postural differences in healthy active athletes are usually of little consequence, as the body has a remarkable ability to compensate for deviations from the norm. Athletic activity can lead to postural adaptations, but these do not necessarily cause injuries. Each individual instance requires careful professional judgement. An athletic trainer should be able to recognize moderate to severe deviations in alignment or posture that may be associated with an injury or painful condition. The ability to recognize these factors allows the athletic trainer to refer the athlete for more definitive diagnosis or develop effective exercise programs designed to increase strength or flexibility and to aid in preparing strategies to change body mechanics or improve poor postural habits.

This evaluation of alignment or posture is also important when an injury alters an athlete's posture. Pain and muscle spasms associated with an athletic injury can change the positioning and posture of an athlete. As long as symptoms persist, normal posture may not be possible. Occasionally a faulty postural habit is established that may continue after the injury has healed. Therefore continuing evaluation of body alignment or posture can serve as a basis for measuring future progress and improving faulty postural habits resulting from injury.

Evaluate the alignment or posture with the athlete standing in shorts or other brief clothing so that the back is bare. For women, this is best performed with the athlete in a two-piece swimming suit. Observe the general body build and development of the athlete. Notice if the athlete can stand evenly with both feet flat on the floor. Occasionally, because of pain, an athlete will be unable to bear weight equally on both feet, and the body weight will be shifted toward one side.

The athlete should be viewed from the back, front, and side. When evaluating injuries to the spine, it is probably most revealing to view the athlete from the back first. Standing behind the athlete, survey the entire spine as well as the relationship of the head, shoulders, and pelvis. Normal alignment of the body when viewed from the rear is illustrated in Fig. 12-10. An imaginary vertical line should bisect the body into symmetric halves. Any irregularities in symmetry should be noted, as they may indicate circumstances that contributed to the injury or painful condition, such as a short leg, muscle weakness, or spinal curvature. Remember, irregularities in symmetry can also result directly from an injury and may be caused by muscle spasms or pain.

Fig. 12-10. Normal alignment of the body when viewed from the back.

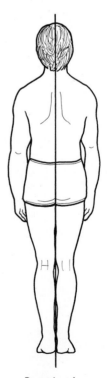

Posterior view

When viewing the athlete's spine from the back, you should first consider the level of the pelvis. The pelvis is the "keystone," or foundation, of the spine. When the pelvis is not level, the spine and upper body must compensate in an attempt to keep the body alignment balanced. Determining the level of the pelvis can be accomplished by several methods. The easiest method is to place your fingertips on each iliac crest and check the horizontal level of your fingers or the relative heights of each anterior superior iliac spine (Fig. 12-11). Another method to determine relative heights of each side of the pelvis would be to palpate both posterior superior iliac spines simultaneously to determine if they are in the same horizontal plane.

Whenever a pelvic obliquity is observed, a discrepancy in leg length should be suspected and evaluated further. A discrepancy in leg length, either actual or functional, can cause an imbalance and contribute to an injury or produce overuse symptoms in the back, pelvis, or lower extremities. To determine if a leg length discrepancy exists, have the athlete lie supine, place both legs in a neutral position, and observe the medial malleoli (Fig. 12-12). If the malleoli do

Fig. 12-11. Palpating anterior superior iliac spines to determine level of pelvis.

Fig. 12-12. Observing alignment of medial malleoli to determine if a leg length discrepancy exists.

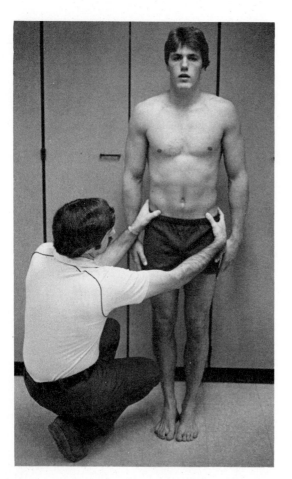

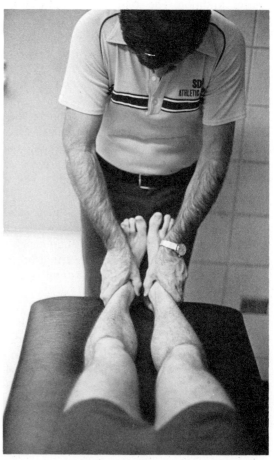

not appear to match, a difference in leg length should be suspected. To determine if there is an actual discrepancy in leg length, measure the distance from the anterior superior iliac spine to the medial malleolus of each ankle and compare (Fig. 12-13). Unequal distances between these bony landmarks indicate an actual difference in leg length. If the length of the legs are the same but the level of the pelvis is uneven, the pelvis is tilted laterally, resulting in one leg being functionally shorter. This pelvic obliquity can be caused by an injury or problem in the back, hips, knees, or feet.

It is doubtful that minor leg length discrepancies cause significant injury symptoms. However, when a leg length discrepancy is encountered, the relevance of the discrepancy to the athlete's symptoms should be investigated further. For example, is pain associated with the condition increased by standing and walking? If not, the difference in leg length is likely to be irrelevant. If pain is produced by standing and walking, perhaps the leg length discrepancy has an effect on the athlete's symptoms and the athlete should be referred for medical evaluation.

The back view can also indicate whether the

Fig. 12-13. Measuring the distance between the anterior superior iliac spine to the medial malleolus. Compare both sides to determine if an actual leg length discrepancy exists.

Fig. 12-14. Athlete with a scoliosis.
(Courtesy Steve Yoneda, California Polytechnic State University.)

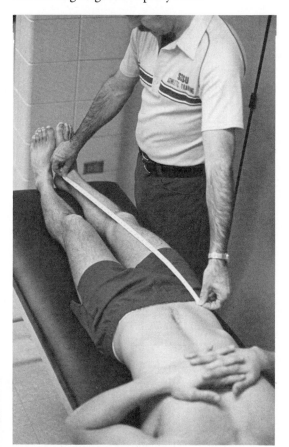

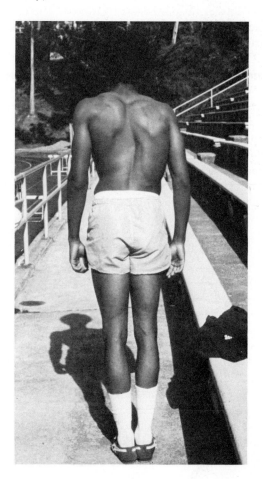

spine appears straight. The spinous processes of each vertebrae should appear in a straight line from top to bottom. Any lateral deviation of the spinal column is called *scoliosis* (Fig. 12-14). It is among the most serious of postural deviations. Later stages of scoliosis can cause asymmetry of the upper extremities, shoulders, thorax, pelvis, and lower extremities. Minor lateral deviations of the vertebral column can result from athletic activity that utilizes one side of the body more than the other, or from symptoms of an acute injury. Unilateral spasm of vertebral muscles caused by the pull of a rope ski tow, for example, would result in such lateral deviation. Lateral deviations that remain after the cessation of injury symptoms, and especially those found in young athletes, should be referred to a physician for further diagnosis and treatment. The early stages of scoliosis can be corrected by proper treatment.

Additional postural alignments that should be viewed from the back of an athlete include positioning of the shoulders and scapulae. Both shoulders should be at an equal height or in the same horizontal plane. Unequal height of the shoulders may result from such conditions as lateral curvature of the spine, unequal development of the shoulder girdle musculature, or injury symptoms. It is important to determine whether the unequal shoulder height is caused by a local injury or by such remote conditions as leg length discrepancy or lateral curvature of the spine. Both scapulae should also be level and positioned an equal distance from the vertebral column. Occasionally, both scapulae will be a greater distance from the vertebral column than is considered normal. This condition results in the scapula pulling away from the rib cage and is called *winged scapula.* It is usually caused by muscular weakness and can generally be improved with an exercise program.

When viewing the back of an athlete, head position is an important consideration in assessing spinal alignment. The head should be held in a level, well-balanced position. Occasionally, because of pain and muscle spasms in the cervical musculature, an athlete's neck may be slightly twisted, resulting in the head being held in an unnatural position. This is called *torticollis,* or wryneck.

When evaluating the alignment or posture of the body, the athlete should also be viewed from the side. Normal alignment of the body when viewed from the side is illustrated in Fig. 12-15. An imaginary vertical line should pass through the ear lobe, tip of the shoulder, greater trochanter of the femur, posterior to the patella, and anterior to the lateral malleolus. This side view of body alignment allows the athletic trainer to analyze the anteroposterior curvatures of the spine. Normal spinal curvatures include a concave curve at the cervical and lumbar spine areas and a convex curve of the thoracic spine.

One of the more common postural deviations

Fig. 12-15. Normal alignment of the body when viewed from the side.

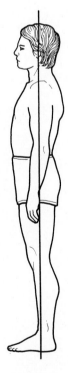

Lateral view

in athletes is an accentuation of the forward curve of the lumbar spine. This is called *lumbar lordosis* and usually results in forward tilting of the pelvis. Lumbar lordosis is usually associated with weakened and elongated abdominal muscles and contracted and tight muscles of the lower back. This muscular imbalance results in tilting the pelvis anteriorly, creating the common swayback or hollow back appearance. Lumbar lordosis can be improved or overcome by an exercise program involving stretching the lower back muscles, strengthening the abdominals, and making a concerted effort to reestablish proper pelvic alignment.

An exaggerated curve in the thoracic spine is called *kyphosis,* which is an abnormal rounding of the upper back (Fig. 12-16). This condition is often associated with *forward shoulders,* in which the shoulders are carried abnormally forward of the imaginary vertical line described previously. These conditions are usually associ-

ated with muscular tightness in the chest and stretched, weakened muscles of the upper back region.

The head should be held in a well-balanced position directly above the shoulders. A common deviation from what is considered normal alignment, is *forward head.* This condition occurs when an athlete carries his or her head in an abnormal anterior position, which can result in weakened cervical extensor muscles and tightened flexor muscles. The forward head may become realigned by development of *cervical lor-*

Fig. 12-17. Wall test to observe anterior posterior alignment of the spine.

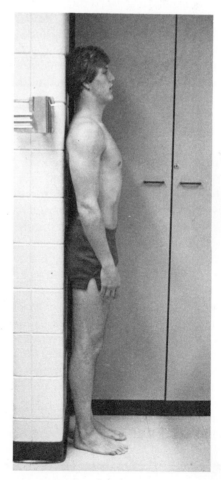

Fig. 12-16. Young athlete exhibiting rounded shoulders (kyphosis).

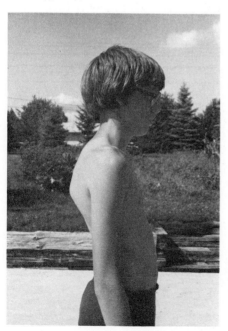

dosis, which is an accentuation of the normal curvature of the cervical spine.

An alternative method of evaluating the alignment of the body is to have the athlete stand with his or her back against a wall (Fig. 12-17). Instruct the athlete to stand straight with the heels within two inches of the wall. The back of the head, scapular area, and buttocks should touch the wall. In this position it is easier to recognize anteroposterior problems such as lumbar lordosis, forward shoulders, or forward head. You can also have the athlete actually participate in the evaluation process. Ask the athlete to place a hand in the small of the back to evaluate spinal curvature in this area. Normally a person should be able to slip a hand in between the wall and the lumbar spine. If there is more room than that and one is able to wiggle the hand around freely, there is probably some degree of lordosis. Using the wall in analyzing posture is an excellent method of allowing athletes to evaluate and monitor their own postural habits.

Palpation

Procedures using palpation were discussed during the history portion of this assessment process. These procedures were used to evaluate whether sensations were intact and to localize painful areas. It is important to use these procedures early in the assessment of spinal injuries to recognize possible spinal cord involvement. Palpation procedures used on spinal injuries not suspected of involving the spinal cord are for the purpose of localizing the injured area.

Tenderness and muscle spasm. Carefully palpate along the spinous processes as well as the paraspinal muscles in an attempt to localize tenderness or muscle spasms associated with injury. It may be helpful to have the athlete hunch the shoulders forward or slightly flex the spine so that the spinous processes are more pronounced (Fig. 12-18). If the athlete can assist in the examination in this way it will highlight anatomic landmarks in the area and help the examiner localize the injury. Even with this type of help, however, it may be difficult to identify the exact

structures involved in an injury, as many of the structures about the spine are deep and not subcutaneous. In addition, there may be a great deal of generalized muscle spasm or referred pain associated with the injury, making it difficult to define exactly which structures are injured. Every effort should be made, however, to localize the painful areas as precisely as possible and correlate this information with active and resistive movements described in the next section.

Stress

Following history, observation and palpation techniques, in the absence of spinal cord involvement, appropriate movement procedures can be very helpful in the assessment of the more common injuries to the spine. It is important to remember that if pain is increased considerably on any attempt to move the spine, or if the ath-

Fig. 12-18. Palpating spinous processes with the spine in flexion.

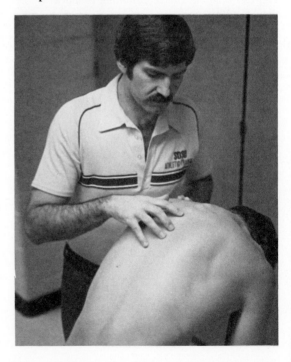

lete bitterly resists moving the spine, he or she should be handled as if there may be serious spinal injury. In these cases the athlete must not be subjected to continued movement or manipulation. Instead, the athlete should be protected from further trauma and referred to a physician.

Active movements. Initially, active movements should be attempted by an athlete complaining of a back injury. Careful movements made by the athete suffering an acute injury to the spine are not likely to cause spinal cord damage, as the athlete will usually cease even the slightest move-

ment on experiencing a significant increase in pain. Do not encourage the athlete to move the spine if pain is increased. The importance of being cautious when evaluating an acute injury to the spine cannot be overemphasized.

Active movements are performed to evaluate the flexibility and range of motion in various segments of the spine and to localize any pain associated with movement. As the athlete performs each of the movements, observe if the motion is performed smoothly and through a normal range of motion. To evaluate the active

Fig. 12-19. Active range of motion of the cervical spine: **A,** flexion, **B,** hyperextension, **C,** lateral bending, and **D,** rotation.

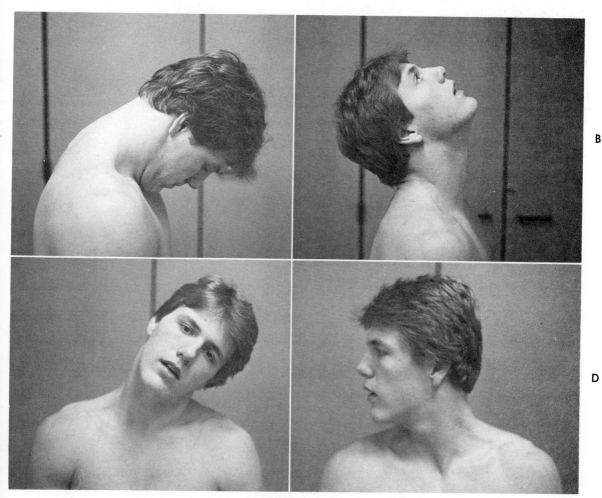

Fig. 12-20. Active range of motion of the trunk: **A,** flexion, **B,** hyperextension, **C,** lateral bending, and **D,** rotation.

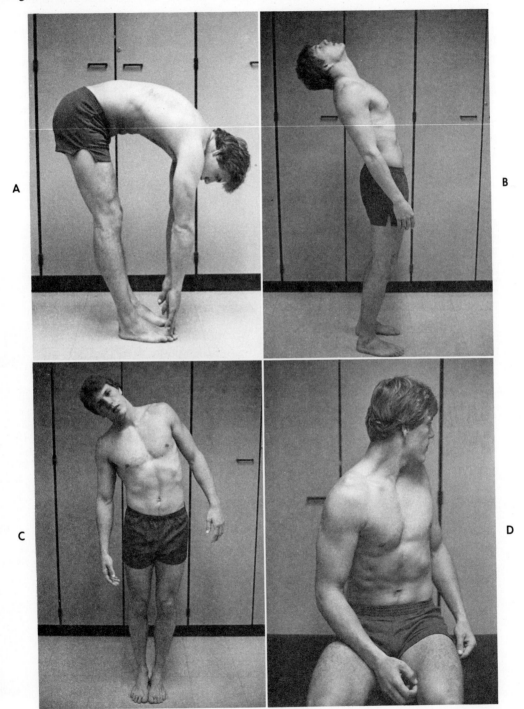

A

B

C

D

range of motion in the cervical spine, ask the athlete to perform each of the basic movements of the neck (Fig. 12-19). To test flexion and extension, ask the athlete to nod the head forward and backward. Normally an athlete should be able to touch the chest with the chin and to look directly upward. To evaluate rotation in the cervical area, ask the athlete to turn his or her head to both sides as far as possible. An athlete should be able to move the head to each side so that the chin is almost in line with the shoulder. Remember to compare motions on each side. To evaluate lateral bending, ask the athlete to move the head from side to side as if to touch the ear to the shoulder. Normally an athlete should be able to tilt the head about 45° toward each shoulder. Again compare motions in each direction and make sure the athlete does not compensate by lifting a shoulder toward the ear.

The active range of motion in the thoracic and lumbar areas of the spine is evaluated simultaneously. Remember, more movement is possible in the lumbar than in the thoracic area, but only a small amount of that movement actually takes place in the spine. As the athlete performs each of the active movements, observe the degree of motion, smoothness of the spinal curve, and symmetry of body areas. To evaluate flexion, ask the athlete to bend forward with the knees straight as if to touch the toes (Fig. 12-20). Although most of this motion occurs at the hip joint, it allows the athletic trainer to observe the movements of the spine. Observe extension as the athlete returns to an upright position. To test hyperextension, ask the athlete to bend backward as far as possible. Normally an athlete can hyperextend approximately 30°. To test lateral bending, ask the athlete to bend to the left and right as far as possible. It may be necessary to stabilize the pelvis, as an athlete may compensate by moving the pelvis. Normally an athlete should have approximately 35° of lateral bending in each direction. To evaluate trunk rotation, ask the athlete to turn the head and shoulders to both sides. Again, it is important to stabilize the pelvis so that the athlete is not turning the hips

to compensate for lack of rotation in the spinal area. One method of stabilizing the pelvis is to have the athlete perform trunk rotation while sitting on a table (Fig. 12-20, *D*).

In addition to evaluating the flexibility of the spine, active maneuvers can be used to evaluate any limitation of motion in body areas that may affect spinal alignment. Certain muscles and muscle groups are frequently found to be shortened in athletes with apparent abnormal spinal alignment. This may be caused by atypical muscle usage during athletic activity or inappropriate posture. If the athletic trainer suspects that shortening of muscles may be a causitive factor in loss of flexibility or decrease in range of motion, muscle groups should be evaluated.

Forward shoulders is usually associated with tight shoulder adductor and internal rotator muscles. To evaluate any limitation of these shoulder motions, have the athlete lie supine. Instruct the athlete to place the hands behind the neck and elbows on the table (Fig. 12-21). Normally an athlete should be able to rest his or her elbows on the table without any strain. If rounded shoulders or kyphosis prevents the elbows from resting on the table, the athlete would probably benefit from an exercise program designed to stretch these muscle groups.

The pelvis is another body area that has a major effect on spinal alignment. Muscular tightness can tilt the pelvis, resulting in compensating curves in the lumbar spine. Hip flexor and hamstring muscle groups are the more common sites of muscle tightness about the pelvis. To evaluate the hip flexors, have the athlete lie in a supine position and instruct him or her to pull one thigh up against the chest (Fig. 12-22). If the hip flexors of the opposite leg are not tight, the extended leg will remain on the table. If the hip flexors are tight, the opposite thigh will be lifted from the table. Repeat the same procedure using the other leg. This procedure is called a *Thomas test*.

The same supine position can be used to quickly evaluate hamstring tightness. Instruct the athlete to raise one leg as high as possible

Fig. 12-21. Evaluating tightness in the shoulder adductor and internal rotator muscles by having the athlete lie supine with hands behind the neck. An athlete should be able to place both elbows on the table.

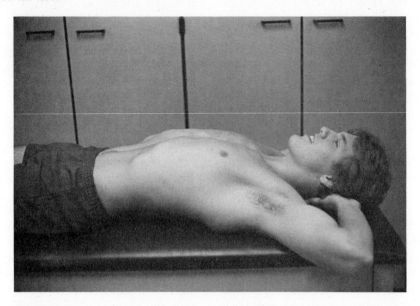

Fig. 12-22. Thomas test. Evaluating tightness in the hip flexor muscles by having the athlete pull one thigh up against the chest. The opposite leg should remain on the table. Compare both legs.

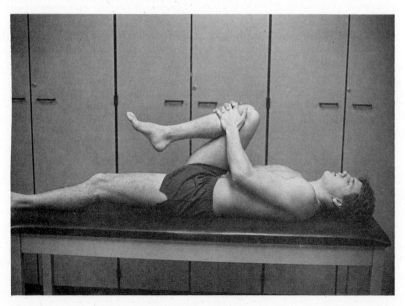

without flexing the knee (Fig. 12-23). The opposite extremity should remain in contact with the table. Repeat the same procedure with the other leg. An athlete should be able to obtain approximately 70° of flexion with each leg. An alternate method of evaluating the hamstrings is to put the athlete in a long sitting position. Instruct the athlete to reach out as far as possible and try to touch the toes without flexing the knees. Tight hamstrings or lack of spinal flexibility can prevent an athlete from touching the toes.

Resistive movements. Applying resistance against spinal motions can serve two main purposes: (1) to assist in determining which structures are involved in spinal injury, and (2) to assess the strength of muscles surrounding and supporting the spine. Both of these functions are important in evaluating acute and chronic spinal injuries affecting the spine. Remember, active motion of an injured muscle against resistance will cause pain or increase severity of existing pain. In addition, applying resistance against active movement allows one to evaluate the relative strength of specific muscles. The strength of muscles surrounding the flexible segments of the vertebral column is extremely important in supporting the spine and keeping the various segments in proper alignment. Muscle weaknesses and imbalances can cause injury symptoms. This is especially true in the lower back.

The muscles about the cervical spine are evaluated by applying resistance against the neck movements described previously. For each movement, manual resistance is applied. This is accomplished by using one hand to stabilize the shoulder or thorax to prevent any substitute motions, and exerting the resistance with the other hand. To evaluate cervical flexion, place the stabilizing hand on the athlete's shoulder and the palm of the resistance hand on the forehead. Instruct the athlete to flex the neck slowly while resistance is increased until the pain is localized or the relative strength of those muscles producing flexion is determined (Fig. 12-24, *A*). To test extension, cup the palm of one hand over the back of the athlete's head, stabilize the thorax

Fig. 12-23. Evaluating tightness in the hamstring musculature by having the athlete raise one leg as high as possible without flexing the knee. An athlete should be able to obtain approximately 70° of flexion with each leg. Compare both legs.

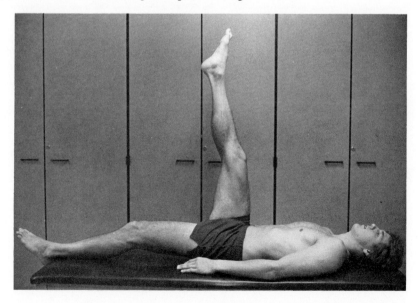

Fig. 12-24. Applying manual resistance against cervical motion: **A,** flexion, **B,** extension, **C,** lateral bending, and **D,** rotation.

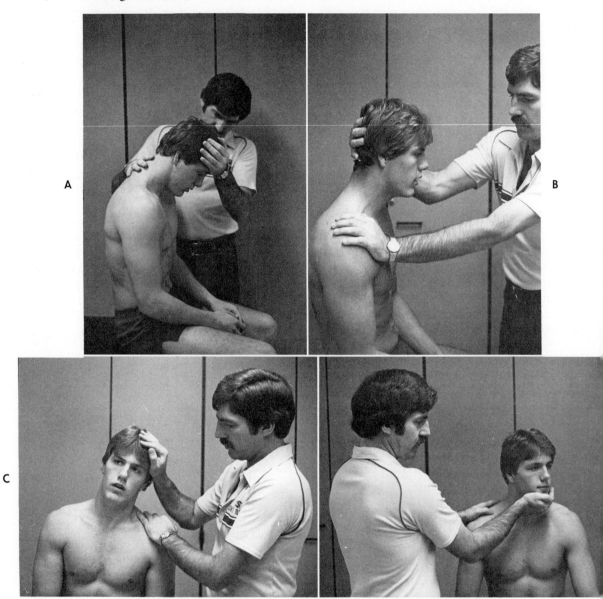

with the other, and instruct the athlete to slowly extend against resistance (Fig. 12-24, *B*). To evaluate lateral flexion of the neck, place the resistance hand against the side of athlete's head and the stabilizing hand on the shoulder on the same side to prevent elevation (Fig. 12-24, *C*). To evaluate rotation of the head to the right, the examiner should stabilize the left shoulder and apply resistance along the right side of the athlete's jaw (Fig. 12-24, *D*). To test rotation to the left, reverse the hand positions.

Applying resistance against trunk movements can be accomplished by resisting motions in the standing position, as described earier. However, it is much easier to apply resistance to trunk movements when the athlete is lying down. In these positions gravity can assist in applying resistance against a particular movement. It must be remembered that movements involving the trunk can be made more or less difficult by varying the weight distribution; for example, placement of the athlete's hands and arms can make the movements easier or harder. Movements can be performed with the hands at the athlete's side, at the abdomen, behind the neck, on top of the head, or extended overhead. Each of these changes in arm position shifts the center of gravity upward and thereby progressively increases resistance. As techniques are refined and "hands on" experience in the assessment process grows, the student athletic trainer will learn a great deal about the practical aspects of functional anatomy and applied kinesiology. Overall body position and the selective positioning of the extremities during the assessment, for example, will not only shift the center of gravity but may also change the angle of attack of secondary and tertiary movers at a joint, thus significantly altering the athlete's response to a particular test. Therefore functional anatomy and principles involving mechanics of motion must be understood and applied by the athletic trainer during the evaluation process.

The abdominals are an extremely important group of muscles that must be considered when evaluating any lower back condition. These muscles are a key factor in lumbar spine support, as they provide anterior stability and active forward flexion of the trunk. Weakness of the abdominals can result in forward tilting of the pelvis, cause an increase in lumbar lordosis, increase the possibility of lumbosacral ligament sprains, and ultimately contribute to lower back pain. The abdominals are one of the most common areas of muscular weaknesses in athletes. To evaluate the strength of the abdominals, have the athlete perform a partial sit-up from the supine position, with knees flexed and feet unsupported (Fig. 12-25, *A*). The hands can be at the side, on the chest, or behind the head, depending on abdominal strength. An athlete with normal abdominal strength should be able to perform this activity with their hands behind their head. Instruct the athlete to raise the head and continue to curl the spine upward until the thoracic spine is lifted from the table, approximately 30° to 40°. Motion up to this point is caused predominately by the abdominals, especially the rectus abdominus muscle, and provides a good test of abdominal strength. Athletes who are recognized as having weakened abdominals should be instructed in an abdominal strengthening program. To evaluate trunk rotation, have the athlete perform the same partial sit-up in a rotated position (Fig. 12-25, *D*). Instruct the athlete to rotate in the other direction. These tests are designed predominately to evaluate the oblique abdominal muscles. When the trunk is rotated to the right, this sit-up uses the right external oblique and left internal oblique muscles. When the athlete rotates the trunk to the left, the action is brought about by the opposite muscles.

In order to apply resistance against extension or hyperextention of the spine, have the athlete lie prone and raise the head and shoulders off the table (Fig. 12-25, *B*). The muscles causing lateral flexion of the trunk are evaluated with the athlete lying on one side and the feet stabilized (Fig. 12-25, *C*). Additional resistance can be applied against these movements as the athlete raises the hands above the head. The athletic trainer can also apply additional resistance against the athlete's upper back or shoulders. Watch the mechanics of these movements to recognize any increase in pain or muscular weaknesses.

Passive movements. Few passive movements are used during the assessment of injuries to the spine, especially injuries to the cervical spine. An athletic trainer should not attempt to passively evaluate the range of motion in an athlete's spine after an injury. The vertebral column may be unstable, and damage to the spinal cord could result. Remember, passive movements are generally more dangerous, and caution must be

used in evaluating injuries to the spine.

In appropriate circumstances, a passive procedure that may assist in evaluating injuries to or conditions of the spine is the straight-leg raising test. This test is designed to reproduce back and leg pain to determine its cause. With the athlete lying supine, grasp the athlete's heel with one hand, place your other hand on his or her knee to prevent it from bending, and lift the leg upward until there is discomfort or tightness (Fig. 12-26). You should be able to raise the leg approximately 70° to 80°. Straight-leg raising may be limited and painful because of tight hamstrings, lumbosacral or sacroiliac joint injury, or a problem with the sciatic nerve. Determine the

Fig. 12-25. Active movements resulting in resistance to specific trunk movements: **A,** flexion, **B,** hyperextension, **C,** lateral bending, and **D,** rotation.

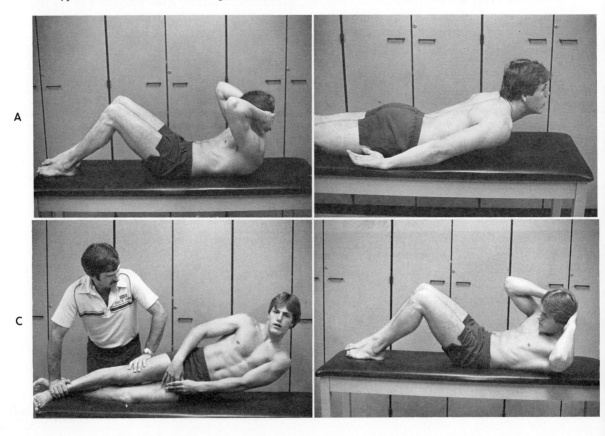

Fig. 12-26. Straight-leg raising to evaluate hamstring tightness, lumbosacral, sacroiliac, or sciatic nerve involvement.

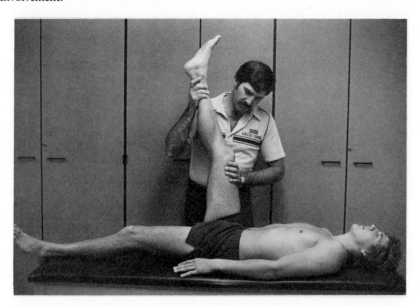

Fig. 12-27. Straight-leg raising with ankle dorsiflexion to determine possible sciatic nerve involvement.

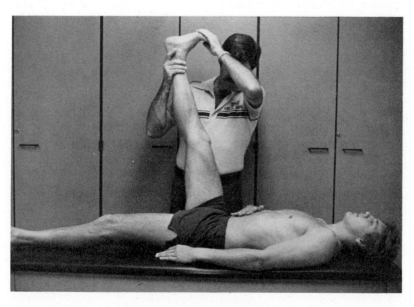

location of the pain. Tight hamstrings will produce pain in the posterior thigh. An injury to the lumbosacral or sacroiliac joints should produce pain in those areas of the spine. Sciatic pain can radiate all the way down the leg. To determine if there is a sciatic nerve problem, drop the leg back down slightly until there is no pain or discomfort. With the leg held stationary, dorsiflex the foot (Fig. 12-27). This maneuver puts no additional stress on the lumbosacral or sacroiliac joints or the hamstrings. It does, however, place additional pull on the sciatic nerve trunk, and increased pain indicates possible sciatic nerve involvement. This athlete should be referred to a physician for further assessment.

Functional movements. Functional movements are used to evaluate the functional abilities of the athlete who has suffered a spinal injury. These are especially important in evaluating athletes who have suffered injuries to the back or neck. The initial functional movements are the same as those described in the stress portion of the assessment process. That is, alignment, flexibility, and strength. The athletic trainer must carefully monitor the treatment and rehabilitation of the injured athlete to ensure that no abnormal alignments, faulty postural habits, or inequality in flexibility and strength occur as an athlete returns to activity. The athlete who returns to active competition with any of these conditions is subject to reinjury and continued problems. Once the athlete can demonstrate normal alignment, flexibility, and strength, he or she should be observed performing movements or activities specific to his or her sport. The athletic trainer must continue to evaluate an athlete who has suffered an injury to the spinal area. Follow-up care is extremely important to ensure rapid and safe return to activity.

Evaluation of findings

The most disastrous and serious athletic injuries which can occur to the spine are fractures or dislocations of the vertebrae with actual or potential damage to the spinal cord. Whenever a severe injury to the spine is recognized or suspected, it is imperative that you make certain the athlete is protected from further trauma to the neural elements. An injury without neurologic involvement must not be converted into one with irreversible spinal cord or peripheral nerve damage by ill-advised evaluation, manipulation, or transportation procedures. The mechanism for a catastrophic injury to the spine is present in most athletic activities. Therefore the assessment of injuries involving the spine are among the most important that you will perform.

The majority of athletic injuries to the spine, however, are not this serious or disastrous and will consist of contusions, sprains, and strains. For most injuries involving the spine, the assessment process will be centered on evaluating the severity of the injury and identifying the structures involved. This usually cannot be accomplished quickly. A complete and accurate evaluation of spinal injuries or related conditions takes considerable time. The information gained during the assessment process is essential in establishing a treatment regime aimed at relieving acute pain and restoring normal flexibility, strength, and proper body mechanics.

When to refer the athlete

When a serious injury to the spine occurs, the athlete must be referred to medical assistance immediately. You must be able to recognize signs and symptoms of severe spinal injuries. Following is a list of conditions or findings that indicate the athlete has a potentially serious spinal injury and should be protected from further trauma and referred to medical assistance.

1. Paralysis—inability to move arms or legs
2. Loss of normal sensations
3. Pain, tenderness, or deformity along the vertebral column
4. Unremitting neck or back pain
5. Weakness noted in the extremities
6. Loss of coordination of the extremities
7. Unusual sensations in the extremities or body surface
8. Doubt regarding the presence of spinal cord involvement

**ATHLETIC INJURY
ASSESSMENT PROCEDURES
SPINE INJURIES**

Primary survey

_____ Responsiveness
_____ Airway
_____ Breathing
_____ Circulation

Secondary survey

_____ History
　　　_____ Paralysis
　　　_____ Sensations
　　　_____ Pain
　　　_____ Mechanism of injury
　　　_____ Previous history
_____ Observation
　　　_____ Motionlessness
　　　_____ Deformities
　　　_____ Signs of trauma
　　　_____ Movements and positions
　　　_____ Alignment of neck and back
_____ Palpation
　　　_____ Tenderness
　　　_____ Muscle spasm
　　　_____ Sensations
_____ Stress
　　　_____ Active movements
　　　_____ Resistive movements
　　　_____ Passive movements
　　　_____ Functional movements

KEY TERMS

abducted scapulae Scapulae are held a greater distance from the vertebral column than is considered normal

anesthesia Loss of feeling or sensation

annulus fibrosus Circumferential ringlike portion of an intervertebral disc, composed of fibrocartilage and fibrous tissue

cauda equina Latin equivalent for *horse's tail;* lower spinal nerve roots descending in the spinal canal from their point of attachment to the spinal cord to the site of their emergence between the vertebrae

cervical lordosis Increased concavity in the curvature of the cervical spine

dermatome Segment or strip of skin supplied by a given spinal nerve

forward head Deviation from normal alignment in which the head is carried in an abnormal anterior position

forward shoulders Deviation from normal alignment in which the shoulders are carried in an abnormal forward position

kyphosis Increased convexity in the curvature of the thoracic spine

lumbar lordosis Increased concavity in the curvature of the lumbar spine

lumbar puncture Piercing of the subarachnoid space in the lumbar region, usually between the third and fourth lumbar vertebrae, for the purpose of withdrawing cerebrospinal fluid

nucleus pulposus Semifluid mass of fine white and elastic fibers that forms the central portion of an intervertebral disc

paraplegia Paralysis of the lower extremities

paresis Slight or incomplete paralysis

paresthesia Abnormal sensation such as burning, prickling, or tingling

quadriplegia Paralysis of all four extremities

sciatica Pain along the course of the sciatic nerve, possibly with associated paresthesia of the thigh and leg and atrophy of calf muscles

scoliosis Lateral curvature or deviation of the spine

spina bifida occulta Defect in the bony spinal canal without involvement of the spinal cord or meninges

spondylolisthesis Forward displacement, or slippage, of one vertebra on another; usually occurring between L_4 and L_5 or L_5 and the sacrum

spondylolysis Defect in the pars interarticularis, or that part of the vertebra between the superior and inferior articular processes

torticollis (wryneck) Contracted state of the cervical muscles, producing an unnatural position of the head

winged scapula Marked projection and upward tilt of the lower angle of the scapula

SUGGESTED READINGS

Arnheim, D.D.: Modern principles of athletic training, ed. 6, St. Louis, 1985, Times Mirror/Mosby College Publishing.

Edgelow, P.I.: Physical examination of the lumbosacral complex, Physical Therapy 59:974-977, 1979.

Hoppenfeld, S.: Physical examination of the spine and extremities, New York, 1976, Appleton-Century-Crofts.

Jackson, D.W., and Wiltse, L.L.: Low back pain in young athletes, Physician Sportsmedicine 2:53-60, 1974.

Keim, H.A., and Kirkaldy-Willis, W.H.: Low back pain, CIBA Clinical Symposia, 32:6, 1980.

Mericer, L.R., and Pettid, F.J.: Practical orthopedics, Chicago, 1980, Year Book Medical Publishers, Inc.

Mueller, F.O., and Blyth, C.S.: Catastrophic head and neck injuries, Physician Sportsmedicine 7:71-74, 1979.

O'Donoghue, D.H.: Treatment of injuries to athletes, ed. 4, Philadelphia, 1984, W.B. Saunders Co.

Roy, S., and Irvin, R.: Sports medicine: prevention, evaluation, management, and rehabilitation, Englewood Cliffs, N.J., 1983, Prentice-Hall, Inc.

Torg, J.S.: Athletic injuries to the head, neck and face, Philadelphia, 1982, Lea & Febiger.

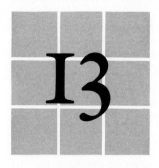

I3 Throat, chest, abdomen, and pelvis injuries

The torso of the body is composed of two major areas: (1) the chest, or thorax, and (2) the abdomen. The boundary between these two is the diaphragm, and each forms a major body cavity containing vital life-sustaining organs. Athletic injuries can occur to either the walls of these cavities or their visceral contents. Superficial injuries involving the cavity walls are much more common during athletic activity and are generally not serious. Fortunately, athletic injuries to the internal contents (viscera) of either of these cavities are not common; however, serious and potentially life-threatening injuries can occur to these vital organs. Athletic trainers must therefore be alert to the possibilities of serious internal injuries resulting from athletic activity.

The chest and abdomen contain organs essential to respiration, circulation, and digestion.

Structures vital to each of these systems pass through the neck. As a result, athletic injuries or related conditions involving the neck can compromise these bodily processes. This chapter discusses injuries involving the anterior neck, or throat (excluding the cervical spine), and the chest, abdomen, and pelvis.

THE THROAT (ANTERIOR NECK)

For purposes of description, the upper limit of the neck is considered to be the lower border of the jaw extending on either side of the mastoid process just behind the ear. The lower limit is defined by the suprasternal notch anteriorly, the clavicles, and a line extending from the acromioclavicular joint on either side to the spinous process of the seventh cervical vertebra posteriorly. The surface characteristics and contour of the neck vary with age, sex, body type, and level of conditioning. The neck is rounded in women, more angular in men. Landmarks such as the thyroid cartilage (Adam's apple) are more conspicuous and defined in the male.

The numerous visceral structures, blood vessels, and nerves found in the neck are relatively exposed and therefore vulnerable to traumatic injury. Because of the functional significance of these anatomic structures, proficiency in assessment of injuries in this area is critically important to the athletic trainer.

Neck muscles

The two major muscles of the neck are the sternocleidomastoid and trapezius muscles. The sternocleidomastoid muscles divide each side of the neck into an anterior and posterior triangle. The athletic trainer should review both the points of attachment and function of the sternocleidomastoid and trapezius muscles in movements of the head and neck. Note in Fig. 13-1 that the sternocleidomastoid muscle arises by two heads: a narrow sternal head from the manubrium of the sternum, and a broader clavicular head from the medial third of the clavicle. The small triangular interval between the two heads is quite noticeable in thin athletes and

Fig. 13-1. Anatomic structures of the neck.

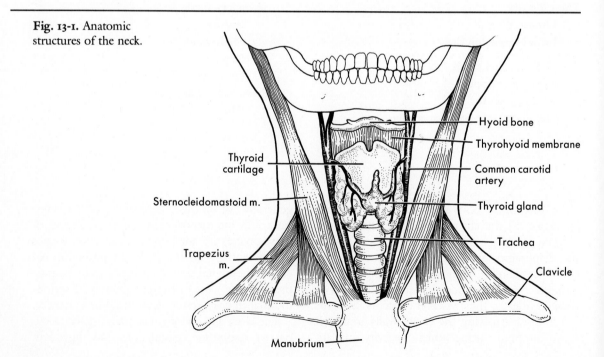

Thyroid cartilage

Sternocleidomastoid m.

Trapezius m.

Manubrium

Hyoid bone

Thyrohyoid membrane

Common carotid artery

Thyroid gland

Trachea

Clavicle

generally appears as a slight depression. The carotid arteries, internal jugular vein, vagus nerve, and portions of the cervical plexus lie beneath the sternocleidomastoid muscle.

Anatomic structures of the neck

The major anatomic structures in the midline of the neck include the hyoid bone, the larynx, the trachea, the thyroid gland, and the more deeply placed pharynx and esophagus. The major blood vessels, important nerves, and many lymph nodes are located on the sides of the neck under or around the sternocleidomastoid muscles. The posterior portion of the neck contains the cervical segment of the spinal cord, the cervical vertebrae, and surrounding musculature, which was discussed in Chapter 12.

Locate the hyoid bone in Fig. 13-1. This unusually shaped little bone is unique in that it does not articulate with any other bone in the skeleton. It lies at the level of the third cervical vertebra just below the mandible. Located in the musculature and soft tissues at the root of the tongue, the hyoid bone is in close proximity to many major structures in the upper neck. It possesses great mobility but is vulnerable to injury in certain kinds of athletic activity.

The larynx (voice box) lies between the root of the tongue and the upper end of the trachea and can be described as the opening into the trachea from the pharynx. It normally extends between the fourth, fifth, and sixth cervical vertebrae but is often somewhat higher in women and during childhood. The larynx consists of cartilage and muscles. The largest cartilage, the thyroid, or Adam's apple, is normally quite smooth and is an easily palpable landmark in front. The cricoid cartilage forms a complete ring around the larynx and is also easily palpable inferior to the thyroid cartilage. The cricoid lies on a level with the sixth cervical vertebra.

The trachea (windpipe) is a tube about 4-1/2 inches (11 cm) long that extends from the larynx to the bronchi in the thoracic cavity. Its diameter measures about 1 inch (2.5 cm) and its walls are composed of smooth muscles in which C-shaped rings of cartilage are embedded. The cartilaginous rings give firmness to the wall of the trachea, preventing collapse and occlusion of the airway, and are incomplete on the posterior surface. The trachea is easiest to palpate just above the manubrium (suprasternal notch) between the sternal attachment of the two sternocleidomastoid muscles.

In most persons the H-shaped thyroid gland is not visible during inspection of the neck. However, occasionally the gland can be palpated when the upper trachea or cricoid cartilage is being examined. The right lobe of the thyroid is larger than the left and is sometimes noticed if the athlete swallows during the examination. If felt, the lobes of the thyroid gland are smooth, nontender, and tend to move freely under the skin.

The pharynx is a tubelike structure approximately 5 inches (12.5 cm) in length, extending from the base of the skull to the esophagus and lying just anterior to the cervical vertebrae. It is made of muscle and lined with mucous membrane. The pharynx serves as a passageway for the respiratory and digestive tracts; both air and food must pass through this structure before reaching their respective tubes.

Lymph nodes in and around the neck are found in serial groups called "chains." There are many chains of lymph nodes in the neck that normally cannot be felt or seen. However, lymph nodes in the neck are often enlarged as a result of head and neck infections. The athlete may complain of "swollen glands" or "lumps."

THROAT INJURIES

Most athletic injuries to the throat are caused by some type of direct blow to the anterior or lateral portions of the neck. This normally results in a contusion with varying degrees of pain, soreness on swallowing, hoarseness, and tenderness to touch. Occasionally the blow results in shortness of breath and the inability to speak, which can cause the athlete to become extremely anxious and apprehensive. A calm and reassuring approach to these athletes is indicated.

Symptoms of this type usually subside rather quickly, but soreness and hoarseness may persist. The athlete should be able to resume activity if normal speech and breathing return. Athletes whose symptoms persist longer than a day should be referred to a physician for a laryngeal examination.

An athletic injury resulting in a fracture of the cartilage of the larynx or trachea would be quite rare. However, this is a serious and potentially life-threatening injury; therefore the athletic trainer must be prepared to recognize and handle such an emergency. Difficulty in breathing, loss of voice, inability to swallow, bleeding from the throat, and crepitation on palpation are signs and symptoms indicating immediate medical attention is required.

A more common complaint that the athletic trainer will have to evaluate is the sore throat. Inflammation or infection of the pharynx is called *pharyngitis.* This condition is indicated by pain on swallowing, dryness, hoarseness, and burning of the throat. If symptoms are severe, persist, and occur along with a fever, chills, and swollen lymph nodes in the neck, strep throat should be suspected, and the athlete should be referred to a physician. *Laryngitis,* an inflammation or irritation of the larynx, is another common complaint. This condition may be indicated by hoarseness, loss of voice, dryness and soreness of the throat, cough, and difficulty in swallowing. A period of yelling may cause vocal strain, resulting in swelling and irritation of the vocal cords. If symptoms persist, a physician should be consulted.

THE CHEST

The chest, or thoracic cavity, is surrounded by a conical bony cage (Fig. 13-2) formed by the sternum and costal cartilages anteriorly, the ribs

Fig. 13-2. Anterior view of thorax (rib cage).

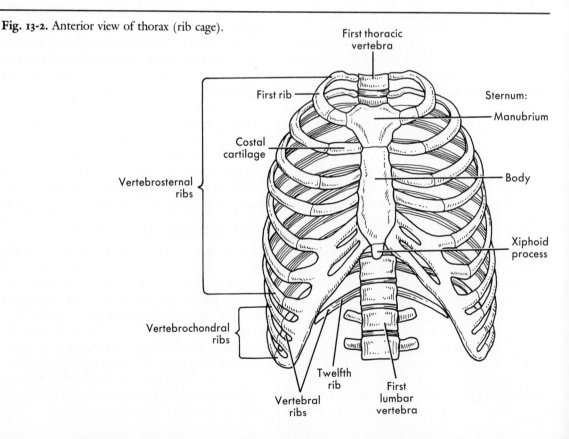

laterally, and the thoracic vertebrae posteriorly. The anatomy of the thoracic skeleton described in Chapter 3 should be reviewed.

Topographic anatomy of the thorax

The athletic trainer must have a sound working knowledge of the topographic, or surface, landmarks of the thorax in order to properly assess an injury to this area. Anatomic assessment guidelines assist in identifying the location of internal structures and in describing the exact location of injury. Review the lines of reference and surface landmarks in Figs. 13-3 to 13-5. Anatomic descriptions of many of the muscles that attach to or are an integral part of the thorax are given in the discussion of shoulder injuries in Chapter 17. Muscles of particular interest and importance at this time are the pectoralis major, serratus anterior, latissimus dorsi, trapezius, rectus abdominis, external oblique, intercostals, and superficial back muscles. Review the points of attachment of these muscles described in Chapter 5.

Fig. 13-3. Anterior view of thorax, indicating **A,** lines of reference and **B,** surface landmarks and placement of internal anatomic structures.

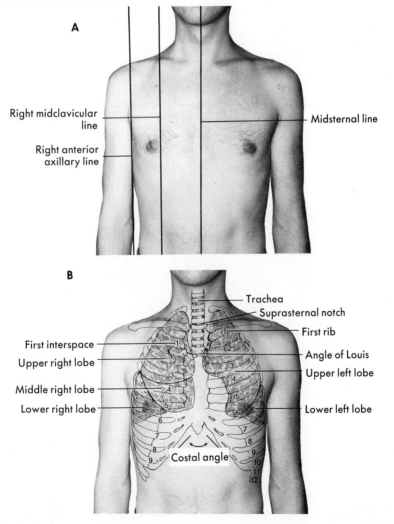

A

Right midclavicular line

Right anterior axillary line

Midsternal line

B

Trachea
Suprasternal notch
First rib
Angle of Louis
Upper left lobe
Lower left lobe

First interspace
Upper right lobe
Middle right lobe
Lower right lobe

Costal angle

Fig. 13-4. Posterior view of thorax, indicating **A,** lines of reference and **B,** surface landmarks and placement of internal anatomic structures.

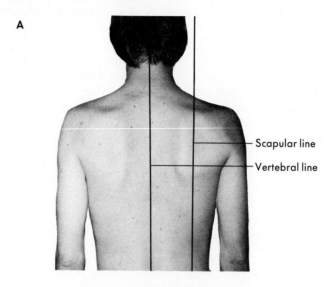

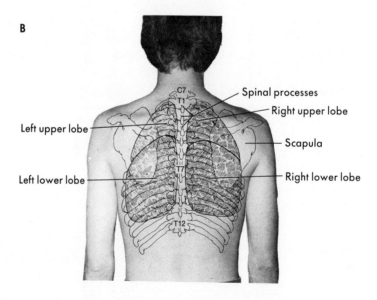

The anterior chest wall is characterized by a shallow midline depression just over the subcutaneous sternum. This shallow median furrow lies between the two pectoralis major muscles and is more prominent in athletes with good muscular definition and limited subcutaneous fat. The anterior axillary line is formed by the lateral border of the pectoralis major. The tooth-like points of origin of the serratus anterior muscle are prominent along the lateral chest wall. The point of origin of the serratus from the fifth rib can be seen just below the pectoralis major. The *sternal angle,* or *Louis's angle,* is the manubriosternal junction just opposite the sternal end of the second rib. It is an extremely useful aid in rib identification and is the most reliable thoracic surface landmark. The lines of reference and surface landmarks should be employed during the assessment process.

The nipple in the male and young female who has not borne children (nulliparus female) lies opposite the fourth intercostal space. In the female the breasts lie over the pectoral muscles and extend from the second to the sixth or seventh rib and from the lateral border of the sternum to beyond the anterior axillary line. The nipples are bordered by a circular pigmented area, the *areola.* Female breast size is determined more by the amount of adipose (fat) tissue around the glandular tissue than by the amount of glandular tissue itself. Although symmetric, they are usually not absolutely equal in size and shape.

Thoracic viscera

The visceral structures contained in the thoracic (chest) cavity (Figs. 13-3 and 13-4) are found in subdivisions called the right and left *pleural cavities* and a region situated between these called the *mediastinum.* Fibrous tissue forms a wall around the mediastinum, completely separating it from the right pleural sac, in which the right lung lies, and from the left pleural sac, which contains the left lung. Contained within the mediastinum are the heart and great vessels, the thymus gland, the trachea and right and left bronchi, the esophagus, the thoracic duct, and other lymphatic vessels and many nerves, arteries, and veins. Thus the only organs in the tho-

Fig. 13-5. Lateral lines of reference.

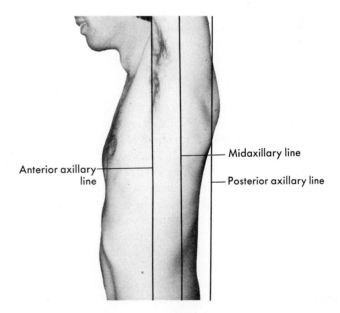

Anterior axillary line

Midaxillary line

Posterior axillary line

racic cavity that are not located in the mediastinum are the lungs.

The mediastinum is commonly subdivided into four parts. The superior portion lies above a horizontal plane that passes through the great vessels above the heart, the anterior portion lies between the sternum and the heart, the middle portion consists of the heart and its pericardium, and the posterior portion is located between the heart and the bodies of the thoracic vertebrae.

Lungs and pleura

Paired conical lungs are the essential organs of respiration. Each lung invaginates and fills its pleural cavity. They extend from the diaphragm to a point about 1/2 to 1 inch (1.5 to 2.5 cm) above the clavicles and lie against the ribs both anteriorly and posteriorly. The medial surface of each lung is roughly concave to allow room for the mediastinal structures and for the heart, but concavity is greater on the left than on the right because of the position of the heart. The primary bronchi and pulmonary blood vessels, bound together by connective tissue to form what is known as the root of the lung, enter each lung through a slit on its medial surface called the *hilum.* Lung tissue is light, spongy in texture, and highly elastic. The right lung contains three lobes, whereas the left lung contains two. The broad inferior surface of each lung, which rests on the diaphragm, is called the base. The pointed upper margin, or apex, projects above the clavicle.

The term "pleura" is used to describe the thin, serous membrane that invests the lungs *(visceral pleura)* and lines the pleural cavity *(parietal pleura)* in which each lung is situated. The visceral pleura adheres so firmly to the lung surface that it is difficult to differentiate from lung tissue.

The parietal layer of the pleura lines the entire thoracic cavity. It adheres to the internal surface of the ribs and the superior surface of the diaphragm, and it partitions the pleural cavities from the mediastinum. A separate pleural sac thus encases each lung. Because the outer surface of each lung is covered by the visceral layer of the pleura, the visceral pleura lies against the parietal pleura, separated only by a potential space (pleural space) that contains just enough pleural fluid for lubrication. Thus when the lungs inflate with air, the smooth, moist visceral pleura adheres to the smooth, moist, parietal pleura, friction is thereby avoided, and respirations are painless. In pleurisy, on the other hand, the pleura is inflamed and respirations become painful.

Mechanism of pulmonary ventilation

The thorax plays a major role in ventilation. Because of the elliptic shape of the ribs and the angle of their attachment to the spine, the thorax becomes larger when the chest is raised and elongated and smaller when it is lowered and shortened. It is these changes in thorax size that bring about inspiration and expiration. Lifting up the chest raises the ribs so that they no longer slant downward from the spine, and because of their elliptic shape, this enlarges both the depth (front to back) and the width (side to side) of the thorax.

Inspiration

Contraction of the diaphragm alone, or of the diaphragm and the external intercostal muscles, produces quiet inspiration. The diaphragm descends as it contracts, making the thoracic cavity longer. Contraction of the external intercostal muscles pulls the anterior end of each rib up and out. This also elevates the attached sternum and increases the depth and width of the thorax. In addition, contraction of the sternocleidomastoid and serratus anterior muscles can aid in elevation of the sternum and rib cage during forceful inspiration. As the thorax enlarges, it forces the lungs to expand along with it because of cohesion between the moist visceral pleura covering the lungs and the moist parietal pleura lining the thorax. As the size of the thorax is enlarged, the pressure inside the chest decreases. This leads to a relative decreased pressure inside the bronchial tubes and alveoli, and thus air moves into the lungs.

Expiration

Quiet expiration is ordinarily a passive process that begins when those pressure changes in the thorax that resulted in inspiration are reversed. It is important to remember that lung tissue is highly elastic and tends to return to its original size during expiration. As the thorax decreases in size, the pressure in the bronchial tubes and alveoli increases, and a positive pressure gradient is established from alveoli to atmosphere. This results in expiration as air flows outward through the respiratory passageways. In forced expiration, contraction of the abdominal and internal intercostal muscles can increase the pressure in the thorax far above that produced by the elastic recoil of lung tissue and assist in the outward flow of air.

CHEST INJURIES

Most athletic injuries to the chest are the result of a direct blow. The majority of these injuries are superficial, involving the chest wall or rib cage. Occasionally, athletic injuries may involve the contents of the chest cavity, such as the lungs, heart or great vessels. These injuries can be life threatening and should be of primary concern to athletic trainers when they occur.

Chest wall

Contusions, or bruises, are the most frequent injuries to the chest wall. They may involve the skin, subcutaneous tissues, muscles, or periosteum of the ribs or sternum. On examination, contusions to the chest wall reveal an area of localized tenderness and possibly swelling. In most instances this type of injury does not cause pain during breathing or restrict motion of the rib cage unless very deep respirations are taken. Occasionally, a breast tissue contusion, especially to the female breast, will result in fatty necrosis and the formation of a firm nodule of fibrous tissue. These are generally of little consequence but should be examined by a physician for further evaluation.

A muscle strain is much more likely to involve muscles attached to the rib cage rather than the intercostal muscles within the chest wall. A number of muscles attach to the chest wall and may be strained by overstretching or sudden violent contractions. Injuries to these muscles are discussed in Chapter 17, because disability associated with them is primarily in the use of the arm. Intercostal muscle strains do not occur frequently because these muscles are well protected and usually do not act forcibly enough to stretch their fibers. The signs and symptoms of an intercostal muscle strain resemble those of a chest wall contusion and require similar treatment.

Another fairly common injury to the chest wall resulting from athletic activity is a rib fracture. These are normally caused by a direct blow to the ribs. Less frequently a rib fracture may be caused by forceful compression of the rib cage. An example of this mechanism would be an athlete who is involved in a "pile-up" or gives a history of the rib cage being crushed or compressed. The bony integrity may be interrupted anywhere along a rib or ribs because of this general compression of the rib cage; however, ribs tend to break just in front of the angle, which is the weakest point. Ribs 4 through 9 are more liable to fracture, as the first three ribs are protected by the shoulder girdle. The lower ribs (10 through 12) also have a greater freedom of movement. Undisplaced fractures, or cracked ribs, are more common in athletic activity than displaced fractures, because the ribs are well stabilized by the attachment of the intercostal muscles and the fixation of each rib to its corresponding thoracic vertebra. Signs and symptoms associated with fractured ribs include severe localized pain, which is usually increased on movement of the ribs, breathing deeply, coughing, and sneezing. An athlete with fractured ribs will generally refrain from breathing deeply by taking rapid shallow breaths. The athlete may also hold the injured side in an attempt to restrict any painful movement of the chest. During gentle palpation and compression of the ribs, the athlete will indicate pain at the fracture site. If the fracture is displaced, there may also be a palpable defect in the rib and crepitation on movement or coughing. Serious complications, such as puncture of thoracic or abdominal visceral structures, can occur as a result of rib fractures.

The mechanisms of injury described for rib fractures are also responsible for costochondral separations. Instead of a rib fracture, there may be a separation or actual dislocation at the articulation between the rib and its articulating cartilage. Signs and symptoms of costochondral separations are similar to rib fractures. In this type of injury, the pain and tenderness are localized over the costochondral junction. If the dislocation is complete, there may be a palpable defect, as the tip of the rib rests anteriorly to the costocartilage. In many cases the dislocation will spontaneously reduce, and the athlete may feel a click or snap as the rib dislocates and then almost immediately relocates after the injury. Occasionally this audible and palpable click can be detected on examination (palpation) or will occur during certain voluntary movements of the rib cage.

Injuries involving only the sternum seldom occur during athletic activity. The sternum can be fractured, however, or the chondrosternal junction may be separated by the same types of trauma that cause rib injuries. The signs and symptoms are similar except that tenderness exists along the sternum or chondrosternal junctions. The sternum is thin at the junction of the manubrium with the body, and if fractures do occur, this will be the area most likely involved. If the upper manubrium should pass behind the body at the point of fracture, the possibility of an airway obstruction exists; the athlete should be monitored very carefully for signs of respiratory distress.

Intrathoracic injuries

Intrathoracic (visceral) injuries or conditions occur very rarely during athletic activity because of the protection provided by the rib cage and the protective equipment required for various sports. However, these types of injuries can occur as the result of severe trauma to the chest or from complications accompanying rib or sternal fractures. An athlete may also suffer an intrathoracic injury as a result of the penetration of a sharp object. Fortunately, this type of injury rarely occurs during athletic activity. Intrathoracic injuries or conditions can develop rather quickly or insidiously over several hours. Therefore the athletic trainer must be alert to recognize immediate and delayed signs and symptoms associated with chest injuries indicating possible intrathoracic involvement.

One of the more common intrathoracic complications after chest injury is a *pneumothorax,* that is, an accumulation of air in the pleural space, that can collapse the lung. This condition may be caused by either trauma or the spontaneous rupture of lung tissue. A traumatic pneumothorax can occur when the lung is punctured by a bone fragment resulting from a rib fracture. When lung tissue is lacerated, air from the lung enters the pleural cavity with each inspiration. As this air is trapped in the pleural cavity, the lung separates from the chest wall. With the air continuing to fill the pleural cavity, the volume of the lung is reduced, and the lung can no longer expand normally. This condition is referred to as a collapsed lung and can result in chest pain and shortness of breath. As the uninjured lung fills with air, the trachea may shift or deviate toward the side of the collapsed lung. If the tear in the lung does not seal itself, the amount of trapped air that cannot escape from the pleural space will continue to increase, and the pressure will continue to build up in the affected pleural cavity. With the increasing pressure, the collapsed lung may be pressed against the uninjured lung and heart, thereby reducing their efficiency. This can develop into a life-threatening situation called a *tension pneumothorax.* A true medical emergency, the tension pneumothorax will usually manifest signs and symptoms of rapidly progressing respiratory distress or breathing difficulty *(dyspnea).* The trachea shifts or deviates away from the affected or injured side because of the increase in pressure. The importance of following (and completing) a predetermined checklist in the assessment of thoracic injuries is critical. Unless such a formal and sequential approach is followed, a serious problem, such as pneumothorax, may be overlooked as attention of both athletic trainer and athlete is focused on a painful but non–life-threatening injury such as a broken rib.

A *spontaneous pneumothorax* occurs in the absence of trauma or injury. This condition is most common in young people between the ages of 15 and 30 and occurs more often in women than men. A spontaneous pneumothorax usually occurs during or immediately after activity when an area of lung tissue ruptures spontaneously, resulting in release of air into a pleural cavity. Spontaneous pneumothorax is characterized by the sudden onset of severe sharp pain in the chest and shortness of breath. It can occur during simple exertions such as coughing.

A *hemothorax* is an intrathoracic condition similar to a pneumothorax except that blood, rather than air, collects in the pleural cavity. Hemorrhage may result from injured blood vessels in the chest wall or within the chest cavity. A hemothorax may also be caused by fractured ribs and may occur spontaneously or in conjunction with a pneumothorax *(hemopneumothorax)*. A small amount of bleeding will cause few if any symptoms. If bleeding is significant, the signs and symptoms are similar to a pneumothorax in that normal lung expansion cannot occur and lung volume is decreased. If bleeding is very severe, the athlete may also show signs of shock from the loss of blood.

Another important sign indicating intrathoracic involvement is coughing of blood or spitting of blood-stained sputum *(hemoptysis)*. This may be one of the first signs of injury to the pulmonary structures and must be distinguished from bleeding of the mouth or nose. On occasion an athlete will complain of spitting up blood hours after a traumatic injury to the chest or abdomen. In these cases it is important to differentiate blood-stained sputum from the vomiting of blood *(hematemesis)*, which may occur as a result of hemorrhage into the digestive tract. Ask the athlete to bare the teeth. True hematemesis will often show as coagulated blood at the gum line. Any episodes of hemoptysis following injury to the chest should not be

ignored. The athlete should be referred to medical attention for further diagnosis.

Any violent blow or compression of the chest may cause additional intrathoracic involvement, such as lung hemorrhaging, heart contusion, laceration of the great vessels, or cessation of breathing. Therefore the athletic trainer must be constantly alert during the assessment process to recognize signs and symptoms indicating intrathoracic involvement and be prepared, if necessary, to provide artificial ventilation and circulation, treat for shock, or refer the athlete to medical attention.

THE ABDOMEN AND PELVIS

The abdomen is that portion of the body torso bounded above by the diaphragm and below by the upper pelvis. The abdominal cavity is continuous with the pelvic cavity and its wall merges with the wall of the pelvis below and the thorax above.

Fig. 13-6. Division of the abdomen into four quadrants. *1*, Right upper or superior, *2*, left upper or superior, *3*, right lower or inferior and *4*, left lower or inferior. Inguinal ligaments are indicated by arrows.

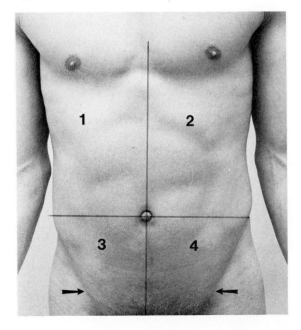

Anatomic mapping

The method of dividing the abdomen into quadrants (Fig. 13-6) or sections for study purposes is discussed in Chapter 2 and should be reviewed. The box below lists the abdominal and pelvic visceral structures located in each of these subdivisions.

Surface anatomy

In the upper abdomen the costal angle (Fig. 13-3) is formed below the xiphoid process by the diverging cartilages of the sixth to eighth ribs. The costal margin on the upper and lateral abdominal wall is usually found at the inferior limit of the tenth costal cartilage. Inferiorly, the ab-

---

VISCERAL STRUCTURES LOCATED IN THE FOUR ABDOMINAL QUADRANTS

Right upper (superior) quadrant

Right lobe of liver
Gallbladder
Right kidney and adrenal gland
Pylorus of stomach
Duodenum (bulb)
Hepatic flexure of large intestine
Small intestine
Distal (upper) half of ascending colon
Right half of transverse colon
Head of pancreas
Proximal portion of right ureter
Blood vessels, nerves, and lymphatics associated
   with the above visceral structures

Right lower (inferior) quadrant

Small intestine
Cecum
Appendix
Proximal half of ascending colon
Portion of urinary bladder
Portion of rectum
Distal portion of right ureter
Reproductive structures:
   Female
      Portion of uterus and vagina
      Right ovary
      Right fallopian tube
   Male
      Portion of right vas deferens
      Right seminal vesicle
      Right ejaculatory duct
      Portion of prostate gland
Blood vessels, nerves, and lymphatics associated
   with the above visceral structures

Left upper (superior) quadrant

Small intestine
Body and fundus of stomach
Spleen
Splenic flexure of large intestine
Tail of pancreas
Left half of transverse colon
Left kidney and adrenal gland
Terminal esophagus
Proximal portion of left ureter
Upper half of descending colon
Blood vessels, nerves, and lymphatics associated
   with the above visceral structures

Left lower (inferior) quadrant

Small intestine
Distal portion of descending colon
Sigmoid colon
Portion of urinary bladder
Portion of rectum
Distal portion of left ureter
Reproductive structures:
   Female
      Portion of uterus and vagina
      Left ovary
      Left fallopian tube
   Male
      Portion of left vas deferens
      Left seminal vesicle
      Left ejaculatory duct
      Portion of prostate gland
Blood vessels, nerves, and lymphatics associated
   with the above visceral structures

dominal wall is bounded by the iliac crest of the hip. The crest ends in front in the anterior superior iliac spine and behind in the posterior superior iliac spine. The inguinal ligament (Fig. 13-6) in the groin marks the separation between the abdominal wall and the lower extremity.

The umbilicus is a prominent but somewhat unreliable midline landmark normally located at the level of the intervertebral disc between the third and fourth lumbar vertebrae. In well-developed athletes the anterior abdominal wall is marked by three vertical lines: the *linea alba,* which marks the midline junction between the rectus abdominis muscles, and the two *linea semilunares,* which define the lateral margins of these muscles.

Abdominal and pelvic anatomy

Division of the abdomen into regions or quadrants makes it easier to locate organs in the abdominopelvic cavity. It is important for the athletic trainer to be able to visualize the placement of these deep visceral structures using external landmarks on the abdominal wall. Recall from Chapter 2 that the abdominal area can be divided into four quadrants if the umbilicus is intersected by a midsagittal and a horizontal (transverse) section, or "cut" (Fig. 3-6). Dividing the area into nine regions permits an even more precise method of describing the location of abdominal and pelvic visceral organs.

Review the major internal abdominal organs and their relationships to bony landmarks in Fig. 13-7. The abdominal cavity contains the liver, gallbladder, stomach, pancreas, intestines, spleen, kidneys, and ureters. The bladder, certain reproductive organs (uterus, uterine tubes, and ovaries in the female; prostate gland, seminal vesicles, and part of the vas deferens in the male), and part of the large intestine (namely, the sigmoid colon and rectum) lie in the pelvic cavity.

Fig. 13-7. Major structures of abdominal cavity.

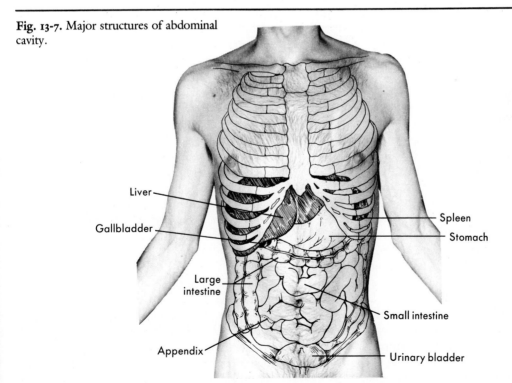

Liver

Gallbladder

Large intestine

Appendix

Spleen

Stomach

Small intestine

Urinary bladder

ABDOMINAL INJURIES

The abdominal area is vulnerable to injury during most athletic activities, especially contact sports. The muscular abdominal wall is the most commonly involved area. Occasionally, the visceral contents of the abdominal cavity may be involved. Intra-abdominal injuries can be very serious, possibly life threatening. Therefore the athletic trainer must be constantly alert to detect signs and symptoms that may indicate intra-abdominal involvement.

Abdominal wall

Because the abdominal wall is predominately muscular, strains are a common injury. Muscle strains of the abdominal wall are usually the result of a sudden violent contraction, overstretching, or continued overuse. Signs and symptoms associated with strains of the abdominal muscles include localized tenderness, muscle spasm, and rigidity. In strain injuries, the pain will be increased or aggravated by active muscle contraction or passive stretching. For this reason, strains of the abdominal muscles tend to be disabling, as these muscles are important when performing most athletic activities. Abdominal strains do not usually involve rupture of the muscle fibers, and recovery is generally rapid. However, when the injury does involve some tearing of muscle fibers or musculotendinous units, the symptoms can be prolonged and quite disabling. This is especially true if the injury occurs where the abdominal muscles attach to the ribs, iliac crests, or pubis. In these instances, the athlete may continue to aggravate the injured area, and the injury can be quite self-limiting.

Contusions are common injuries to the abdominal muscles, as this area can be subjected to direct blows during many types of athletic activity. Because of the resiliency of the abdominal wall, muscle contusions in this area are generally not severe. No rigid background exists on which an external blow can impact to cause this type of injury. The greatest danger of impact-type trauma to the abdominal wall is injury to the visceral contents within the cavity. Direct blows to the bony attachments of the abdominal muscles can be quite severe. For example, a blow to the crest of the ilium can cause both a crushing type of injury, resulting in a localized muscle contusion, and tearing of some fibers at the point of muscle attachment to bone. This injury, commonly called a hip pointer, can be very disabling. Athletes will complain of severe and agonizing pain that is aggravated by any type of movement, such as turning, twisting, laughing, coughing, or going to the bathroom. In such cases the athlete should be treated symptomatically, that is, kept inactive until the symptoms subside.

Sideache

Another common condition involving the abdominal wall is a sideache, or "stitch in the side." The sharp pain and muscle spasms associated with this condition usually occur along the lower rib cage or in the upper abdominal muscles and are often associated with running activities. In many cases the pain will be increased on inspiration, making deep breathing very uncomfortable. Most sideache attacks are short lived, and pain is relieved after cessation of the activity. A sideache also appears to respond well to stretching of the involved side. Several theories have been advanced to explain why an athlete may experience a sideache. Current theories point to local anoxia (lack of oxygen) of the involved muscles or spasm of the diaphragm as causative factors. Athletes who experience repeated sideaches may need additional evaluation to determine possible causes contributing to the condition. Level of conditioning, current training program, eating habits, or elimination routines may also be causative factors.

Hernia

The protrusion of abdominal viscera through a portion of the abdominal wall is called a **hernia**. These conditions, while generally not caused by an athletic injury, can be aggravated by athletic activity. Intra-abdominal pressure, which increases during weight training or strenuous athletic activity, can produce the signs and symptoms associated with a hernia. The areas of the abdominal wall most susceptible to hernias are the inguinal and femoral canals. The inguinal canal is the point at which the spermatic cord containing blood vessels, nerves, and the vas deferens of the male reproductive system leaves the abdominal cavity and enters the scrotum. In the female, the round ligament of the uterus passes through the canal and terminates in the labia majora. The femoral canal is the point at which the femoral blood vessels and nerve pass from the abdominal cavity into the lower extremity. These two openings are protected by muscular control, much like the shutter of a camera. These openings may be congenitally weak or weakened by continued intra-abdominal pressure, resulting in abdominal viscera being forced through these canals and out of the abdominal cavity. The resulting hernia can range from a minor problem to a severe abdominal wall defect. Symptoms associated with a hernia are pain and prolonged discomfort as well as a feeling of weakness or pulling in the groin. A protrusion may also be felt in the groin, which will increase on coughing. In almost every case an athlete with a hernia experiences only minor pain and discomfort, which is tolerated well during athletic activity. However, in a severe hernia, there is always the danger of incarceration of the protruding viscera with the possibility of occluding the blood supply to the tissue. This is called a *strangulated hernia* and needs immediate medical attention. Any time the signs and symptoms of a hernia are increased by athletic activity, the athlete should be referred to a physician.

Intra-abdominal injuries

Athletic injuries involving the contents of the abdominal cavity occur infrequently. The musculature of the abdominal wall provides adequate protection for the intra-abdominal viscera from most injuries. However, serious athletic injuries to the intra-abdominal contents do occur and can become life threatening. These injuries are usually associated with contact or collision sports and occur as the result of some type of direct trauma to the abdomen or lower back. The structures most often associated with serious intra-abdominal injuries are the solid organs such as the kidneys, spleen, and liver, all organs rich in blood supply. Occasionally the hollow organs, mesentery, peritoneum, or female reproductive organs are involved in an athletic injury. Intra-abdominal injuries or conditions can develop quickly or insidiously over a period of time. Therefore the athletic trainer must be alert to recognize signs and symptoms, such as shock, that may indicate possible intra-abdominal involvement.

The most common intra-abdominal injury is a blow to the *celiac plexus* (solar plexus), more commonly known as having the "wind knocked out." This network of nerves lies deep in the upper middle region of the abdomen. A blow to this area can cause a transitory paralysis of the diaphragm. Although an athlete may become very anxious, this injury is usually of very short duration, and no treatment is necessary because the condition responds to a few moments of rest and reassurance. If complete recovery does not occur within minutes, and pain, tenderness, and signs of shock appear, intra-abdominal injury should be suspected. The athlete should be referred to a physician for further evaluation or treatment. It is important to remember that the signs and symptoms associated with significant intra-abdominal injuries will persist.

Signs and symptoms associated with an injury to the abdominal viscera depend on the organ involved, severity of the injury, and the resulting amount of hemorrhaging. For the most part, the abdominal organs are insensitive to pain because they contain few pain fibers. Therefore an injury to the organ itself may cause little if any pain or tenderness unless the covering capsule is involved. An exception to this is the liver, which has a good network of nerves; an injury to the liver will cause acute pain. More often it is hemorrhaging into the capsule of an organ or into the peritoneal cavity that causes pain. For example, bleeding into the capsule surrounding one of the kidneys will cause pain or point tenderness.

Injuries to the hollow organs are extremely uncommon, as an athlete's stomach, intestines, and bladder are generally empty during athletic activity. A hollow organ injury may not produce symptoms unless some of the contents within come into contact with the peritoneum and cause irritation or the organ becomes distended. A common example of this is the appendix. Many times the symptoms associated with appendicitis are not present until the organ distends or ruptures. Hollow organs are more susceptible to an athletic injury when they are full of food or waste products. When these hollow structures are injured, the resulting signs and symptoms are similar to those associated with injuries to solid organs. Additional signs that may indicate an injury to one of the hollow organs are black *tarry stools,* bright red blood in the fecal discharge, or bloody vomitus (hematemesis).

Another important symptom that must be remembered when evaluating abdominal injuries is referred pain. Many injuries affecting abdominal viscera will cause pain to be felt in a part of the body removed from an injured area. For example, an injured spleen may cause pain in the left shoulder and upper arm *(Kehr's sign).* An injury to the liver may refer pain to the right shoulder, and an injury to one of the kidneys may be felt high in the posterior costovertebral angle as well as radiating forward. Table 13-1 lists the common referral sites for pain corresponding to injured viscera. It is not necessary for the athletic trainer to remember all the referral sites of pain. However, it is important to understand the phenomenon of referred visceral pain, which often accompanies an intra-abdominal injury, and to be able to recognize this symptom.

The "visceral pain" that arises in an injured abdominal organ is generally poorly localized at the actual site of injury. Instead, referred pain is felt at a distant site (Table 13-1) that is innervated by the same spinal segment as the injured visceral structure. Although the exact mechanism of referred pain is still unknown, the most ac-

cepted theory suggests that visceral pain fibers synapse with neurons in the spinal cord that receive pain fibers from the skin in the referred area. When a visceral structure is injured and pain fibers are stimulated, the pain sensations spread to neurons that normally conduct pain sensations from the skin, and the athlete has the feeling that the pain sensations actually originate in the skin of the referred pain area. The location of the referred pain on the body surface is in the same dermatome of the segment from which the injured visceral organ was originally derived during embryonic development. Some types of referred pain also result from reflex muscular spasm. A bruised ureter, for example, will cause reflex spasm of the lumbar muscles on the side of injury.

Among the solid organs, the kidneys are the most frequently injured, followed by the spleen and liver. When these organs are injured during athletic activity, the mechanism is usually some type of direct blow to the abdomen or back. The primary danger of any solid organ injury is the possibility of severe hemorrhaging into the abdominal cavity. Bleeding can occur rapidly or very slowly and insidiously. Occasionally the

Table 13-1. Referred visceral pain

Organ	Area of body to which pain may be referred
Appendix	Right lower quadrant, umbilicus
Bladder	Lower abdomen and upper thighs
Diaphragm	Anterior shoulders
Esophagus	Along sternum, left upper thorax
Heart	Base of neck, left jaw, and left shoulder and arm
Intestines	Back (backache or sharp pain in the back), umbilicus
Kidney	High in the posterior costovertebral angle and radiating forward around the flank
Liver	Right shoulder
Pancreas	Directly behind pancreas
Spleen	Left shoulder and upper third of arm
Ureter	Costovertebral angle, radiating to lower abdomen, testicles (male), and inner thigh

bleeding will stop a short time after the injury, only to start again hours, days, or possibly weeks later. Therefore the athletic trainer must be alert for delayed symptoms occurring with abdominal injuries. The injured athlete must also be made aware of possible delayed symptoms that, if they occur, should be reported immediately.

The signs and symptoms associated with an injury to a solid organ usually include pain, localized tenderness, rebound tenderness, abdominal rigidity, nausea, and vomiting. If hemorrhaging is severe, the athlete will also exhibit signs of blood loss or shock. These signs include pallor, rapid pulse, low blood pressure, dizziness, and fainting. An injury to the kidneys usually produces blood in the urine *(hematuria)*. The amount of blood in the urine may be such that it is easily recognized on inspection or so minor that the urine looks normal *(microscopic hematuria)*. Therefore, following a suspected injury to the kidneys, all urine passed should be checked visually as well as microscopically for blood.

Athletic trainers should also be alert for signs and symptoms that may indicate the presence of an infection or inflammatory process in the gastrointestinal or genitourinary systems. The presence of these complaints are normally not associated with an athletic injury but indicate the athlete should be referred to a physician for further diagnosis. Signs and symptoms that may be associated with gastrointestinal conditions include vomiting, difficulty in swallowing *(dysphagia),* diarrhea, and the passage of blood in the stool. Signs and symptoms that may be associated with genitourinary conditions include the sensation of pain, burning or itching on urination *(dysuria),* blood in the urine, frequent urinations, and urethral discharge.

THE GENITALIA
Male

The external genitalia in the male consist of the scrotum and penis (Fig. 13-8). The scrotum is a skin-covered pouch suspended from the perineal region. Internally it is divided into two sacs

Fig. 13-8. Sagittal section through male penis.

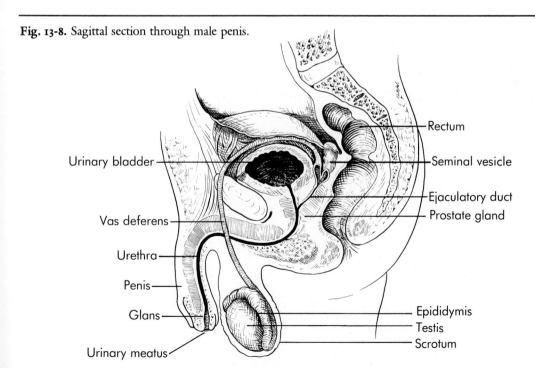

Urinary bladder

Vas deferens

Urethra

Penis

Glans

Urinary meatus

Rectum

Seminal vesicle

Ejaculatory duct

Prostate gland

Epididymis

Testis

Scrotum

by a septum, each sac containing a testis, epididymis, and lower part of a spermatic cord. The testes are small ovoid glands somewhat flattened from side to side. The left testis is generally located about 1 cm lower in the scrotal sac than the right. Both testes are suspended in the pouch by attachment to scrotal tissue and by the spermatic cords, which ascend from the scrotum and enter the abdomen by passing through the inguinal canals. The muscular vas deferens, a component of the spermatic cord, can be palpated through the scrotal wall as a firm and rounded cord.

The penis is composed of three cylindrical masses of erectile, or cavernous, tissue, enclosed in separate fibrous coverings and held together by a covering of skin. The two larger and uppermost of these cylinders are named the corpora cavernosa penis, whereas the smaller, lower one, which contains the urethra, is called the corpus cavernosum urethrae (corpus spongiosum).

The distal part of the corpus cavernosum urethrae overlaps the terminal end of the two corpora cavernosa penis to form a slightly bulging structure, the glans penis, over which, in the uncircumcised male, the skin is folded doubly to form a more or less loose-fitting, retractable casing known as the prepuce or foreskin. The open-

Fig. 13-9. Sagittal section through female pelvis.

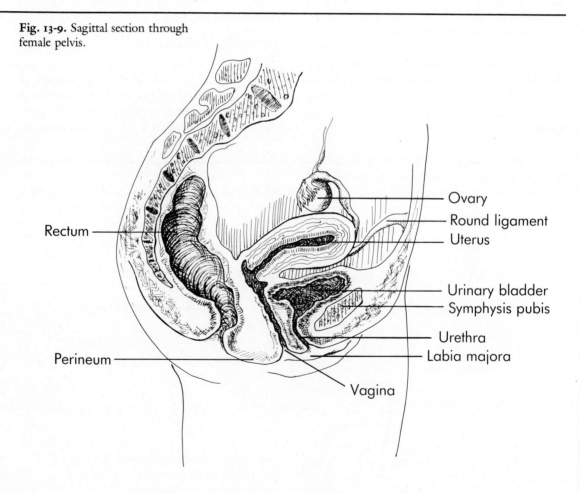

Rectum

Perineum

Ovary

Round ligament

Uterus

Urinary bladder

Symphysis pubis

Urethra

Labia majora

Vagina

ing of the urethra at the tip of the glans is called the external urinary meatus.

Female

The term "vulva" is used to describe those structures that, together, constitute the female external genitalia (Fig. 13-9). The vulva consists of the mons pubis, labia majora, labia minora, clitoris, urinary meatus (external orifice), and vaginal orifice. Ducts from the greater vestibular (Bartholin's) and lesser vestibular (Skene's) glands also open into the vulva.

The mons pubis is a skin-covered pad of fat over the symphysis pubis. Pubic hair appears on this structure at puberty. The labia majora (large lips) are covered with pigmented skin and hair on the outer surface and are smooth and free from hair on the inner surface.

The labia minora (small lips) are located within the labia majora and are covered with modified skin. These two lips come together anteriorly in the midline. The area between the labia minora is the vestibule.

The clitoris is a small organ composed of erectile tissue, located just behind the junction of the labia minora, and homologous to the corpora cavernosa and glans penis. The prepuce, or foreskin, covers the clitoris, as it does the glans penis in the male. The urinary meatus (urethral orifice) is the small opening of the urethra, situated between the clitoris and the vaginal orifice. The vaginal orifice is located posterior to the external urinary meatus.

GENITALIA INJURIES

Athletic injuries to the genitalia, and especially to the internal reproductive organs, are extremely uncommon. The female reproductive structures, being almost entirely internal and well protected by the bony pelvis and abdominal musculature, are seldom injured. Occasionally the vulva is injured as the result of a fall astride some object such as a balance beam or uneven parallel bar. The resulting injury is normally a contusion and should be treated as any other

injury of this nature. Contusions should be treated with a cold pack to minimize hemorrhaging, and lacerations should be referred for suturing to minimize scarring. Even relatively small lacerations involving the skin-covered muscular region (perineum) between the vaginal orifice and the anus are potentially dangerous and should always be referred to a physician for treatment. In women the perineum and perineal body form an important support structure in the pelvic floor and, if weakened, may result in partial uterine or vaginal prolapse.

A much more common injury is to the external genitalia of the male athlete. The testes are fairly vulnerable to injury during many types of athletic activity. These injuries usually occur as the result of a direct blow to the scrotum. The resulting contusion can range from very mild to an extremely painful, nauseating, and disabling injury for the athlete. In most cases, pain from these injuries is short lived. Occasionally there will be a significant amount of bleeding associated with a testicular contusion, which requires the application of an ice pack to the scrotal area. An athlete may also complain of a drawing sensation as the muscles attached to the testes go into spasm. Two methods of reducing testicular spasm are commonly used. One is to instruct or assist the athlete in bringing both knees up toward his chest (Fig. 13-10, *A*). This assists in relaxing the muscle spasms and reducing discomfort. Another maneuver often used by athletic trainers is illustrated in Fig. 13-10, *B*. With the athlete sitting on the floor, lift him about 2 to 3 inches and drop him to the floor. This results in a mild jolt to the genitalia and may assist in relaxing the testicular muscle spasm. Some caution should be employed in using this drop technique, especially if pain persists. The signs and symptoms associated with most genital injuries normally subside in a few minutes and require no further evaluation. However, if symptoms do persist or develop in time, the athlete should be referred to medical assistance for further evaluation and treatment.

Fig. 13-10. Methods of reducing testicular spasm. **A,** Bringing both knees up to the chest; **B,** lifting seated athlete a few inches and dropping him to the ground.

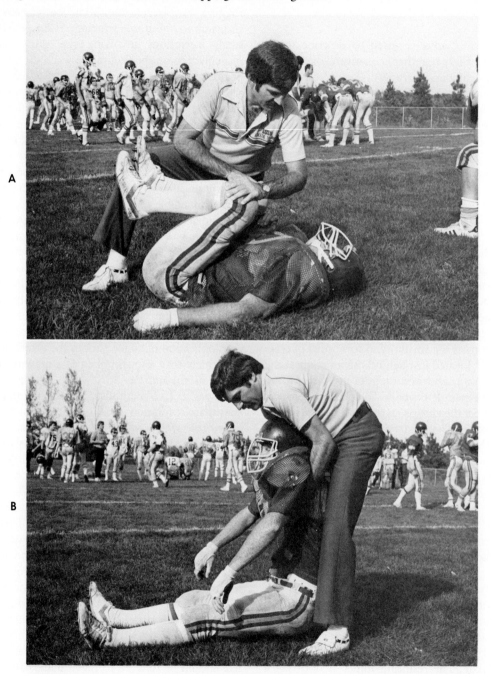

ATHLETIC INJURY ASSESSMENT PROCESS

Potentially serious and life-threatening injuries involving the chest or abdomen can occur during athletic activity. The chest contains the heart and lungs, our most vital life-sustaining organs. Any trauma to the chest that seriously compromises the function of these organs can pose an immediate threat to survival. The abdomen contains several organs richly supplied with blood, trauma to which can cause severe and possibly fatal hemorrhaging. Although most athletic injuries involving the chest and abdomen are not serious or life threatening, the possibility always exists. Therefore the athletic trainer must be aware of the possible types of abdominal injuries that can occur and be alert for signs and symptoms indicative of life-threatening situations to ensure appropriate assessment and emergency treatment.

Primary survey

During the primary survey, evaluation of the respiratory and circulatory status of the athlete is of utmost importance. As has been stated previously, you must be sure the athlete has a patent (unobstructed) airway, is breathing, and has a pulse. An athlete suffering from a significant injury to the chest may have difficult or labored breathing (dyspnea). This can be a serious condition and terrifying for the athlete. The athletic trainer must have a calm and reassuring approach to these athletes to help them relax and breathe more easily. Assisting these athletes may include (1) making certain the airway remains clear of blood and vomitus, (2) helping the athlete find the most comfortable position for breathing, (3) being ready to help the athlete control vomiting, (4) being prepared to provide artificial ventilation and circulation if necessary, and (5) providing prompt transportation to emergency medical services. Once these conditions or problems are under control, you can proceed to the secondary survey.

Secondary survey

The evaluation of athletic injuries to the chest and abdomen is of major importance because of the possibility of internal bleeding or involvement of internal organs. As previously mentioned, most athletic injuries affect the chest or abdominal wall. It is important, however, for the athletic trainer to determine as quickly as possible if there are any associated intrathoracic or intra-abdominal injuries. An athlete exhibiting signs and symptoms that may indicate internal involvement should be referred to medical attention immediately. A "wait and see" approach should not be practiced, as an internal injury can quickly develop into a serious and complicated condition. Follow-up examinations are also important to detection of slowly developing intrathoracic or intra-abdominal problems. For example, an injured spleen may splint itself only to go into a delayed hemorrhage hours or days after the injury. For this reason, it is important that the athlete who has suffered direct trauma to the chest or abdomen and does not initially exhibit signs and symptoms indicating internal injuries be instructed to immediately report further complications that may develop. This is also true for the athlete whose signs and symptoms subside only to recur. Signs and symptoms that may indicate internal involvement are discussed throughout this chapter and listed on p. 339.

Another important point to remember is that athletes who have suffered acute trauma to the abdomen, or in whom intra-abdominal involvement is suspected, should not be allowed to eat or drink anything after the injury. The ingestion of food or fluids may aggravate the symptoms, and if surgery is required, the presence of food in the digestive tract will make the operation more dangerous. In addition, the athlete should not be given any medication for the pain because some of the symptoms may be masked. A physician examining the athlete must know both the location and the intensity of the pain.

History

The history of an injury to the chest or abdomen is extremely important as an indication of both the nature of the injury and what has happened since the injury occurred. Begin by determining the mechanism of injury. Most injuries to the chest and abdomen occur during contact sports and are caused by some type of direct trauma, such as a direct blow or forcible contact with an object or another athlete. Question the athlete to get a detailed description of how the injury occurred. Was there a direct blow, and if so, by what? How large was the area of contact? Attempt to determine the severity of the blow or force. In addition to the mechanism, determine the location of the injury. Was the trauma to the back, chest, or abdominal area? Attempt to localize the site of the trauma as precisely as possible.

Next, question the athlete about any pain associated with the injury. Ask the athlete to localize the painful or tender areas. How severe is the pain? Is it constant or intermittent? Is the pain increased during respiration or movement? Does the athlete feel the pain is located in the chest or abdominal wall, or does he or she believe it is deeper, or inside the cavity? Does there appear to be any radiating or referred pain? Remember, an injury involving a visceral organ may cause no other symptom than referred pain. Correlating the mechanism of injury to the exact location of all painful areas and realizing that visceral pain may be referred are very important in assessing injuries of the chest and abdomen.

Inquire about any additional symptoms the athlete may have experienced. Does the athlete express any crepitation that may accompany a fractured rib or costochondral separation? Does he or she feel any tightness, cramping, or rigidity of the abdominal muscles, which may indicate peritoneal irritation? Is there a pulling sensation in the groin or abdominal musculature? Does the athlete feel nauseated? Does the athlete complain of trouble with breathing? Allow the athlete to describe his or her impression of the injury. Does the athlete think the injury is of a serious nature?

If the athlete was not evaluated immediately after the injury, inquire about what has happened to any signs or symptoms since the injury first occurred. Have they improved, deteriorated, or stayed about the same? Has the athlete urinated or defecated since the injury? If so, was there any indication of blood in the urine or stool? If the athlete failed to check or has not yet eliminated, he or she should be instructed to look for blood after the next episode of elimination. Remember, blood in the urine or stool should be reported immediately. Inability to urinate after abdominal trauma should also be reported.

Additional information that may be important to you or the physician assessing abdominal trauma concerns the status of the hollow organs before and after the injury. Was the athlete participating on a full stomach? Was the bladder full or empty? If a period of time has elapsed since the injury, has the athlete recently eaten? Did the symptoms appear worse or better after eating?

Observation

Observations made during assessment of chest and abdomen injuries can be very beneficial in determining the site, nature, and severity of the injury. These observations begin as soon as you see the athlete and continue throughout the assessment process. If the athlete is seen immediately following the trauma or remains lying on the court or field, the initial observations are concerned with assessing the respiratory and circulatory systems as described during the primary survey. Once the adequacy of these systems is assured, observations are concerned with evaluating all signs and symptoms associated with the injury. It is extremely important to watch for the development of signs that may indicate intrathoracic or intra-abdominal involvement.

Begin by noting the position of the injured athlete. If the athlete remains lying on the court or field, notice if the athlete is moving about. Remember, if an athlete hurts, he or she will usually not want to perform any movement that will increase the pain. Is the athlete holding an area of the chest or abdomen? Does the athlete have his or her knees drawn up toward the chest? This position takes stress off the abdominal muscles and is generally more comfortable for a person who has suffered an injury to the abdomen. The athlete may also be taking rapid shallow breaths in an attempt to avoid pain caused by thoracic or abdominal movement. If the athlete is up and moving around, notice his or her gait and willingness to move. Is the athlete leaning toward or favoring one side of the body? Does the athlete appear to be in much pain during movement? Is the athlete avoiding any position or movements that may increase the pain? These initial observations can be very helpful in determining which further assessment procedures will be used.

When evaluating trauma to the torso, and especially the chest, monitor the athlete's respiratory rate and rhythm. Does either appear to be abnormal or irregular? Is the athlete having a difficult time breathing or catching his or her breath? If the athlete has had the "wind knocked out," normal breathing will return rapidly, and most signs and symptoms will subside quickly. However, if signs and symptoms persist, additional intrathoracic or intra-abdominal involvement must be suspected and the injury must be evaluated further. Note if the breathing appears to be painful or if the athlete is holding an area of the chest wall. Does the athlete avoid taking any deep breaths, which may increase the pain? While observing the rate and rhythm of the respirations, inspect the chest for symmetry of movements. Both sides of the chest should move equally with each breath. Also look at the trachea to note any change in position. Normally the trachea lies in the midline of the neck and does not move during respirations. Also note the symmetry of the abdomen. Does there appear to be any abnormal distention or protrusion? Are there overlying contusions? Does the abdomen appear to be rigid? Any signs that may indicate intrathoracic or intra-abdominal involvement must be carefully and continually monitored.

Bilateral symmetry of the neck should be judged with the head centered and muscles relaxed. Look for head tilting, muscle shortening, and masses. Inspect the anterior and posterior chest, noting the general shape of the thorax and its symmetry (Fig. 13-11). Observe the skin color and integrity, looking for cyanosis, pallor, or for obvious signs of traumatic injury. To do this, clothing or equipment should be removed. Look for deformities, contusions, abrasions, bleeding, or swelling. These observations can indicate the site of the trauma and provide important clues as to which structures may be involved. These signs may also indicate the severity of the direct trauma. Are there any areas of ecchymoses about the abdomen, which may suggest internal hemorrhaging? Periumbilical ecchymosis (Cullen's sign) is indicative of intraperitoneal bleeding; flank ecchymosis (Grey-Turner's sign) points to retroperitoneal hemorrhage. Do the painful areas correlate with the site of trauma? That is, are the injured structures lying immediately below the site of trauma, or is pain expressed at an area away from the direct

Fig. 13-11. Inspecting the anterior chest and abdomen.

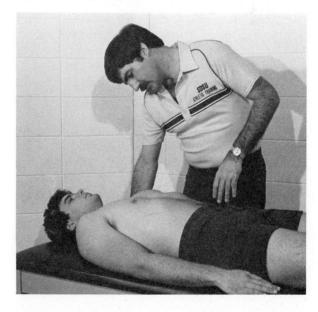

trauma? Examples of the latter could be forceful compression of the rib cage, resulting in a fracture or separation away from the site of direct trauma as well as referred visceral pain.

In addition to these observations, an athlete with an injury to the chest or abdomen should be watched particularly for signs of impending shock or internal involvement. Signs of shock include pallor, cool clammy skin, and a weak, rapid pulse. These signs and symptoms, along with others that suggest hemorrhaging or additional internal complications, are important to recognize. The rapidity with which the signs and symptoms develop following a torso injury is extremely important. Signs and symptoms developing quickly indicate a medical emergency requiring immediate attention by a physician. Remember, an athlete may appear to be doing well but may actually have a serious internal condition that becomes symptomatic hours or even days after the injury. Therefore you must continue to observe and reassess the health status of athletes who suffer trauma to the chest or abdomen.

Palpation

Careful palpation techniques can be beneficial in evaluating injuries to the chest or abdomen. They can be used to confirm or investigate those findings or suspicions gained during the history and observation portions of the assessment process. Remember to begin all palpation techniques very gently to elicit the athlete's cooperation and to avoid inflicting any unnecessary pain.

When palpating the chest, gently feel the site of the trauma as well as all painful areas expressed by the athlete (Fig. 13-12). Locate as precisely as possible the tender areas. Note the anatomic structures you are palpating, such as along a rib, between two ribs, at the costochondral junction, or along the sternum or trachea. Do you feel any obvious deformities, crepitation, or swelling? Remember, if an obvious deformity or injury is recognized, it is not necessary to continue the assessment process; the appropriate

treatment or transfer procedures should be initiated. Rib or costochondral injuries that are not obvious but suspected because of the site of the pain, can be evaluated by stress procedures described later.

You can also evaluate the symmetry of respirations by placing your hands on the athlete's rib cage. Anteriorly place the tips of your thumbs on the xiphoid process and spread your hands over the lower rib cage (Fig. 13-13). Posteriorly, place your thumbs along a lower thoracic spinous process and spread your hands over the posterior lateral rib cage. Both hands should move equally with each breath. If one side does not move as much, and the athlete exhibits signs of breathing difficulty, there may be intrathoracic involvement. In addition, you should palpate the trachea during respirations to note any shifting that may accompany an intrathoracic condition such as pneumothorax.

Palpation of the abdomen should be performed with the athlete lying supine and as relaxed as possible. It is best to have the athlete's arms along either side of the torso, rather than

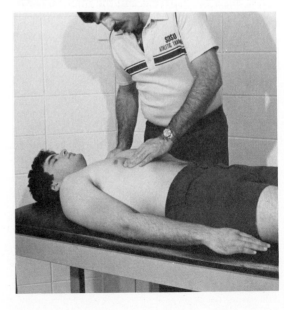

Fig. 13-12. Palpating site of trauma on the chest.

behind the head. The hips should be flexed. The place where the examination is conducted should be sufficiently warm so the athlete does not shiver. Instruct the athlete to relax and breathe quietly and slowly. Everything should be done to avoid tensing the abdominal muscles. If these muscles are contracted or tense, it is difficult to accurately palpate the abdomen. Also avoid using cold hands or quick pokes into the abdomen, as both can cause the athlete to tighten, or guard, the abdominal muscles. Palpation techniques should be performed with the flats of the fingers with the palm of the hand lying lightly on the abdomen (Fig. 13-14).

Palpate the abdomen gently so as not to cause unnecessary pain or further injury. It is a good practice to palpate the uninjured areas of the abdomen to begin with, to gain the athlete's cooperation and assist in relaxing the abdominal muscles. Feel for any tightness or muscle rigidity. Remember, peritoneal irritation is indicated by a rigid abdomen. However, an athlete with tenderness in the abdomen may guard the painful area by tightening or contracting the abdominal muscles. This rigidity can be distinguished from peritoneal rigidity by careful palpation; voluntary guarding of the muscles by the athlete can be relaxed, whereas peritoneal rigidity cannot. Continue to palpate the tensed area while instructing the athlete to relax and breathe slowly. If you feel a relaxation of the muscle rigidity, it is voluntary guarding. Occasionally, distracting the athlete may also help overcome the voluntary guarding. A truly rigid abdomen resulting from peritoneal irritation will not be affected and may feel boardlike.

Rebound tenderness is also present with peritoneal irritation. This is elicited by putting firm pressure on the abdomen and then quickly releasing the pressure. The release of pressure will cause a sharp severe pain. For example, rebound tenderness in the lower right quadrant of the abdomen is a classic sign of acute appendicitis. It is normally unnecessary to perform this procedure and cause the athlete additional pain. However, it is important to understand that this phenomenon does occur with peritoneal irritation and that an athlete may experience this sudden stabbing pain with any unexpected movement, such as coughing or being jolted.

If the abdomen is not rigid and tense, you can continue palpating for tenderness in each of the

Fig. 13-13. Feeling for symmetry of respirations.

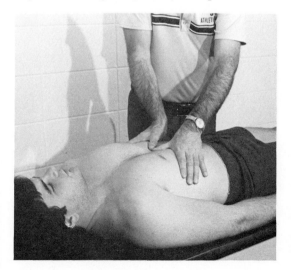

Fig. 13-14. Palpating an athlete's abdomen.

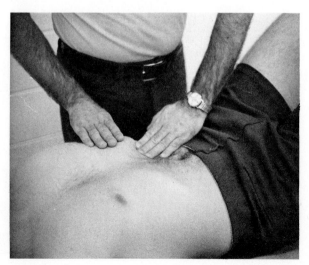

four quadrants. Feel about the spleen, liver, and kidneys. Locate any areas of tenderness. Remember to palpate gently to begin with; then, if there is no pain, you can proceed with deeper palpation. While palpating, feel for masses, swelling, protrusions, or other deficits in the continuity of the abdominal wall. If the athlete suffered a blow to the crest of the ilium, palpate along this bony ridge (Fig. 13-15).

Stress

The majority of the assessment process to evaluate injuries to the chest and abdomen is completed by following the history, observation, and palpation procedures described above. Very few stress maneuvers are performed. When stress techniques are utilized they are used to assist the assessment of injuries to the chest or abdominal walls.

Active movements. Assessment of injuries to the neck includes an evaluation of active motion (see Chapter 12). Evaluate the normal range of motion of the neck for flexion, hyperextension, lateral bending, and rotation. In checking for adequacy of lateral bending movements, make certain that the athlete moves the side of the

head toward the shoulder, not the shoulder up to the ear. Look for ratchety or tremulous movements. Is there pain associated with any movement or at any particular point during movement? Is muscle spasm apparent? Is there a limited range of motion? Always remember, *never* initiate passive range of motion assessment techniques in the presence of a traumatic neck injury.

The integrity of the abdominal wall, which is composed primarily of muscles, can be further evaluated by having the athlete actively contract the abdominals. Remember, pain associated with a muscle strain is usually aggravated by active contraction or stretching of the muscle. When an abdominal muscle strain is suspected, instruct the athlete to perform a series of range of motion exercises for the trunk. The normal range of motion of the trunk in flexion, hyperextension, lateral bending, and rotation is discussed and illustrated in Chapter 12. Can the athlete perform these movements? Is there pain associated with any active movement or at any particular point during motion? Is there a limited range of motion?

Resistive movements. Resistance can be applied against these active movements to further

Fig. 13-15. Palpating crest of the ilium.

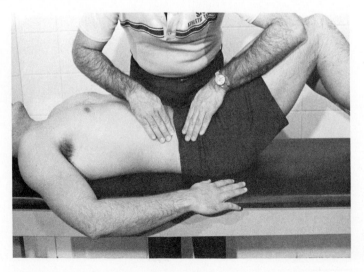

evaluate the integrity of the contractile unit. With cervical motion, resistance is easily applied manually, as described in the previous chapter. For trunk movements, instruct the athlete to perform a partial sit-up (Fig. 13-16, *A*). If pain is increased significantly, note the exact location. The oblique muscles may be better evaluated by having the athlete perform some twisting of the trunk during the sit-up (Fig. 13-16, *B*). Another point to remember is that performing a sit-up will increase the intra-abdominal pressure, which may also increase the symptoms associ-

Fig. 13-16. Athlete performing partial sit-up **(A)** to stress the abdominal muscles and **(B)** with trunk rotation to apply more resistance to the oblique muscles.

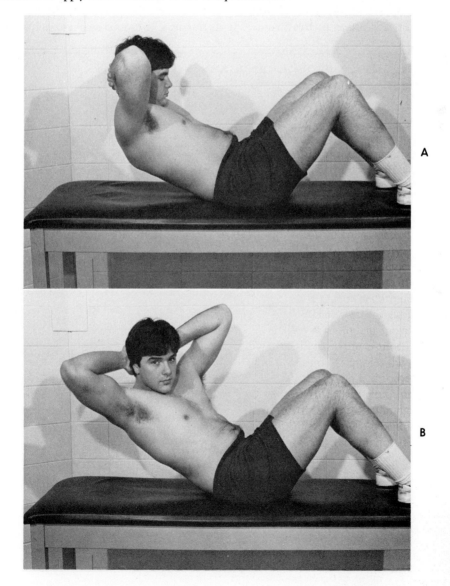

A

B

ated with a hernia or other internal injury.

Passive movements. The integrity of the chest wall, composed primarily of the ribs, sternum, and rib cartilages, can be further evaluated by applying passive stress to these structures. When a bone or costochondral injury is not obvious but is indicated or suspected, you can apply stress to the structures by gently compressing the rib cage. If a fracture is suspected along the lateral side of the rib cage, apply gentle compression in an anteroposterior direction (Fig. 13-17, *A*). Each rib can be stressed in this manner. If

pain is increased at the suspected site, the continuity of the rib is probably interrupted and referral is indicated. Remember, a bruise or other injury to the intercostal muscles does not result in a significant increase of pain during this maneuver. If pain is expressed along the costochondral margin, apply gentle compression on the rib cage in a transverse direction (Fig. 13-17, *B*). Again, stress can be applied to each rib. If pain is increased at the costochondral junction, the athlete has probably suffered a separation at this area. It cannot be overemphasized that these

Fig. 13-17. Applying compression to the rib cage. **A,** Anteroposterior compression to evaluate bony integrity. **B,** Transverse compression to evaluate costochondral junctions.

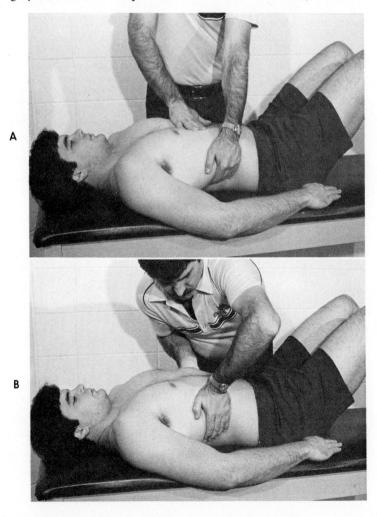

passive stress maneuvers must be performed gently to begin with so as not to cause any additional damage. They are only performed after thorough history, observation, and palpation.

Evaluation of findings

As stated earlier, the majority of athletic injuries to the chest and abdomen involve the walls of these two major body cavities. Occasionally the visceral contents of these cavities are also injured. Visceral injuries can develop into serious, possibly life-threatening, conditions. When evaluating injuries to the chest or abdomen, the athletic trainer must also be alert for signs and symptoms that may indicate an intrathoracic or intra-abdominal injury, and be prepared to provide emergency care if necessary as well as refer the injured athlete to a physician or medical facility.

When to refer the athlete

Whenever intrathoracic or intra-abdominal involvement is indicated or suspected, the athlete should be referred to medical assistance immediately. Prolonged periods of watching and waiting can allow internal conditions to become more serious. Therefore the athletic trainer must be constantly alert for signs and symptoms that may indicate internal injuries. It must also be remembered that internal complications may develop hours, days, or possibly weeks after significant trauma to the chest or abdomen. An athlete may appear to be doing very well, only to have delayed symptoms develop later. For this reason, any athlete suffering what appears to be severe trauma to the chest or abdomen, but who does not show signs of internal complications, should be instructed to immediately report any unusual signs and symptoms that may develop later. These signs and symptoms can be listed on a medical follow-up sheet similar to the one on p. 340. This sheet can be given to the athlete with instructions to follow immediately should any of the signs and symptoms develop. Following is a list of conditions or findings that indicate the athlete with a chest or abdominal injury should be referred to medical attention.

Throat injuries or conditions
Persistent soreness, hoarseness, or loss of voice
Difficulty in breathing
Inability to swallow
Bleeding from the throat
Crepitation on palpation
Suspected inflammation or infection of throat structures
Doubt regarding the nature and severity of the throat injury or condition
Chest injuries
Difficult or labored breathing
Shortness of breath—inability to catch breath
Severe pain in chest
Diminished chest movement on affected side
Shifting or moving of trachea with each breath
Vomiting or coughing up blood
Suspected rib fracture or costochondral separation
Signs of shock
Doubt regarding the nature and severity of the chest injury
Abdominal and pelvic injuries
Severe pain in abdomen
Presence of what appears to be radiating or referred pain
Tenderness, rigidity, and spasm of the abdominal muscles
Blood in the urine or stool
Signs of shock
Rebound tenderness
Prolonged discomfort, sensation of weakness or pulling in groin
Superficial protrusion or palpable mass
Increasing nausea
Vomiting
Any perineal laceration (women)
Doubt regarding the nature and severity of the abdominal injury

---

SOUTH DAKOTA STATE UNIVERSITY TRAINING ROOM

This is a medical follow-up sheet for your health and safety. Signs of a chest or abdominal injury may not appear immediately following trauma but can develop hours after the injury. The purpose of this fact sheet is to alert you to the symptoms of significant chest or abdominal injuries which may develop several hours after you leave the training room.

If you experience one or more of the following symptoms, medical help should be sought:

Chest injuries
  Difficulty in breathing
  Shortness of breath—inability to catch breath
  Pain increasing in chest
  Vomiting or coughing up blood
Abdominal injuries
  Pain or discomfort increasing in abdomen
  Rigidity and spasm of abdominal muscles
  Blood in the urine or stool
  Vomiting
  Increasing nausea
  Painful urination

The appearance of any of the above symptoms tells you that you may have sustained a significant chest or abdominal injury that *requires medical attention*. If any of these symptoms appear, contact Jim Booher, Barb Moran, or Dr. Bruce Lushbough, or report to the Brookings Hospital Emergency Room.

REMEMBER: Your health depends on how much you care about proper medical attention.

THE SDSU ATHLETIC TRAINING STAFF

KEY TERMS

celiac (solar) plexus Largest of the abdominal plexuses, supplies the viscera in the abdominal cavity; it lies in the upper middle region of the abdomen

dysphagia Difficulty in swallowing

dyspnea Labored breathing

dysuria Sensation of pain, burning, or itching on urination

hematemesis Vomiting of blood

hematuria Blood in the urine

hemopneumothorax Presence of both blood and air in the pleural cavity

hemoptysis Coughing up blood or blood-stained sputum

hemothorax Blood in the pleural cavity

hernia Protrusion of abdominal viscera through a portion of the abdominal wall

hypoxia Low oxygen content, deficiency of oxygen in the inspired air

Kehr's sign Referred pain to the left shoulder and upper arm resulting from an injury to the spleen

laryngitis Inflammation or irritation of the larynx indicated by hoarseness, dryness, soreness, and difficulty in swallowing

pharyngitis Inflammation of the pharynx (throat) indicated by pain on swallowing, dryness, burning, and hoarseness

pneumothorax Accumulation of air in the pleural cavity

spontaneous pneumothorax Pneumothorax occurring without apparent cause

strangulated hernia Herniated portion of viscera that has become incarcerated or tightly constricted and is likely to become gangrenous

tachypnea Abnormally rapid shallow breathing

tarry stool Blood in the fecal discharge

tension pneumothorax Condition in which air continues to be drawn into the pleural cavity and cannot escape; pressure continues to rise on the affected side, pushing the collapsed lung against the heart and unaffected lung

---

ATHLETIC INJURY ASSESSMENT CHECKLIST
THROAT, CHEST AND ABDOMEN INJURIES

Primary survey

_____ Airway
_____ Breathing
_____ Circulation

Secondary survey

_____ History
        _____ Mechanism of injury
        _____ Location of injury
        _____ Pain
        _____ Sensations
        _____ Progression of signs and symptoms
_____ Observation
        _____ Position and movements
        _____ Respiratory rate and rhythm
        _____ Symmetry
        _____ Signs of trauma
_____ Palpation
        _____ Tenderness
        _____ Deformities
        _____ Swelling
        _____ Crepitation
        _____ Symmetry
        _____ Muscle rigidity
        _____ Rebound tenderness
_____ Stress
        _____ Active range of motion
        _____ Resistive movements
        _____ Passive stress on rib cage

ADDITIONAL READINGS

American Academy of Orthopaedic Surgeons: Emergency care and transportation of the sick and injured, ed. 3, Chicago, 1981, The Academy.

Arnheim, D.D.: Modern principles of athletic training, ed. 6, St. Louis, 1985, Times Mirror/Mosby College Publishing.

Budassi, S.A., and Barber, J.M.: Mosby's manual of emergency care: practices and procedures, St. Louis, 1984, Times Mirror/Mosby College Publishing.

Grant, D., and others: Emergency care, ed. 3, Bowie, Md., 1982, Robert J. Brady Co.

Kuland, D.N.: The injured athlete, Philadelphia, 1982, J.B. Lippincott Co.

Malasanos, L., and others: Health assessment, ed. 3, St. Louis, 1985, Times Mirror/Mosby College Publishing.

O'Donoghue, D.H.: Treatment of injuries to athletes, ed. 4, Philadelphia, 1984, W.B. Saunders Co.

The Nurse's Reference Library: Assessment, Springhouse, Pa., 1982, Internal Communications, Inc.

Warner, C.G.: Emergency care, assessment and intervention, ed. 3, St. Louis, 1982, The C.V. Mosby Co.

U N I T

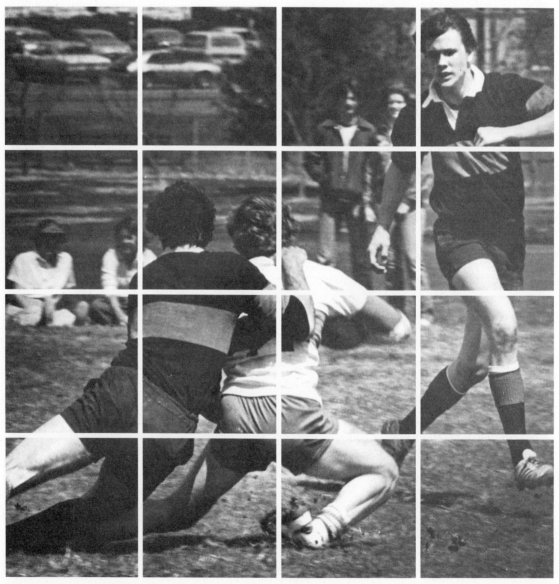

Ankle fracture and dislocation.
(Courtesy Cramer Products, Inc., Gardner, Kan.)

F I V E

Athletic injuries of the lower extremities

The lower extremities are complex functioning units extremely important to almost every type of athletic endeavor. There are few athletic activities that do not require the use of the lower extremities in one manner or another. Because of its high and diversified utilization, this area of the body is continually subjected to many traumatic stresses. Athletes involved in running and jumping are especially at risk. All sports participants are, however, susceptible to sustaining some type of injury to this area of the body. Considered as a functioning unit, the lower extremity is impaired more frequently and is subject to more injury-related conditions or problems than any other area of the body. Athletic trainers are constantly called on to handle injuries and disorders involving the lower extremities. The professional athletic trainer must continue to improve and broaden assessment skills related to evaluation and treatment of injuries to this important area of the body.

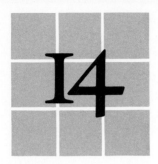

I4 Foot, ankle, and leg injuries

The feet, ankles, and legs form the foundation for the body. Just as buildings and structures are only as strong as their foundations, athletes are only as sturdy and effective as their base of support.

The body's foundation originates with the feet, which support the body weight in a myriad of positions and function over a multitude of surfaces and contours. Most athletic activity begins with and is dependent on the feet. As such, the feet continually bear the brunt of physical stresses and rapidly changing forces thrust on them from all directions. The ankle joint is the fulcrum between the foot and leg, and as such is also subjected to tremendous amounts of physical stress and many types of potentially damaging forces. The leg is the functional unit that transmits muscular power to the foot and ankle. Combined, the leg, ankle, and foot constitute the area of the body most frequently involved with athletic injuries. Therefore athletic trainers must possess the knowledge and skills necessary to accurately assess and effectively manage athletic injuries of the foot, ankle, and leg. This effective management begins with a fundamental understanding of the anatomy, functional mechanics, and possible mechanisms of athletic injury involving this region of the body.

ANATOMY OF THE FOOT AND ANKLE

The structure of the foot is similar to that of the hand, with certain differences that adapt it for locomotion and supporting weight. The skeleton of the foot is composed of tarsal, metatarsal, and phalangeal bones (Fig. 14-1). The word "tarsus" is a collective term used to describe the seven bones that constitute the midfoot and hindfoot: talus, calcaneus, navicular, cuboid, and the three cuneiform bones. Although the calcaneus, or heel bone, is the largest and strongest tarsal, it supports only about half

Fig. 14-1. Bones of the ankle and foot, dorsal view.

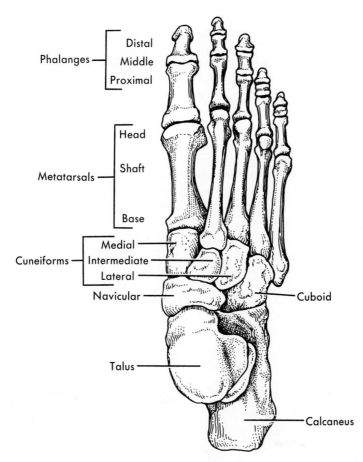

of the total weight transmitted from the talus during walking or running. The remaining weight is transmitted evenly to the other tarsals.

The calcaneus projects backward behind the ankle, thus providing leverage for the *triceps surae,* (gastrocnemius and soleus muscles), which inserts on its posterior surface. The lateral surface of the calcaneus is almost entirely subcutaneous. It can be palpated easily just distal to the lateral malleolus and can be followed forward from the back of the heel for approximately 2 inches. The upper surface of the calcaneus has articular facets for the talus, the largest being the medially projecting ledge called the *sustentaculum tali.* Between the talus and the calcaneus is the important subtalar joint, and at the anterior ends of these bones is the transverse tarsal joint. These two joints allow inversion and eversion to occur. The upper end of the talus is called the *trochlea.* It is this bony process that articulates with the tibia and fibula. The anterior end of the talus articulates with the navicular bone. The navicular has a rather large process (tuberosity) on its medial side. The tuberosity of the navicular can be palpated quite easily as a prominence about an inch diagonally below and in front of the medial malleolus. It lies about midway between the back of the heel and the base of the great toe and serves as a useful landmark during the assessment process. Practice locating these bony landmarks in the healthy, noninjured foot. The more practical experience you have in mentally visualizing underlying anatomic structures, the more accurate you will become in identification of specific types of injury in this complex area.

The *metatarsus* consists of five bones named and numbered 1 to 5 from the medial to the lateral position. The metatarsals resemble the metacarpals of the hand; each has a proximal base, a body, or shaft, and a distal head. Identify the proximal and distal points or articulation of the metatarsals in Fig. 14-1. The bases of the first three metatarsals articulate with the cuneiforms, whereas the fourth and fifth articulate with the cuboid. The head of each metatarsal articulates

with the base of its corresponding proximal phalanx. Note also in Fig. 14-1 that the body (shaft) of the first metatarsal is thicker than the other four—a structural adaptation that permits it to bear more weight.

Like the fingers, there are 14 phalanges in the toes—three for each digit except the big toe, which has two. The phalanges are designated as proximal, middle, and distal. Normally the tarsals and metatarsals play the major role in the functioning of the foot as a supporting structure, with the phalanges being relatively unimportant. In the hand, where manipulation rather than support is the main function, the reverse is true.

Accessory bones

Accessory bones occur in both the hands and feet but are of much greater practical importance in the feet. Over 20 types of accessory bones can be found in the feet, and they occur in about 25% of the population. They are easily mistaken on x-ray film for bone fragments, which would indicate a fracture. For this reason physicians will sometimes conduct radiographic examinations of both feet when only one foot is injured. As a group, accessory bones are divided into two classes: (1) sesamoids and (2) true accessory bones, which are almost always bilateral in their appearance (hence the need for examining both feet by radiography).

Arches

The bones of the feet are held together in such a way as to form springy lengthwise and crosswise arches. The longitudinal and transverse arches (Fig. 14-2) of the feet provide a highly stable and resilient base to bear the body's weight and also yield as weight is applied to aid in absorbing the shocks associated with walking and running. The longitudinal arch has an inner (medial) portion and an outer (lateral) portion, both of which are formed by the tarsals and metatarsals. The medial longitudinal arch is sometimes referred to as the "arch of movement." It is high, easily seen in most persons, and is made up of the calcaneus, talus, navicular, the three cuneiforms, and the first, second, and third metatarsals. In the medial longitudinal arch the principal weight-bearing points are the heel and the metatarsal heads. The apex of this arch is the talus.

The calcaneus and cuboid, plus the fourth and fifth metatarsals, shape the lateral longitudinal arch. The cuboid is the apex of this arch. It is low, however, and permits the outer border of the foot to touch the ground along its entire length. The longitudinal arch is formed by the placement of the metatarsals and tarsals. The result is a convexity formed on the top (dorsum) of the foot and a concavity on the sole (plantar aspect). Strong ligaments and tendons from muscles originating in the leg normally hold the bones of the foot firmly in their arched positions, but it is not uncommon for these to weaken, causing the arches to flatten, a condition aptly called fallen arches, or flatfeet.

The transverse arch is perpendicular to the length of the foot. Essentially, there is a series of transverse arches across the plantar surface of the foot. The talonavicular joint forms the highest part of this arch on the medial side and the calcaneocuboid joint the highest part on the lateral side. Anterior to the peak of the transverse arch, the plantar surface becomes successively less arched. Athletic trainers occasionally manage painful transverse arch conditions occurring just proximal to the metatarsal heads. This area is frequently referred to as the metatarsal arch.

Joints

The many interlocking bones of the ankle and foot result in the formation of numerous joints. The joints of the foot (Fig. 14-3) are generally subdivided into five major groups: (1) tarsal, (2) tarsometatarsal, (3) intermetatarsal, (4) metatarsophalangeal, and (5) interphalangeal. The joints of the foot are listed in the box on p. 348.

Fig. 14-2. Arches of the foot.
(From Arnheim, D.D.: Modern principles of athletic training, ed. 6, St. Louis, 1985, Times Mirror/Mosby College Publishing.)

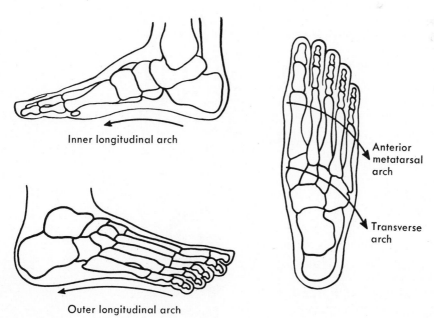

Inner longitudinal arch

Anterior metatarsal arch

Transverse arch

Outer longitudinal arch

JOINTS OF THE FOOT

Tarsal
    Proximal intertarsal joints
        Subtalar (talocalcaneal)
        Talocalcaneonavicular
    Transverse intertarsal joints
        Calcaneocuboid
        Talonavicular
    Distal intertarsal joints
        Cuneonavicular
        Intercuneiform
        Cuneocuboid
Tarsometatarsal
Intermetatarsal
Metatarsophalangeal
Interphalangeal

The tarsal joints are further subdivided into proximal, transverse, and distal intertarsal groups. The proximal intertarsal joints, that is, the subtalar (talocalcaneal) and talocalcaneonavicular, are of particular importance and practical significance to the athletic trainer.

The subtalar joint is the point of articulation between the talus and the calcaneus. This is a diarthrotic, gliding type of joint with a capsule and a synovial membrane. The subtalar joint is not the only point of articulation between the talus and calcaneus; inversion and eversion movements of the foot on the talus occur simultaneously at both the subtalar and talocalcaneonavicular joints. A limited range of inversion and eversion are extremely important to the athlete. They enable the body to move sideways over the foot while the foot itself remains fixed. The mus-

Fig. 14-3. Joints of the foot. *A,* Tarsal, *B,* tarsometatarsal, *C,* intermetatarsal, *D,* metatarsophalangeal, and *E,* interphalangeal.

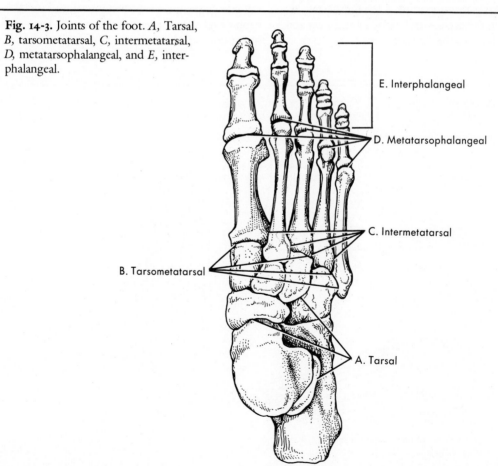

E. Interphalangeal

D. Metatarsophalangeal

C. Intermetatarsal

B. Tarsometatarsal

A. Tarsal

cles producing inversion are the tibialis anterior and tibialis posterior. Eversion movements are produced by the peroneus longus, brevis, and tertius muscles.

As the name implies, the talocalcaneonavicular joint is really a complex of synovial joints between the talus, navicular, and calcaneus bones. In addition, the calcaneonavicular, or spring ligament also enters into the formation of this important and frequently injured joint. The spring ligament attaches the calcaneus to the navicular bone and limits the flattening of the medial longitudinal arch of the foot.

The distal intertarsal, tarsometatarsal, and intermetatarsal joints are all plane-type, synovial joints. Although several of them form single joint cavities, they are, individually, of only limited importance to the athletic trainer. As a group these joints permit only limited gliding movements. The joint between the medial cuneiform and the metatarsal of the great toe is somewhat unique in that it allows a greater range of plantar flexion and dorsiflexion to occur. Some rotary movements are also available at this joint.

The arrangement of the metatarsophalangeal and interphalangeal joints is on the same basic plan as in the hand. Metatarsophalangeal joints are of the ellipsoid type. They permit plantar flexion, dorsiflexion, and some abduction and adduction. The interphalangeal joints are classified as hinge joints and permit only flexion and extension.

Foot types

The structure and alignment of the foot is an extremely important consideration whenever assessing injuries to the lower extremities, and especially when evaluating overuse injuries. The shape of the foot is subject to as many individual variations as any other area of the body. These variations are the culmination of the development of the foot and result from a variety of causes, such as functional demands, structural deformities, injuries, heredity, body type, and postural faults. Significant foot variations are considered the most common form of physical impairment among athletes. Before an athletic trainer can recognize variations of the foot that may predispose an athlete to injuries, he or she must have a conception of what is considered to be a "normal" foot. An accurate definition of the ideal or normal foot is elusive. However, there are criteria established for a normal foot, and the athletic trainer should be familiar with these characteristics and alert to any significant variations. These criteria are listed in the box below.

Most people have varying degrees and types of deviation from the ideal foot type. These deviations seldom cause problems in normal everyday activities. However, because of the nature of

---

CRITERIA FOR A NORMAL FOOT

1. The anatomic contours should appear in neutral positions.
2. The calcaneus should be centrally located below the leg and perpendicular to the floor.
3. The medial border of the foot should lie in a reasonably straight line from the heel to the great toe.
4. Each toe should be flexible and in straight alignment.
5. The medial longitudinal arch should form a gentle, smooth curve.
6. A normal range of active motion at the ankle joint should be available.
7. There should appear to be good tone and balanced strength of the leg muscles.
8. During weight bearing, the contact of the foot should be distributed between the heel and the ball of the foot. All metatarsal heads should rest firmly on the floor.
9. The feet should be asymtomatic under most conditions. That is, the athlete with what is considered normal alignment and structure of the feet should have a very low incidence of injury symptoms when following a sensible training program. Of course, this precludes traumatic injuries such as those caused by twisting or collision.

sporting activities, these variations are magnified and become much more significant in athletes. The greater the degree of variation, the more susceptible an athlete is to problems. Also, the greater the continued repetitive nature of the athletic activity, the more susceptible an athlete is to developing overuse problems. For example, runners who train many miles a week are more susceptible to overuse injuries caused by variations in their feet than are athletes participating in sports requiring less constant running. Therefore the athletic trainer should be able to recognize a foot that is more susceptible to overuse injuries. The athletic trainer should also be alert to signs about the feet and shoes that may indicate malalignment or imbalance conditions. These signs include such things as excess callus formation on the foot, blisters, clawed toes, bunions, and shoes that wear unevenly.

There are three foot types commonly associated with overuse injuries: (1) the pronated foot, (2) the cavus foot, and (3) Morton's foot. The athletic trainer should be able to recognize each of these foot types and understand something about the mechanics associated with each. Again, the athletic trainer is not expected to be an expert on evaluating foot types; however, he or she should be able to recognize gross abnormalities of the foot. Recognizing these foot types can provide the athletic trainer with sufficient information to refer the athlete to a foot specialist, or plan treatment strategies designed to alleviate the symptoms.

Pronated foot. Pronation of the foot is a combination of abduction, dorsiflexion, and eversion. These motions take place in the tarsal joints and especially the subtalar joint. Some pronation is normal, but excessive pronation, or hyperpronation during weight bearing, is a common condition found in athletes who exhibit overuse problems of the feet and legs. In fact, this defect is considered to be the most common cause of chronic overuse injuries in runners. *Pes planus* is commonly associated with foot pronation; however, the two are separate deviations. Pes planus, or flatfoot, is a static structural abnormality in

which the position of the bones relative to each other has been altered, resulting in a lowering of the longitudinal arch.

The hyperpronated foot is considered to be a very flexible foot with excessive motion at the subtalar joint. When the foot pronates, the weight line falls to the medial side of the foot, the medial longitudinal arch depresses, and the toes tend to be directed outward (Fig. 14-4). Other common signs of a pronated foot include an inward tilting of the heel, causing a medial curving of the Achilles tendon and a more pronounced medial malleolus. These deviations result in an abnormal relationship between the talus, calcaneus, and tarsal articulations with each foot strike, and a variety of chronic overuse syndromes in the foot, leg, and knee can result.

The amount of pronation of the foot can range from quite mild to very severe. The mildly

Fig. 14-4. Pronated foot.

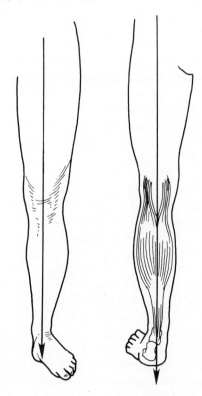

pronated foot may present as a generalized postural fatigue, especially with running activities. This malaligned foot may cause fatigue and pain in the arch as well as mild **bunions** (Fig. 14-5) and possibly **hammertoes**. The moderately pronated foot has increased mobility and poorer shock-absorbing qualities at heel strike. The toes are more unstable, and the intrinsic muscles fatigue more quickly. There is a higher incidence of overuse injuries such as plantar fascial strains, heel bruises, calcaneal spurs, bursitis, tendinitis, and stress fractures. The severely pronated foot is a hypermobile flatfoot with very little longitudinal arch visible during weight bearing. All the symptoms are accentuated and occur frequently during athletic activity. The athlete with severely pronated feet may even exhibit pain and symptoms without athletic activity.

Cavus foot. The cavus foot (pes cavus) has a high longitudinal arch with limited tarsal motion (Fig. 14-6). This is considered to be an in-

flexible foot that does not adequately absorb shock or easily adapt to various surfaces. The cavus foot is usually associated with heavy callus formation on the ball of the foot or heel caused by additional stresses placed on these areas. Clawing of the toes and pain along the bottom of the foot or under the metatarsal heads is typical. Lateral tilting of the calcaneus, or rearfoot varus, is often associated with this type of foot. In addition, the cavus foot transmits increased shock to the ankle, leg, knee, thigh, hip, or back, creating an increased incidence of overuse injuries.

The cavus foot can range from a flexible foot to one that is very rigid. The flexible cavus foot has a high arch when it is not bearing weight. The toes also appear to be mildly clawed when there is no weight on the foot, but straighten out during weight-bearing. The flexible cavus foot has somewhat limited shock-absorbing qualities, which predisposes it to overuse injuries such as plantar fasciitis, heel bruises, Achilles tendinitis, shin splints, and stress fractures. The flexible cavus foot may progress to a rigid cavus foot deformity despite treatment strategies.

As the cavus foot becomes rigid, the high arch and claw toes become less flexible. The arch will flatten only mildly and the claw toes do not straighten completely with weight-bearing. This foot has more callus build-up, and frequent

Fig. 14-5. Bunion (hallucis valgus).

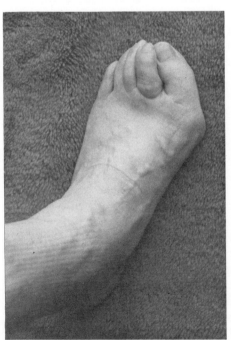

Fig. 14-6. Cavus foot with a rigid high arch.

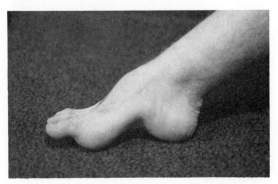

complaints of pain under the metatarsal heads because of the increased abnormal stresses transmitted to this area are common. Dorsiflexion of the ankle is limited to a greater degree, and the intrinsic muscles of the foot are tighter. This type of foot is called a semiflexible or moderate cavus foot. This foot has more limited shock-absorbing properties, which results in more stress being transmitted to the lower extremity and lower back. There is also a related increase in overuse injuries.

The rigid cavus foot is the most difficult foot to manage. This foot has a very high longitudinal arch and clawed toes at rest and when bearing weight. It has a tight plantar fascia, and painful calluses usually develop under the metatarsal heads. The rigid cavus foot does not absorb shock well, adapts to surfaces very poorly, and is inadequately suited for athletic activity. Athletes with this type of foot are more susceptible to sprained ankles, Achilles tendon problems, arch conditions, stress fractures, and a variety of overuse injuries.

Morton's foot. Morton's foot is characterized by a short first toe and longer second toe. This can result from a shortened first metatarsal and a normal second or a normal first metatarsal and shortened second. Normally the second metatarsal is just slightly longer than the first, which usually absorbs more stress than any of the other metatarsals during weight-bearing. When the first metatarsal is significantly shorter, the foot must adapt to this abnormal condition. The great toe does not bear weight until later in the gait cycle, and the second metatarsal must absorb more stress during weight-bearing. This can increase the incidence of overuse injuries. The foot may attempt to compensate for this by pronating or rolling inward so that the first metatarsal can more quickly contact the surface. The magnitude of overuse problems associated with excessive pronation was previously discussed.

An accurate diagnosis of Morton's foot normally involves a radiographic study. However, the athletic trainer should be familiar with the common signs that may indicate Morton's foot.

A rough estimate of the length of the metatarsals can be observed while the athlete flexes the toes. The head of the first metatarsal will sit back farther than the second. When the second metatarsal is longer, there often will be a callus buildup under the head of the second metatarsal as the result of increased stress to this area. The athlete may complain of pain in the ball of the foot or longitudinal arch during or after activity. This pain may be a burning type of pain accompanied by numbness or tingling. Pain may also be elicited by pressure applied under the first and second metatarsal heads.

Ankle joint

The term "ankle" is used to describe the region of transition between leg and foot. It consists of the ankle joint and those structures that surround it. The skin about the ankle is normally thin and loosely attached to the underlying parts. If edema occurs, fluid will accumulate in the loose tissue spaces, and the skin will "pit" or become indented, when pressure is applied by the fingertips during palpation.

The medial and lateral malleoli, which are the distal ends of the tibia and fibula, respectively, can be palpated at the ankle. However, the lateral one is less prominent, lies farther back, and extends more distally than the medial. The distal tip of the lateral malleolus projects a half inch below and behind its palpable bony prominence. The ankle joint is located about one-half inch above the tip of the medial malleolus, which serves as the most prominent of the medial bony landmarks in this region. The Achilles tendon is the prominent landmark at the back of the ankle. It is important to realize that blood vessels, nerves, and tendons, which all have a vertical orientation in the leg, must turn forward and assume a horizontal orientation in order to enter the foot. Although specialized connective tissue bands (retinacula) hold these structures against the bones of the ankle and foot to prevent "bowstringing," they are still vulnerable to injury in this area.

The ankle joint is a uniaxial, diarthrotic hinge

joint. It is often described as a three-sided box-like or mortise joint. The ankle joint is designed for weight bearing and has great strength and stability. The top and sides of the box-shaped socket are formed by the medial and lateral malleoli and the distal articular surface of the tibia. This socket articulates with the trochlea of the talus below (Fig. 14-1).

The active movements permitted at the ankle joint include dorsiflexion and plantar flexion. In dorsiflexion the forepart of the foot is raised and the angle between the front of the leg and the top of the foot is decreased; in plantar flexion the foot is lowered and the angle is increased as the toes are pointed downward. If the foot is forcibly plantar flexed, the talus will be pushed forward and become prominent just in front of the lateral malleolus. In the normal range of movement, the two malleoli project downward and tightly grasp the sides of the talus. As a result, only very slight lateral or medial movement is possible.

The principal dorsiflexor of the ankle is the tibialis anterior, assisted by the extensor digitorum longus and the extensor hallucis longus. The principal plantar flexors are the gastrocnemius and soleus. The tibialis posterior, flexor hallucis longus, and flexor digitorum longus also assist in plantar flexion at the ankle joint.

Ankle ligaments

The bones that compose the ankle are held together by a strong fibrous capsule that is attached to the articular margins of the tibia and fibula above and to the talus below. In addition to the capsule, the distal ends of the tibia and fibula are tightly bound to each other by ligaments at the distal tibiofibular articulation just above the ankle. The capsule of the ankle joint proper is subdivided into four ligaments: (1) anterior, (2) posterior, (3) medial (deltoid), and (4) lateral. The requirement of free movement in flexion and extension results in the anterior and posterior ligaments of the capsule being loose and weak. The medial (deltoid) and lateral (collateral) ligaments of the capsule are tight and

---

CAPSULE OF THE ANKLE

Anterior ligament
Posterior ligament
Collateral ligaments
  Medial (deltoid) ligament
  Lateral ligament
    Anterior talofibular ligament
    Posterior talofibular ligament
    Calcaneofibular ligament

---

very strong. The individual components of the articular capsule are listed in the box above.

The deltoid, or medial collateral, ligament is triangular, thick, and very strong. Its apex is attached to the medial malleolus and its base to bones and ligaments in the foot. It supports the talus and braces the spring ligament between the calcaneus and navicular bones, thus helping to preserve the medial longitudinal arch of the foot. In extreme and forced eversion of the foot, the deltoid ligament may tear away from or fracture the medial malleolus rather than tear or rupture itself.

The lateral collateral ligament comprises three separate ligaments. These three components of the lateral ligament are not as strong as the single deltoid ligament on the medial side of the ankle; as a result, sprains occur more frequently when the ankle is turned inward (inverted).

FOOT AND ANKLE INJURIES

Athletic injuries involving the foot and ankle are very common and vary widely in terms of structural damage or functional loss. Because of the high utilization of the foot in most types of athletic activity, acute traumatic injuries are as prevalent as overuse injuries. Injuries involving an athlete's feet are often magnified in severity because the feet are weight-bearing structures. A relatively minor injury of the foot can impair an athlete's performance as dramatically as a major injury to another body area. Unfortunately, athletes often abuse or neglect their feet until conditions or symptoms interfere with their performance. Proper and adequate care should be given all injuries and athletic-related conditions of the feet, no matter how minor they may appear. This discussion of the more common foot injuries includes injuries to the ankle joint.

Contusions

Contusions about the foot resulting from various types of direct impacts are common occurrences in athletics. The skin over the dorsum of the foot is thin and only loosely attached to the underlying structures. Further, the subcutaneous placement and exposed nature of most structures near the dorsum of the foot make them susceptible to contusion injuries. Injuries in this area tend to be painful even if actual tissue damage is minor. However, all direct trauma to the dorsum of the foot should be evaluated for the presence of significant damage to underlying structures such as bones, tendons or nerves. In most instances, although painful initially, such injuries are not serious. Contusions that do not heal promptly must be reevaluated periodically.

Contusions to the plantar, or weight-bearing, surface of the foot can be particularly bothersome and handicapping. These injuries, common to the plantar aspect of the heel and ball of the foot, are normally caused by direct trauma such as repeated pounding on a hard surface, a faulty spike or cleat, stepping on an object, or even a wrinkle in the athlete's sock. The subcutaneous tissue between the bones of the foot and the thick plantar skin becomes bruised and inflamed. This injury, often called a *stone bruise,* or heel bruise, may become quite painful and disabling during weight bearing and athletic competition. Localized tenderness at the site of trauma may persist until weight bearing is relieved. Contusions of this type may develop into a chronic inflammatory process and recur throughout the athletic season.

Strains

Strains involving the foot are common occurrences in athletics. These injuries may involve the intrinsic muscles, the tendons and tendinous attachments of the extrinsic muscles, and the *plantar aponeurosis* (plantar fascia). Strains may occur to any of the intrinsic muscles of the foot as a result of excessive overuse or violent stresses applied to muscles during athletic activity. Symptomatically, these injuries usually cause cramping or fatigue of the involved muscles and are painful during resistive movements. Symptoms normally subside when activity is reduced or discontinued.

Athletic trainers are called on more often to manage strains involving the extrinsic muscles of the foot or those muscles that originate about the leg. These injuries are discussed in more detail along with injuries of the leg. Because the tendons and tendinous attachments of these extrinsic muscles are in and about the foot and ankle, injuries involving these structures produce symptoms similar to foot and ankle sprains. Therefore each must be accurately evaluated. Strains of these extrinsic tendons cause tenderness at the site of injury and increased pain on active and resistive contractions of the muscle or muscles involved.

Another common strain of the foot occurs to the plantar aponeurosis or fascia. These strong bands of fibrous connective tissue originate on the calcaneal tuberosities and insert into the sides of the metatarsal heads and into the flexor digital tendon sheaths. This tough fascia surrounds the soft tissue structures of the sole of the foot and acts as one of the primary supports for the longitudinal arch. It is often described as a "tie rod" for the longitudinal arch because it serves to connect its ends and prevent their spread. The plantar fascia is subjected to many stresses and forces during athletic activity, which may result in a strain injury that often becomes chronic and is commonly called *plantar fasciitis.* The pain associated with this type of an injury can be acute and quite handicapping. In many cases the pain is most severe when the athlete first puts weight on the foot, as when getting out of bed in the morning or at the beginning of activity. The pain generally diminishes during activity, only to increase when activity stops or when the athlete is "cooling down." Point tenderness is usually towards the calcaneal end of the aponeurosis and very often over the medial tuberosity of the calcaneus. Occasionally the pain can be reproduced by having the athlete stand on the toes. Plantar fasciitis is often aggravated by excessive pronation of the foot, obesity, or an abnormally high arch. Occasionally a forward prolongation of the calcaneal tuberosity, termed a *heel spur,* may be present on a radiograph of plantar fasciitis. However, heel spurs may be present with or without any painful symptoms.

Sprains

Injuries involving the ligaments or ligamentous capsules surrounding the various joints of the foot are common in athletic activity. This is especially true of the ankle joint. Sprains frequently result from forced motion at a joint, especially torsion movements, which can stress any of the supporting ligaments and cause various degrees of damage. Although it must be remembered that the human body is a chain-linkage system, sprains will be discussed in three segments corresponding to divisions of the foot: (1) forefoot, (2) midfoot, and (3) hindfoot, which includes the ankle joint. An injury in any one of these segments can cause problems or affect the others.

Forefoot. The forefoot is composed of the metatarsals and phalanges. This part of the foot is used in the pushing-off phase of the gait cycle and as such is subjected to stresses that may result in various types of sprains. The interphalangeal and metatarsophalangeal joints are most often injured by extreme dorsiflexion or plantar flexion forces. The most common site for this type of an injury is to the metatarsophalangeal joint of the great toe, which is sometimes referred to as a *turf toe.* A sprain of this joint can be debilitating in that the great toe is very important in weight bearing, and the proximal joint must bear the brunt of every step. Symptomatically, sprains about the toes will present

tenderness at the site of injury and an increase in pain on reproduction of the stress that caused the injury. In addition, there are normally varying amounts of swelling, stiffness, and soreness surrounding the articulations. Depending on the amount of ligamentous damage, there may be varying amounts of instability associated with the injury. If instability is recognized, the athlete should be referred to medical assistance. Various instability tests are discussed in the assessment portion of this chapter.

The metatarsal bones are joined by a complex mechanism of ligaments. Occasionally the ligaments and supporting tissues of the metatarsal heads will be injured. The mechanism of injury is varied but usually is associated with prolonged activity on hard surfaces or with overuse. Physical findings normally include tenderness and swelling under the heads of the metatarsals and pain upon weight bearing. Sprains involving the tarsometatarsal joints sometimes occur as a result of a twisting mechanism or direct stress, such as the athlete stepping on someone or something. This type of forefoot sprain can also be very disabling because of the increased tenderness and pain upon weight bearing. Occasionally return to full activity may take up to 4 weeks or longer with this type of injury.

Midfoot. The midfoot is composed of the navicular, cuboid, and three cuneiform bones. These midtarsal joints are supported by a strong ligamentous system that is rarely injured. However, midfoot sprains can result from severe twisting mechanisms or forceful direct trauma that causes a subluxation of the involved tarsals. These sprains produce tenderness at the site of injury, and quite often weight bearing is extremely painful. Midfoot sprains can prevent an athlete from normal activity for a considerable length of time.

Hindfoot. The hindfoot is composed of the calcaneus and talus. These bones serve as attachments for the medial and lateral ligaments supporting the ankle joint; therefore injuries to the hindfoot will include sprains of the ankle.

Ankle sprains are among the most commonly

treated injuries occurring to athletes. The frequency of ankle injuries results from the anatomic structure, the weight-bearing function, and the violent forces applied to this joint during high-speed athletic activity. As previously discussed, the talus fits into a mortise formed by the distal ends of the tibia and fibula. The medial and lateral malleoli project downward to articulate with the sides of the talus. The talus is narrower posteriorly than anteriorly. This anatomic fact explains the slight looseness or increased amount of motion of the ankle joint in plantar flexion. The talus fits more snugly into the mortise during dorsiflexion. The ankle joint is designed to function as a hinge joint permitting only dorsal and plantar flexion. Ankle injuries occur when this joint is forced to the extremes of motion or in an abnormal direction.

One of the most common mechanism of injury occurs when the ankle is forced laterally, or inverted. Because of the shorter medial malleolus, inversion occurs more readily than eversion. In fact, during forced inversion, the short medial malleolus may become a fulcrum, causing

Fig. 14-7. Common mechanism of ankle sprain.

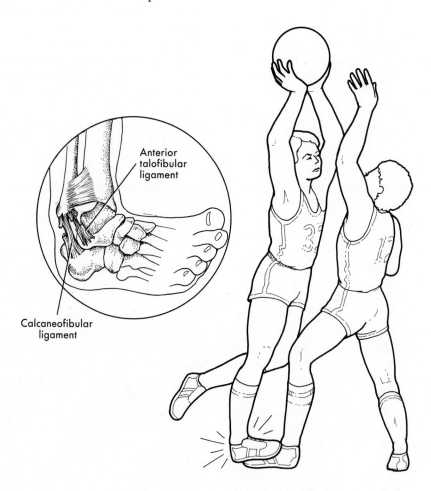

Anterior
talofibular
ligament

Calcaneofibular
ligament

further inversion. Most athletic activity predisposes a participant to inversion injuries. This occurs because most cutting and turning maneuvers are initiated from the foot opposite the direction of the turn. For example, if an athlete wants to cut right, the maneuver begins with a lateral push-off from the left foot, which forces the ankle into inversion, external rotation, and plantar flexion. This stresses the lateral ligament complex, which in athletics is the most frequently injured ligament structure in the body. Additional factors that accentuate the ankle's normal tendency to go into inversion occur if the foot strikes an irregular or uneven surface, such as coming down on another athlete's foot (Fig. 14-7).

The opposite mechanism of injury, forced eversion, occurs much less frequently during athletic activity. This can occur when the leg is hit laterally with the foot fixed. Because the lateral malleolus is as long as the talus is high, it is very difficult for the lower end of the fibula to act as a fulcrum during this type of an injury. This fact, along with the strength of the medial ligaments, explains why athletic trainers seldom see isolated injuries to the deltoid ligament. Sprains to the medial side of the ankle are often severe and involve additional structures such as a fractured fibula.

Additional mechanisms causing ankle sprains are forced dorsiflexion, plantar flexion, and rotation of the leg when the foot is firmly fixed. As the foot is forced into dorsiflexion, the broad part of the talus is located firmly between the malleoli and may force them apart, thus injuring the ligaments of the distal tibiofibular joint. A similar injury can result from forced rotation of the leg with the foot firmly fixed. In these cases the shape of the talus acts as a fulcrum forcing the tibia and fibula apart.

In light of the many and varied mechanisms that can cause ankle sprains, it is easy to understand the importance of an accurate history in evaluation of these injuries. The information gained in a thorough history assists the athletic trainer in focusing on those anatomic structures that might be involved. A good history always includes a review of the forces and stresses associated with the injury and a careful evaluation of the athlete's description of what happened. Significant ankle sprains are almost always accompanied by immediate pain and difficulty in bearing weight. Localized tenderness will be exhibited over the ligaments involved, and there may or may not be swelling initially. Ankle motion may or may not be restricted. It is important to evaluate the severity of the sprain before swelling develops and motion is restricted. On initial evaluation, the athletic trainer must attempt to recognize an unstable ankle, which should be referred to a physician for additional diagnostic assessment.

Dislocations

Dislocations of the foot and ankle are uncommon in athletic activity. This is largely because

Fig. 14-8. Athlete with fracture-dislocation of left ankle.
(Courtesy Dr. James Garrick, Center for Sports Medicine, St. Francis Memorial Hospital, San Francisco)

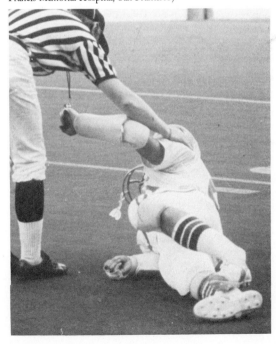

the feet are usually covered by some type of athletic footwear that supports and protects this area of the body from dislocating forces. More frequent dislocations occur to the toes when the athlete is not wearing any type of footwear. These dislocations are usually readily reduced by traction and produce periods of disability similar to severe sprains. Severe injuries, such as third-degree sprains of the forefoot or midfoot, may result in separation of the metatarsals or tarsals with significant ligament damage. The only symptom may be a painful, swollen foot. Radiographic studies are important in evaluating a swollen foot to assess bone and joint relationships. These types of injuries should be managed by a physician skilled in management of foot injuries. Occasionally the ankle is dislocated during athletic activity (Fig. 14-8). An ankle that remains displaced is normally easily recognized and should be splinted and the athlete referred to medical assistance *immediately*.

Fractures

Fractures of the bones composing the foot and ankle are relatively common in athletics and result from both acute trauma and overuse. The forefoot, composed of the long bones of the metatarsals and phalanges, is by far the most common area for fractures in the foot. These fractures can result from a direct blow to the area or by indirect trauma produced when harmful forces are transmitted along the shaft of these bones. Symptomatically these fractures demonstrate point tenderness over the injured site and increased pain during longitudinal stress. Swelling, discoloration, crepitation, and deformity may also be present. Fig. 14-9 shows a fracture of the middle phalanx of the second toe.

The current emphasis on cardiovascular fitness and long-distance running has increased the incidence of overuse injuries, including stress or fatigue fractures. These types of fractures may involve any bone in the foot, but more commonly involve the second, third, or fourth metatarsal. These fractures, commonly called *march fractures,* occur with repetitive trauma. Exces-

sive foot pronation or a high and rigid arched foot may contribute to the incidence of stress fractures. Symptomatically, stress fractures often exhibit a gradual increase in forefoot pain that is aggravated by activity and relieved by rest. X-ray films may be negative initially. If symptoms persist, the foot should be reexamined by radiography in a few weeks. At that time callus formation may indicate the presence of a stress fracture.

Fractures involving the midfoot and hindfoot during athletic activity are not nearly as common as those in the forefoot. When fractures do occur in these areas of the foot, they are usually associated with severe torsion or compression forces and result in major foot injuries. Fractures about the ankle are usually to the medial or lateral malleoli. These are caused by the same forces that cause ankle sprains and present a clinical picture of tenderness and swelling in the area of the malleolus. Malleolar fractures are often recognized by the associated instability exhibited during lateral or medial stress.

Fig. 14-9. Fracture of the middle phalanyx of the second toe.
(Courtesy Bruce Johnson, A.T.,C., Orthopedic Clinic, Grand Forks, N.D.)

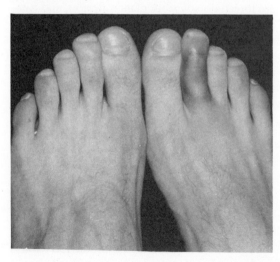

ANATOMY OF THE LEG

The leg is that part of the anatomy from the knee to the ankle. It is composed of the tibia and fibula, which furnish points of attachment for both thigh and leg muscles and transmit the body weight to the ankle and foot.

Tibia and fibula

The tibia is the larger and stronger and the more medially and superficially located of the two lower leg bones. It can be divided into a shaft separated by proximal and distal ends. The larger proximal end is prismatic in shape and overhangs the shaft. It consists of a tuberosity and medial and lateral condyles (Fig. 14-10). The expanded proximal end provides a good weight-bearing surface for the distal end of the femur. The subcutaneous tibial tuberosity can be palpated on the anterior aspect of the bone just below the condyles, about an inch from the top of the bone in most adults. In addition to the tibial tuberosity, both condyles of the tibia can be readily palpated at the sides of the bone. The condyles form most of the proximal end of the bone. The anterior border of the tibial shaft (shin) can be easily palpated because it is located very near the surface of the skin. Usually the shaft can be palpated from the tibial tuberosity

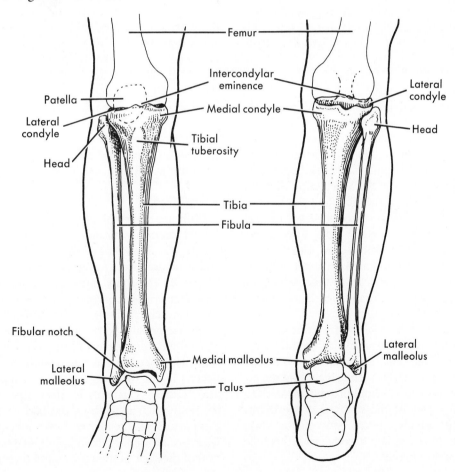

Fig. 14-10. Right tibia and fibula.

to the medial malleolus. In some athletes, however, the shin may be somewhat indistinct in its lower third. The distal (lower) end of the tibia projects medialward and downward as the medial malleolus of the ankle.

The fibula, the lateral of the two leg bones, is long and slender and lies parallel to the tibia. It is attached proximally and distally to the lateral aspect of the tibia but does not bear any weight. With the tibia it aids in forming the ankle joint and also serves as the site of attachment for muscles. Like the tibia it can be divided into proximal and distal ends and a shaft. It is the pointed distal end of the fibula that forms the lateral malleolus. As you can see in Fig. 14-10, the lateral malleolus descends about 1.5 cm beyond the medial malleolus of the tibia. Distally the fibula articulates not only with the tibia but also with the talus. The latter fits into a boxlike socket (ankle joint) formed by the medial and lateral malleoli.

Tibiofibular joints

The two leg bones articulate with each other at their proximal and distal ends. Additionally a very strong interosseous membrane joins the bones throughout their length. The proximal (superior tibiofibular) joint is a diarthrotic (synovial) joint that permits some gliding movements. It is formed by the articulation between the lateral condyle of the tibia and the head of the fibula. The joint is surrounded by a tough fibrous capsule reinforced by both anterior and posterior ligaments. The actual capsule surrounding the joint is much stronger in front than behind, and in about 10% of the population the synovial membrane of the joint is continuous with that of the knee joint.

The inferior tibiofibular joint is a fibrous articulation between the lateral malleolus and the inferior end of the tibia. It is a strong joint reinforced by numerous ligaments, including the anterior and posterior tibiofibular ligaments. Occasionally a part of the synovial cavity of the ankle joint extends upward between the lower end of the tibia and fibula, converting this joint into a diarthrotic joint.

Muscles of the leg

The muscles of the leg are divided by thick fascial sheaths into four distinct compartments. The anterior compartment contains the tibialis anterior, extensor hallucis longus, and extensor digitorum muscles as well as the deep peroneal nerve and the anterior tibial artery. The lateral compartment contains the peroneal muscles and the superficial peroneal nerve. The deep posterior compartment contains the tibialis posterior, flexor digitorium longus, and flexor hallucis longus muscles as well as the tibial nerve and the posterior tibial artery. The superficial posterior compartment contains the gastrocnemius, soleus, and plantaris muscles. Excessive pressure developing within these compartments can give rise to injury symptoms described later.

The largest tendon in the body, the Achilles, is the common attachment for the gastrocnemius and soleus muscles. This tendon runs from approximately two thirds of the way down the lower leg, where it attaches the calf muscles to the calcaneus. Two bursae surround the Achilles attachment, the superficial subcutaneous between the skin and the Achilles tendon and the deep retrocalcaneal between the calcaneus and the tendon. Either of these bursae can be irritated during athletic activity.

Alignment of the lower extremity

With any injury involving the lower extremity, and especially those of a chronic or overuse nature, it is important to appraise the alignment and structure of the lower extremity as a whole. The lower extremity functions optimally when each segment is in proper alignment and there are no structural abnormalities. This area of the body is especially susceptible to injuries resulting from malalignment and structural abnormalities. These conditions can produce abnormal stresses in the musculoskeletal structures of the lower extremity as well as affect other areas of the body, such as the hips and back. The alignment and structure of the lower extremities is therefore an important indicator of the soundness of the skeletal framework and muscular system in this area.

Evaluating the alignment of the lower extremities can be accomplished while the athlete is sitting or lying down with both legs in an extended and neutral position. However, it is usually easier to observe alignment when the athlete stands with his or her feet together. An important advantage of having the athlete stand is that most abnormal conditions are magnified with weight bearing and therefore more easily recognized. The athlete should be viewed from the front, side, and back. During the initial evaluation it is important to observe the pelvic area and the spine in addition to the lower extremities, as abnormalities may be manifested in these body areas. While viewing the athlete, look for any obvious malalignments or structural faults. The common malalignment problems of the lower extremity are listed in the following box. Those conditions involving the knee are discussed in more detail in Chapter 15.

When observing an athlete, an important consideration is the length of the legs. A discrepancy in leg length, either actual or functional, can cause an an imbalance and produce symptoms of overuse syndromes in the lower extremities, pelvis, or back. Whenever a difference in the level of the hips is observed, a discrepancy in leg length should be suspected. Determining leg length discrepancies was previously discussed and illustrated in Chapter 12 along with spinal alignment but is reviewed in this chapter. To determine if the hips are level, have the athlete stand and look to see if both anterior superior iliac spines are in the same horizontal plane. If the iliac spines appear to be uneven, a difference in the length of the athlete's legs may be present. With the athlete lying down, place both legs in a neutral position and observe the medial malleoli. If the malleoli do not appear to match, a difference in leg length should be suspected. To determine if there is an actual discrepancy in leg length, have the athlete lie supine with both legs in a neutral position. Measure the distance from the anterior superior iliac spines to the medial malleoli of both ankles. Unequal distances between these bony landmarks indicate an actual difference in

---

COMMON MALALIGNMENTS OF THE LOWER EXTREMITY

Thigh

Leg length

Knee

Genu varum
Genu valgum
Q angle
Patella alta
Squinting patella
Genu recurvatum

Leg

Internal tibial torsion
External tibial torsion

Ankle

Ankle varus
Ankle valgus

Foot types

Pronated foot
Pes cavus
Morton's foot

Toe deformities

Bunions
Hammertoes

---

leg length. If the legs are the same length but the iliac spines appear to be uneven, the pelvis is tilted laterally, resulting in one leg being functionally shorter. This may be caused by a problem in the back, hips, knees, or feet. A common observation of the athlete with a leg length discrepancy is toeing outward of the foot on the short leg side. This causes the foot to pronate, which is the body's way of adapting to a shortened leg. The foot on the longer leg will be carried in a more straightforward, natural position. Leg length discrepancies may or may not cause problems for an athlete or produce symptoms. In many cases, minor differences in leg length remain asymptomatic.

The normal alignment of the lower extremity when viewed anteriorly with the athlete standing is illustrated in Fig. 14-11. When observing the lower extremity from the front, three landmarks are important: (1) the anterior superior iliac spine, (2) the patella, and (3) the web space between the first and second toes. The lower extremity of the athlete is considered to be in normal alignment when these three landmarks appear to be in a straight line. This straight vertical alignment results in a mechanically straightforward position of the feet during walking and running. This position allows the most efficient and powerful action of the leg muscles in propulsion of the body. When these three landmarks do not lie in a straight line, a malalignment is indicated. The greater the deviation from a straight line, the greater the degree of

Fig. 14-11. Normal alignment of the lower extremity when viewed anteriorly.

Fig. 14-12. Normal alignment of the lower extremity when viewed laterally.

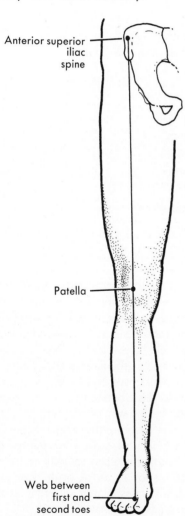

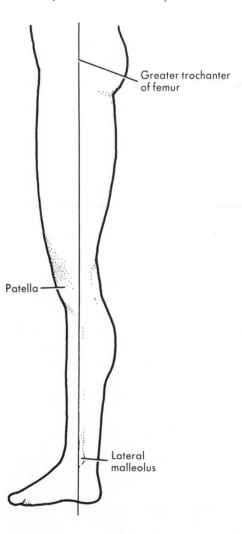

malalignment. Any deviation from a straight line imposes abnormal stresses on the joints, ligaments, tendons, and muscles of the lower extremities and feet.

The normal alignment of the lower extremity when viewed laterally is illustrated in Fig. 14-12. When observing the lower extremity from the side, three landmarks are again important: (1) the greater trochanter of the femur, (2) the patella, and (3) the lateral malleolus. The lower extremity is considered in normal alignment when an imaginary vertical line extends from the greater trochanter, posterior to the patella and anterior to the lateral malleolus. The most common fault in lateral alignment of the lower extremity is hyperextension of the knee (Fig. 14-13). This is also known as *genu recurvatum* or

back knee. Some degree of genu recurvatum should be considered normal in certain persons. However, a severe form of alignment discrepancy of this type can contribute to stability problems in the vulnerable knee joint. Hyperextension of the knee can result from structural defects, muscular imbalance, and compensation for functional faults.

Viewing an athlete from the back is extremely

Fig. 14-14. Alignment of the lower extremity when viewed posteriorly. **A,** Diagram showing normal alignment; **B,** photograph showing bilateral curvature of the Achilles tendons medially.

Fig. 14-13. Hyperextension of the knee.

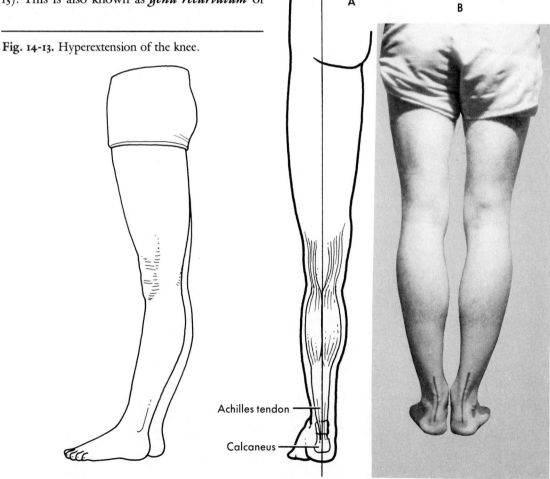

Achilles tendon

Calcaneus

A

B

useful in determining the alignment of the spine and pelvic area, as was discussed in Chapter 12. This posterior view can also be used to evaluate the alignment of the knees. In assessment of the lower extremity, this view is most useful in observing alignment between the leg and foot. The midline of the Achilles tendon should extend downward to the calcaneus without curving medially or laterally (Fig. 14-14). The midline of the calcaneus should also be perpendicular to the surface on which the athlete is standing. Any deviation from this line is usually associated with a malalignment of the foot and is discussed with the various types of feet (see p. 350).

Mechanics of the foot, ankle, and leg

The mechanics of a body area involve the function of that part during motion and the forces acting upon it. To further understand the function of the lower extremity and conditions that may contribute to overuse injuries, the athletic trainer should possess basic knowledge of the mechanics involved. Understanding these mechanics allows the athletic trainer to more accurately evaluate injuries affecting the lower extremities. The mechanical function of the foot and ankle reflects the mechanics of the entire lower extremity.

The alignment and structure of the lower extremity is certainly an indication of the functional relationship and mechanical efficiency of each segment. Variations and abnormalities observed while the athlete is sitting or standing will also be present during activity. In fact, these conditions may be further magnified and more easily recognized during motion because of additional stress applied to the area. Thus observing an athlete who is walking or running can help the athletic trainer determine if there are functional reasons for the athlete's particular injury. A complete examination of the lower extremity, designed to recognize all possible conditions that may contribute to overuse injuries, will many times include an observation of the athlete walking or running.

Walking and running gaits are divided into two major phases: (1) the stance phase and (2) the swing phase. The stance phase begins with the foot in contact with the ground and is subdivided into three basic portions: (1) foot strike, beginning at the time the foot touches the ground; (2) midstance, when the weight is directly over the foot; and (3) push off, when the body is being propelled forward. The swing phase begins when the foot is off the ground and the leg is moving to another point of contact. One cycle of gait is from foot strike until that same foot strikes the ground again. During walking one foot is always in contact with the ground, and there is a period of time when both feet are simultaneously in contact with the ground. Running differs in that there is a period of time when neither foot is in contact with the ground.

To understand and correlate the function of the foot and ankle during walking and running, the athletic trainer should first have an understanding of what is considered by experts to be normal mechanical function. It is important to remember that any variations observed while the athlete is walking will also occur when the athlete is running and performing other types of athletic activity. When watching an athlete walk, the athletic trainer should first look for the previously described characteristics of normal standing alignment of the lower extremity. The same criteria for neutral positions and straight alignments are used to determine if the athlete's feet, ankles, and legs appear to be mechanically sound. The characteristics of normal standing alignment should be present at midstance during walking and running.

In addition to observing the athlete at midstance, the athletic trainer should be aware of some normal functions of the foot and be alert for any deviations that may occur during the cycle. The foot needs to be flexible on contact and rigid on push off. This is accomplished by pronation and supination during weight bearing. Immediately after heel strike, the foot begins to pronate. This pronation unlocks the midtarsal joints, dampens the shock of heel strike, and allows the forefoot to become more flexible to adapt to various surfaces. This is very important in dissipating the constant stress of foot contact and serves to absorb shock. As the body moves over the fixed foot into midstance, the foot begins to supinate. This supination locks the midtarsal joints, stabilizes the forefoot, and provides a rigid lever for push off. The foot usually remains in supination during the swing phase until the next heel strike. These motions are necessary for the foot to change from a mobile adapter at foot strike to a rigid lever at push off.

Difficulties can arise when pronation continues past midstance and into the propulsive phase. This limits the effectiveness of the propulsive action. Excessive and prolonged pronation also flattens the medial longitudinal arch and transfers abnormal stresses and torques to the lower extremities. This can lead to overuse syndromes, fatigue, and a less efficient athletic performance.

To discuss all the components involved with the complicated mechanics of the foot, ankle, and leg is beyond the realm of this text. We recommend that athletic trainers seek additional information concerning the mechanics of the foot, ankle, and leg. We also recommend that athletic trainers continue to develop their assessment skills by observing and analyzing the various foot mechanics of their athletes.

Circulation and nerve supply

The femoral artery in each lower extremity enters the leg at the back of the knee as the popliteal artery. The popliteal becomes the posterior tibial artery as it courses between the knee and ankle. The peroneal and anterior tibial arteries branch off the posterior tibial artery in the lower leg near the ankle. It is the anterior tibial artery that is continued beyond the line of the ankle joint, as the dorsalis pedis. The posterior tibial divides into the lateral and medial plantar arteries, which anastomose with the dorsalis pedis in supplying blood to the foot.

Blood from the foot is returned by both su-perficial and deep veins. The great saphenous vein enters the lower leg from the foot just in front of the medial malleolus and then ascends from this constant anterior position along the medial surface of the leg. The small saphenous vein enters the lower leg by passing behind the lateral malleolus and then upward under the skin of the back of the calf to empty into the popliteal vein behind the knee.

The sciatic nerve enters the lower extremity and divides into two terminal divisions called the tibial and common peroneal nerves. The tibial is the larger of the two divisions. After passing between the heads of the gastrocnemius it descends to the ankle, providing branches to the leg musculature, knee, and ankle joints. Branches of the tibial nerve are distributed to the skin of the heel and sole of the foot. In addition, digital branches of the tibial nerve supply the deep muscles of the foot and adjacent sides of the toes. Branches terminate in the base of the toes and structures around the nails.

The common peroneal nerve, the smaller of the two sciatic divisions, divides into superficial and deep branches. Both branches have muscular and cutaneous components. The muscles on the anterior surface of the leg are supplied by the deep peroneal, those on the lateral surface by the superficial peroneal. The superficial branch of the peroneal nerve also provides sensory innervation to the dorsum of the foot and digits, except for the area between the great and second toes. An interosseous branch of the deep peroneal nerve supplies the metatatarsophalangeal joint of the great toe and the skin between the great and second toes.

Occasionally one of the digital nerves becomes pinched or squeezed between the metatarsal heads. The nerve responds by swelling, which is called a neuroma. This condition occurs more commonly with repetitive trauma, especially in a hypermobile foot, and is referred to as *Morton's neuroma*. The nerve between the third and fourth metatarsal is affected most often. A sharp, burning pain is present in the region of the third web space and is accentuated by activity. The pain may radiate into the third and fourth toes. Tight shoes aggravate the condition, and the pain is often relieved by removing the shoe. The condition is recognized by squeezing the ball of the foot together, which drives the metatarsals against the swollen nerve, or palpating directly between the metatarsal heads.

LEG INJURIES

Injuries involving the leg are common in all athletic activities. Many of the injuries which occur to the distal portion of the leg were discussed along with ankle injuries. Those athletic injuries occurring to the proximal portion of the leg are discussed in the following chapter on knee injuries. In addition to the high incidence of athletic injuries occurring about the ankle and

knee joints, the leg proper is also subject to a significant amount of athletic related trauma.

Contusions

The lower leg is exposed to various types of direct trauma during athletic activity and is therefore subjected to frequent contusions. Contusions occur most often over the shin, where the anteromedial tibia lies subcutaneously (Fig. 14-15). Bone periosteum is extremely sensitive, and a blow to this area of the leg can be very painful and disabling. There is hardly ever a doubt as to the mechanism of injury, that is, a history of direct impact. Contusions to the shin are often associated with abrasions or lacerations resulting from the direct trauma. Once the possibility of direct bone injury has been eliminated by the evaluation process, the area should be treated using standard treatment procedures and protected from further trauma.

Contusions can also involve the muscular areas of the leg. A possible complication of a severe contusion to any of the leg muscles is significant swelling within the various compartments. In these closed spaces, swelling is not only uncomfortable but may also lead to a compartment syndrome, which is discussed in greater detail later in this section. Another possible complication of a direct blow to the leg is damage to the peroneal nerve. This nerve is particularly vulnerable as it passes around the head of the fibula. A severe blow to this area may cause peroneal nerve injury, with pain radiating throughout the distribution of the nerve. Transient tingling and numbness to the lateral surface of the leg or dorsal surface of the foot may remain for a period of time. Occasionally peroneal nerve damage will result in loss of function to the dorsiflexors and evertors of the foot, resulting in *foot drop*. These symptoms are often temporary and recovery is usually complete.

Strains

The lower leg is the site of origin for the primary muscles responsible for transmitting power to the foot and ankle. The explosive and repet-

Fig. 14-15. Contusion to the shin of a gymnast who hit the right leg on the uneven parallel bars. Note swelling and ecchymosis of the right leg. Note also the hyperextension of the opposite knee.

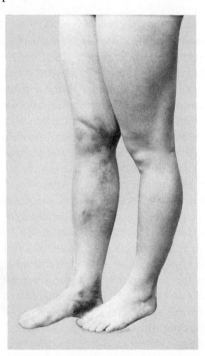

itive nature of various athletic activities subjects these muscles to extremely dynamic forces. Frequent and powerful use of the leg muscles commonly results in injuries. Strains can occur anywhere along these contractile units and normally result from a violent contraction, overstretching, or continued overuse.

The most common leg strains occur to the calf muscles because of the forcible contractions of these muscles during most athletic activities. Strains usually occur in the area of the musculotendinous junction or at the insertion of the Achilles tendon into the calcaneus. These injuries may result from repetitive overuse or a single violent contraction. However, acute strains to the Achilles tendon have a tendency to become chronic and frequently are complicated by tendinitis. *Achilles tendinitis* (Fig. 14-16) is a

Fig. 14-16. Chronic Achilles tendinitis. Note swelling of left Achilles tendon.
(Courtesy Dr. James Garrick, Center for Sports Medicine, St. Francis Memorial Hospital, San Francisco)

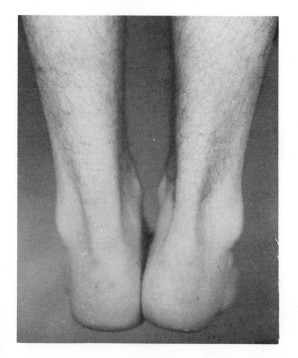

common disorder, especially in distance runners. The Achilles tendon is surrounded by a sheath of loose areolar and adipose peritendon tissue, which contains lubricating fluids. Inflammation between the tendon and its sheathlike covering can result in a thickening of the surrounding tissue and loss of the smooth gliding movements. This inflammation can cause tenderness on palpation along the tendon and an increase of pain with activity. Many times there is also swelling along the tendon, crepitation with movement, and a stiffness or lack of normal motion. In addition, the retrocalcaneal bursa can become inflamed.

Contractile and connective tissue components in the calf muscles may be partially or completely ruptured during athletic activity. This can result from a single violent contraction or repeated strains. Serious tears occur most frequently in the musculotendinous junction, through the tendon itself, or at the tendinous attachment to the calcaneus (Fig. 14-17). Any calf strain should be evaluated for the possibility of Achilles tendon rupture. Symptomatically, calf strains will produce tenderness at the site of injury and an increase in pain on active contraction, resistive movements, and passive stretching. A complete rupture should be readily recognized, as there is often a palpable gap in the tendon and loss of function of the calf muscle. The athlete will also exhibit a positive Thompson test, which is described and illustrated on p. 382.

Other muscles of the leg can also be strained during athletic activity. The more common of these are the tibialis anterior, which is the primary muscle for dorsiflexion, the tibialis posterior, whose tendon passes immediately behind the medial malleolus, and the peroneus longus and peroneus brevis, which are the lateral muscles of the leg. These two peroneal muscles pass downward in close conjunction and enter a common synovial tendon sheath above the ankle and pass behind the lateral malleolus. Occasionally these tendons become dislocated from their fixation behind the malleolus and may cross over the distal end of the fibula. The most common mechanism of peroneal tendon dislocation is hyperdorsiflexion of the ankle, as with going forward over the tips of skis. An athlete with this type of an injury must be referred to a physician, as surgery may have to be performed to correct the damage. Injury to the leg muscles may occur to any part of these contractile units from origin to insertion. Therefore symptoms may be present in the leg, about the ankle, or in the foot and include tenderness at the site of injury and increased pain on active and resistive movements.

A term unique to the leg is *shin splints,* which is a catch-all for chronic painful conditions. Shin splints most often occur early in a training program or after training has been discontinued for a period of time and then resumed. It appears to be associated with repetitive activity on hard surfaces or forcible excessive use of the leg muscles. There is much disagreement as to the exact nature and cause of this extremely common condition. However, shin splints are considered to be an overuse syndrome generally limited to the musculotendinous components. Pain associated with shin splints may occur anywhere in the leg and occasionally will become totally disabling. Tenderness is most often found along the medial border of the tibia, which is the origin for the tibialis posterior muscle. There may be any number of causes of shin splints, such as muscle inflexibility, a fallen longitudinal arch, a pronated foot, ill-fitting footwear, training techniques and playing surfaces. All evaluations of shin splints must take into consideration all possible causes

Fig. 14-17. Complete rupture of Achilles tendon.
(Courtesy A.G. Edwards, A.T.,C., University of Nevada–Las Vegas)

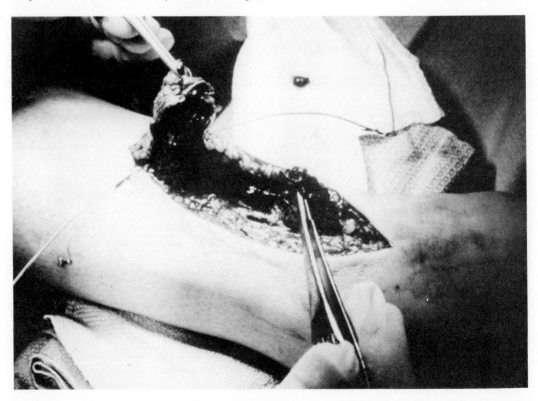

of the pain and discomfort in the athlete's leg and rule out stress fractures and ischemic disorders. Treatment procedures must emphasize the correction or modification of possible causes. There is no one best treatment for shin splints, and athletic trainers cannot simply treat the symptoms. This overuse syndrome certainly emphasizes the importance of a thorough and accurate injury assessment.

Other important conditions that must be recognized by athletic trainers and properly managed are *compartment syndromes.* These are disorders of the extremities in which increased tissue pressure compromises the circulation to the muscles, nerves, and blood vessels within the space and distal to the compartment. Compartment syndromes are more common in the lower leg, where four natural compartments exist. The superficial posterior compartment is a more loosely contained space not subjected to the constriction forces placed on the anterior, deep posterior, and lateral compartments. The anterior compartment is more frequently involved, followed by the deep posterior. The tight binding of fascia that forms these compartments does not allow for significant swelling within their confines.

Compartment syndromes can develop whenever there is swelling within these tightly closed spaces. Swelling may be caused by excessive exercise, overuse, contusion, localized infection, or overstretching of a particular muscle group. Anything that causes an inflammatory response or uncontrolled swelling may result in increased pressure within a compartment and a subsequent condition termed "compartment syndrome." Another possible cause of compartment syndrome is muscle hypertrophy. As muscles in these tightly confined compartments become bigger as a result of repetitive use or exercise, the relative space decreases, which may give rise to constriction forces. Depending on the cause of the condition there may be sudden or gradual onset of symptoms in the involved leg. There will be swelling accompanied by point tenderness and pain in the affected muscle group. In the later stages, numbness, weakness, and the inability to use the affected muscle may develop. Regardless of how or why the symptoms develop, it is important to recognize them early and

Fig. 14-18. Compression test performed on the deep posterior compartment of the leg. A catheter is inserted into the compartment to record internal pressure.

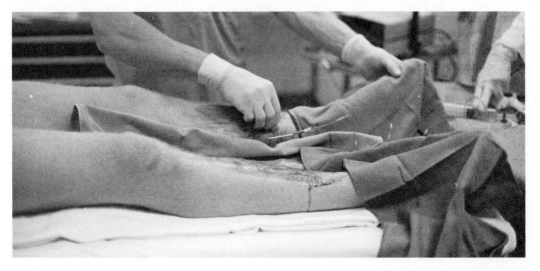

seek medical attention quickly. Any delay in treatment may result in permanent neurologic disability. Acute compartment syndromes with severe pain as the result of muscle and nerve ischemia should be readily recognized. However, many compartment syndromes develop slowly, with symptoms similar to shin splints, stress fractures, muscle strains, or cramps. Any athlete with lower leg symptoms that do not respond to treatment should be reevaluated frequently. Athletes complaining of a constant aching pain that does not completely disappear with rest and becomes more intense with activity should be referred to medical assistance. Compression tests within the involved compartment

may be required to diagnose the presence of compartment syndromes (Fig. 14-18).

Fractures

The tibia and fibula are very susceptible to fractures associated with athletic activity (Fig. 14-19). The tibia, which is not fractured nearly as often as the fibula, can be fractured as the result of a direct blow, a twisting force, or occasionally from repetitive overuse, which produces a stress fracture. Acute tibial fractures are usually readily recognized, as this is the weight-bearing bone in the leg and symptoms are normally severe enough to mandate radiographic studies. Stress fractures may be indicated by local tenderness

Fig. 14-19. Fracture of the left tibia and fibula. Picture was taken at the moment of fracture.

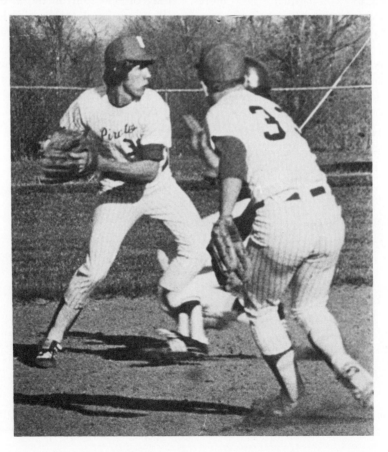

over the bone and persistent aching pain. The fibula is normally fractured by a direct blow to the outside of the leg and is also prone to stress fractures. Because this is not a weight-bearing bone, the athlete may not exhibit severe disability and may be able to walk or even finish a practice or contest. Symptomatically, fractures of the fibula reveal tenderness at the site of injury, local swelling, and increased pain on any manipulation of the bone. The tenderness and swelling might be mistaken for a contusion because the athlete is able to walk. A fracture of the lower fibula that also involves the tibial articulation is called *Pott's fracture.* This type of fracture usually results in a chipping off of a portion of the medial malleolus or a rupture of the deltoid ligament.

ATHLETIC INJURY ASSESSMENT PROCESS

As segments of the lower extremity, the foot, ankle, and leg form a complex unit that must function efficiently and in proper alignment for optimum athletic performance. The lower extremities are the functional basis for many of the important motor skills required for most athletic activity. They allow athletes to run, jump, cut, push, throw, strike, deliver a blow, and perform in numerous other ways. Athletic activities place tremendous demands and physical stresses on the lower extremities, which can result in various types and degrees of severity of injuries to the foot, ankle, and leg. In addition, with the intensity of modern training techniques and the growing interest in physical fitness, there is a continuing increase in overuse injuries affecting the lower extremities of athletes in all sports.

Secondary survey

In assessing athletic injuries involving the foot, ankle, and leg, the athletic trainer must take into consideration the functional interrelationships of the lower extremity as a whole. The many factors that can predispose or increase the frequency of athletic injuries to the lower extremities must be considered individually and as a group. Among the more common factors that can influence injuries to the lower extremities are malalignments, structural abnormalities, faulty foot and leg mechanics, improper training techniques, and footwear problems. All of these factors can be interrelated and affect one another; for example, faulty foot mechanics can cause an injury to the knee or hip. Therefore a comprehensive assessment of any injury occurring to one segment of the lower extremity should include an evaluation of the entire lower extremity in an attempt to recognize all the associated and potentially interrelated factors.

It is important to remember that deviation from proper alignment and normal function in one area of the body may cause a compensation in another area. The greater the deviation, the greater the susceptibility to problems and symptoms of injury. However, not all malalignments, abnormalities, or functional faults result in injuries or produce symptoms. The body has the remarkable ability to adapt to or compensate for the various stresses and demands imposed on it. Many athletes with varying degrees of malalignments, structural abnormalities, or functional faults perform quite well athletically without overt problems or complications.

The athletic trainer is not expected to be able to evaluate all the various alignmental, structural, and functional problems that may be present in the lower extremity. Some of these conditions will be minor and only detected by someone highly specialized in their recognition. However, the more information the athletic trainer possesses concerning these factors, the more proficient he or she will become in assessing injuries to the lower extremity. The ability to recognize these factors allows the athletic trainer to develop more effective exercise programs designed to increase strength and flexibility and also aids in preparing strategies to change mechanics, training techniques, or shoes. It is important for the athletic trainer to continually develop assessment skills to be able to accurately recognize conditions and problems in the lower extremities. An athletic trainer should be able to recognize factors that predispose an athlete to various types of injuries.

History

The history component of the assessment of foot, ankle, or leg injuries should first determine if the problem is an overuse syndrome or acute traumatic injury. As was previously mentioned, both types of conditions commonly occur to this area of the body. An overuse injury is suggested when the etiology of the injury is of gradual onset. This type of injury may begin as a nagging pain during activity or may only be apparent after a workout. On the other hand, an acute traumatic injury occurs suddenly. Questioning the athlete helps the athletic trainer to quickly distinguish between an acute injury and an overuse syndrome and also assists in determining the questions that should be asked to complete the evaluation.

To begin the questioning, ask the athlete to describe, as clearly as possible, the primary complaint or complaints. Allow the athlete enough time to thoroughly describe the manner in which the injury occurred, factors surrounding the disorder, and any symptoms associated with the injury. By allowing the athlete to talk freely about the incident, many questions will be answered. When the athlete is finished relating the chain of events surrounding the injury, you should ask pertinent questions to clarify the situation and complete a thorough history.

Overuse syndromes. The foot and leg are especially susceptible to overuse injury, particularly in activities requiring innumerable repetitions of the same action, such as running or jumping. It is not enough to merely treat the symptoms that result from an overuse injury. The athlete will then continue to perform using the same mechanisms that produced the problems, thus causing the symptoms to reappear. The athletic trainer must attempt to recognize factors that may be causing the problem and implement appropriate treatment procedures to alleviate or improve conditions producing overuse syndromes. With overuse injuries the history is ex-

tremely important in attempting to determine possible causes or conditions. The history-taking process can be quite time-consuming in assessing overuse injuries, but its importance cannot be overemphasized. Many conditions that contribute to an overuse injury can be recognized only by completing a careful history.

Overuse injuries may first be noticed as an inconvenience to the athlete. The area may be bothersome and painful only before or after athletic activities, but not during actual participation. These types of injuries are many times ignored by the athlete until they become more serious and begin to affect performance. Overuse injuries may progress to a point at which the athlete's activity must be severely limited or ended. Therefore a thorough history should include how and when the symptoms first appeared. Question the athlete at length about all symptoms associated with the injury. When do the symptoms occur? Where are they located? How have they progressed and what activities decrease or increase the severity of these symptoms? Is the athlete ever symptom free?

During the early stages of an overuse injury, athletes will often treat themselves. These treatments may improve the athlete's condition, alleviating the symptoms or at least preventing them from getting worse. However, when the symptoms do become more severe and the athlete reports the overuse injury, the history should include the treatment procedures the athlete used to correct or alleviate the symptoms. Did any of the techniques used help or aggravate the condition?

Also question the athlete about any previous injuries to the area. If the current problem is a foot injury, ask about previous injuries to other components of the lower extremity. Has the athlete ever exprienced a similar injury? If the area has been injured before, obtain as much information as possible about all previous injuries. What was the nature of the previous injury? Is the current injury an aggravation or recurrence of that injury? What treatment procedures were used with any previous injuries? The more information gained pertaining to previous injuries, the better the athletic trainer can evaluate the nature and status of the current injury.

To complete the history of an overuse injury, the athletic trainer should ask questions about the athlete's training program and footwear and any recent changes in either. The training program includes many factors, such as training routines, strength and flexibility exercises, and playing surfaces. All of these can contribute to or cause an overuse syndrome, and the athletic trainer must consider the importance of each factor.

Training is essentially preparing the body to adapt to a stressful situation, in this case, athletic activity. When more stress is placed on a body part than it is accustomed to tolerating, the symptoms of an overuse syndrome may begin. Overuse syndromes are often the result of errors in training methods, changes in training routines, or an overzealous training program. Therefore it is very important to question the athlete about his or her training methods. How long has the athlete been training? Has there been a dramatic change in the workout pattern, such as a rapid increase in mileage or speed? The body must adapt to increases in stress, and drastic changes may bring about overuse syndromes. Modern training methods impose tremendous stresses on the body. With these additional stresses, it is easy to understand why there has been an increase in overuse syndromes affecting the feet and legs of athletes involved in all sports activities.

In addition to the training routine, is the athlete doing any strength or flexibility exercises? Is weight training a part of the overall routine? If the athlete is on a strengthening program, is it designed to increase strength or endurance? Is the athlete overtraining certain muscle groups and causing a muscle imbalance? For example, distance runners tend to overdevelop their posterior muscles. This can result in a muscle imbalance between tightened calf and hamstring muscles and weakened anterior leg muscles. Also question the athlete about flexibility routines he

or she may be following. Many times it is helpful to ask the athlete to demonstrate how he or she is stretching. Lack of flexibility in the foot or ankle can be a factor in overuse injuries. Evaluating possible muscle imbalances and flexibility problems will be discussed in greater detail later in the assessment process.

Another important factor that can contribute to overuse syndromes is the surface or terrain on which the athlete has been training. Question the athlete concerning the types of surfaces being used for training. Has the athlete been training on a very hard surface, such as cement or asphalt? Continuous training on hard surfaces can place tremendous stresses on the structures of the lower extremity. Has the athlete been working out on an indoor track with tight corners or banked curves? These conditions can place abnormal stress on the legs and contribute to overuse syndromes. Has there been any changes in surfaces or terrains? For example, has the athlete started running on hills after spending much time training on flat surfaces? Has the athlete gone from a grass field to a hard court? Overuse injuries can be related to abrupt changes in surfaces or terrain, and proper training should include a gradual transition.

It is also important to question the athlete concerning footwear. Shoes can help or hinder an athlete. Athletic footwear has become as specific as the sports themselves. Athletic shoes are made for a variety of surfaces, sports, and types of foot mechanics. There is no one best type of shoe for any athletic activity. A shoe that works well for one athlete may cause pain for another athlete involved in the same sport. For example, a shoe that is good for controlling a hypermobile foot may cause trouble in a high-arched, rigid foot. It is not our intent to go into detail about the advantages and disadvantages of the various types of shoes and the modifications that may be necessary for their use by certain athletes. However, the athletic trainer evaluating overuse injuries of the foot or leg must consider the shoes as a possible source of the problem. It is recommended that athletic trainers learn as much as possible about the various types of shoes. Answers to the following questions may indicate that the shoes have contributed to the overuse syndrome. Do the shoes fit the athlete correctly and comfortably? Has the athlete recently changed the type or brand of shoes? Is the athlete wearing new shoes? Are the old shoes in need of repair? Perhaps the athlete has allowed the shoes to wear down too much. For example, the more a shoe wears down along its outer edge, the more weight is placed on the outside of the foot during activity. Overuse injuries may be related to abnormal shoe wear. Is the athlete wearing shoes that were designed for the activity? For example, an athlete wearing shoes designed for tennis may develop problems if these shoes are worn for long distance running. An athlete training in a running shoe with a cushioned heel may develop symptoms on changing to racing spikes with no heel. Any change in footwear may place unaccustomed stresses on parts of the foot or leg and contribute to overuse injuries.

During the history portion of the assessment process, strive to gain as much information as possible concerning the nature of the injury, the training history, and the athlete's shoes. This information, along with that gained during the physical examination that follows, will allow you to arrive at possible causes or contributing conditions for the overuse syndrome. Information is vital to planning treatment strategies designed at improving or eliminating overuse syndromes.

Acute traumatic injury. An acute traumatic injury to the foot, ankle, or leg will present an entirely different history to the athletic trainer than that of an overuse injury. The athlete will normally report that the injury occurred suddenly and will be able to describe a definite mechanism of injury. Encourage the athlete to describe in detail those events surrounding the traumatic injury and then question the athlete to collect further information to complete the history. The information pertinent to this history can be divided into three main areas: (1) the mechanism of injury, (2) signs and symptoms related to the

injury, and (3) any previous injuries to the same body area.

Ask the athlete to describe and demonstrate if possible the mechanism of injury. How did the injury occur? What activities was the athlete participating in at the time of the injury? Was the athlete running, jumping, cutting, or twisting? Was there a direct blow related to the injury? Did the ankle turn in or out? What was the position of the foot at the time of injury? Was an irregular surface involved, such as a hole in the playing field or landing on another player's foot? The athletic trainer should gain as much information as possible in order to have an accurate impression of the mechanics involved in causing the injury.

Have the athlete describe as specifically as possible any signs and symptoms associated with the injury and their behavior since the injury occurred. Ask the athlete to detail the location of pain and any tender areas. What movements or activities increase the pain? Is there a loss of motion, function, or strength associated with the injury? Is there any swelling associated with the injury? How soon after the injury did the swelling occur? For example, rapid swelling in the *sinus tarsi* is usually a sign of at least a second-degree sprain of the anterior talofibular ligament. However, swelling is not directly related to the severity of injury. For example, a rapidly ballooning ankle may be a simple reflection of minimal ligament stretching with involvement of a blood vessel. Also question the athlete about any sensations associated with the injury. Did he or she hear or feel anything at the time of injury, such as a popping or snapping sensation? If the athlete reports a snap or pop at the time of injury, keep the possibility of a fracture in mind, but remember that a torn ligament can also cause these sensations. Does the athlete have the sensation of the foot or ankle giving way or being unstable? Listen to the athlete's description of all signs, symptoms, and sensations associated with the injury, as well as his or her impressions concerning the injury. This valuable information is necessary to determine the nature of the injury and the structures involved.

Question the athlete about any previous injuries to the foot, ankle, or leg. Has the athlete experienced a similar injury or problem to this area of the body? Obtain as much information as possible about any previous injuries. Remember, the more information gained concerning previous injuries, the better the athletic trainer can evaluate the nature and status of the current injury.

Observation

Valuable information can be gained during the observation portion of the assessment process. The observation begins as soon as you see the injured athlete and continues throughout history, palpation, and stress segments of the injury evaluation. If you observe the athlete walking, notice his or her gait pattern. Does the athlete limp or seem to favor one leg? If the athlete is sitting or lying down, notice the alignment, contours, and position of the legs. Does either leg appear to be in an abnormal position? Is the athlete holding a certain area of the foot, ankle, or leg? Observe the athlete's attitude and behavior concerning the injured area. Assessing chronic overuse syndromes can be enhanced by observing the athlete's gait pattern and footwear (Fig. 14-20). Does the athlete appear to have

Fig. 14-20. Evidence of pronated feet by observing an athlete's footwear.

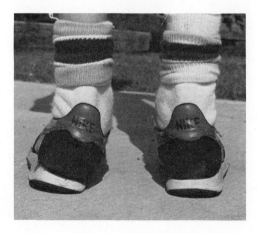

normal function or mechanics of both lower extremities? Do the shoes appear to be worn abnormally or unevenly? Always ask the athlete to show you his or her shoes when evaluating a chronic or overuse condition.

The foot and ankle are easily inspected. Shoes, socks, and any tape should be removed from the injured area. If the athlete is in considerable pain, attempt to calm the athlete and elicit his or her cooperation before removing any clothing. During this time, continue talking with the athlete and observe what you can.

Once shoes and socks are removed, inspect the injured area carefully. Look for any obvious deformities and signs of swelling. Notice the appearance of the skin for any signs of trauma. Remember to always compare the injured area to the contralateral uninjured area, to note any differences in symmetry or contour.

If the injury to the foot, ankle, or leg is of an acute traumatic nature, you can proceed to the palpation portion of the assessment process. However, if the injury is an overuse syndrome, continue to inspect the injured area as well as the entire lower extremity in an attempt to recognize all possible contributing factors. A complete observation of this area of the body includes an examination of the athlete during non-weight bearing, weight bearing, and walking. In each of these situations, those criteria discussed previously as considered normal for alignment, foot structure, and functional mechanics should be individually sought. All deviations from normal should be recognized and their possible contribution to overuse syndromes appreciated. Whenever the foot, ankle, or leg is involved in a chronic or overuse injury, the athlete's shoes should also be inspected.

The athletic trainer should be alert to recognize signs about the feet which may indicate abnormal conditions. These include such signs as excess callus formation, blisters, clawed toes, bunions, and corns. Each of these signs is an indication of adjustments being made in the feet as the result of abnormal stresses, faulty mechanics or poorly fitting shoes.

Palpation

Palpation procedures can be used to evaluate the adequacy of circulation and nerve supply to the lower extremity. These important functions should be assessed with any major injury involving the lower extremity. Circulation can be evaluated by feeling for peripheral pulses, namely the dorsalis pedis on the dorsum of the foot and the posterior tibial behind the medial malleolus. Another method of evaluating circulation is to squeeze a small area of the athlete's foot or toe between your fingers to cause blanching, then release the pressure and observe how rapidly normal color returns. Immediate return indicates good arterial supply. Nerve impairment can be assessed by evaluating sensations over the leg, foot, and toes and noting the ability to actively contract the extrinsic and intrinsic muscles of the foot.

Palpation of the injured area is used to further identify specific structures involved in the injury. This is accomplished by accurately locating all areas of associated tenderness and swelling. The bones and ligaments composing the foot and ankle are easily accessible to palpation, as most structures are subcutaneous. If the underlying anatomy is clearly understood, tenderness can be readily identified with those anatomic structures suspected of being injured. Therefore palpation, combined with a careful history and observation, can be quite informative in identifying those structures involved in the injury.

Palpation of the foot, ankle, and leg should be conducted with the area as relaxed as possible. This can be accomplished by having the athlete sit with both legs dangling over the edge of the table or sit back on the table with both legs supported. As with most athletic injuries, the integrity of the bony anatomy is usually evaluated first, followed by an assessment of damage to the soft tissues. Carefully palpate the bones and bony landmarks about the site of injury, noting any points of tenderness. If you elicit any pain or crepitation as you feel these bony areas, the suspicion of a possible fracture should be increased. Remember to begin palpation gently and in-

crease pressure until you are satisfied that no fracture line pain or crepitation exists. Gently palpate the various ligaments and other soft tissues suspected of being injured, again noting specific areas of tenderness. Tenderness must be carefully outlined and precisely identified to accurately identify the underlying structures that may be damaged. The specific structures to be palpated will be determined by the information gained during the history and observation. Procedures used to palpate the various anatomic structures about the foot, ankle, and leg are discussed briefly in the following pages, as are the common athletic injuries that may be indicated by tenderness. Pay particular attention to the bony landmarks.

Toes. In palpating the injured toes of an athlete, it is important to locate the point tenderness precisely. The structures of the toes are very superficial, and it is usually easy to localize the pain. Notice whether the tenderness is located in one of the phalanges or primarily at a joint or articulation (Fig. 14-21). This information, com-

---

Fig. 14-21. Palpating great toe.

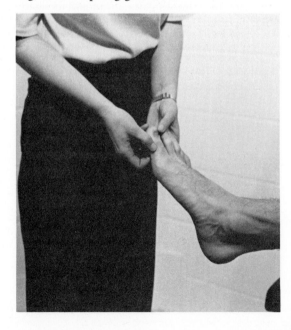

bined with the stress procedures described later, will allow you to distinguish between a fracture and a sprain of the toes.

Medial aspect of the foot and ankle. Along the medial aspect of the foot, you can palpate the head of the first metatarsal bone and the meta-tarsophalangeal joint (Fig. 14-22, *A*). A sprained or jammed toe would cause pain in this area. This is also the site of hallux valgus or bunion formation. The first metatarsal can be palpated along its entire shaft to the first metatarsocunei-form joint (Fig. 14-22, *B*). This is the insertion

Fig. 14-22. Palpating medial aspect of the foot and ankle: **A,** first metatarsophalangeal joint, **B,** metatarsocuneiform joint, **C,** navicular tubercle (under index finger), and **D,** deltoid ligament just inferior the medial malleolus.

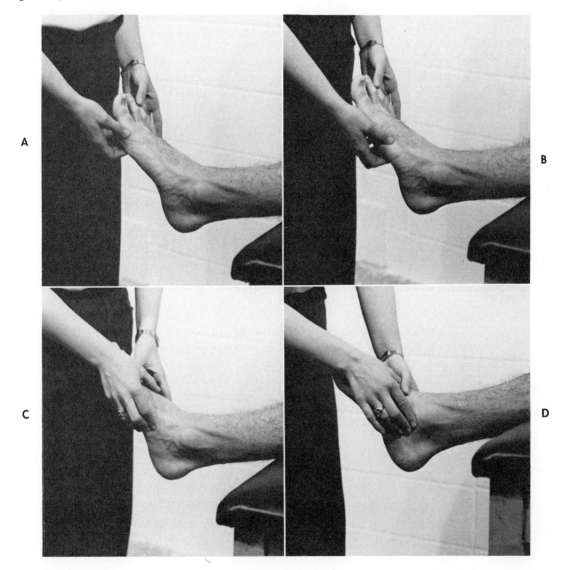

of the tibialis anterior muscle. Continuing to palpate proximally, the next bony landmark would be the navicular tubercle (Fig. 14-22, *C*). Immediately proximal to the navicular bone is the talus, which is not readily palpable, and above that the medial malleolus. The medial malleolus is the major bony landmark on the medial ankle. Its entire surface should be thoroughly palpated. Pain elicited as you palpate the medial malleolus should raise your suspicion of a possible fracture. Tenderness elicited with palpation just inferior to the medial malleolus or along its edge may indicate a sprain to the deltoid ligament (Fig. 14-22, *D*). The depression lying between the posterior aspect of the medial malleolus and the Achilles tendon contains the tendons of the tibialis posterior, flexor digitorium longus, and flexor hallucis muscles, as well as the posterior tibial nerve and artery. Tenderness expressed in this area may indicate a strain of these muscle tendons or an inflammation of the synovial lining protecting them (Fig. 14-23).

Fig. 14-23. Palpating the flexor tendons lying posterior the medial malleolus.

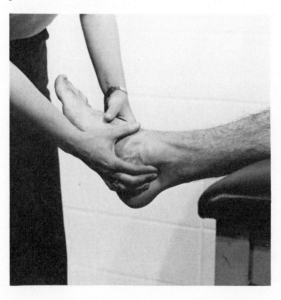

Lateral aspect of the foot and ankle. Along the lateral aspect of the foot, you can palpate the head of the fifth metatarsal bone and the metatarsophalangeal joint (Fig. 14-24, *A*). This is the site of a *bunionette,* or tailor's bunion, which is a bunionlike enlargement of this joint caused by excessive friction or lateral pressure to this area. The fifth metatarsal can be palpated along the entire shaft to its flared base (styloid process) (Fig. 14-24, *B*). The peroneus brevis muscle has its insertion on this process. Tenderness in this area may be caused by an avulsion of the tendon's insertion, fracture of the styloid process, or an inflamed bursa over the process. Proximal to the styloid process lies a bony depression in the cuboid containing the tendon of the peroneus longus muscle. Continued palpation proximally will bring you to the calcaneus. A bony landmark on the lateral calcaneus is the peroneal tubercle, which separates the peroneus brevis and longus tendons as they pass around the calcaneus. The peroneus brevis lies above the tubercle, whereas the peroneus longus lies below. These tendons are surrounded by synovium and held to the tubercle by a retinaculum. Tenderness identified by palpating the peroneal tubercle may indicate tenosynovitis. Just above the peroneal tubercle lies the lateral malleolus, which is the major bony landmark on the lateral ankle (Fig. 14-24, *C*). The entire surface of the lateral malleolus should be palpated, and any pain caused by palpation should raise your suspicion of a possible fracture. The lateral collateral ligaments of the ankle attach to the lateral malleolus, and tenderness elicited on palpation of these ligaments is usually indicative of an inversion sprain. The anterior talofibular ligament is the ligament most commonly sprained. It is most easily palpated in the sinus tarsi (Fig. 14-24, *D*). This concavity just in front of the lateral malleolus is commonly filled with edema after an ankle sprain. The calcaneofibular ligament is palpable directly beneath the lateral malleolus (Fig. 14-24, *E*), whereas the posterior talofibular ligament can be palpated from the posterior edge of the lateral malleolus (Fig. 14-24, *F*).

Fig. 14-24. Palpating the lateral aspect of the foot and ankle: **A,** fifth metatarsophalangeal joint, **B,** styloid process of fifth metatarsal, **C,** lateral malleolus, **D,** talofibular ligament in the sinus tarsi, **E,** calcaneofibular ligament, and **F,** posterior talofibular ligament.

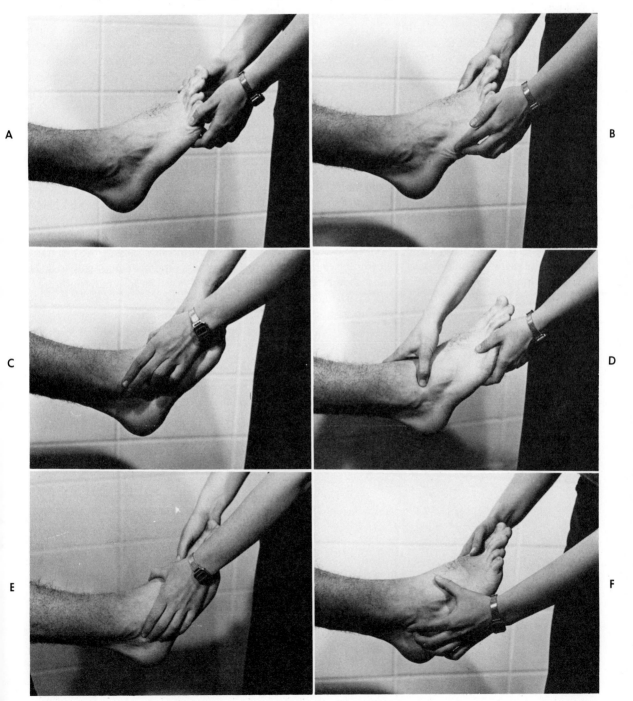

Dorsal aspect of the foot. The dorsum of the foot is subcutaneous and easily palpated. You can feel the lengths of the second, third, and fourth metatarsals as well as the metatarsophalangeal and tarsometatarsal joints (Fig. 14-25, A). To palpate the main tendons on the dorsum of the foot, palpation should be combined with active or resisted motion. For example, to palpate the tibialis anterior tendon, ask the athlete to dorsiflex and invert the foot. The tendon should then become quite prominent as it crosses the ankle joint and can be easily palpated to its insertion on the first cuneiform and metatarsal (Fig. 14-25, B). The tendon of the extensor hallucis longus muscle can be more easily palpated when the great toe is actively extended. The tendons of the extensor digitorum longus muscle can be palpated when the toes are actively extended. The dorsalis pedis artery lies between the extensor hallucis longus tendon and the extensor digitorum longus tendon. The pulse of this artery is usually easy to detect and is used to evaluate circulation distal to the knee as previously described.

Plantar aspect of the foot. The plantar surface of the foot is usually more difficult to palpate because of the thickened skin, calluses, fascial bands, and pads of fat. To palpate the plantar surface, have the athlete sit back on a table with the leg extended and supported and the sole of the foot facing you. Each of the metatarsal heads can be palpated separately by squeezing them between your thumb and forefinger or palpating with your fingers on the dorsal surface (Fig. 14-26, A). Pain beneath the metatarsal heads, especially the second and third, is referred to as *metarsalgia.* This usually indicates abnormal pressure being applied to this area of the foot and can result from a variety of conditions. The transverse (metatarsal) arch of the foot is located directly behind the metatarsal heads, and pain in the area may indicate a fallen or weakened arch. Also, with increased pressure or abnormal stress, callosities may form under any of the metatarsal heads. Tenderness and swelling palpated between the metatarsal heads may indicate a neuroma in this space.

The plantar aponeurosis, or plantar fascia, can also be palpated along the sole of the foot (Fig. 14-26, B). Point tenderness along these fibrous

Fig. 14-25. Palpating the dorsal aspect of the foot: **A,** first metatarsophalangeal joint and **B,** anterior tibialis muscle and tendon.

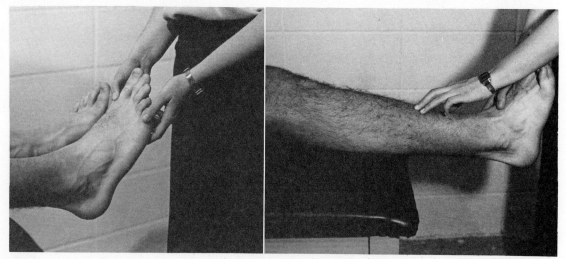

A

B

bands may indicate plantar fasciitis. Point tenderness is usually found at the proximal portion of the arch (Fig. 14-26, *C*). A plantar fascia problem may be aggravated by a coexistent heel spur and/or bursitis. If either of these conditions are present, the point tenderness will be located directly over the medial process of the tuberosity of the calcaneus. An athlete suffering from a bruised heel will express pain during palpation of the plantar aspect of the calcaneus (Fig. 14-26, *D*). Another test used to evaluate the integrity of the bones of the heel and ankle is percussion of the plantar surface of the heel. This impacts the calcaneus, talus, tibia, and fibula together. If the athlete expresses pain in one of these bones, you should suspect a fracture. Remember to percuss

Fig. 14-26. Palpating the plantar aspect of the foot. **A,** Metatarsal heads, **B,** plantar aponeurosis along sole of the foot, **C,** proximal attachment of plantar aponeurosis, and **D,** plantar aspect of calcaneus.

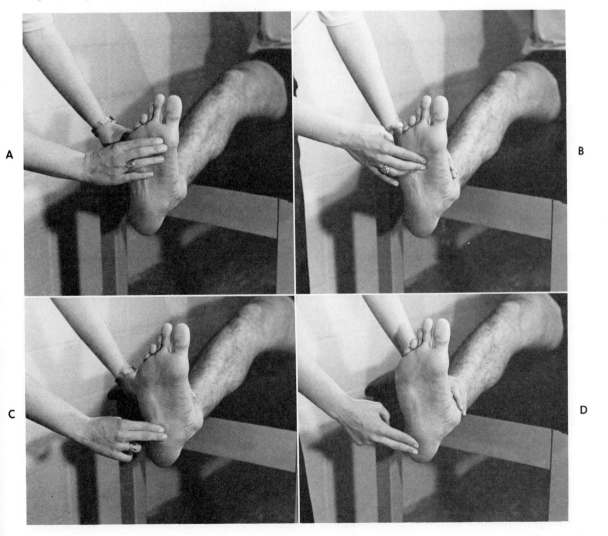

A

B

C

D

gently at first and increase intensity to the athlete's tolerance.

Posterior aspect of the leg. The posterior compartment of the leg contains the gastrocnemius and soleus muscles and their common tendon, the Achilles, which is attached to the calcaneus. With the athlete in a prone position, and the foot hanging free over the edge of the table, the gastrocnemius can be palpated along its entire course (Fig. 14-27, *A*). Locate tender areas and feel for any tightness or swelling, which may be associated with a strain or contusion. It is easier to denote swelling and compare symmetry by palpating both calves at the same time.

The Achilles tendon can be palpated from about the lower one third of the calf to the calcaneus (Fig. 14-27, *B*). A strain of the Achilles tendon or an inflammation of the peritendon tissue causes pain on palpation of the involved area. Retrocalcaneal bursitis causes pain when you palpate the tissue just anterior to the Achilles tendon (Fig. 14-27, *C*). If the Achilles tendon has been ruptured, there is often a palpable gap or defect. To further evaluate the continuity of the Achilles tendon, the ***Thompson test*** should be performed. This is accomplished with the athlete prone or kneeling, with the feet extended beyond the edge of the table. Squeeze both

Fig. 14-27. Palpating posterior aspect of leg. **A,** gastrocnemius muscle, **B,** Achilles tendon, **C,** test for retrocalcaneal bursitis, and **D,** Thompson test.

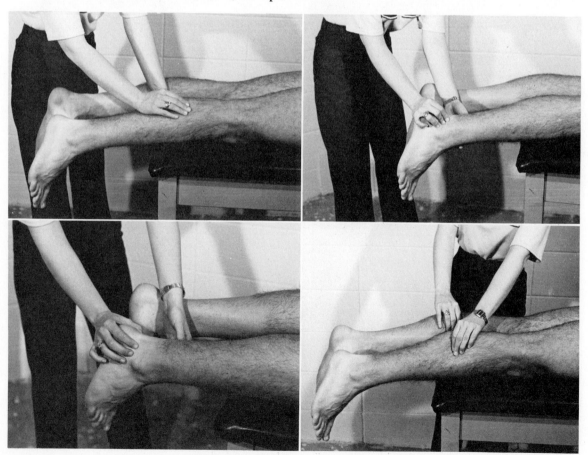

calves just below their widest circumference (Fig. 14-27, *D*). The test is positive when the foot on the injured side fails to plantar flex.

Lateral aspect of the leg. The lateral aspect of the leg includes the fibula and the lateral compartment containing the peroneal muscles. The fibula should be carefully palpated whenever a fracture is suspected (Fig. 14-28, *B*). Locate any existing areas of tenderness. If tender, the fibula can then be stressed above or below the point tenderness to evaluate the integrity of the bone. This can be accomplished by gently lifting or pushing on the fibula away from the painful area (Fig. 14-28, *A*). If pain is always expressed at the same site as the palpable tenderness during these maneuvers, the athlete should be treated as if he or she has a fractured fibula. If the bony integrity appears normal, the athlete has probably suffered a contusion at the site of the palpable tenderness.

The muscles within the lateral compartment can also be palpated. Depending on the mechanism of injury, tenderness expressed during palpation combined with pain on active and resistive eversion is used to recognize involvement of the peroneal musculature and the possibility of lateral compartment syndrome.

Anterior aspect of the leg. The anterior compartment of the leg contains the tibialis anterior, extensor hallucis longus, and extensor digitorum muscles. These muscles can be palpated along their entire course. It is easier to locate these muscles during mild resistance to the action in which each muscle is involved. For example, it is easiest to palpate the tibialis anterior during mild resistance to dorsiflexion and inversion, as previously explained. During this maneuver the tendon of the tibialis anterior can be easily identified and palpated. Knowing the area of point tenderness, the mechanism of injury, and the location of pain with active and resistive motion, you will be able to determine the involvement of these muscles. Remember the importance of early recognition in the development of anterior compartment syndrome and immediate referral if suspected.

Medial aspect of the leg. The medial aspect of the leg contains the subcutaneous anteromedial surface of the tibia called the shin. The entire length of this surface of the tibia is easily palpated. Pain expressed along either the anteromedial or anterolateral border of the tibia is commonly classified as "shin splints." Understanding the

Fig. 14-28. Palpating lateral aspect of leg. **A,** Gently lifting the fibula; **B,** distal fibula.

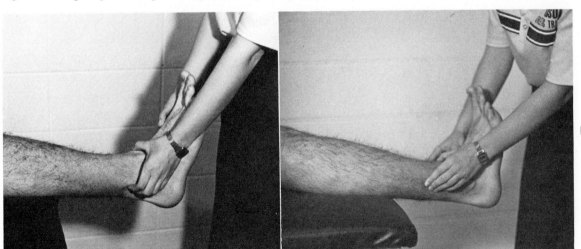

A   B

underlying anatomy allows you to determine which structures may be involved by identifying the areas of point tenderness.

Stress

After history, observation, and palpation procedures, stress maneuvers are used to complete the assessment process conducted by the athletic trainer. The precise stress maneuvers used depend on which joints and structures appear to be involved in the injury. Not all of the maneuvers described in this section will be used with any particular foot, ankle, or leg injury. The athletic trainer will select the appropriate maneuvers based on information gained during the assessment process up to this point.

Active movements. Active movements are performed to evaluate the range of motion of the foot and ankle joints as well as to begin testing the integrity of the muscles responsible for these motions. Ask the athlete to perform each movement through as great a range of motion as possible and to express any sensations or feelings experienced during movement. With foot and ankle motion, it is best to always have the athlete perform active movements with both extremities at the same time. This will provide you with an immediate reference for comparing the injured

Fig. 14-29. Active motion of the foot and ankle. **A,** Toe flexion, **B,** foot inversion, **C,** dorsiflexion and **D,** plantar flexion.

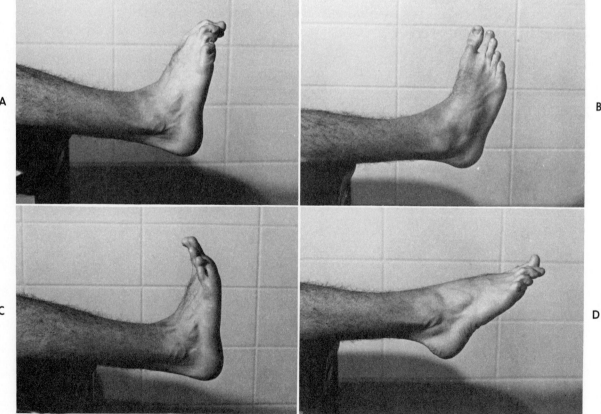

side to the uninjured. Whenever an athlete expresses pain upon active movement, attempt to localize this pain as precisely as possible. For example, does the pain appear to be in a bone, at a joint, along a tendon, or in a muscle? Remember, pain located in contractile tissue should be further evaluated using resistive movements, whereas pain in noncontractile tissue should be further evaluated using passive movements. These procedures are described later.

To evaluate the active motion of the toes, instruct the athlete to flex and extend all the toes on both feet (Fig. 14-29, *A*). Is the range of motion limited or restricted on the injured side? Does the athlete express any pain, discomfort, or other sensations during these movements?

To evaluate subtalar motion, ask the athlete to invert and evert both feet (Fig. 14-29, *B*). Does the range of motion appear to be equal on both sides? It is more difficult to accurately evaluate active inversion and eversion than other motions about the foot and ankle. However, if there is a distinct and obvious difference between the motions on either side, further evaluations should be carried out. What types of sensations are ex-

pressed by the athlete while performing these movements? Remember, pain or swelling associated with a sprained ankle may severely restrict active inversion and eversion.

To evaluate ankle motion, instruct the athlete to dorsiflex and plantar flex both feet (Fig. 14-29, *C* and *D*). Again, does the range of motion appear to be equal on both sides, and does the athlete express any pain during these movements? To specifically test for dorsiflexion, which is many times restricted, the following procedure should be performed. With the athlete sitting and the legs supported, passively move both feet until each foot is at a right angle to the leg (Fig. 14-30, *A*). Instruct the athlete to dorsiflex the feet, bringing both feet toward the knees (Fig. 14-30, *B*). If the athlete has normal dorsiflexion, he or she should be able to dorsiflex the feet between 15° and 20°. Many times an athlete with an overuse syndrome, such as shin splints, will have little if any dorsiflexion. To determine if the lack of dorsiflexion is caused by tightness in the gastrocnemius or soleus muscles, perform the same procedures with the athlete sitting on the table with his or her legs hanging

Fig. 14-30. To specifically test for dorsiflexion, passively move both feet to 90° (**A**) and instruct the athlete to dorsiflex (**B**).

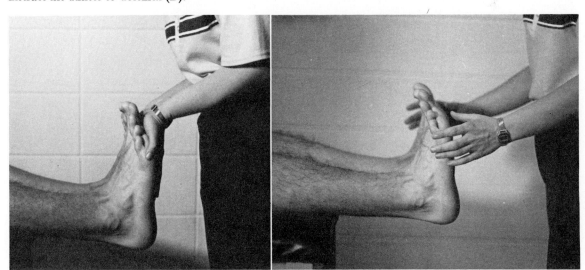

A

B

down. Flexing the knee relaxes the gastrocnemius and tests the flexibility of the soleus muscles. A stretching routine can then be initiated once the tight muscles are identified.

An alternate method of quickly checking ankle and foot motion is to have the athlete stand on his or her toes and then on the heels (Fig. 14-31). This can be accomplished while you are evaluating the weight-bearing alignment as described previously. Although these tests do not allow precise measurement of each motion, they do indicate functional abilities and provide a quick test. If the athlete is unable to perform these procedures, further evaluation is indicated.

Resistive movements. Resistive movements are used to further evaluate the integrity of the contractile tissues. Manual resistance applied against active motion can accurately identify specific painful areas, allowing one muscle to be differentiated from another. Resistive movements are also used to compare muscular strength between extremities. Resistive procedures are potentially the most informative maneuvers used in assessing muscle injuries. To accurately use resistive movements in the injury evaluation process, you must have a general understanding of the underlying muscular anatomy as well as the movement for which each muscle is responsible.

It is important that you explain exactly what you want the athlete to do during resistive movements and how you are going to apply resistance. Because of the limited range of motion in the foot and ankle, most resistive maneuvers are usually performed as an isometric contrac-

Fig. 14-31. Checking ankle motion by instructing athlete to (**A**) raise up on toes and (**B**) then on heels.

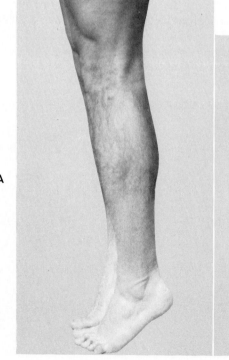
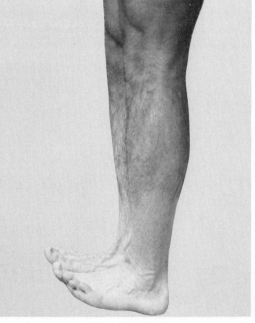

tion. In other words, the athlete is instructed to perform a certain movement, and manual resistance is provided against that movement. The intensity of the resistance should be determined by the athlete's tolerance.

To evaluate the integrity of the tibialis anterior muscle, instruct the athlete to dorsiflex the foot as resistance is applied to the dorsal aspect of the foot (Fig. 14-32, *A*). The tendon of the tibialis anterior should be visually and palpably prominent on the anterior aspect of the ankle. Palpate the muscle as you perform this resistive maneuver.

The other two muscles in the anterior compartment are evaluated in a similar manner. The integrity of the extensor hallucis longus muscle

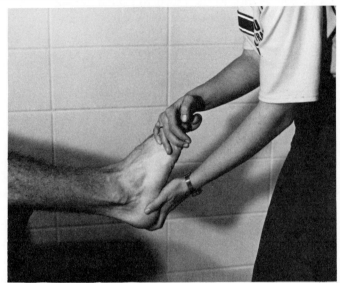

Fig. 14-32. Applying manual resistance against the muscles in the anterior compartment: **A,** the anterior tibialis by dorsiflexion of the foot, **B,** the extensor hallucis longus by extension of the great toe, and **C,** the extensor digitorum by extension of the other four toes.

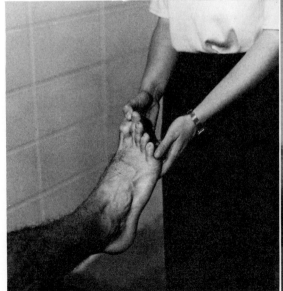

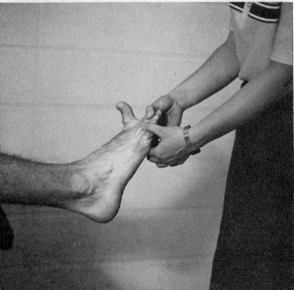

is evaluated by applying resistance against extension or dorsiflexion of the great toe (Fig. 14-32, B). The extensor digitorum longus muscle is evaluated by putting manual resistance against extension of the other four toes (Fig. 14-32, C). The tendons of these muscles should become prominent on the dorsum of the foot.

The muscles in the lateral compartment, the peroneus longus and brevis, are evaluated simultaneously. Instruct the athlete to plantar flex and evert the foot. Resistance is then applied against the lateral aspect of the fifth metatarsal bone (Fig. 14-33). The tendons of the peroneal muscles should become prominent as they pass around the lateral malleolus, run on either side of the peroneal tubercle, and continue to their respective insertions.

The three muscles in the deep posterior compartment, whose tendons pass under the medial malleolus, can also be individually tested. The flexor hallucis longus muscle is evaluated by applying resistance against flexion of the great toe (Fig. 14-34, A). To manually test the integrity of the flexor digitorum longus muscle, resistance is applied to the plantar surface of the distal phalanges as the athlete attempts to flex the toes (Fig. 14-34, B). The tibialis posterior is evaluated while resistance is applied against the medial aspect of the first metatarsal bone during plantar flexion and inversion (Fig. 14-34, C). The tendon of this muscle should be prominent and palpable as it comes around the medial malleolus and inserts into the navicular tubercle.

The gastrocnemius and soleus muscles can be evaluated by applying resistance against plantar flexion. This is accomplished by applying resistance to the ball of the foot and instructing the athlete to plantar flex or point the toes as far as possible (Fig. 14-35). As mentioned earlier, to isolate the soleus muscle, flex the knees during this maneuver. Remember, to compare the relative strengths of these muscles, or any of those discussed in this section, always repeat each of the resistive procedures on the uninjured foot.

Passive movements. Passive movements are maneuvers performed completely by the athletic trainer while the athlete relaxes the contractile tissues as much as possible. These procedures can be used to evaluate the range of motion as well as the integrity of the noncontractile tissues

Fig. 14-33. Applying manual resistance against the muscles in the lateral compartment by resisting eversion of the foot.

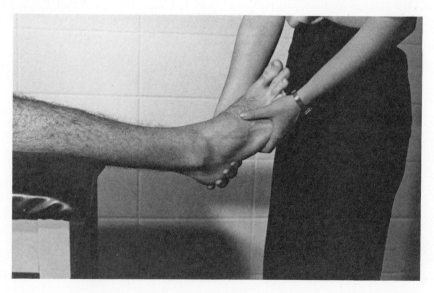

about the foot and ankle. Remember, begin passive movements gently so as not to aggravate the injury or increase the pain and lose the athlete's cooperation. The intensity or force used with each passive maneuver can then be increased depending on the athlete's tolerance and the severity of the injury. It may also be beneficial to

perform passive procedures on the uninjured side first, to elicit the athlete's cooperation and provide you with a point of reference.

Passive maneuvers can be used to evaluate the integrity of the bones in the foot. If the symptoms cause you to suspect a possible fracture to the phalanges or metatarsals, longitudinal stress

Fig. 14-34. Applying manual resistance against the muscles in the deep posterior compartment: **A,** the flexor hallucis longus by flexion of the great toe, **B,** the flexor digitorum longus by flexion of the other four toes, and **C,** the tibialis posterior by plantar flexion and inversion.

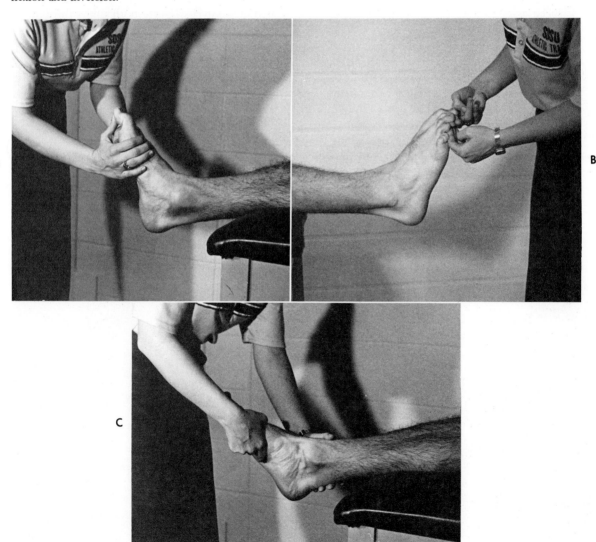

should be applied to these bones. This can be accomplished by stabilizing the foot with one hand and with the other hand applying stress directly along the long axis of the bone or bones suspected of being fractured (Fig. 14-36). The stress should be very gentle to begin with and then increased, depending on the athlete's tolerance. If the bone integrity is intact, there should be no pain associated with this type of a stress procedure. However, if a fracture is present, the athlete will usually express pain at the fracture site during longitudinal stress.

To assess the integrity of the ligaments supporting these bones, valgus and varus stresses should be applied. If the symptoms raise your suspicion of a possible sprain of the supporting ligaments and the bony integrity appears intact, apply forces that will stress the ligaments. For example, to evaluate the integrity of the supporting structures around one of the interphalangeal or metatarsophalangeal joints, support the bone on either side of the joint and gently apply lateral force (Fig. 14-37). Pain or instability with

this type of a maneuver indicates a sprain of the supporting structures.

Passive range of motion of the foot or ankle is many times evaluated in conjunction with injuries to this area of the body. Remember to always compare the passive range of motion on the injured side to the uninjured side. For this reason, it may be easier to perform these passive maneuvers on both feet or ankles at the same time. Each of the toes can be passively moved through a complete range of motion. Dorsiflexion and plantar flexion of the ankle can be evaluated by passively moving both ankles through as great a range of motion as possible. Remember, pain or swelling associated with an acute injury may greatly limit the motion available.

The passive motion available during inversion and eversion should be evaluated in conjunction with assessing the integrity of the ligaments supporting the ankle. Stabilize the tibia with one hand and grip the foot with the other. Alternately invert and evert both feet (Fig. 14-38). Locate any pain or instability associated with these

Fig. 14-35. Applying manual resistance against the gastrocnemius and soleus muscles by resisting plantar flexion.

Fig. 14-36. Applying a longitudinal compression stress to the great toe.

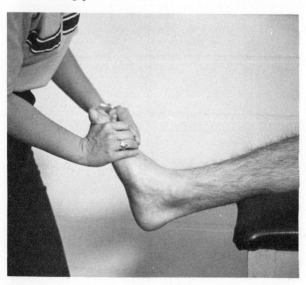

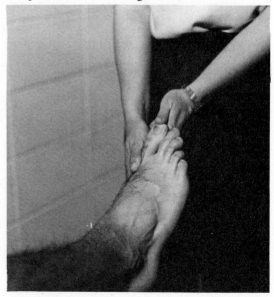

movements. Pain along the course of one of the lateral ligaments that increases with inversion suggests that the ligament is sprained. Pain expressed in one of the components of the deltoid ligament during eversion also suggests a ligament sprain. Compare the amount of inversion and eversion of both ankles in an attempt to recognize any instability. Unless there is obvious instability, it is often difficult to assess the degree of instability associated with a sprained ankle. Stress radiographs may be required to accurately measure the instability present at the ankle joint (Fig. 14-39).

Another procedure that should always be performed on a suspected sprained ankle is the *anterior drawer test.* This tests the integrity of the anterior talofibular ligament, which is the ligament most commonly injured in the ankle. This procedure is performed with the injured ankle in a relaxed, and slightly plantar flexed, position. The athletic trainer stabilizes the lower leg by placing one hand on the anterior aspect of the

tibia and grips the calcaneus in the palm of the other hand. The calcaneus is then lifted forward while the tibia is kept steady (Fig. 14-40). If the anterior talofibular ligament is intact, there should be no anterior movement of the talus in relation to the tibia. If, however, the anterior talofibular ligament is ruptured, the drawer test will be positive and the talus will slide forward from under the tibia. You may feel a distinct "clunk" as the talus slides out and back again. Whenever this anterior drawer test is positive, the athlete should be referred to a physician.

Fig. 14-38. Passively inverting **(A)** and everting **(B)** the foot.

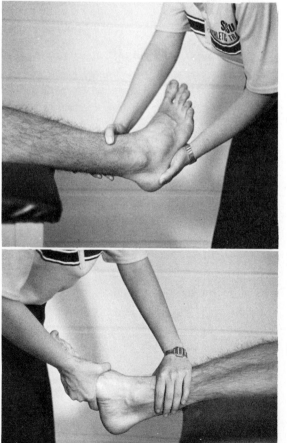

A

B

Fig. 14-37. Applying a transverse (varus) stress to the metatarsophalangeal joint of the great toe.

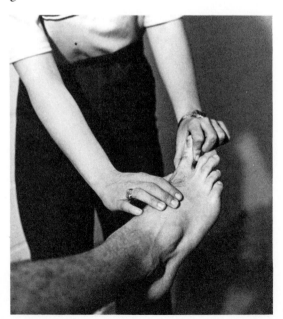

Functional movements. Functional movements can be very helpful in evaluating injuries to the foot, ankle, and leg. This is especially true for the overuse syndromes, because these injuries are many times the result of functional problems. Some of the more commonly used functional movements have been previously discussed, such as having the athlete bear weight, alternately rising on the toes and heels, and walking. Additional functional tests include asking the athlete to hop on the injured leg, jog, sprint, run figure-of-eight patterns, and perform cutting, starting, and stopping activities. These procedures are used to localize pain or instability and to recognize any functional factors that may be associated with the injury. Symptoms associated with an overuse injury are sometimes present only during activity, and these functional procedures may be necessary to reproduce the symptoms and assist in a comprehensive assessment.

Occasionally these same functional activities are used during the initial evaluation of an acute traumatic injury of the foot, ankle, or leg. This is particularly true when the assessment process completed to this point has produced few definitive signs and symptoms. The athlete may be asked to perform functional activities or replicate the mechanism of injury as closely as possible to assist in identifying any structures that may be involved. Pain or instability may be demonstrated in this manner.

All restrictions placed on an athlete's participation are determined by the level of functional activity at which that athlete can perform. If the athlete can perform the functional activities described without pain and disability, the athlete can return to full athletic activity. Functional movements should therefore always be used on follow-up evaluations to determine at what level of activity the athlete can safely perform. As an athlete recovers from a foot, ankle, or leg injury, the intensity of functional activity should be increased according to the limits of pain and range of motion.

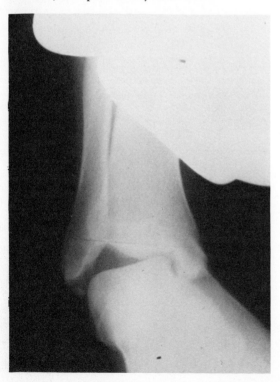

Fig. 14-39. Stress radiograph of ankle. Note how the joint opens laterally under stress.

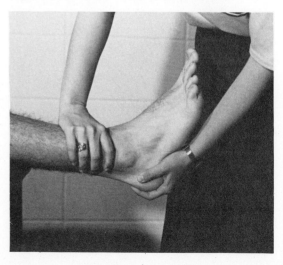

Fig. 14-40. Anterior drawer test for ankle.

ATHLETIC INJURY ASSESSMENT CHECKLIST
FOOT, ANKLE, AND LEG INJURIES

Secondary survey

_____ History
- _____ Primary complaint
- _____ Mechanism of injury
- _____ Pain
- _____ Sensations
- _____ Previous injuries
- _____ Training program
- _____ Surface or terrain used for training
- _____ Footwear

_____ Observation
- _____ Obvious deformity
- _____ Swelling
- _____ Contours
- _____ Alignment
- _____ Foot types
  - _____ Pronated foot
  - _____ Cavus foot
  - _____ Morton's foot
- _____ Mechanics and functioning
- _____ Gait pattern
- _____ Abnormal conditions
  - _____ Excess callus formation
  - _____ Blisters
  - _____ Clawed toes
  - _____ Bunions
  - _____ Corns
  - _____ Footwear

_____ Palpation
- _____ Circulation
- _____ Sensations
- _____ Tenderness
- _____ Swelling
- _____ Deformity

_____ Stress
- _____ Active movements
  - _____ Range of motion
  - _____ Associated symptoms
- _____ Resistive movements
  - _____ Pain
  - _____ Strength
- _____ Passive movements
  - _____ Bony integrity
  - _____ Ligament integrity
  - _____ Range of motion
- _____ Functional movements
  - _____ Functional abilities

Evaluation of findings

The foot, ankle, and leg are the most frequently injured areas of the body during athletic activity. Because of the utilization of the lower extremities in most sports, tremendous amounts of physical stress and force are thrust on these portions of the body. Acute traumatic injuries to these structures are as prevalent as overuse syndromes, and both can result from or be influenced by a host of factors such as malalignments, structural abnormalities, faulty mechanics, improper training techniques, and footwear problems. An accurate and comprehensive assessment of an injury occurring to any segment of the lower extremity therefore should include an evaluation of all possible associated factors.

When to refer the athlete

Many injuries or conditions involving the foot, ankle, or leg can be accurately assessed and managed without medical referral. Other injuries to these structures require medical assistance for an accurate assessment and proper treatment. Occasionally these injuries must be referred to someone highly specialized in their diagnosis. The athletic trainer must therefore continue to develop assessment skills necessary to evaluate injuries involving these structures, to be able to recognize signs and symptoms that indicate the

---

Gross deformity

Suspected fracture or dislocation

Significant swelling

Significant pain, especially within the compartments of the leg

Persistent pain within the compartments of the leg

Decreased circulation, motor function, or sensations in the leg or foot

Significant loss of motion of the foot

Joint instability

Suspected malalignment or structural abnormalities

Any doubt regarding the severity or nature of the injury

---

athlete should be referred for further diagnosis. The following list of conditions can be used to determine if medical referral is indicated.

KEY TERMS

anterior compartment syndrome Pain and tenderness in the anterior compartment caused by swelling within this tightly closed space; in later stages, numbness and inability to dorsiflex the foot develop

anterior drawer test Test of integrity of anterior talofibular ligament; with athlete's ankle relaxed one hand stabilizes the leg as the other lifts anteriorly while cupping the calcaneus

bunion (hallux valgus) Abnormal enlargement of the metatarsophalangeal joint of the great toe, usually the result of chronic irritation and pressure from poorly fitted shoes and characterized by soreness, swelling, and lateral displacement of the great toe

bunionette Bunionlike enlargment of the metatarsophalangeal joint of the little toe; also called *tailor's bunion*

cavus foot (pes cavus) Inflexible, high-arched foot that does not adequately absorb shock or easily adapt to various surfaces

compartment syndromes Condition in which increased tissue pressure compromises the circulation to the muscles and nerves within one of the osseofascial compartments; they may be acute or chronic

footdrop A condition in which the foot hangs in a plantarflexed position because of a lesion on the peroneal nerve

forefoot Area of the foot composed of the metatarsals and phalanges

genu recurvatum Knee hyperextension; also called *back knees*

hammertoe Toe permanently flexed at midphalangeal joint, resulting in clawlike appearance

heel spur Bony projection at the plantar aspect of the calcaneal tuberosity, which may accompany or result from severe cases of plantar fascitis

hindfoot Area of the foot composed of the calcaneus and talus and including the ankle joint

march fracture Stress fracture of one of the metatarsals; name caught on during World War II, when many soldiers unaccustomed to being on their feet received fatigue fractures after walking long distances

metatarsalgia   Pain or tenderness beneath the metatarsal head, more commonly the second and occasionally the third

metatarsus   Structure consisting of the five metatarsal bones

midfoot   Area of the foot composed of the navicular, cuboid, and three cuneiform bones

Morton's foot   Is characterized by a short first and longer second metatarsal

Morton's neuroma   Swelling of one of the digital nerves when squeezed or pinched between the metatarsal heads; the nerve between the third and fourth metatarsal heads is most often involved

pes planus (flatfoot)   Static structural abnormality in which the relative position of the foot bones have been altered, resulting in a lowering of the longitudinal arch

plantar aponeurosis   Strong bands of fibrous connective tissue originating on the calcaneal tuberosity and inserting near the metatarsal heads, they act as primary supports for the longitudinal arch; also called *plantar fascia*

plantar fasciitis   Overuse syndrome that involves an inflammatory reaction at the insertion of the plantar fascia (aponeurosis) into the calcaneus

Pott's fracture   Fracture of the lower fibula that involves the tibial articulation and usually a chipping off of a portion of the medial malleolus or a rupture of the deltoid ligament; also called Dupruytren's fracture

pronated foot   Flexible foot that exhibits excessive pronation, which is a combination of dorsiflexion, eversion, and abduction at the subtalar joint

shin splints   Catch-all term for chronic pain and discomfort in the leg, generally limited to musculotendinous involvement

sinus tarsi   Concavity or space between the calcaneus and talus

stone bruise   Persistent contusion on the plantar aspect of the foot; also called a *heel bruise* when located under the calcaneus

sustentaculum tali   Medially projecting ledge on the upper surface of the calcaneus and the largest articular facet for the talus

tarsus   Collective term used to describe the seven bones that constitute the mid- and rear foot: talus, calcaneus, navicular, cuboid, and the three cuneiforms

Thompson test   Test to indicate the integrity of the Achille's tendon; with the athlete's legs extended and the feet hanging over the table, each calf muscle is squeezed. Normally, the foot will react by plantar flexing; if the Achilles tendon is ruptured, there will be no movement of the foot

triceps surae   Name given to the gastrocnemius and soleus muscles, which share the same tendon of insertion

trochlea   Pulley-shaped surface of the talus that articulates with the tibia and fibula

turf toe   Sprain of the metatarsophalangeal joint of the great toe, normally caused by extreme dorsiflexion or plantar flexion

SUGGESTED READINGS

American Academy of Orthopaedic Surgeons: Symposium on the foot and leg in running sports, St. Louis, 1982, The C.V. Mosby Co.

American Academy of Orthopaedic Surgeons: Symposium on the foot and ankle, St. Louis, 1983, The C.V. Mosby Co.

Birnbaum, J.S.: The musculoskeletal manual, New York, 1982, Academic Press, Inc.

Brody, D.M.: Running injuries, CIBA Clinical Symposia 32:2-36, 1980.

Clinics in Sports Medicine: Symposium on, Ankle and foot problems in the athlete, Torg, J.S., (editor) Vol. 1:1, 1982, W.B. Saunders Co.

Ellison, A.E.: Skiing injuries, CIBA Clinical Symposia, 29:1, 1977

Henry, J.H.: Soft tissue injuries of the foot, Athletic Training, 16:173-177, 1981.

Hoppenfeld, S.: Physical examination of the spine and extremities, New York, 1976, Appleton-Century-Crofts.

Jesse, J.: Hidden causes of injury, prevention and correction for running athletes and joggers, Pasadena, 1977, The Athletic Press.

Klenerman, L.: The foot and its disorders, Oxford, 1976, Blackwell Scientific Publications, Ltd.

Krissoff, W.B., and Ferris, W.D.: Runner's injuries, Physician Sportsmedicine, 7:53-64, 1979.

Latin, R.W., and Kauth, W.O.: Lower leg compartment syndromes, Athletic Training 14:78-80, 1979.

Nicholas, J.A.: Ankle injuries in athletics, Orthop. Clin. North Am. 5:153-175, 1974.

O'Connor, P., and Kersey, R.D.: Achilles peritendinitis, Athletic Training 15:159-166, 1980.

O'Donoghue, D.H.: Treatment of injuries to athletes, ed. 4, Philadelphia, 1984, W.B. Saunders Co.

Subotnick, S.I.: Podiatric sports medicine, Mount Kisco, N.Y., 1975, Futura Publishing Co.

Zang, K.: Traumatic ankle conditions, Mount Kisco, N.Y., 1976, Futura Publishing Co.

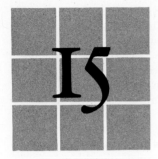

Knee injuries

The knee joint is often described as the largest and most complex joint in the human body. It is also one of the more superficial, more frequently injured, and more difficult to evaluate of the joints. The knee joint is the fulcrum of the body's longest lever and is subjected to tremendous torsional forces and loads during athletic activity. As a result, this vulnerable joint is the site of many athletic injuries.

ANATOMY OF THE KNEE

Examining the knee joint in an articulated skeleton, it is apparent that the bony components alone are not capable of providing the support required for weight bearing and athletic activity. The joint is made up of articulations between the vertically apposed ends (condyles) of the femur and tibia and between the patella and femur (Fig. 15-1). The bones alone articulate in a precariously unstable way. It is the compensating reinforcement provided by the joint capsule, cartilages, ligaments, and numerous muscle tendons that provides the knee with the security and stability so essential for successful performance in athletic activity.

Movements

The knee is a hinge-type diarthrotic (freely movable) joint. As a uniaxial joint, movements of the knee are primarily restricted to flexion and extension. It is important to realize, however, that as a biologic joint the knee is not totally limited in its movement around a fixed axis, as is the pin of a door hinge. In addition to flexion and extension, some rotation of the knee is also possible, especially when the joint is flexed.

Full flexion occurs at about 130° and is limited by contact between the calf and thigh. In the standing position (full extension), the knee is fixed and rigid. The rigidity results in part because the medial condyle of the tibia, which is larger than the lateral one, slides forward on the medial femoral condyle. This results in external (lateral) rotation of the tibia, which causes a "screwing" of the opposing bones firmly together. For flexion to occur, the fully extended knee must be "unscrewed." Thus slight internal (medial) rotation of the leg on the femur is the first step in flexion. This is brought about by contraction of the popliteus muscle, which is described later.

Structures

The anatomic components of the knee include the articular (joint) surfaces of the femur, tibia, and patella; the articular capsule lined with its synovial membrane comprising the synovial cavity; two cartilages called the medial and lateral menisci (singular, meniscus); the cruciate, collateral, and several other ligaments; and numerous muscle tendons and bursa (Figs. 15-1 to 15-4). Any combination of these structures may be injured during athletic activity.

Following is a brief description of the anatomic components of the knee. Because of the complexity of this body area, the common athletic injuries are discussed with each of these

Fig. 15-1. Right knee viewed from the front. Patella has been removed.

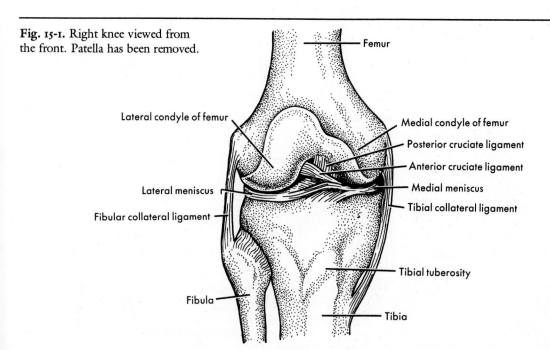

Femur

Lateral condyle of femur

Medial condyle of femur

Posterior cruciate ligament

Anterior cruciate ligament

Lateral meniscus

Medial meniscus

Fibular collateral ligament

Tibial collateral ligament

Tibial tuberosity

Fibula

Tibia

anatomic structures. The common mechanisms of injury and the frequent signs and symptoms denoting the various athletic injuries are also discussed.

Synovial cavity

The *synovial cavity* of the knee is the largest joint space in the body. The space surrounds the articulating bony condyles, extends upward be-hind the patella, and then communicates with the suprapatellar bursa (Fig. 15-5). This large joint space extends three finger-breadths (4 to 6 cm) above the superior edge of the patella. The joint cavity also extends behind the posterior portion of each femoral condyle and under the tendon of the popliteus muscle. The knee joint cavity normally contains 1 to 3 ml of synovial fluid. The volume may be greatly increased as a

Fig. 15-2. Right knee viewed from behind.

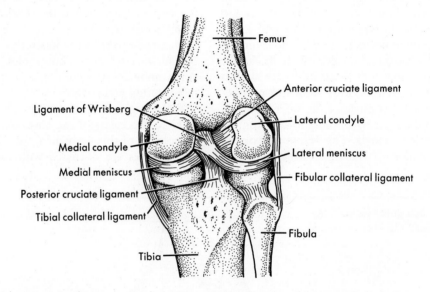

Fig. 15-3. Right tibia viewed from above.

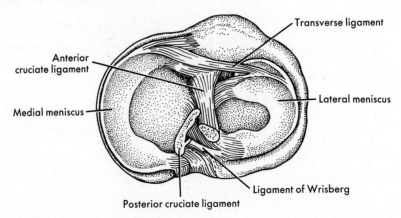

result of an athletic injury that causes hemorrhage into the joint cavity or by inflammation of the synovial membrane (synovitis), which increases the production of synovial fluid. This increased volume is called *joint effusion.* The contours of the joint will adapt to this increased fluid. This is a very important sign in evaluating injuries to the knee and is discussed in more detail on p. 413. The volume capacity of the joint cavity is reduced when the knee is extended by compression of the gastrocnemius muscle against the posterior femoral condyles. In addition, when the knee is fully flexed, the quadriceps tendon compresses the suprapatellar pouch, again reducing the capacity of the joint cavity. Therefore the athlete with a joint effusion will frequently hold the injured knee in 30° to 45° of flexion, at which point the volume of the joint cavity is the greatest; consequently the injured knee is less painful.

The synovial cavity is reinforced by a thin, strong articular capsule that surrounds the knee joint and is strengthened by several ligaments and muscle tendons. The patella is located in the tendon of the quadriceps femoris muscle and serves to replace a portion of the capsule in front. This joint capsule provides some stability for the knee in each direction and may be stretched or torn in injuries caused by abnormal motion such as sprains.

Menisci

The medial and lateral menisci are crescent-shaped pads of fibrocartilage attached to the flat top of the tibia. Because of their concavity, they form a shallow socket for the condyles of the femur. These semilunar cartilages enhance the total stability of the knee, assist in the control of normal knee motion, and provide shock absorption against compression forces between the tibia and femur. The *medial meniscus* is larger and more oval or C-shaped in outline than the lateral meniscus. The medial cartilage is also more firmly fixed to the tibia and capsule than its lateral counterpart; as a result it is much more frequently injured than the lateral cartilage. Be-

Fig. 15-4. Sagittal section through the knee joint.

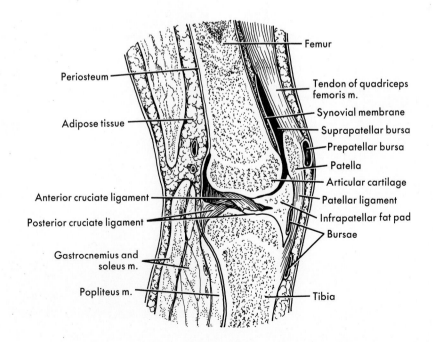

Periosteum

Adipose tissue

Anterior cruciate ligament

Posterior cruciate ligament

Gastrocnemius and soleus m.

Popliteus m.

Femur

Tendon of quadriceps femoris m.

Synovial membrane

Suprapatellar bursa

Prepatellar bursa

Patella

Articular cartilage

Patellar ligament

Infrapatellar fat pad

Bursae

Tibia

cause of its attachments to the medial collateral ligament, the medial meniscus may also be injured in conjunction with a sprain of this ligament.

The *lateral meniscus* is smaller and more round or O-shaped. It is not as firmly attached to the tibia and is not connected to the lateral collateral ligament. Therefore the lateral meniscus has greater freedom of movement and is not injured nearly as often as is the medial cartilage.

Meniscal tears are the most common of all knee injuries. The menisci are frequently injured or torn as they become trapped, pinched, or crushed between the femoral condyles and the tibial plateaus. The damage sustained by the menisci can be quite varied, ranging from a very small tear along the periphery of the cartilage to a large longitudinal tear resulting in a displaced segment of the cartilage. This type of longitudinal tear is generally referred to as a *bucket handle* tear. The menisci are often injured by twisting activities during weight bearing but also can be

Fig. 15-5. Synovial cavity. **A,** Diagram showing relationship of synovial joint space, suprapatellar pouch, and related anatomical structures in the knee. **B,** Arthrogram of knee joint showing radiopaque dye in the joint cavity. Note that dye extends above level of patella, filling suprapatellar pouch.

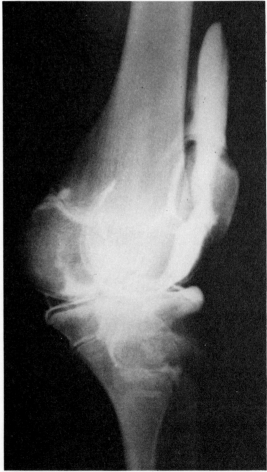

B

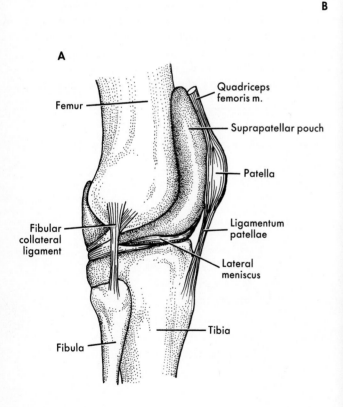

A

Femur

Quadriceps femoris m.

Suprapatellar pouch

Patella

Fibular collateral ligament

Ligamentum patellae

Lateral meniscus

Tibia

Fibula

damaged by direct blows to the knee or chronic trauma. Tears around the periphery of the meniscus or to the ligamentous attachments may heal because of the blood supply to this area. Tears involving the avascular body of the meniscus will not heal and usually result in persistent symptoms.

On initial evaluation it is often difficult to recognize a cartilage injury, as symptoms may be limited or vague. Experienced athletic trainers stress the importance of a careful and accurate history concerning meniscal injuries. In many cases the suspicion of meniscal damage is made by history alone. Along with the mechanism of injury, the athlete may relate a popping or tearing sensation felt at the time of injury, followed by pain. The pain is usually localized along the medial or lateral joint line. The athlete may also complain that the knee "gives out" or buckles. Walking up and down stairs is frequently difficult, and squatting may be painful. The swelling associated with a damaged meniscus is usually caused by synovial irritation and occurs gradually over several hours. The maximum amount of swelling is frequently seen the day after a meniscus injury.

Two classic symptoms of meniscal injuries, which seldom occur with the initial injury, are *"clicking"* and *"locking."* Clicking is an audible or palpable sensation often caused by a torn meniscal fragment rubbing against a femoral condyle. This clicking may become more evident with time as the torn edges of the injured cartilage harden. Locking is the mechanical blockage of the complete range of motion. This is usually caused by some type of internal derangement. The most common cause of locking of the knee results from a fragment of an injured meniscus becoming caught between the femoral condyle and tibial plateau, thus restricting complete extension. Athletic trainers must always be aware of pseudolocking, in which the athlete cannot complete the range of motion and believes the knee is locked. This effect can be caused by hamstring spasms or swelling. If the athlete had normal range of motion immediately after an injury

and the loss of extension developed over a period of time, the restricted motion is probably caused by pseudolocking effect.

The acute symptoms of a meniscal injury may subside within a few days, only to recur when activity is resumed. The athletic trainer should suspect meniscus damage when indicated by history and recurrent episodes of effusion and disability. Various manipulative tests that place stress on each meniscus to assess their integrity are described later in this chapter.

Cruciate ligaments

The cruciate ligaments are relatively short but strong, rounded bands that cross each other, forming an *X* within the joint capsule. They are located between the articular surfaces of the tibial and femoral condyles and are named according to their tibial attachments (Fig. 15-3). The role of the cruciate ligaments is complex; however, their primary function is to provide anteroposterior stability. They also function to stabilize the knees from rotational stresses, excessive hyperextension, and abduction and adduction forces. These ligaments are most taut when the knee is in full extension, but some fibers of both cruciates are always tight throughout the full range of motion.

The *anterior cruciate ligament* attaches to the anterior part of the tibia, between its condyles, then crosses upward and backward to attach on the posterior aspect of the lateral condyle of the femur. This ligament is primarily responsible for preventing anterior tibial displacement on the femur or, from a more functional standpoint, prevent posterior femoral displacement on a fixed lower leg. The anterior cruciate ligament can be injured in a number of ways. Often an injury results from a twisting maneuver during weight bearing (Fig. 15-6). The anterior cruciate is often injured along with the medial collateral as a result of a lateral blow to the knee (Fig. 15-7). Injury to this ligament can also occur as a result of forced hyperextension or a direct blow to the back of the tibia that drives the tibia forward. The athlete with an anterior cruciate liga-

Fig. 15-6. Possible mechanism of knee injury involving cutting, twisting, or turning activity during weight bearing on a fixed foot.

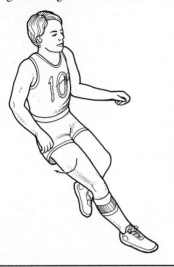

ment injury will many times describe feeling a "pop" in the knee, will be unable to continue activity, and will have a bloody effusion *(hemarthrosis)* within the first few hours. Loss of normal motion may be almost immediate as a result of this hemorrhaging.

The *posterior cruciate ligament* attaches posteriorly to the tibia and lateral meniscus, then crosses upward, forward, and inward to attach to the anterior aspect of the femur's medial condyle. This ligament is primarily responsible for preventing posterior tibial displacement on the femur or anterior femoral displacement on a fixed lower leg. The posterior cruciate is shorter than the anterior cruciate and is located nearer the center of the joint. It is believed that the posterior cruciate functions as the axis around which rotation of the knee takes place. Experimental work has shown the posterior cruciate

Fig. 15-7. Classic knee injury occurring in football as a blow is delivered to the outside of the knee. Note on the insert the potential injury to the medial collateral and cruciate ligaments. The anterior cruciate ligament is more vulnerable to injury than the posterior cruciate.

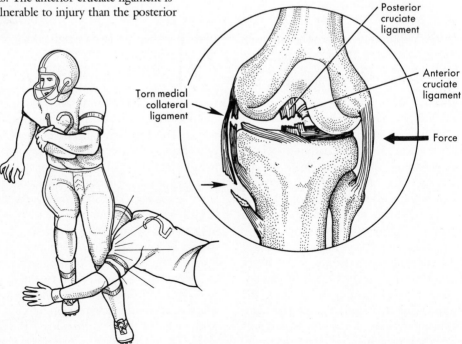

ligament to be twice as strong as the anterior cruciate or medial collateral ligaments, which may account for its not being injured as frequently. The posterior cruciate may be injured by a direct force against the tibia, that drives it backward in relation to the femur. This ligament may also be injured, in conjunction with other supporting structures, from excessive hyperextension, hyperflexion, or abduction forces.

Collateral ligaments

The collateral ligaments reinforce the joint capsule on the medial and lateral side. The primary purpose of the collateral ligaments is to provide lateral stability, or prevent abnormal movement of the knee from side to side.

The *medial collateral ligament* (sometimes called the tibial collateral ligament) is a strong, flat band that extends from the medial (adductor) tubercle of the femur to the tibia, where it attaches to the medial condyle and medial surface of the shaft. Anatomically, this 8 to 9 cm long ligament can be subdivided into a number of distinct segments. However, from a functional standpoint, it is usually divided into two layers of fibers—superficial and deep. The superficial layer extends the full length of the ligament and passes deep to the pes anserinus before inserting into the tibia. The fibers of the deep layer (sometimes called the medial capsular ligament) are much shorter. They originate on the adductor tubercle of the femur just below the superficial layer, but extend downward only to the upper tibial margin. Fibers from the deep layer of the medial collateral ligament blend into and fuse with both the joint capsule and medial meniscus. The primary function of the medial collateral ligament is to provide stability against valgus forces or to prevent abnormal movements to the inside. The ligament is tightest on complete ex-

Fig. 15-8. Mechanism of knee injury as the right knee is forced into valgus with external rotation of the tibia.
(Courtesy Bill Oakes, Northern Iowan.)

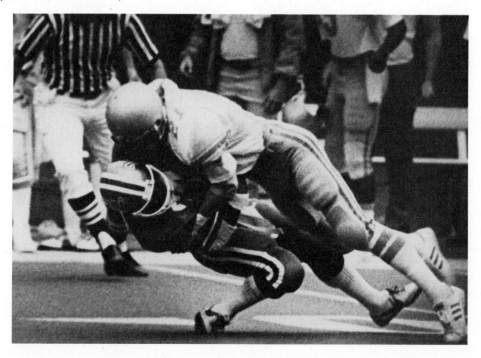

tension; however, because it is a flat band, some of the fibers provide support throughout the range of motion.

The medial collateral is the most frequently injured ligament in the knee. The most common cause of injury is a blow to the outside of the knee, which stresses the medial structures as shown in Fig. 15-7. Fig. 15-8 shows another mechanism of knee injury as the joint is forced into valgus without a lateral blow. Because the superficial and deep layers are in effect anatomically separate structures, they often stretch or tear at different levels during injury. The medial collateral ligament can also be injured during rotational stresses on the knee (Fig. 15-6). This mechanism most commonly results in an injury to the femoral attachment of the medial collateral ligament.

The *lateral collateral ligament* (sometimes called the fibular collateral ligament) is a rounded, pencil-like cord about 5 cm long. It passes from the lateral condyle of the femur to the head of the fibula just anterior to its apex. There is no attachment between the lateral meniscus and the lateral collateral ligament. The tendon of the biceps femoris muscle splits on either side of the ligament. Unlike its medial counterpart, the lateral collateral ligament is not a part of the joint capsule and plays a less significant role in joint stability. It is tight and contributes to stability mainly in extension of the knee; it becomes slack during flexion.

Much of the lateral support of the knee is provided by a broad tendon called the *iliotibial band*. This tendon is the distal attachment of the tensor facia lata muscle, which originates at the iliac crest and posterior aspect of the sacrum. As it passes over the thigh in the region of the greater trochanter it condenses into a broad tendon called the iliotibial band. As it passes down the lateral aspect of the thigh it attaches indirectly to the distal femur just above the lateral condyle through an intramuscular septum. It then crosses the knee and inserts into the upper (proximal) end of the tibia at the *tubercle of Gerdy*. The iliotibial band is many times considered to be the true lateral collateral ligament. It serves as a strong static stabilizer of the lateral side of the knee. There is no connection between the joint capsule and the fibular collateral ligament or iliotibial band. Portions of the iliotibial band are commonly transplanted during surgery to help correct anterolateral rotatory instability of the knee.

Muscles

In addition to providing movement, the muscles about the knee contribute much in the way of support and stability for the joint. These muscles and their tendinous attachment are susceptible to injury because of the explosive muscular action required during most athletic activity (Fig. 15-9). The most important muscles acting on the knee can be classified as the extensors (quadriceps) and the flexors (hamstrings, gastrocnemius, and popliteus). Some of these muscles also serve as internal and external rotators of the tibia.

Extensor muscles. The main muscle of the extensor group is the quadriceps femoris, which comprises the rectus femoris, vastus medialis, vastus lateralis, and vastus intermedius (Fig. 15-10). All four muscles converge into a common tendon that attaches to the patella and then extends downward to insert into the tibial tuberosity. Collectively this unit is called the *quadriceps*

Fig. 15-9. Possible mechanism of injury involving explosive muscular action.

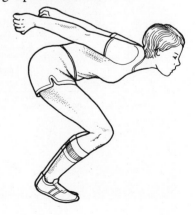

mechanism or *extensor mechanism* and is the site of many athletic injuries. Injuries can occur at any point along this mechanism at any time during explosive muscular activity or result from direct trauma. Overuse syndromes often involve components of the quadriceps mechanism.

A common site for strains or ruptures of the quadriceps mechanism is at the insertion point on the upper pole of the patella. Injuries of this type usually result from a sudden violent contraction of the musculature. Findings usually include tenderness and swelling at the insertion site, with pain when the quadriceps mechanism is subjected to stress. Additional strains involving the quadriceps are discussed in more detail in Chapter 16.

Flexor muscles. The flexor muscles of the knee include the hamstrings, sartorius, gracilis, gastrocnemius, and popliteus (Fig. 15-10). The hamstrings are actually three muscles, the biceps femoris, the semimembranosus, and the semitendinosus. The biceps femoris, or lateral hamstring, is composed of two heads, which attach to the head of the fibula. This muscle assists in stabilizing the posterior and lateral capsule and externally rotates the lower leg during knee flexion.

The semimembranosus attaches to the posterior side of the medial tibial condyle. It assists in stabilizing the medial and posterior capsular structures and internally rotates the tibia during knee flexion. The semitendinosus joins the sartorius and gracilis muscles to form a common tendon called the *pes anserinus*. Their attachment is on the medial aspect of the tibia (Fig. 15-10), and they assist in medial stability along with the medial capsule and medial collateral ligament. These muscles also internally rotate the lower leg

Fig. 15-10. Muscles and structures about the knee joint.

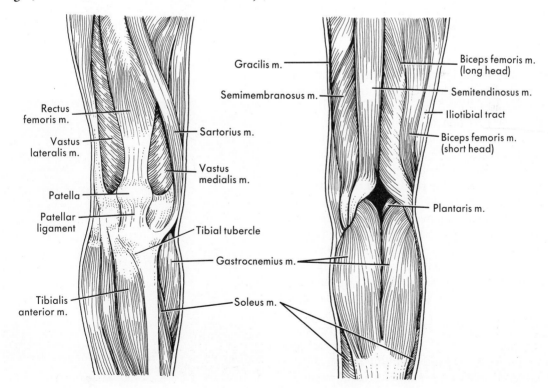

when the knee is flexed. Portions of this tendon are commonly transplanted during surgery to help correct anteromedial rotatory instability. Injuries involving the hamstring muscles are discussed in Chapter 16.

The gastrocnemius muscle is essentially a plantar flexor of the ankle but does originate above the knee and therefore has some effect on the joint. The two heads of the muscle attach to the medial and lateral epicondyles of the femur and then quickly unite and continue down the leg to their insertion on the calcaneus. The two heads can be palpated above the femoral condyles. They form the inferior border of the popliteal space.

The popliteus muscle is located on the posterior surface of the knee. It takes its origin from the lateral condyle of the femur and is inserted into the back of the tibia near its upper end. The popliteus is a weak knee flexor but, as previously discussed, is primarily responsible for the very important internal rotation of the tibia required to begin knee flexion.

Bursae

There are 13 bursae, which serve as pads around the knee joint: four anteriorly, four laterally, and five medially. Bursae usually become injured and inflamed as a result of direct trauma or constant friction between supporting structures. Most of the bursae around the knee are not injured frequently; the one most commonly injured is the prepatellar bursa, which lies between the front of the patella and the skin. This is the largest bursa in the knee and is usually injured by direct trauma. *Prepatellar bursitis* is a common problem in athletes who suffer repeated knee trauma, such as falling on the knee or getting hit on the patella. The condition is usually easy to evaluate because of the large amount of fluid between the skin and the patella (Fig. 15-11).

The most common bursa affected by running is the anserine bursa. This lies between the pes anserine tendon insertion and the medial collateral ligament. *Anserine bursitis* is usually caused

by constant friction or perhaps by an external blow to the area. The symptoms may be confused with an injury to the medial collateral ligament. However, it should be distinguishable following an assessment of the area.

Occasionally a swelling in the popliteal space on the posterior part of the knee may indicate a *popliteal cyst,* or *Baker's cyst.* This is normally a distension of the gastrocnemius-semimembranosus bursa. However, these terms also apply to an inflammation and herniation of the synovial membrane in the popliteal region. Such a cyst presents itself as a large, soft, painless mass in the popliteal space. This bursa may communicate with the joint cavity, and the swelling may come and go. This type of bursitis may be the result of chronic trauma to the knee, internal derangement, recurring joint effusion, or simply asymptomatic swelling behind the knee.

Patella

The patella is a flat, triangular bone located in front of the knee joint. Its posterior surface articulates with the femur. It covers and protects the anterior aspect of the knee and increases the

Fig. 15-11. Prepatellar bursitis.

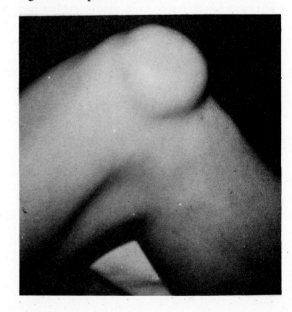

angle of pull, and therefore the leverage, of the quadriceps muscle. The posterior surface of the patella is divided by a ridge into two articular areas, or facets. The ridge articulates with a groove on the patellar surface of the femur.

Normally the patella is ossified from several centers. By 3 or 4 years of age they coalesce to form a single center, which completes ossification about the age of puberty. In rare instances the ossification process results in two or three separate patellar components, or ossicles. This condition is called *bipartite* or *tripartite* patella. If it exists, the condition is almost always bilateral. This fact helps exclude the possibility of the condition being mistaken for a fracture.

Injuries involving the patella. The athletic trainer should be familiar with a number of conditions that may involve the patella. The kneecap may fully dislocate (Fig. 15-12) or, more commonly, sublux during activity. Movement is almost always lateral as the patella slides over the lateral femoral condyle. Recurrent dislocations or subluxations of the patella are usually associated with (1) congenital or (2) developmental deficiencies in the quadriceps mechanism. Congenital deficiencies include a shallow patellar groove, abnormal patella, a laterally displaced patellar tendon attachment (Q angle, which is described later), laxity of the patella, and genu valgum (knock-knees). Women are more prone to this problem because of their wider bony pelvic structure and internally angulated femurs. In both men and women displacement of the patella is most likely to occur with the knee flexed between 20° and 45°. The dynamic forces of the quadriceps coupled with external rotation of the foot results in an increased Q angle. Developmental deficiencies have to do with the supporting muscles that guide the patella and influence the mechanics of knee motion. Underdevelopment of the vastus medialis muscle and atrophy secondary to other injuries or disuse are frequently associated with patellar dislocation.

It may be difficult to differentiate symptoms produced by recurrent subluxation of the kneecap because the symptoms are similar to other internal derangements of the knee. The athlete will frequently describe the knee as "giving

Fig. 15-12. Dislocated patella.

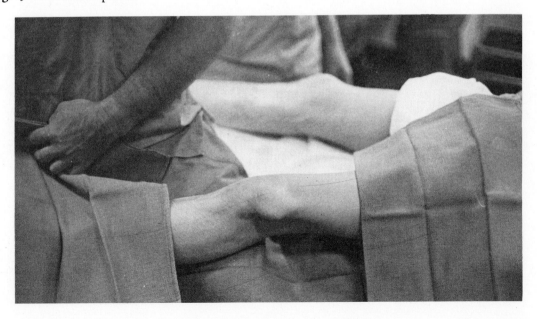

way," popping, or catching. In addition, there will normally be tenderness on the medial or lateral edges of the patella, and the athlete will resist any attempt to move the kneecap. The apprehension test, which is described on p. 416, remains one of the most significant evaluative maneuvers to test a subluxating patella. Fig. 15-13 is a radiograph showing subluxation of the patella when taken using a "sunrise view" procedure.

Acute dislocation of the patella can also occur with a direct blow against the medial aspect of the kneecap or a sudden valgus stress to the knee. Deformity is usually obvious, as the patella is displaced laterally and the knee held in slight flexion. Spontaneous reduction of an acute subluxation of the patella should be evidenced by the history and a positive apprehension test.

Chondromalacia patellae is a degenerative process that results in a softening (degeneration) of the articular surface of the patella. The symptoms associated with chondromalacia of the patella are a common cause of knee pain in athletes. Chondromalacia is usually caused by an irritation of the patellar groove, with subsequent changes occurring in the cartilage on the posteri-

or surface of the patella. There are many factors that may contribute to chondromalacia. It can be caused by direct trauma to the patella, malalignment and recurrent subluxations discussed previously, internal derangement, quadriceps muscle imbalance, increased Q angle, or abnormal anatomy of the patella or femoral groove. The symptoms of chondromalacia often show an insidious onset and progress slowly. The athlete will complain of pain arising from behind or beneath the kneecap, especially during activities that require flexion of the knee, such as climbing stairs, kneeling, and jumping or running. The athlete may also complain of the knee buckling during activity, a grating or grinding feeling with movement, an aching pain after vigorous exercise, or pain after sitting a prolonged time with the knees flexed. This is sometimes referred to as the *"movie sign."* On evaluation of the knee, there is usually tenderness along the edges of the patella, especially under the medial facet, discomfort on compressing the kneecap into the femoral groove, and pain on contraction of the quadriceps against patellar pressure. The athlete may also exhibit swelling, crepitus, and a positive apprehension test.

Fig. 15-13. Sunrise view radiograph showing a patellar subluxation.

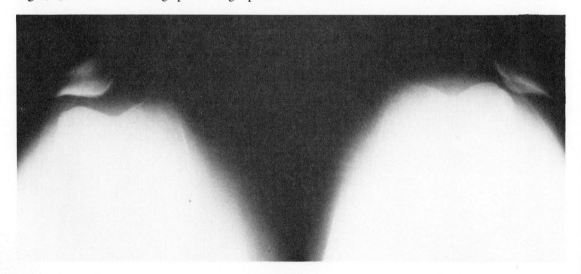

Patellar tendinitis (jumper's knee) is a condition found in many athletes involved in repetitive jumping activities. It is an inflammatory response to repeated stress or irritation at the patellar tendon insertion. It is normally characterized by pain localized at the distal pole of the patella; however, pain can also occur at the proximal pole of the patella. The athlete will complain of pain or discomfort during activity, which may become progressively worse with excessive quadriceps action. The athlete will usually experience aching after exercise, and occasionally swelling may occur. On examination of the knee, the athlete will have point tenderness with palpation at the tendon insertion and pain during resistive movements involving knee extension.

Other common athletic-related conditions

Osgood-Schlatter syndrome is a condition involving the growing tibial tuberosity of adolescents. It occurs in young athletes when the attachment of the epiphysis of the tibial tuberosity to the shaft (diaphysis) of the bone is the weakest link in the extensor mechanism. Repeated stresses on the patellar tendon cause a minor avulsion of the tibial tuberosity, leading to an inflammatory reaction. Osgood-Schlatter syndrome is aggravated by running, jumping, or kneeling. The young athlete will have pain on active use of the quadriceps, which will normally limit activity. On evaluation the athlete may have local swelling, tenderness with direct pressure on the tuberosity, and pain on resistance to quadriceps action. Osgood-Schlatter syndrome is a self-limiting condition an athlete will eventually grow out of; however, an enlarged tibial tuberosity often remains (Fig. 15-14). Occasionally, symptoms may persist into adulthood.

Athletic trainers should be familiar with three additional conditions that may affect the knee: chondral and osteochondral fractures and osteochondritis dissecans. These conditions can occur in other joints in the body but most commonly occur in the knee. Chondral fractures involve the articular cartilage, and osteochondral fractures involve the underlying bone and also the articular cartilage. These fractures result from acute trauma and are caused by direct stresses applied to the articular surfaces of the femur, tibia, or patella. The result may be an acute contusion to the articular surface with fissuring of the cartilage, which can be likened to the cracking of an egg shell. The fracture can be incomplete, so that no fragment is actually dislodged, or complete, with a loose piece of cartilage separated from the underlying bone to produce a loose body within the joint (Fig. 7-24, *J*). These fractures may be difficult to evaluate or differentiate from cartilage injuries and may go completely unrecognized. If the fracture is complete and there is one or more cartilage fragments (commonly referred to as *"joint mice"*) within the joint, the symptoms will be similar to a meniscal injury. Fragments of this type may cause clicking, catching, or locking sensations.

Osteochondritis dissecans is a condition of unknown cause in which a segment of subchondral bone undergoes avascular necrosis. The most common site for this condition is the lateral surface of the medial femoral condyle. It is believed

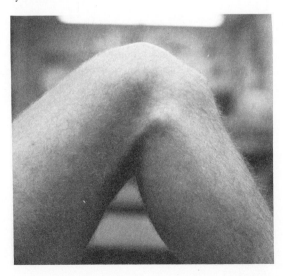

Fig. 15-14. Note enlarged tibial tuberosity remaining as a result of Osgood-Schlatter syndrome.

that osteochondritis dissecans is the result of loss of circulation to the area, which may be the result of recurrent trauma. This may be initiated by a chondral or osteochondral fracture. This condition may also be difficult to evaluate. Symptoms may consist of pain, stiffness, and swelling that are made worse with activity. There may be a medial joint line tenderness and a limited range of motion. Osteochondritis dissecans may also give rise to a loose body within the joint. These conditions should be suspected and the athlete referred to medical assistance when the athlete has persistent symptoms in an otherwise normal-appearing knee.

ATHLETIC INJURY ASSESSMENT PROCESS

All too often the evaluation of a knee injury begins in a haphazard or unstructured manner, and the athlete is seen for definitive diagnosis and treatment too late for an ideal result to be obtained. A careful, comprehensive, and systematic evaluation of every knee injury should be done promptly and completely so that an accurate assessment with definitive care can be achieved. It is not proper to simply rest an injured knee and then wait and hope for improvement to occur. An in-depth assessment must be made if a knee injury is of any significance.

Secondary survey

Initial assessment of any knee injury must be carried out promptly and competently by a person skilled in at least the techniques of a preliminary knee examination. If findings in any way raise questions as to the stability or function of the knee, it is imperative that the athlete be referred to someone who has expertise in knee injuries. It is the responsibility of the physician to arrive at an absolute diagnosis of the knee injury and prescribe, in conjunction with the athletic trainer, a program of care and periodic assessment to evaluate the injury and subsequent recovery. By evaluating knee injuries in a careful, systematic manner, problems that arise from a neglected or poorly treated knee can be minimized.

The remainder of this chapter presents a common approach to evaluating an injured knee. Actual assessment procedures are described and explained. The examination of an injured knee should follow logical, sequential procedures designed to evaluate the various structures about the knee; however, each athletic trainer must develop his or her own techniques of evaluating a knee, which includes adding or deleting procedures depending on the pathology of the knee injury. All evaluative procedures discussed in this chapter will seldom if ever be used on any one knee injury. Those procedures used with each injury will be determined by the information gained during the systematic assessment process.

History

The history is an extremely important aspect of the knee evaluation. This phase of the assessment process will help distinguish between the acute, chronic, and overused knee injuries as well as indicate which structures may be injured and suggest which additional evaluative procedures should be used. The history should be completed as the first step in this assessment process and should include information concerning previous injuries, history of the present injury, and the postinjury course, if appropriate.

Previous injury. An important aspect of the history-gathering process is determining whether there has been any previous difficulty with the knee. If so, obtain as much information as possible about this previous injury, including the nature of the injury, the treatment, and the extent of rehabilitation. Had symptoms completely subsided before the onset of the present injury? Had full functional capabilities been regained? Was the knee weakened or susceptible to certain types of trauma because of earlier injuries? Are symptoms of the current injury similar to those of any previous injuries? All previous injuries should be documented, as should their postinjury course. If there has been previous surgery performed on the knee, it is essential to have accurate, detailed information as to the pathology, surgical procedures performed, and any evidence of injury to other structures at that time. In addition, it is important to inquire about any significant injuries to the opposite or uninjured knee, because it will be used as a baseline for comparison during the assessment.

Present injury. Next, question the athlete and develop a history of the present injury. Was the onset gradual? There may be a history of specific injury to the knee, with symptoms spontaneously arising during or after activity. This may reflect chronic or overuse conditions such as chondromalacia, tendinitis, or bursitis. Was the onset sudden? If the injury occurred as the result of direct trauma, ask the athlete to describe or demonstrate the mechanism of injury. It is important to detail the mechanism of injury, as this can indicate which anatomic structures may have been injured. What types of stresses were applied to the knee? Was the athlete twisting so that rotation was involved in the injury? Did marked flexion or hyperextension occur at the time of injury? If the knee was hit, where was the blow delivered and what were the positions of the foot, knee, and hip at the time of injury? All these factors are extremely important to document when taking the current history. Take the time required to ask questions and listen attentively.

Common symptoms associated with knee injuries should be evaluated in some detail, as they will help in differentiating between various injuries. Have the athlete describe any symptoms as specifically as possible. Ask for specifics concerning the nature and behavior of the symptoms. How long did these symptoms last, and were they constant, intermittent, or changing? First, is there pain, and if so, where? Localization of pain may help indicate the type of injury; however, in many knee injuries pain is poorly localized. This is especially true just after an acute injury. Is the pain constant or intermittent? Determine what types of activity produce the pain.

Is there swelling associated with the knee injury? The presence or absence of swelling within

the knee is a very significant aspect of the history. When swelling occurs, it is important to determine how soon the swelling developed after the injury. Swelling that occurs in the first 2 hours after an injury usually indicates blood in the joint cavity (hemarthrosis). This condition is often associated with a more serious injury such as cruciate ligament involvement, osteochondral fracture, or a peripheral meniscal tear. Gradual swelling occurring over 12 to 24 hours suggests synovial irritation, which may accompany a more minor meniscal injury or ligament sprain. Swelling that occurs after activity and goes away with 1 or more days rest may indicate an overuse process or an internal derangement of some kind.

Is there a loss of motion? If so, what type of motion loss? Is the athlete unable to extend the knee or unable to fully flex the knee, or are both extremes of motion limited? Loss of motion may be caused by pain, swelling, or protective muscle spasms around the knee. Loss of motion may also be the result of locking of the knee, which prevents the athlete from fully extending the knee. Locking is a symptom associated with internal derangement of the knee and is usually caused by a loose body within the knee or a displaced fragment of a torn meniscus. Find out if the locking is intermittent or if the knee has been locked ever since the onset of the injury. Intermittent locking or catching suggests a loose body or dislodged fragment of meniscus that periodically becomes caught between the articular surfaces of the tibia and femur. Constant locking suggests a larger displaced bucket-handle tear of the meniscus.

In addition to questions concerning the symptoms associated with the injured knee, find out about any sensations the athlete has experienced. Did he or she feel or hear anything at the time of the injury, such as a popping, snapping, grinding, catching, or buckling sensation? Does the athlete complain of weakness in the injured knee? The feeling that the knee may give out during activity is another symptom that may be associated with internal derangement. These descriptions of sensations associated with a knee injury should never be ignored. Find out the athlete's impressions of the injury and use this information during the assessment.

Post-injury course. It is unfortunate that in many cases an injured knee is not evaluated immediately after the injury, which is the ideal time for assessment. In these instances, it is important to determine what has happened to the knee since the injury. Did the athlete continue activity without difficulty, developing soreness later, or did he or she have to stop activity immediately? Can the athlete walk, run, or climb stairs without pain or complications? Has there been any clicking, locking, or giving way of the knee? Has there been any change in the symptoms since the injury? What makes the symptoms better or worse? All these findings concerning the postinjury course should be carefully documented and later correlated with all data obtained as a result of the complete knee evaluation.

The information gained during the history portion of the assessment process is extremely important in selecting the appropriate evaluative procedures to be used in examining an injured knee. Knowing the mechanism of injury, the symptoms expressed by the athlete, and conditions associated with the injury, coupled with an understanding of the anatomy of the area, will allow you to visualize those structures that may be injured and need to be evaluated.

Observation

The visual inspection of an injured knee begins as soon as you see the athlete. Watch the athlete's attitude about the injured knee and willingness to move and use the extremity. If the athlete walks on the injured knee, what is the gait pattern? Can the athlete bear full weight on the knee? Does the athlete limp? If so, how much? Does the athlete require assistance to walk?

As soon as possible, get the athlete to a place where clothing, equipment, and tape can be removed from both legs so that a complete inspection is possible and evaluation or assessment can

continue. If possible, have the athlete stand with both feet together to observe the alignment and position of the knees. Terms used to describe any angulation between the tibia and femur are "valgus" and "varus." These terms refer to the body part distal to the joint in question. *Valgus* means an angulation outward, or away from the midline of the body, whereas *varus* indicates an angulation of the distal part toward the midline (Fig. 15-15). An athlete with knock knees is said to have *genu valgum,* whereas an athlete with bowlegs has *genu varum.* Women tend to have more valgus angle than men. Also view the extended knees from the side. Is there any evidence of hyperextension of the knees *(genu recurvatum)?* Women also tend to have more hyperextension than men. Remember, an athlete who has an injury may not be able to completely extend the knee. Compare the injured knee to the uninjured knee to note any difference in symmetry and alignment.

Also observe the alignment of the patellae. Do they appear symmetric and level? Do the patellae face forward when the feet are pointed straight ahead or do they appear to face each other *(squinting patellae)* (Fig. 15-16). A technique used to evaluate the alignment of the patellae is to measure the *Q angle.* The Q angle is formed by a line from the anterior superior iliac spine to the midpatella and another line from the midpatella to the tibial tubercle (Fig. 15-17). An angle of 15° or less is considered normal. An angle greater than 20° is considered excessive and may be associated with an unstable extensor mechanism and patellar instability.

Inspect the knee for any signs of trauma such as abrasions, contusions, or deformity. These signs may indicate areas of stress and give important clues as to the mechanism of injury. For example, a bruise on the outside of the knee indicates that the supporting structures on the inside of the knee may have been subjected to stress and injured by a blow to the outside of the knee. Therefore the integrity of the supporting structures on the side of the knee opposite any signs of trauma should always be evaluated.

Notice the contour of the legs. Are there signs of swelling? The swelling may be generalized over the entire area, which will mask the normal contour of the knee (Fig. 15-18). As was previously discussed, an athlete with marked effusion usually holds the knee in some degree of flexion rather than complete extension, because in flexion the volume of the joint capsule is greater. Localized swelling about the knee is normally at the site of the injury or over the bursae, such as over the patella (prepatellar bursitis), or over the tibial tubercle (infrapatellar bursitis). Also look at the contours of the musculature above the knee for any visible atrophy. Atrophy of the thigh will usually be present if the knee injury is a chronic problem. A convenient method to document atrophy is to measure thigh circumference at the same level in both legs. Another method used to reveal atrophy is to note the character of the muscle tone during maximal contraction of the quadriceps. Look specifically at the size and tone of the vastus medialis. It is the most superficial of the quadriceps muscles and the most sensitive to disuse. The involved leg may have noticeably decreased muscle size and tone.

Palpation

After completing the history and inspection of the knee, palpation can assist in locating specific structures involved in the injury. Remember, it is a good practice to begin palpation away from

Fig. 15-15. Valgus and varus angulation of the leg. **A,** Genu valgus, or knock knees, and **B,** genu varus, or bowlegs.

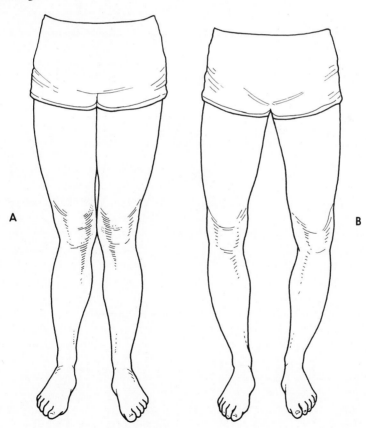

Fig. 15-16. Squinting patellae.

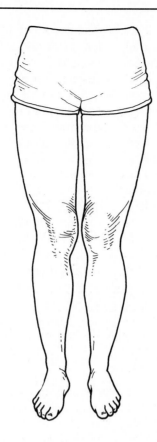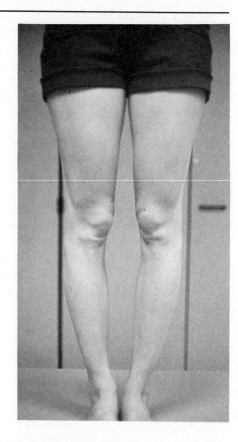

Fig. 15-17. Q angle of the patella. An angle of 15°
or less is considered normal.

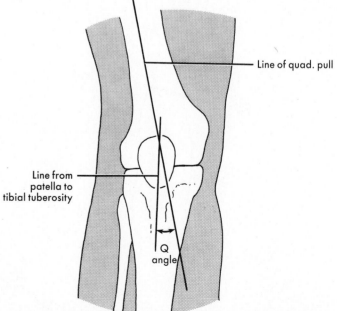

Line of quad. pull

Line from
patella to
tibial tuberosity

Q
angle

the suspected area of injury. This promotes co-operation from the athlete. Take care not to overlook any unsuspected injuries. It is usually easier to palpate the knee when it is in a flexed position because the supporting structures are more relaxed and anatomic landmarks more distinct. However, certain palpation techniques require that the knee be extended.

Begin the palpation portion of a knee evaluation by localizing any pain or swelling. To localize pain, gently palpate various areas about the knee to elicit tenderness or pain. Remember, tenderness is normally present at the site of an injury. Swelling may also be localized at the site of an injury. Evaluate any localized swelling by gently feeling for fluid that lies between the skin and the underlying structures. Swelling may also be within the knee joint capsule (effusion), or diffused outside the joint capsule. Diffuse swelling outside the knee joint usually indicates injuries to structures outside the joint capsule or

an injury involving the capsule, allowing the fluid to escape from the knee joint into the surrounding soft tissue.

An athlete with marked effusion will usually demonstrate a ***ballotable patella.*** With the leg relaxed, push the patella down and posteriorly and then release it quickly (Fig. 15-19). The large amount of fluid under the patella will cause it to rebound or appear to be floating. In palpating for minor effusion, gradually run one hand down the thigh, ending just above the kneecap to "milk" the suprapatellar pouch (Fig. 15-20). Then feel for fluid on each side of the knee at the joint line. If there is fluid within the joint capsule, you will feel a fluid wave on one side of the joint as you push on the opposite side.

Careful palpation of all specific structures suspected of being involved in an injury can provide valuable assessment information. Procedures used to palpate the various structures about the knee, as well as the common injuries

Fig. 15-18. Examples of generalized swelling of knee masking normal contours.

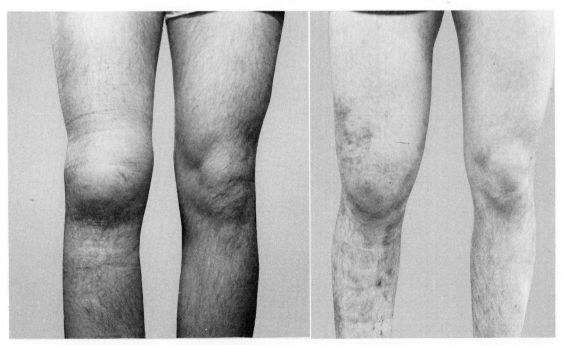

that may be indicated by tenderness expressed or swelling located during these procedures, are discussed below.

The patella is a good point of reference to begin palpating around the knee. The patella is best palpated with the leg in extension and the athlete relaxed. Prepatellar bursitis may be indicated by superficial swelling and tenderness over the kneecap. Place your fingers on either side of the kneecap and move it up, down, and from side to side to determine if tenderness exists. Push the kneecap against the femur as you repeat these same moves to evaluate the articulating surfaces of the patella and the trochlear grove of the femur (Fig. 15-21, A). Pain on compression against the femur may indicate chondromalacia or a chondral fracture. Another test for evaluating the underside of the kneecap is the *patella femoral grinding test* (Fig. 15-21, B). Push the patella distally and ask the athlete to contract the quadriceps as you apply pressure on the kneecap. It is a positive test if pain occurs. This test is more accurate with the knee in about 20° of flexion. An important point to remember is that a vigorously performed patella femoral guiding test can be extremely uncomfortable, even on a normal knee. If done forcefully, this test may be the last part of the assessment for which the athlete is going to be cooperative.

The *apprehension test* will indicate if the athlete has a patella that is prone to dislocating or subluxing. While palpating the patella, push it outward, attempting to dislocate it laterally (Fig. 15-22). If the patella is not prone to dislocating and the extensor mechanism is stable, there will be no reaction or pain. However, if the extensor mechanism is weakened from previous injury, such as a subluxation or dislocation, the athlete will become apprehensive about lateral movement of the patella. This test should be performed with the knee flexed to about 20°.

Palpate just above the patella in the extensor mechanism and on up into the quadriceps muscles. Feel both thighs at the same time to compare the symmetry and definition of the quadriceps (Fig. 15-23). Note any defects that indicate tears or ruptures. Tenderness in the muscle in-

Fig. 15-19. Ballotable patella.

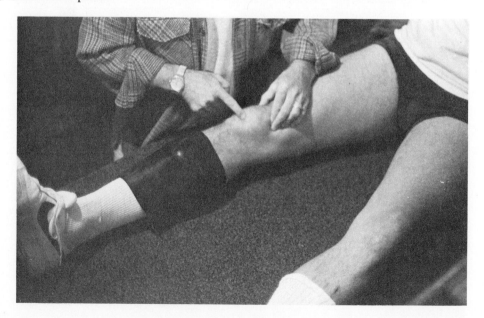

dicates a posssible strain and should be evaluated further by resistive stress.

Also palpate the lower end of the patella and the point of attachment of the patellar tendon to the tibial tuberosity. Local swelling and tenderness here indicates patellar tendinitis, or jumper's knee. To assess this injury, "wing" the patella by pushing down on the upper end of the kneecap with one hand, then palpate the inferior pole using the index finger of your other hand (Fig. 15-24).

Continue palpation along the length of the patellar tendon for any defects, swelling, and tenderness. Swelling and tenderness below the

Fig. 15-20. Palpating for effusion in the knee joint. **A,** Milking down suprapatellar pouch; **B,** feeling for fluid wave.

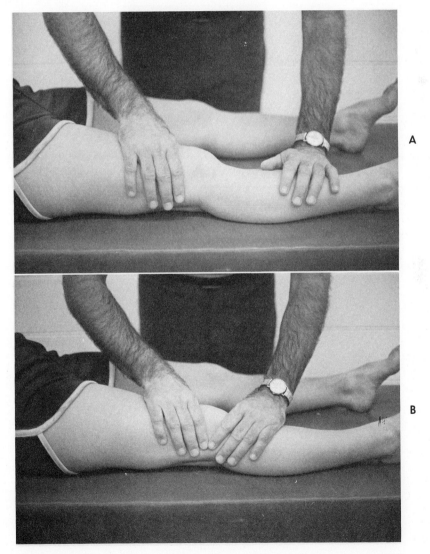

A

B

patellar tendon may be infrapatellar bursitis. Remember, the insertion of the patellar tendon at the tibial tuberosity is the site for Osgood-Schlatter syndrome in young athletes, which will produce point tenderness on palpation.

To palpate the medial aspect of the knee, begin at the joint line for orientation. This is most easily located by having the knee flexed and feeling for the soft depression just inside the patellar tendon (Fig. 15-25). The joint line is between the upper edge of the tibial condyle, called the tibial plateau, and femoral condyle above. You can follow this line between the femur and tibia all the way around to the back of the joint. Tenderness

Fig. 15-21. Evaluating the articulating surfaces of the patella and the trochlear groove of the femur. **A,** Pushing the patella against trochlear groove; **B,** patella femoral grinding test.

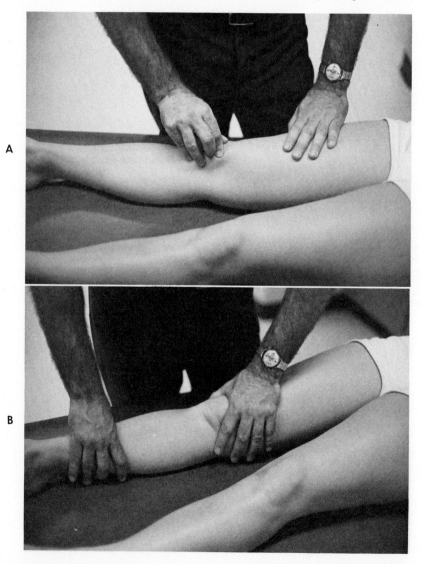

Fig. 15-22. Apprehension test for subluxing patella.

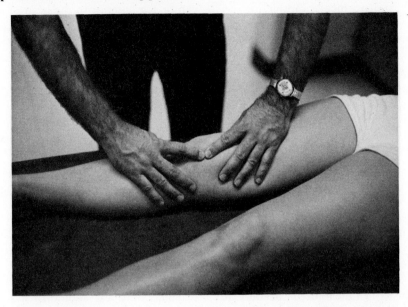

Fig. 15-23. Palpating quadriceps.

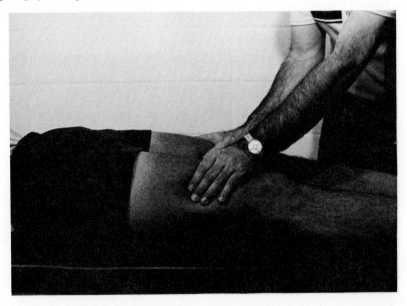

along this line may indicate an injury to the medial collateral ligament, medial capsule, or medial meniscus. Next gently palpate along the course of the medial collateral ligament between the proximal attachment on the adductor tubercle to the distal insertion below the pes anserinus. Tenderness at the proximal portion of the adductor tubercle may indicate an avulsion of the attachment of the vastus medialis, often associated with patellar dislocation.

To palpate the lateral aspect of the knee, begin at the front soft depression just lateral to the patellar tendon (Fig. 15-26) and palpate along the lateral joint line. Tenderness along the joint line in this area may indicate an injury to the lateral collateral ligament, lateral capsule, or lateral meniscus. The lateral collateral ligament is more distinguishable than the medial collateral. To augment the palpation of this ligament, have the athlete place the foot of the injured extremity on top of the uninjured knee (Fig. 15-27). This relaxes the iliotibial band and stretches the lateral collateral ligament, making it easy to palpate along its entire length. The tubercle of Gerdy,

which is the attachment for the iliotibial band, can be felt anterior to the head of the fibula.

In the posterior aspect of the knee, palpate the lateral and medial hamstring insertions. Feel along these tendons (Fig. 15-28) for any defects or tenderness that may indicate a strain. It is easier to palpate the hamstring tendons during resisted flexion of the knee. The two heads of the gastrocnemius muscle are also palpable at their origin just above the femoral condyles when the athlete flexes the knee against resistance. These are not as distinguishable as the hamstring tendons. The popliteal space can be palpated between the hamstring tendons and the heads of the gastrocnemius muscle. A swelling in this area may indicate a popliteal, or Baker's, cyst. This area is easier to palpate when the athlete's knee is extended (Fig. 15-29).

In addition to palpating for tenderness and swelling, note any additional indicators of injury. Feel for any change in skin temperature. A noticeable increase in peripheral skin temperature about the knee indicates an inflammatory process. A noticeable decrease in peripheral skin

Fig. 15-24. Palpating for patellar tendinitis.

Fig. 15-25. Palpating medial joint line.

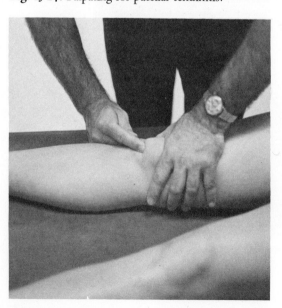

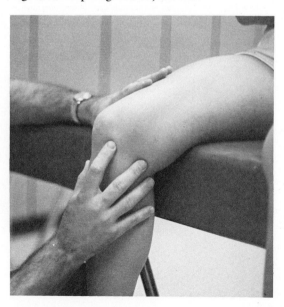

Fig. 15-26. Palpating lateral joint line.

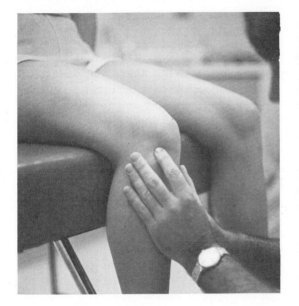

Fig. 15-27. Palpating medial lateral collateral ligament.

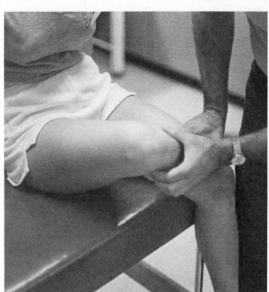

Fig. 15-28. Palpating hamstring tendons.

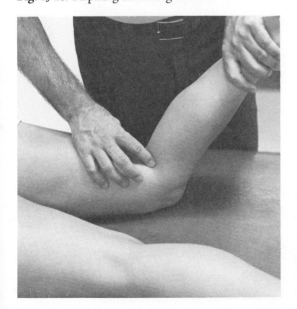

Fig. 15-29. Palpating popliteal space.

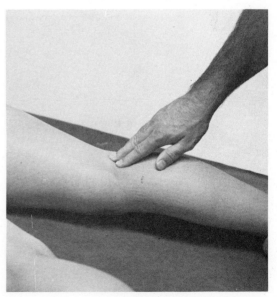

temperature below the knee may indicate the blood flow has been compromised by the injury. Also evaluate the circulation below an injured knee by feeling for a pulse. Whenever ligamentous injuries are of significant severity, consideration must be given to the possibility of vascular injury. The popliteal, posterior tibial, or dorsalis pedis pulses may be used to evaluate the circulation below the knee. Absence of a pulse below the knee after a significant injury indicates an immediate need for referral of the athlete to a physician or medical facility. Changes in skin texture (smooth or tight skin) may signal early edema before actual swelling is evident.

Stress

Stress tests should not be attempted until the history, observation, and palpation steps in the assessment are completed and you have some indication of the nature of the injury. This section will present the more common stress maneuvers that can be used to examine an injured knee. Not all of these procedures will be used on any one knee; the athletic trainer must select the appropriate maneuvers based on information obtained during the initial steps of the assessment sequence.

Before performing any of the manipulative tests, make sure the athlete is as relaxed as possible. It is easier to perform many of these stressful procedures with the athlete lying down. Relaxation is more apt to occur if you talk to the athlete and explain what you are going to do. Performing stress tests on the uninvolved knee first will demonstrate to the athlete what the tests are like and give you a bilateral comparison. Always remember to begin any stress procedures gently and carefully.

Active movements. Active movements should be performed first to evaluate the integrity of the contractile elements and discover any limitation of motion. Ask the athlete to flex and extend each knee. Is there limitation of motion? Most knee injuries are associated with a temporary lack of complete flexion. However, a lack of complete extension is usually a more significant sign and requires further evaluation. The lack of extension can be caused by swelling, muscle spasms, or locking. Does the athlete complain of any pain during active motion? If so, where? If

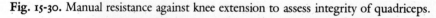

Fig. 15-30. Manual resistance against knee extension to assess integrity of quadriceps.

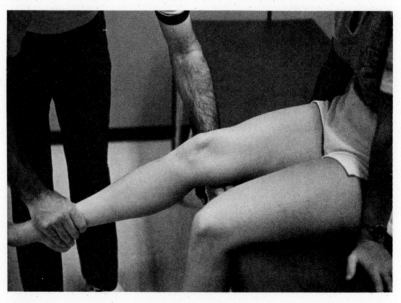

pain appears to be in the muscles, tendons, or musculotendinous junctions, further evaluation of these contractile tissues should follow using resistive movements.

Resistive movements. Resistive movements are used to further evaluate the integrity of contractile tissues. Manual resistance against knee extension, or asking the athlete to hold the knee in extension while attempting to force the knee into flexion (Fig. 15-30), will allow you to assess the integrity of the extensor mechanism. Manual resistance against flexion, or asking the athlete to hold the knee in some degree of flexion while attempting to force the knee into extension (Fig. 15-31), will allow you to assess the integrity of the flexor musculature. Pain with any resistive maneuvers is an indication of an injury to contractile tissue. For example, pain expressed on resistance to flexion coupled with previously identified point tenderness in the hamstring musculature indicates a strain in the hamstrings.

Passive movements. Passive movements are used to evaluate the integrity of the noncontractile tissues about the knee. Therefore all passive

---

Fig. 15-31. Manual resistance against knee flexion to assess integrity of hamstrings.

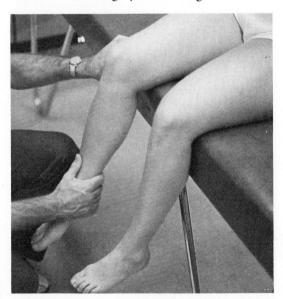

movements should be performed with the contractile units as relaxed as possible, which can be very difficult with an acute knee injury. If the athlete contracts the muscles about the injured knee, or if the muscles are in spasms during passive tests, accurate results are hard to achieve. The athletic trainer must reassure and calm the injured athlete to get him or her as relaxed as possible before initiating any passive stress tests or maneuvers. The time necessary for completing the history, observation, and palpation portion of the assessment process can greatly assist in attaining this goal. Proper positioning of the athlete and use of proper passive stress test techniques are important to ensure an accurate evaluation. The athlete should remain relaxed. Remember, all passive maneuvers should be performed gently to begin with, so as not to aggravate the injury and lose the athlete's cooperation. The intensity of force used with each of these maneuvers can then be increased on repeated tests, depending on the athlete's tolerance and the severity of the injury.

Passive procedures are used to locate instability in the supporting structures about the knee and to evaluate the degree of any laxity that may be present. Passive maneuvers are potentially the most informative procedures used in the assessment of knee injuries. Unfortunately, these maneuvers are also the most difficult to perform and are often subject to misinterpretation. Assessing joint instability is especially difficult for those persons first learning to perform passive stress tests. It takes much practice for anyone to become skilled in using these procedures. All stress tests should be performed consistently so you can become skilled in comparing the findings in any knee injury with those observed in previous injuries. If tests are performed differently each time, the evaluation will often be inaccurate and the findings inconsistent. Each athletic trainer must develop his or her own expertise in evaluating knee injuries and continue to refine the necessary techniques based on experience and knowledge. Following is a discussion of various passive stress tests that can be used to evaluate knee injuries and provide a basis for developing an individualized knee evaluation process.

Instability of ligamentous structures is determined by comparing the degree of separation, or movement, of the injured knee with that of the uninjured knee. The importance of constant comparison of the injured knee with the uninjured knee cannot be overemphasized. Instability, or the difference in movement between both knees, is normally rated according to the following scale: 0 indicates no difference in movement or separation; 1+, a mild instability, indicates the difference in separation between the injured knee and the uninjured knee is less than 0.5 cm; 2+, a moderate instability, indicates a difference of 0.5 to 1 cm; and 3+, a severe instability, indicates more than 1 cm difference between the two knees (Figs. 15-33 and 15-36). An important point to remember is that a negative test does not necessarily mean the supporting structures are intact. There are several factors that may prevent a passive stress test from being positive even when the ligament is ruptured. As already mentioned, muscle spasm, improper positioning, and improper techiques may compromise an accurate assessment. Joint effusion, meniscal tear, incomplete ligament tears, and the combined support of secondary ligaments can also interfere with an accurate test. In addition, the forces applied manually by the athletic trainer during an evaluation are very small compared to the amount of force placed on the knee during activity. An athlete may complain of instability during activity that cannot be demonstrated by passive evaluation techniques.

Stability and support of the knee joint involves many ligamentous and capsular structures that restrain abnormal motion. The primary support in one direction is provided by one or two ligaments, whereas other ligaments provide less important secondary restraints. Most knee injuries of any consequence involve more than one structure. Seldom is there an isolated ligament rupture. Therefore there are many possible laxities or instabilities that can result from in-

juries to various combinations of the supporting structures about the knee. Instabilities are named according to the movement of the tibia in relation to the femur and are listed in the box below. Straight instabilities refer to abnormal motion in one plane around one axis. Rotatory instabilities refer to abnormal motion in two or more planes around two or more axes. It is not the responsibility of the athletic trainer to evaluate precisely each instability that may exist. However, anyone responsible for evaluating an injured knee should be able to recognize instabilities when they are present and be able to refer the athlete to a physician skilled in the examination and care of knee injuries.

Medial (valgus) instability is evaluated by applying stress to those structures that support the medial side of the knee. The test most commonly used is called the **abduction stress test.** The athlete should be in a supine position with both legs supported by a table or ground to assist with relaxation and to avoid muscle contractions. During the actual test, it may be advantageous to lower the leg over the side of the table so that the thigh remains supported in an effort to keep the thigh muscles relaxed. To perform the abduction stress test, place one hand on the lateral side of the knee and place the other hand above the ankle. Then gently apply lateral stress against the ankle, and medial stress (valgus or abduction force) against the knee in an at-

---

INSTABILITIES OF THE KNEE

Straight instabilities

Medial
Lateral
Anterior
Posterior

Rotatory instabilities

Anteromedial
Anterolateral
Posterolateral
Combinations

tempt to open the knee joint on the inside. Repeat the test, increasing the stress gradually up to the point of pain. In this manner, the maximum instability can usually be demonstrated without evoking muscle spasms. Look for any separation or laxity at the medial joint line. The abduction stress test should be done with the knee first in complete extension and then in about 30° of flexion (Fig. 15-32). Medial laxity in complete extension usually reflects a more serious knee injury because the posterior capsule and the posterior cruciate ligament add to the stability of the knee when the leg is straight. Testing the knee in 30° of flexion slackens the poste-

Fig. 15-32. Abduction stress test to assess integrity of structures that support the medial side of the knee **A,** in complete extension and **B,** in approximately 30° of flexion.

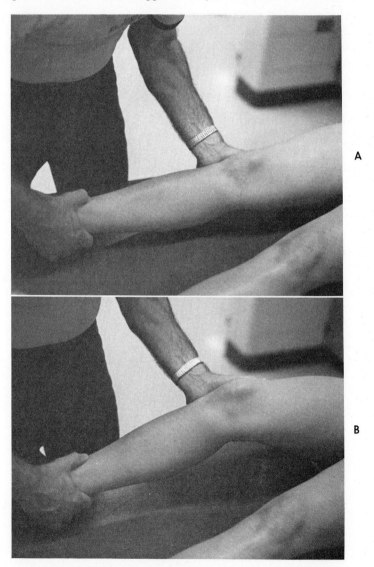

A

B

rior capsule and posterior cruciate ligament, which places more stress on the medial collateral ligament and medial capsule. Laxity or pain reflects an injury to these structures. Fig. 15-33 represents the rating scale for medial instability.

Lateral (varus) instability, instability of those structures supporting the outside or lateral aspect of the knee, is evaluated by means of the **adduction stress test.** As is shown in Fig. 15-34, the hand position is reversed from the abduction test so that one hand is placed on the inside of the knee and the other above the ankle. Medial stress is applied against the ankle and lateral stress (varus or adduction force) against the knee

in an attempt to open the knee joint on the outside. Look for any separation or laxity at the lateral joint line. Instability present in complete extension again indicates a more severe injury. The structures that may be involved include the lateral collateral ligament, the lateral capsule, and possibly the cruciate ligaments. Instability noted on flexion of the knee but not in complete extension, suggests that a rotatory instability exists. Injuries of this type are discussed on pp. 429 to 434.

Anterior instability can be evaluated in several ways. The most commonly used method is called the anterior **drawer test.** This test is best

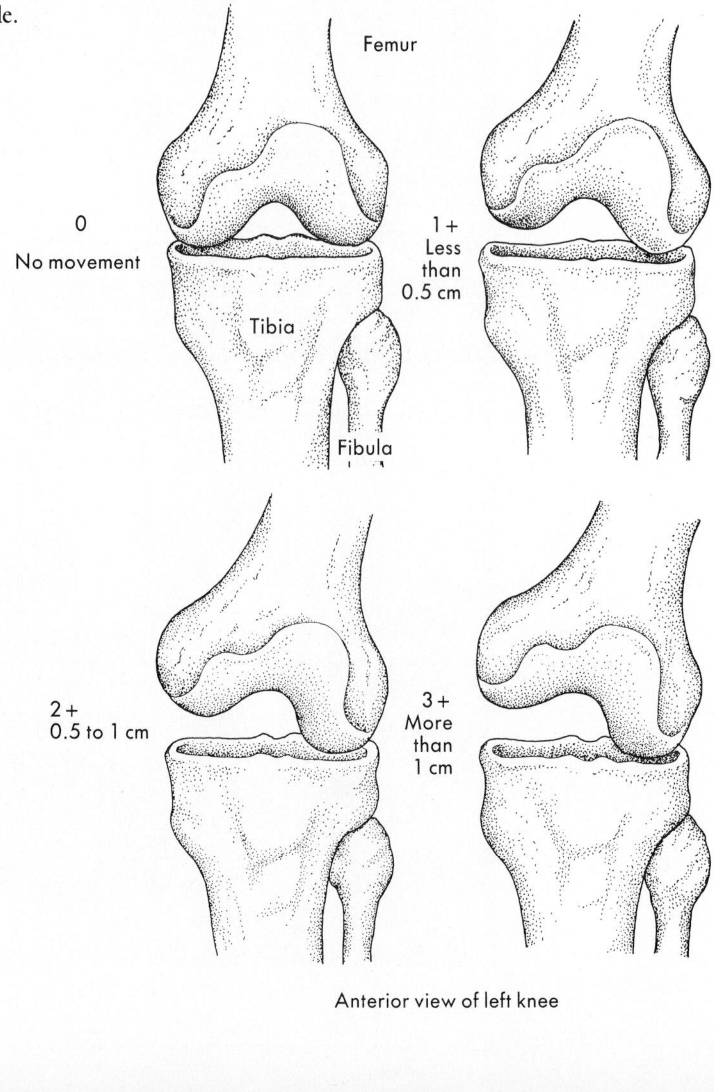

Fig. 15-33. Medial instability rating scale.

Femur

0
No movement

1+
Less than 0.5 cm

Tibia

Fibula

2+
0.5 to 1 cm

3+
More than 1 cm

Anterior view of left knee

Fig. 15-34. Adduction stress test to assess integrity of structures that support lateral side of knee.

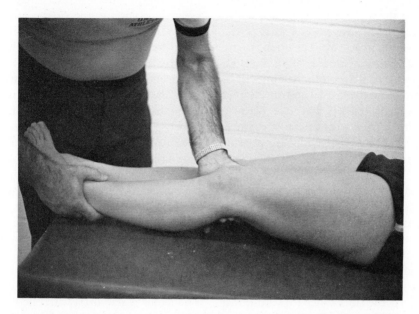

Fig. 15-35. Anterior drawer test to assess anterior stability. **A,** Knee flexed to 90° and foot flat on table; **B,** athlete sitting with knee hanging over edge of table and foot supported.

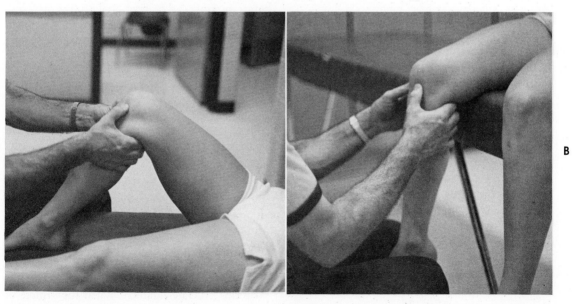

performed with the athlete in a comfortable, relaxed, supine position. The hip is flexed approximately 45°, and the knee about 80° to 90°, with the foot resting flat on the table (Fig. 15-35, *A*). The foot should be in a neutral position, facing straight ahead. Sit on the athlete's foot to stabilize it and cup your hands around the upper tibia, with your thumbs on the medial and lateral joint lines. Some athletic trainers prefer to perform the anterior drawer test with the athlete sitting and the knee hanging over the edge of the table (Fig. 15-35, *B*). The foot is them stabilized between the knees of the examiner and raised slightly to reduce the effects of gravity. If the foot is not supported, tension is applied to the remaining structures and the test is much more difficult to evaluate. Palpate the hamstring tendons with your fingers to make sure the muscles are relaxed. Gently pull the tibia forward. A slow steady pull is more effective than a jerk, which can elicit pain. If the tibia slides forward under the femur, a positive anterior drawer sign is present. Fig. 15-36 represents the rating scale for anterior instability. Instability indicates an injury involving the anterior cruciate ligament and possibly the joint capsule or the medial collateral ligament. Any instability noted should be evaluated for rotatory instability, which will be explained later.

Another test used to evaluate anterior instability is ***Lachman's test,*** which is normally more reliable than the anterior drawer test. It is particularly useful when muscle relaxation is a problem, because the hamstrings and the iliotibial band have little effect on the outcome. When the knee is flexed 90°, as with the anterior drawer test, the hamstrings directly oppose forward movement of the tibia. If the athlete contracts the hamstrings, or if the muscles are in spasm, there may not be any abnormal movement even though an instability exists.

Lachman's test is performed with the athlete supine on the table and the knee flexed 10° to 15°. The femur is stabilized with one hand while the other grasps the upper tibia with the thumb along the joint line, as shown in Fig. 15-37, *A*. When an athlete's leg is too large or the evaluator's hands too small to grasp the tibia in one hand, the tibia can be held between the arm and the chest of the evaluator as shown in Fig. 15-37, *B*. The tibia is then lifted forward and any instability noted.

Posterior instability is usually evaluated in conjunction with the anterior instability tests. It is presented separately only for instructional purposes. The posterior drawer test or Lachman's test is used to evaluate posterior instability. Positioning the athlete is the same as for anterior instability, except now the force applied to the tibia is directed backward, or posteriorly. An important point to remember before evaluating an athlete for posterior instability is the starting position of both knees. Whenever there is increased instability of any kind after an injury, the neutral or starting position becomes more difficult to define. This is especially true for the posterior cruciate ligament when the athlete is supine. Compare normal lateral contours with both knees flexed 90° and the feet flat on the

---

Fig. 15-36. Anterior instability rating scale.

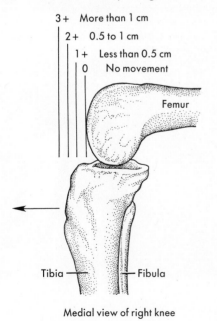

3+ More than 1 cm

2+ 0.5 to 1 cm

1+ Less than 0.5 cm

0 No movement

Femur

Tibia Fibula

Medial view of right knee

table. If posterior instability exists, the starting position may shift posteriorly because of gravity, and there will be a backward sag, or concave appearance, on the injured side when compared to the uninjured side. The results of posterior stress applied to the tibia in this abnormal starting position may be interpreted as negative, whereas anterior stress applied would bring this tibia to its normal position and may be falsely interpreted as a positive anterior drawer sign. When the lateral contours are normal at the start of a test and a positive posterior drawer sign (Lachman's sign) occurs, an injury to the posterior cruciate ligament has probably occurred.

Rotatory instabilities are abnormal anteropos-

Fig. 15-37. Lachman's test to assess anterior stability. **A,** Leg held in hand; **B,** leg held between arm and body of trainer.

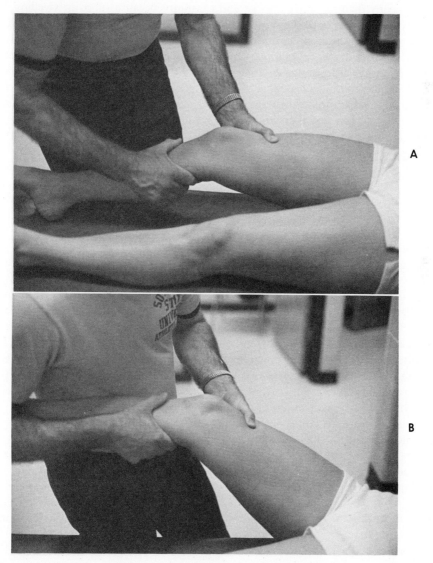

A

B

terior movements combined with internal or external rotation of the tibia. Tests for these rotatory instabilities are among the most complex procedures to perform and interpret. They are used to assist in completing a more thorough examination of an injured knee. The most common rotatory instabilities are anteromedial and anterolateral. Posterior rotatory instabilities have also been described. They are severe injuries normally associated with rupture of the posterior cruciate ligament. Fortunately, they occur less frequently than the anteromedial and anterolateral types. The basics of the more common anterior rotatory tests are presented in this text for general knowledge and for those more highly skilled in knee evaluations.

Rotatory instability should be evaluated initially in conjunction with the anterior and posterior drawer tests. Whenever a drawer test is positive and instability is noticed or felt, it is important to observe the movement of the tibia in relation to the femur. Watch and feel the medial and lateral tibial plateaus at the anterior joint line. Rotatory instability is indicated whenever both plateaus do not move equally. Does one of the tibial plateaus displace more anteriorly than the other during the anterior drawer test? For example, anteromedial rotatory instability is recognized by observing that the medial tibial plateau has a greater displacement forward than the lateral plateau during the anterior drawer test.

To test for *anteromedial rotatory instability,* repeat the anterior drawer test with the athlete's tibia in external rotation (Fig. 15-38, *A*). When the tibia is externally rotated, the cruciate ligaments unwind from each other and more stress is applied to the medial structures such as the medial capsule and the medial collateral ligament. Anteromedial rotatory instability is indicated if the medial tibial plateau rotates and displaces anteriorly from beneath the medial femoral condyle.

To test for *anterolateral rotatory instability,* which occurs more frequently, repeat the anterior drawer test with the tibia internally rotat-

ed (Fig. 15-38, *B*). The cruciate ligaments are tightened as the tibia is internally rotated. In addition, additional stress is placed on the posterolateral capsule, the iliotibial band, and lateral collateral ligament. Anterolateral rotatory instability is indicated if the lateral tibial plateau rotates and displaces anteriorly from beneath the lateral femoral condyle.

There are additional tests used to evaluate anterolateral rotatory instability of the knee. Normally these tests are not used on an acute knee injury because of pain, swelling, or protective muscle spasms. They may be used on follow-up assessments or under anesthesia to evaluate the presence of anterolateral rotatory instability. These tests, if positive, involve subluxating and relocating the anterolateral aspect of the tibial condyle from under the lateral femoral condyle at approximately 30° of flexion.

The *lateral pivot shift test* starts with the leg in an extended position with internal rotation of the tibia and valgus stress at the knee (Fig. 15-39, *A*). If positive, this produces a subluxation of the lateral aspect of the tibial condyle, and as the knee is flexed to around 30° there is a sudden visible, palpable, and audible reduction of the subluxation (Fig. 15-39, *B*).

The *Slocum test* is a modification of the lateral pivot shift test that begins with the athlete lying on the uninjured side. The uninjured leg is flexed at the hip and knee. Again the tibia of the injured leg is internally rotated, valgus force is applied to the knee, and the knee is flexed (Fig. 15-40, *A*). As the knee is flexed approximately 30°, the subluxation will reduce visibly, palpably, and audibly if an anterolateral rotatory instability is present (Fig. 15-40, *B*).

Another test for anterolateral rotatory instability is the *jerk test.* This begins with the knee in 90° flexion, a valgus force at the knee, and the tibia internally rotated. The leg is then extended, and if the test is positive, there is a "jerk" when the tibial condyle subluxes at about 30° and another "snap" or "pop" as relocation occurs as the knee is extended.

The presence of an audible click or sudden

jump as these maneuvers are performed is usually indicative of anterolateral rotatory instability. However, there are conditions, such as a torn meniscus, which may give a false positive test. These procedures are normally used by those athletic trainers more highly skilled in evaluating knee injuries.

Posterolateral rotatory instability occurs when the lateral tibial plateau displaces backward in relation to the lateral femoral condyle. This is a serious injury resulting from damage to the *arcuate complex,* which consists of the arcuate ligament, the popliteal tendon, the lateral collateral ligament, and the posterior third of the capsular ligament. The resulting instability can be recognized by two specific tests, the postero-

Fig. 15-38. Anterior drawer test for rotatory instability. **A,** Anteromedial test with athlete's leg externally rotated; **B,** anterolateral test with athlete's leg internally rotated.

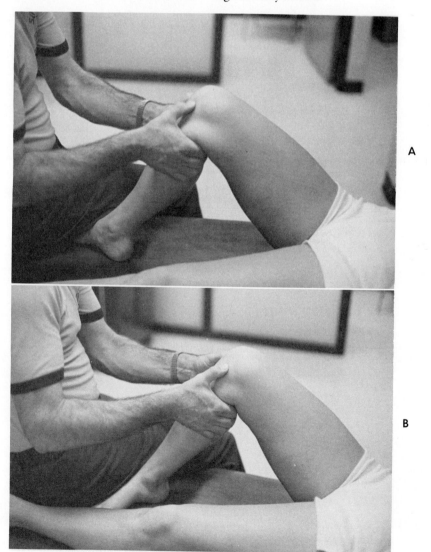

A

B

Fig. 15-39. Lateral pivot shift test. **A,** Leg extended with internal rotation of the tibia and valgus stress at the knee; **B,** knee flexed to approximately 30°. If this test is positive, there will be a subluxation of the lateral aspect of the tibial condyle.

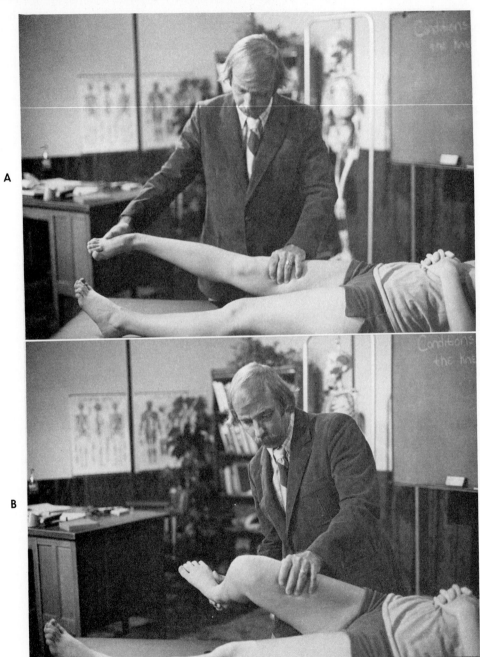

Fig. 15-40. Slocum anterolateral rotatory instability test. **A,** Athlete lying on the uninjured side with the tibia internally rotated and a valgus force applied to the knee; **B,** knee flexed approximately 30°. If this test is positive, there will be a subluxation of the lateral aspect of the tibial condyle.

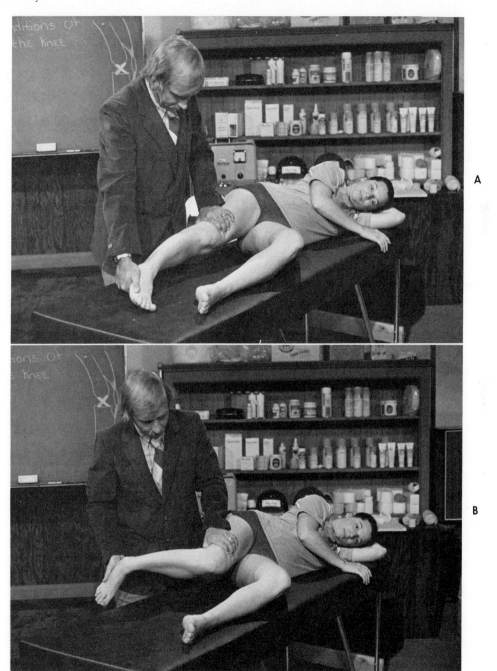

A

B

lateral drawer test and the external rotational recurvatum test. The posterolateral drawer sign is only positive when the posterior drawer test is performed with the tibia in external rotation. This same test would be negative with the tibia internally rotated because of an intact posterior cruciate ligament. The *external rotational recurvatum test* is performed with both legs extended and the feet held by the heels (Fig. 15-41). The test is positive if the tibia shows excessive hyperextension and external rotation.

Meniscus tests. There are also passive stress tests that can be performed to detect an injury to a meniscus. Point tenderness along the joint line, especially in the absence of a positive abduction or adduction stress test, may indicate an injury to the meniscus. If so, further evaluation should be carried out. With the presence of significant ligament instabilities, it may be extremely difficult to recognize an associated meniscus injury. Specific meniscal tests need not be performed at this time, and the athlete should be treated for the ligament laxity. The torn meniscus may then

be recognized on further diagnostic tests by the physician or picked up on repeated evaluations by the athletic trainer.

All of the meniscal tests are founded on the same mechanical basis, attempting to trap or pinch the injured meniscus between the articular surfaces of the femur and tibia by performing various circumduction or rotatory maneuvers. The torn meniscus may cause pain or a clicking or snapping sensation during these procedures. The *McMurray test* is performed with the athlete supine and the hip and knee flexed maximally. Hold the athlete's heel in one hand and palpate the medial and lateral joint lines with the thumb and index finger of the other hand (Fig. 15-42, *A*). Internally and externally rotate the tibia with the hand holding the heel to loosen the knee joint and ensure that the athlete is relaxed. With the tibia in external rotation, apply a gentle medial (valgus) force to the knee and extend the leg passively while feeling and listening for any clicking or snapping (Fig. 15-42, *B*). This maneuver will evaluate the integrity of the me-

Fig. 15-41. External rotational recurvatum test for posterolateral rotatory instability. The test is positive if the tibia shows excessive hyperextension and external rotation.

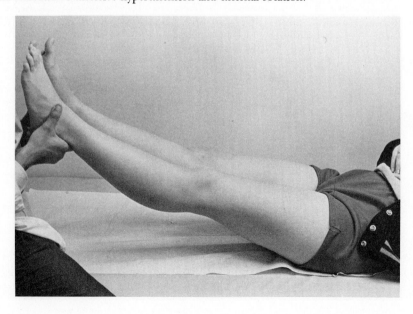

dial meniscus. To test the lateral meniscus, repeat the test with the tibia in internal rotation and apply a lateral (varus) force during extension.

Another test that can be used to evaluate a meniscus is *Apley's compression test*. Have the athlete lie prone (on the stomach) with the injured knee flexed to 90°. Apply pressure on the heel in an attempt to compress the articular surfaces of the tibia and femur while rotating the tibia (Fig. 15-43, *A*). While continuing to maintain compression, extend the leg in an attempt to

Fig. 15-42. McMurray test to test the integrity of the menisci. **A,** Hip and knee flexed while palpating the joint lines; **B,** to test the medial meniscus, externally rotate the tibia and apply a valgus force to the knee as it is passively extended.

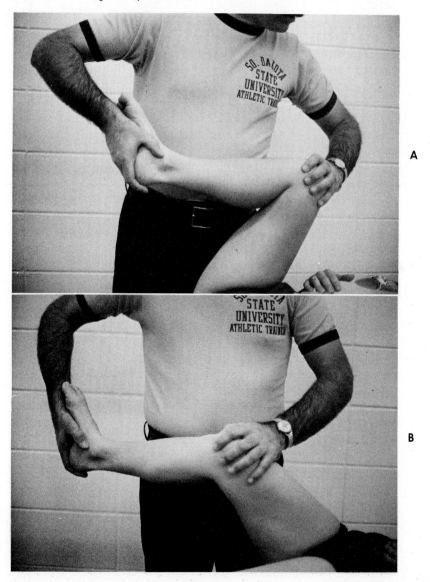

A

B

elicit pain as the meniscus becomes entrapped between the articular surfaces (Fig. 15-43, *B*). Pain or clicking may indicate an injured meniscus.

Apley's distraction test can also be performed at this time to differentiate between a meniscal and ligamentous injury. Stabilize the athlete's thigh by putting your knee on the back of his or her thigh and pull up on the leg to distract the knee joint (Fig. 15-44). While maintaining traction on the leg, rotate the tibia internally and externally to stress the medial and lateral liga-

Fig. 15-43. Apley's compression test for assessment of meniscal integrity. **A,** With the knee flexed to 90°, apply pressure on the heel while rotating the tibia; **B,** maintain compression as the leg is passively extended.

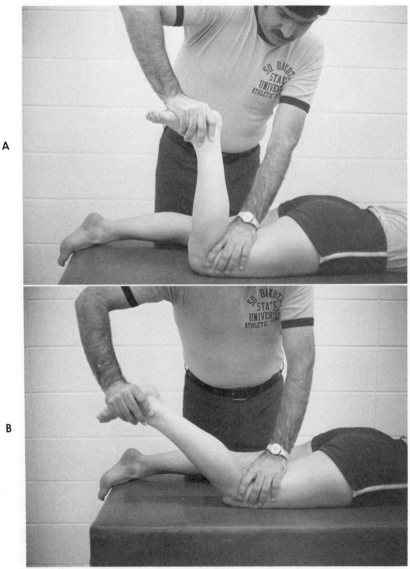

ments while reducing pressure on the menisci. If the athlete has suffered ligamentous injury, this maneuver should elicit pain. If the athlete has suffered only a meniscal injury, this maneuver should not elicit any additional pain.

Functional movements

Functional movements are used primarily to determine when an injured athlete can safely return to activity. However, functional tests can also be used during the initial assessment process in an attempt to localize pain or instability. There will be times when the evaluation will not demonstrate a significant injury or problem with the knee, yet the athlete will continue to complain of pain and instability. In these instances the evaluation should continue and include functional tests.

One method of using a functional test is to ask the athlete to reproduce the injury-producing event as closely as possible to assist in identifying those structures that may be involved. Pain or instability may be demonstrated in this manner when passive tests are negative.

Ask the athlete to squat, bounce up and down, or duck walk. Continue to increase the intensity of the functional activities in an attempt to demonstrate pain or instability. Have the athlete run at various speeds, run figure eights, and perform cutting, starting, stopping, and jumping maneuvers. The inability to perform these functional activities, or pain associated with them, will assist in identifying injuries or conditions requiring further diagnostic tests.

Evaluation of findings

The nature and severity of knee injuries can be extremely difficult to accurately evaluate. A significant knee injury is usually quite easy to recognize and identify. However, less serious knee injuries present the athletic trainer with a difficult and challenging task. The following questions must be considered when evaluating an injured knee. How seriously injured is the knee? Should the athlete be referred for further diagnosis? When can the athlete safely return to activity? Many times these are not easy questions to answer. The degree of success in answering these questions and accurately evaluating knee injuries is directly related to the level of skill and experience of the person performing the assessment. This chapter has presented basic evaluative procedures and techniques, as well as guidelines to assist athletic trainers in assessing knee injuries.

When to refer the athlete

Not all knee injuries require referral to a physician or medical facility. Some injured knees, providing they are accurately evaluated, can be properly cared for without seeking addi-

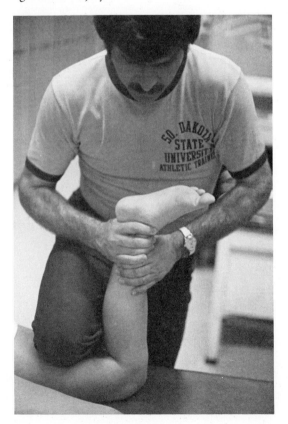

Fig. 15-44. Apley's distraction test to differentiate between meniscal and ligamentous injury.

ATHLETIC INJURY ASSESSMENT CHECKLIST
KNEE INJURIES

Secondary survey

———— History
———— Previous injury
———— Nature
———— Treatment
———— Extent of rehabilitation
———— Similar symptoms
———— Surgery
———— Present injury
———— Onset
———— Mechanism of injury
———— Pain
———— Swelling
———— Loss of motion
———— Locking
———— Sensations
———— Postinjury course
———— Continued activity
———— Symptoms
———— Sensations
———— Observations
———— Bear weight
———— Limp
———— Alignment
———— Q angle
———— Signs of trauma
———— Swelling
———— Atrophy
———— Palpation
———— Tenderness
———— Swelling
———— Effusion
———— Tests
———— Patella femoral grinding
———— Apprehension
———— Skin temperature and texture
———— Pulses
———— Stress
———— Active movements
———— Range of motion
———— Pain
———— Resistive movements
———— Pain
———— Strength
———— Passive movements
———— Pain
———— Instability

ATHLETIC INJURY ASSESSMENT CHECKLIST
KNEE INJURIES—cont'd

_____ Medial
_____ Abduction stress
_____ Lateral
_____ Adduction stress
_____ Anterior
_____ Drawer test
_____ Lachman's test
_____ Posterior
_____ Drawer test
_____ Lachman's test
_____ Anteromedial rotatory
_____ Drawer test (tibia externally rotated)
_____ Anterolateral rotatory
_____ Drawer test (tibia internally rotated)
_____ Lateral pivot shift
_____ Slocum test
_____ Jerk test
_____ Posterolateral rotatory
_____ Posterior drawer test (tibia externally rotated)
_____ External rotational recurvatum test
_____ Meniscal test
_____ McMurray test
_____ Apley's compression test
_____ Apley's distraction test
_____ Functional movements
_____ Replicate mechanism of injury
_____ Functional activities
_____ Jogging
_____ Running
_____ Figure of eights
_____ Cutting
_____ Jumping
_____ Starting and stopping
_____ Squatting
_____ Bounce up and down
_____ Duck walk

tional medical assistance. However, because of the complexity of the joint and the importance of early care, injuries involving the knee frequently require referral and further assistance for an accurate assessment. There are guidelines that can assist in determining if a knee injury is significant and if referral or further assessment is indicated. The following list of conditions or findings in box on p. 440 indicate the athlete should be withheld from further activity until an accurate assessment of the knee is completed and the cause of the condition has been determined.

Gross deformity

Significant swelling and especially an early he-marthrosis

Loss of motion

Joint instability

Significant pain

Abnormal sensations such as clicking, popping, grating, or weakness

Locked knee

Any doubt regarding the severity or nature of the injury

KEY TERMS

abduction stress test Passive procedure used to evaluate medial stability

adduction stress test Passive procedure used to evaluate lateral stability

anterolateral rotatory instability Anterior displacement of the lateral tibial plateau with respect to the femur during testing of the knee

anteromedial rotatory instability Anterior displacement of the medial tibial plateau with respect to the femur during testing of the knee

Apley's compression test Test to evaluate the integrity of the menisci; with the athlete lying prone and the injured knee flexed 90°, pressure is applied to the heel in an attempt to entrap a torn meniscus between the articular surfaces

Apley's distraction test Test to differentiate between a meniscal and ligamentous injury; with the athlete lying prone and the injured knee flexed 90°, pull up and rotate on the tibia in an attempt to distract the knee joint. If a ligamentous injury has occurred, this maneuver should elicit pain

apprehension test Test to evaluate if the athlete has subluxed or dislocated the patella; with the leg flexed about 20°, push the patella laterally and note the reaction of the athlete. Normally there will be no reaction or pain; apprehension about lateral movement of the kneecap indicates possible subluxation

arcuate complex Complex formed by the arcuate ligament, the popliteal tendon, the lateral collateral ligament, and the posterior third of the capsular ligament

ballotable patella Palpatory procedure for evaluating marked effusion of the knee; when the patella is pressed down and released quickly, the large amount of fluid under it causes the kneecap to rebound or appear to be floating

chondromalacia patellae Degenerative process that results in a softening or degeneration of the articular surface of the patella

drawer test Passive procedure used to evaluate anterior and posterior stability with the knee flexed 90°

external rotational recurvatum test Test for posterolateral rotatory instability in which both legs are held extended by the heels; a positive test results in the tibia showing excessive hyperextension and external rotation

genu recurvatum (knee hyperextension) Angulation of leg posteriorly (backward) from the midline of the body

genu valgus (knock knees) Angulation of lower leg laterally (away) from the midline of the body

genu varum (bowlegs) Angulation of lower leg medially (toward) the midline of the body

hemarthrosis Accumulation of blood in the joint cavity

jerk test Test for anterolateral rotatory instability in which the knee is flexed to 90°, the tibia is internally rotated, and a valgus stress is applied to the knee; audible and palpable sublux of the lateral tibial plateau at approximately 30° to 40° on passive extension and relocation as it approaches complete extension indicates a positive test

joint effusion Accumulation of fluid in a joint cavity

jumper's knee (patellar tendinitis) Inflammatory response to repeated stress or irritation at the patellar tendon insertion

Lachman's test Passive procedure used to evaluate anterior and posterior stability with the knee flexed 10° to 15°

lateral pivot shift test Test for anterolateral rotatory instability; with the leg extended, the tibia internally rotated, and a valgus stress at the knee, the knee is passively flexed. If the test is positive, the lateral tibial plateau subluxes immediately and relocates again at approximately 30° to 40°

McMurray test   Test to evaluate the integrity of the menisci; the athlete's hip and knee are flexed maximally, and as the leg is passively extended the tibia is rotated as valgus or varus force is applied to the knee

Osgood-Schlatter syndrome   Condition involving the epiphysis of the tibial tuberosity in adolescents

osteochondritis dissecans   Condition of unknown cause in which a segment of subchondral bone undergoes avascular necrosis

patella femoral grinding test   Test to evaluate the integrity of the underside of the knee cap; the patella is pushed manually against the femoral condyles and the athlete is asked to contract the quadriceps as pressure is maintained

posterolateral rotatory instability   Occurs when the lateral tibial plateau displaces backwards in relation to the lateral femoral condyle

Q angle   Angle formed by a line from the anterior superior iliac spine to the midpatella and another line from midpatella to the tibial tuberosity; an angle of 15° or less is considered normal

Slocum test   Test for anterolateral rotatory instability similar to the pivot shift except the athlete is placed on his or her uninjured side

squinting patellae   Patellae that appear to face inward when the feet are pointed straight ahead

valgus   Bent outward; denoting a deformity in which the angulation of the distal part is away from the midline of the body

varus   Bent inward; denoting a deformity in which the angulation of the distal part is toward the midline of the body

SUGGESTED READINGS

American Academy of Orthopaedic Surgeons: Symposium on the athlete's knee: surgical repair and reconstruction, St. Louis, 1980, The C.V. Mosby Co.

Arnheim, D.D.: Modern principles of athletic training, ed. 6, St. Louis, 1985, Times Mirror/Mosby College Publishing.

Davies, G.J., and Larson, R.: Examining the knee, Physician Sportsmedicine, 6:49-67, 1978.

Davies, G.J., and others: Knee examination, Physical Therapy 60:1565-1574, 1980.

Davies, G.J., and others: Mechanisms of selected knee injuries, Physical Therapy 60:1590-1595, 1980.

Derscheid, G.L., and Malone, T.R.: Knee disorders, Physical Therapy 60:1582-1589, 1980.

Detnbeck, L.C.: Function of the cruciate ligaments in knee stability J. Sports Medicine 2:217-221, 1974.

Ellison, A.E.: Skiing injuries, CIBA Clinical Symposia 29:1, 1977.

Hoppenfeld, S.: Physical examination of the spine and extremities, New York, 1976, Appleton-Century-Crofts.

Hughston, J.C., and others: Classification of knee ligament instabilities. Part I. The medial compartment and cruciate ligaments J. Bone Joint Surg. 58:159-179, 1976.

McCluskey, G., and Blackburn, T.A.: Classification of knee ligament instabilities, Physical Therapy 60:1575-1577, 1980.

Mercier, L.R., and Pettid, F.J.: Practical orthopedics, Chicago, 1980, Year Book Medical Publishers, Inc.

Noyes, F.R., and others: Knee sprains and acute knee hemarthrosis, Physical Therapy 60:1596-1601, 1980.

O'Donoghue, D.H.: Treatment of injuries to athletes, ed. 4, Philadelphia, 1984, W.B. Saunders Co.

Paulos, L., and others: Patellar malalignment, Physical Therapy 60:1624-1632, 1980.

Roy, S., and Irvin, R.: Sports medicine: prevention, evaluation, management, and rehabilitation, Englewood Cliffs, N.J., 1983, Prentice-Hall, Inc.

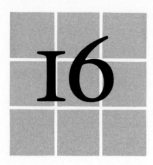

16

Thigh and hip injuries

The thigh and hip present contrasting characteristics in relation to the incidence of athletic injuries. The thigh muscles are subjected to extreme stresses during most athletic activity and are very vulnerable to impact forces, especially during contact sports. As a result of these factors, the thigh is among those areas of the body more commonly injured during athletics. The hip, on the other hand, is one of the strongest and most stable joints in the body; athletic injuries to this joint are relatively uncommon.

However, athletic injuries occurring to the thigh and hip are similar in that most injuries involve the musculotendinous unit.

It is important to re-emphasize that the study of assessment procedures should always begin with a careful review of appropriate regional anatomy. The major skeletal components of the thigh and hip are reviewed in Fig. 16-1. It is particularly important to note the anatomic landmarks on the femur and bony pelvis. Such bony prominences provide for the attachment of major muscles and also serve as palpation reference points during the assessment process.

The muscles of the thigh and hip are illustrated in Fig. 16-2. The muscles are listed by function in the box on p. 445. Table 16-1 lists the origin and insertion of each muscle. Because the majority of athletic injuries to the thigh and hip are muscular in nature, each major muscle is illustrated separately. The more common athletic injuries occurring to the thigh and hip are also discussed.

ANATOMY OF THE THIGH

The femur, the long single bone of the thigh, is surrounded by thick musculature. The proximal portion of the femur is discussed in more detail later in this chapter along with the hip. The distal femur was previously discussed in conjunction with the knee. The major muscles of the thigh, the quadriceps and hamstrings, are illustrated in Figs. 16-3 and 16-4. These muscles were also discussed in Chapter 15 in relation to their function about the knee joint. During

Fig. 16-1. Major skeletal components of the thigh and hip.

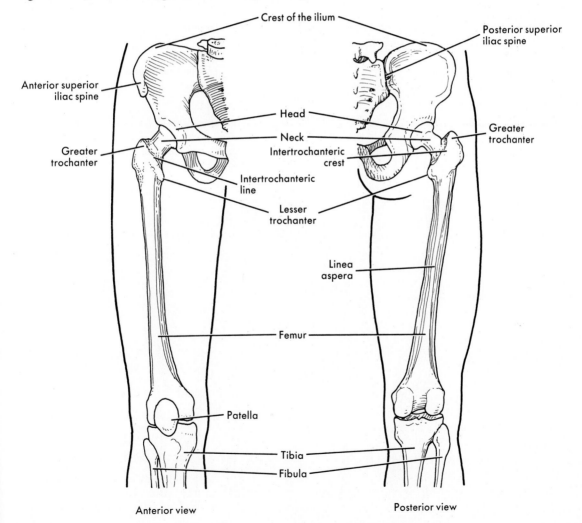

Crest of the ilium

Posterior superior iliac spine

Anterior superior iliac spine

Head

Neck

Greater trochanter

Intertrochanteric crest

Greater trochanter

Intertrochanteric line

Lesser trochanter

Linea aspera

Femur

Patella

Tibia

Fibula

Anterior view

Posterior view

athletic activity, these muscles are subjected to many stresses that may result in injury.

INJURIES TO THE THIGH
Contusions

Contusions are a common thigh injury. Contusions to the anterior thigh, or quadriceps muscle group, occur frequently and are often the result of a direct blow, as illustrated in Fig. 16-5. This type of injury, commonly called a *Charley horse,* occurs frequently during contact activities. Symptoms of a contusion may range from mild tenderness with little restriction of motion

to marked pain, swelling, and disability. A potentially serious assessment problem with thigh contusions is delayed or silent bleeding within the injured muscle that may continue for varying periods of time. In these cases the full extent of the injury may not be recognized for 12 to 24 hours. Frequently the athlete will continue activity during this time, and only after re-evaluation the following day will the severity of the injury be recognized. The signs and symptoms of a muscle contusion will depend on the severity and location of the injury, but usually there are varying degrees of pain, tenderness, swelling,

Fig. 16-2. Muscles of the thigh and hip.

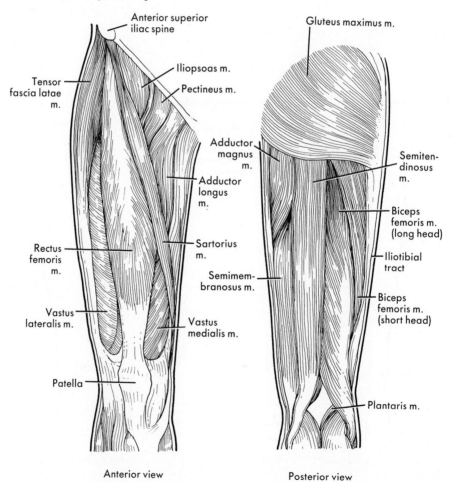

Anterior view

Posterior view

MUSCLES ACTING ON THE HIP JOINT

Flexion

Psoas major
Iliacus
Pectineus (secondary)
Rectus femoris (secondary)
Sartorius (secondary)
Adductors (secondary)

Extension

Gluteus maximus
Biceps femoris (long head)
Semitendinosus
Semimembranosus

Abduction

Gluteus medius
Gluteus minimus
Tensor fasciae latae (secondary)
Sartorius (secondary)

Adduction

Adductor longus
Adductor brevis
Adductor magnus
Pectineus (secondary)
Gracilis (secondary)

Medial rotation

Iliopsoas
Gluteus medius (anterior fibers)
Tensor fasciae latae
Gluteus minimus (anterior fibers)

Lateral rotation

Obturator internus
Obturator externus
Gemelli
Quadratus femoris
Sartorius (secondary)
Piriformis (secondary)

Table 16-1. Muscles acting on the hip joint—points of attachment

Muscle	Origin	Insertion
Psoas major	Lumbar vertebrae (transverse processes)	Lesser trochanter of femur
Iliacus	Upper two thirds of iliac fossa	Tendon of psoas major and body of femur
Pectineus	Tubercle of pubis	Femur—lesser trochanter to linea aspera
Rectus femoris	Anterior inferior iliac spine Groove above acetabulum	Base of patella
Sartorius	Anterior superior iliac spine	Upper tibia
Gluteus maximus	Iliac crest/sacrum/coccyx	Iliotibial band of fascia lata
Biceps femoris (long head)	Tuberosity of ischium	Head of fibula
Semitendinosus	Tuberosity of ischium	Body of tibia (medial surface)
Semimembranosus	Tuberosity of ischium	Medial condyle of tibia
Gluteus medius	Ilium (outer surface)	Greater trochanter of femur (lateral surface)
Gluteus minimus	Ilium (outer surface)	Capsule of hip joint Greater trochanter (anterior border)
Tensor fasciae latae	Iliac crest Anterior superior iliac spine	Iliotibial band
Adductor longus	Pubic symphysis and pubic crest	Linea aspera (middle portion)
Adductor brevis	Inferior ramus of pubis	Linea aspera (upper portion)
Adductor magnus	Inferior ramus of pubis	Linea aspera (lower portion)
Gracilis	Symphysis pubis	Body of tibia
Obturator internus	Ischium	Greater trochanter
Obturator externus	Rami of pubis Ramus of ischium	Trochanteric fossa of femur
Gemelli	Spine of ischium	Greater trochanter
Quadratus femoris	Tuberosity of ischium	Greater trochanter
Piriformis	Sacrum	Greater trochanter

Fig. 16-3. Quadriceps femoris group of thigh muscles.

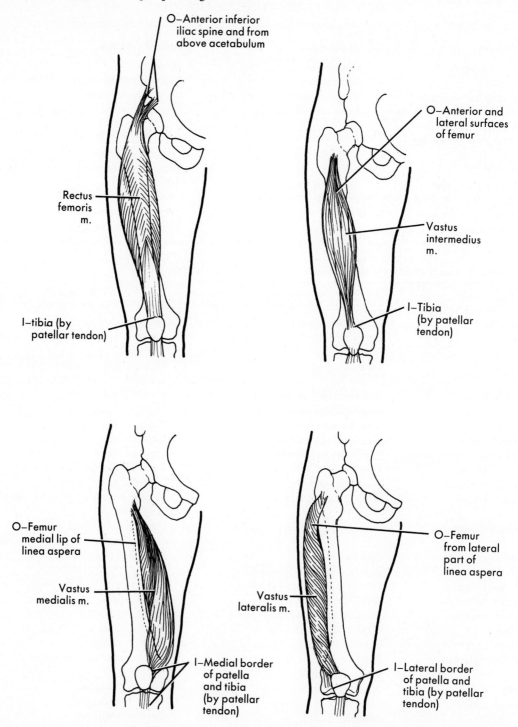

Fig. 16-4. Hamstring group of thigh muscles.

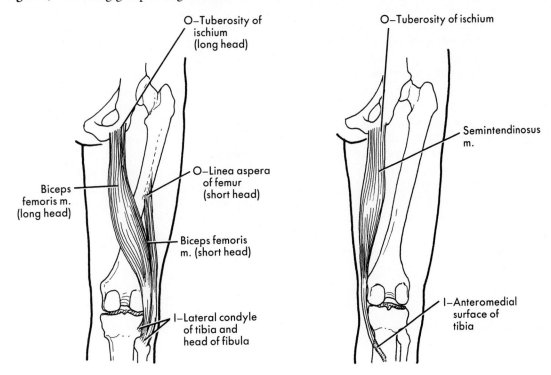

O–Tuberosity of
ischium
(long head)

O–Tuberosity of ischium

Biceps
femoris m.
(long head)

O–Linea aspera
of femur
(short head)

Biceps femoris
m. (short head)

Semintendinosus
m.

I–Lateral condyle
of tibia and
head of fibula

I–Anteromedial
surface of
tibia

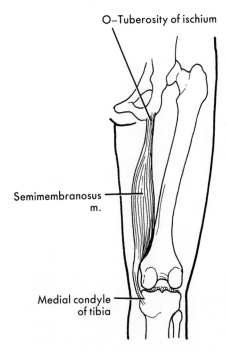

O–Tuberosity of ischium

Semimembranosus
m.

Medial condyle
of tibia

and restricted motion or function. The signs and symptoms associated with thick-muscle injuries are often less localized than in other more subcutaneous areas of the body. As with the thigh strain, the signs and symptoms of a thigh contusion are intensified by active and resistive motion.

A complication to be aware of when dealing with thigh contusions is *myositis ossificans,* which was described in Chapter 7. Myositis ossificans can occur anywhere in the body but more frequently involves the quadriceps. The bony deposits may occur as a separate piece or pieces of bone lying entirely within the muscle or by direct attachment to the femur. This complication

seldom develops as a result of a single injury; it is more likely to occur after chronic irritation, such as continued use of the injured quadriceps or repeated trauma to the thigh. Whatever the reason, the hematoma fails to resolve, resulting in myositis ossificans (Fig. 16-6). It is important for the athletic trainer to recognize the possibility of myositis ossificans after a severe thigh contusion or repeated bruising. This condition should always be suspected if hematoma formation does not promptly resolve and pain, a palpable mass within the muscle, and loss of motion persists for 2 to 3 weeks. When this occurs, the athlete should be withheld from activity until symptoms subside. It is important that athletes suffering from severe thigh contusions be evaluated frequently.

Strains

Muscle strains are another common thigh injury. The type of sudden violent contractions or stretching of muscles associated with running and jumping activities frequently results in strains (Fig. 16-7, *A*). Conditions which may contribute to muscles strains are lack of flexibility, fatigue, inadequate warm-up, muscle weaknesses, deficiency in the reciprocal action of opposing muscles, or imbalance between quadriceps and hamstring strength. The severity of thigh strains may range from muscle cramps to complete tears, or ruptures. The hamstrings are strained more frequently than the quadriceps. This type of injury tends to recur and frequently becomes a chronic problem. The signs and symptoms most commonly associated with thigh strains are pain, tenderness, muscle spasm, and loss of function, motion, or strength. Usually these signs and symptoms are intensified by both active and resistive motion. In moderate to severe strains, the athlete often experiences a pop or snap in the musculature, with immediate pain and loss of function. There may be a palpable gap within the torn fibers or a lump resulting from the contraction of ruptured muscle tissue or hematoma. Ecchymosis may appear a few days after the injury as blood collects under the skin (Fig. 16-7, *B*).

Fig. 16-5. Quadriceps muscle contusion caused by a direct blow.

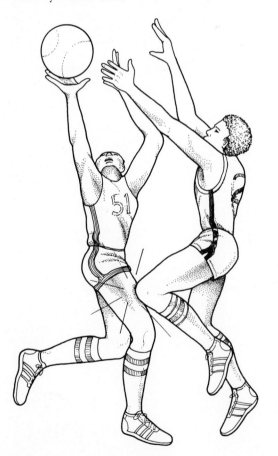

Fig. 16-6. Myositis ossificans. **A,** Calcification in quadriceps muscle after a thigh contusion; **B,** no external evidence of calcification apparent.

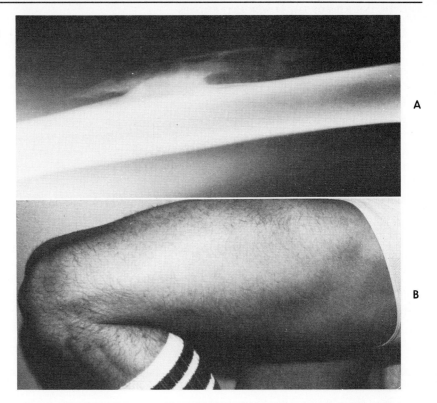

Fig. 16-7. Muscle strain. **A,** Runner suddenly straining a hamstring muscle as a result of a violent contraction. **B,** Ecchymosis five days following a hamstring strain.
(Courtesy Dr. James Garrick, Center for Sports Medicine, St. Francis Memorial Hospital, San Francisco)

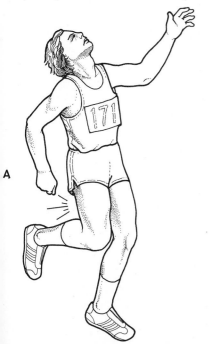

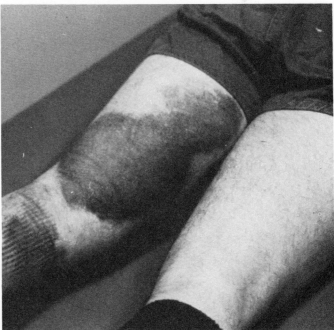

Fractures

Fractures to the shaft of the femur occur infrequently during athletic activity. When they do occur, it is normally the result of a tremendous force, such as a violent direct blow, or excessive rotatory stress. Most of the time the ankle, leg, or knee will give way before the femur fractures during a traumatic episode. When the femur is fractured, disability or loss of function is usually immediate, accompanied by a significant amount of pain. Because of the strength of the musculature surrounding the femur, bony displacement, causing an overriding of the bone fragments, may occur. This can cause a shortened limb on the fractured side. Additional signs and symptoms may include deformity or abnormal rotation of the thigh, swelling of the soft tissues, and shock. Athletes with fractured femurs should be immediately immobilized and referred to medical attention.

ANATOMY OF THE HIP
Hip joint

The hip joint, made up of the head of the femur and the acetabulum, is perhaps the best example of a diarthrodial ball-and-socket joint in the body. Like the shoulder joint, the hip is multiaxial. The hip, however, is modified in several ways to increase its stability. As a result of these modifications, the hip is less mobile than the shoulder and shows less freedom of movement. The articulation of the hip occurs between the cup-shaped acetabulum of the innominate, or pelvic, bone and the smooth, globular head of the femur (Fig. 16-8). The depth of the acetabulum is increased by a triangular rim of fibrocartilage called the *acetabular labrum,* which forms an incomplete ring around the margin of the socket. The labrum actually turns into the acetabular cavity and embraces the head of the femur. The stability of the hip is largely the result of the shape of the head of the femur and the deep acetabular socket into which the femoral head fits. Stability is also effected by the powerful and dense ligaments, especially those located in front of the joint.

Articular (fibrous) capsule

The articular, or fibrous, capsule that encloses the hip joint is quite dense and very strong. The capsule is attached above to the bony margin of the acetabulum and to the acetabular labrum.

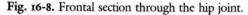

Fig. 16-8. Frontal section through the hip joint.

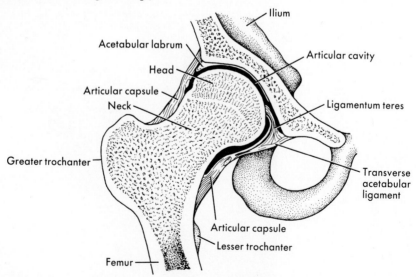

The thickest part of the capsule is located at the anterosuperior aspect of the joint and provides the greatest resistance in the standing position. On the femur, the capsule is attached to the junction between the neck and trochanters and to the intertrochanteric line (Fig. 16-8). The articular capsule is strengthened by the iliofemoral, ischiofemoral, and pubofemoral ligaments. The coarse exterior of the capsule is covered by numerous muscles and is separated in front from the psoas major by a bursa, which may communicate with the joint space.

The synovial membrane of the hip joint lines the articular capsule and covers the portion of the femoral neck contained within the capsule. The synovial membrane is reflected over the rim of the acetabular labrum above and covers the fat pad near the inferior exit of the socket at the acetabular notch below. The ligamentum teres, which permits blood vessels and nerves to pass to the head of the femur, is covered by a sheath of synovial membrane.

Ligaments

The *iliofemoral ligament* is a strong, thick, inverted Y-shaped ligament at the front of the hip that merges with and strengthens the joint capsule (Fig. 16-9). It is shorter in women than in men. Functionally, the iliofemoral ligament is the most important hip ligament. The stem of the inverted Y is attached to the anterior inferior iliac spine. The two divergent bands of the inverted Y fan out and attach to the whole length of the intertrochanteric line of the femur. The iliofemoral ligament becomes taut in full extension of the hip and helps prevent inadvertent hyperextension of the trunk (falling over backward) while standing. It is the iliofemoral ligament that allows us to remain in an erect position without continuous muscular exertion and subsequent fatigue.

The *pubofemoral ligament* is a triangular band of fibers that strengthens the medial and inferior portion of the joint capsule. It arises from the superior ramus of the pubic portion of the innominate bone and a portion of the acetabular rim. Note in Fig. 16-9 that fibers in the apex of the ligament extend down to reach the neck of the femur, where they blend with the lower medial fibers of the iliofemoral ligament. The pubofemoral ligament is tight in extension and also limits abduction of the hip.

Fig. 16-9. Anterior hip.

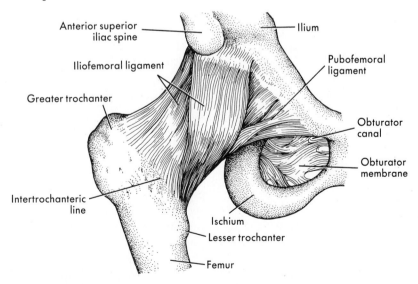

The triangular *ischiofemoral ligament* lies on the posterior aspect of the joint capsule. It extends from the ischium of the innominate bone below and behind the capsule to the trochanteric fossa of the femur. It is the ischiofemoral ligament and posterior part of the fibrous capsule that help limit medial rotation of the hip.

The *ligamentum teres* is the ligament to the head of the femur. It is a short (about 3.5 cm long) but strong band that extends from the wall of the acetabulum to a roughened depression (*fovea*) on the head of the femur. The ligamentum teres is completely covered by a sleeve of synovial membrane and serves as a bridge permitting blood vessels and nerves to enter the head of the femur. This ligament becomes taut in adduction of the femur, when the thigh is semiflexed, and relaxed when the limb is abducted.

The acetabular labrum is a triangular or horseshoe-shaped ridge of cartilage that is deficient below at the *acetabular notch*. The transverse ligament of the acetabulum bridges this notch and completes the circular ring around the socket. In crossing the acetabular notch the ligament creates an opening (foramen) through which blood vessels and nerves can enter the joint space.

Movements

The hip joint allows flexion, extension, abduction, adduction, rotation, and circumduction. As a multiaxial joint the hip permits flexion and extension through a transverse axis, adduction through an anteroposterior axis, and medial and lateral rotation through a vertical axis.

Forward movement about a transverse axis (flexion) is limited to about 90° when the knee is extended because of tension of the hamstrings. With the knee flexed, the range of motion in flexion at the hip is very free (about 120° to 130°), limited only by contact between the thigh and abdomen. Extension of the hip is limited to about 30° (hyperextension) by the iliofemoral and pubofemoral ligaments.

Adduction and abduction of the hip are movements about an anteroposterior axis. Adduction, movement towards the midline, is limited by the opposite limb and by the ischiofemoral ligament and the ligamentum teres. With one leg crossed over the other, the athlete should be able to achieve about 20° of additional adduction. Abduction, movement away from the midline, is a relatively free movement to about 45° and is limited by the pubofemoral ligament, the medial portion of the iliofemoral ligament, and by tension of the adductor muscles.

Lateral and medial rotation of the hip are movements that occur about a longitudinal axis. Lateral, or external, rotation turns the anterior surface of the thigh laterally. Lateral rotation of the hip is a powerful movement and is free through about 45°. It is limited by tension of the front of the capsule and by the lateral band of the iliofemoral ligament. Medial, or internal, rotation, the weakest movement at the hip, is possible through approximately 35°. It is limited by tension on the posterior fibers of the joint capsule.

Muscles

The primary muscles of the hip are illustrated in Figs. 16-10 through 16-14. Review the location and function of these muscles in Tables 16-1 and 16-2. As with the thigh, most athletic injuries of the hip involve the musculature.

INJURIES TO THE HIP
Contusions

The massive hip area is vulnerable to direct blows, resulting in contusions. One of the more common contusions is to the iliac crest, commonly called a **hip pointer**. The iliac crest extends from the anterior superior iliac spine to the posterior superior iliac spine. This crest is the most subcutaneous area of the hip and is especially susceptible to injury during contact sports. A contusion to the iliac crest can involve the hip muscles that originate along its outer border or the abdominal muscles that insert along its upper and inner border. Fig. 16-15 shows ecchymosis resulting from a hip contu-

Fig. 16-10. Muscles that adduct the thigh.

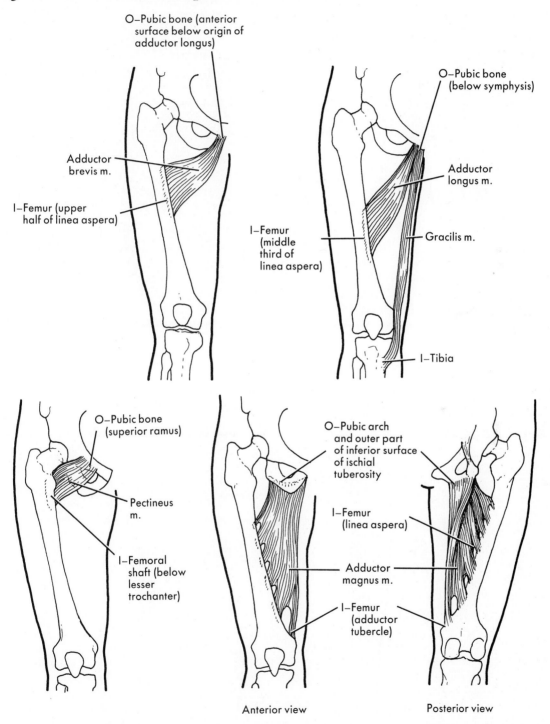

O–Pubic bone (anterior surface below origin of adductor longus)

Adductor brevis m.

I–Femur (upper half of linea aspera)

O–Pubic bone (below symphysis)

Adductor longus m.

I–Femur (middle third of linea aspera)

Gracilis m.

I–Tibia

O–Pubic bone (superior ramus)

Pectineus m.

I–Femoral shaft (below lesser trochanter)

O–Pubic arch and outer part of inferior surface of ischial tuberosity

I–Femur (linea aspera)

Adductor magnus m.

I–Femur (adductor tubercle)

Anterior view

Posterior view

Fig. 16-11. Iliopsoas muscle.

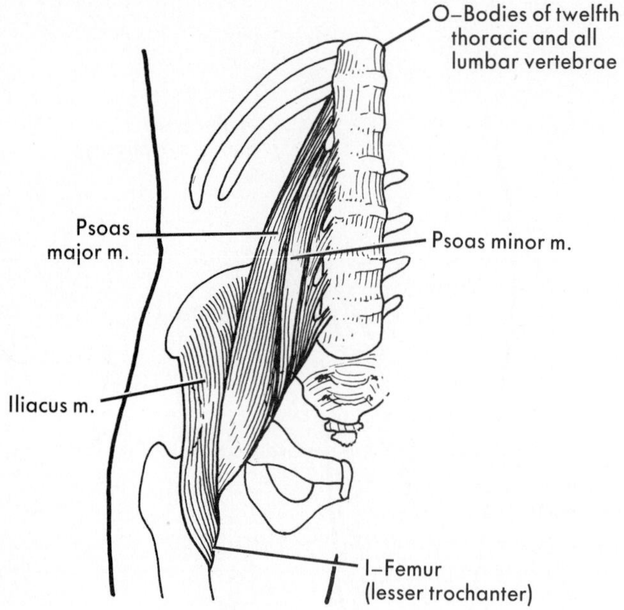

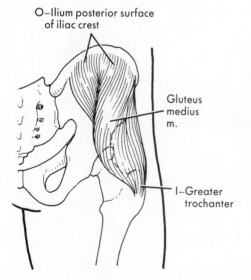

O–Bodies of twelfth thoracic and all lumbar vertebrae

Psoas major m.

Psoas minor m.

Iliacus m.

I–Femur (lesser trochanter)

Fig. 16-12. Gluteus maximus muscle.

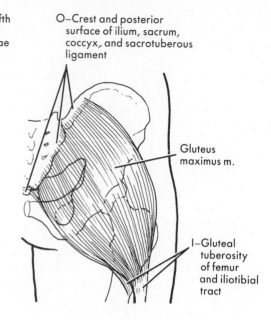

O–Crest and posterior surface of ilium, sacrum, coccyx, and sacrotuberous ligament

Gluteus maximus m.

I–Gluteal tuberosity of femur and iliotibial tract

Fig. 16-13. Gluteus medius muscle.

O–Ilium posterior surface of iliac crest

Gluteus medius m.

I–Greater trochanter

Fig. 16-14. Gluteus minimus muscle.

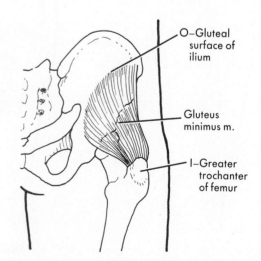

O–Gluteal surface of ilium

Gluteus minimus m.

I–Greater trochanter of femur

sion. The hip and abdominal muscles can also be strained or avulsed along their attachment to the iliac crest. This may result from forced lateral flexion during contraction of these muscles. The athletic trainer can usually determine if the injury is primarily a contusion or if the muscular attachments are strained by careful scrutiny of active movements during the assessment process. If the injury is primarily a bruise, active movements of the hip should not increase the pain dramatically. However, if the injury is a strain involving the muscle attachments, active movements utilizing the involved muscle will significantly increase the pain. Look for voluntary guarding by the athlete. For example, active hip abduction resulting in increased pain below the crest of the ilium may indicate a strain to the gluteus medius muscle. It may be difficult to determine the severity of injuries about the crest of the ilium, and the athlete is normally treated

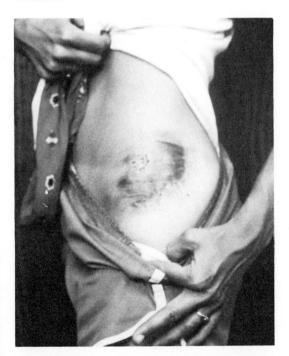

Fig. 16-15. Ecchymosis resulting from a hip contusion.

symptomatically, that is, kept inactive until the symptoms subside or referred to a physician if the symptoms persist or are of a severe nature.

Another area of the hip region vulnerable to contusions lies over the greater trochanter of the femur. The bony trochanter is covered only by the trochanteric bursa and tensor fascia latae muscle. The function of the bursa is to lessen friction as the tensor fascia latae slides over the trochanter during movement. A direct blow to the trochanter may contuse the muscle or lead to trochanteric bursitis. Friction within the bursa caused by the tensor fascia latae muscle constantly gliding over the trochanter can also result in bursitis. Palpating the greater trochanter will cause pain with both a contusion and trochanteric bursitis. However, if the bursa is inflamed, movements forcing the tensor fascia latae muscle over the trochanter will cause pain. Chronic trochanteric bursitis with thickening of the bursal walls can cause a condition known as a *"snapping hip."* As the tensor fascia latae slides back and forth over the trochanteric bursa, an audible and palpable snap will occur. This condition is more common in women because they have a wider pelvis and a more prominent trochanter.

Strains

Of the hip muscles, those in the groin are injured most frequently during athletic activity. The groin is considered to be the body area lying between the thigh and abdominal wall. The muscles in this region consist of the hip adductors (Fig. 16-10) and flexors (Fig. 16-11). Groin muscle strains are common in all athletic activities that involve running, especially those characterized by sudden bursts of speed requiring explosive or almost violent types of muscular contractions. Injuries to groin muscles may also be caused by sudden, unexpected overstretching of the muscles as well as by forced extension or abduction during muscle contraction. In case of injury the athlete may report feeling a sudden twinge or tearing sensation in the groin. In other instances, initial symptoms may be mild and the athlete may not notice or report the injury until after activity is completed. The signs and symptoms of a groin strain are similar to those of other muscle strains. To determine which muscles are involved and the severity of the injury, the athletic trainer must use active and resistive movement tests during the assessment process.

The other muscles about the hip are not strained nearly as often or as severely as those in the groin. However, these muscles can be strained by the same mechanisms responsible for thigh and groin muscle injuries. In most cases signs and symptoms will also be similar to those described for thigh and groin strains. The athletic trainer must be familiar with the various active and resistive assessment procedures used to determine specific muscle injury. These procedures are also used to evaluate the functional integrity of individual muscles. Procedures used to evaluate the hip muscles are illustrated and described later in this chapter as part of the assessment process.

Sprains

Any of the supporting ligaments of the hip joint may become stretched or torn as a result of some type of violent movement that forces the hip to exceed the normal range of motion in any direction. Hip sprains, however, are uncommon and seldom serious. When they do occur, the athlete may express pain in the hip at the limits of motion restricted by the sprained ligament. In addition, pain may be expressed during circumduction of the hip. If the pain is severe enough, the athlete may be unable to circumduct the hip.

An athlete may suffer from traumatic synovitis of the hip caused by either a direct blow to the greater trochanter or a sprain. However, it is difficult to recognize effusion of the hip joint or actually identify a distention of the joint capsule. Traumatic synovitis should be suspected in an athlete with an undiagnosed painful hip, a limp, and complaints of general soreness in the hip during movement. The athlete will also complain of pain during palpation over the greater trochanter.

A possible complication of synovitis is avascular necrosis of the femoral head. This is especially true in preadolescent athletes. In this condition the hip joint is filled with an excess of synovial fluid as the result of the inflammatory process. The pressure from this increased synovial fluid may occlude the blood supply to the femoral head. Young athletes complaining of continued or severe pain in the hip should be carefully evaluated and referred to a physician for assessment of avascular changes.

Dislocations

Dislocations of the hip as the result of athletic activity are rare, although they are more likely to occur than hip fractures. A hip dislocation normally occurs only after a violent force is directed along the femur when the hip is flexed. With this type of injury, the athlete has severe pain and is totally disabled immediately. Because the hip usually dislocates posteriorly, the athlete normally assumes a characteristic position of flexion, adduction, and internal rotation of the hip. The greater trochanter appears quite prominent, and the knee of the dislocated extremity rests on the uninvolved extremity. This type of injury is easily recognized and requires medical attention immediately. The primary danger or complication of a hip dislocation is the possibility of damage to the blood supply to the head of the femur.

Fractures

Fractures about the hip as the result of athletic activity occur very infrequently. The neck of the femur in young athletes is very resilient and rarely fractures. If the femoral neck should be fractured by a violent force, the athlete usually assumes a characteristic position of external rotation and abduction of the thigh. The athlete normally exhibits shortening of the involved extremity and severe pain. This type of injury should be readily recognized and the athlete should be referred to medical attention.

In adolescent athletes, the epiphyses about the proximal femur may be fractured or separated. This can occur to the greater trochanteric epiphysis, in which part of the greater trochanter is completely or incompletely avulsed. Another area of epiphyseal plate fracture occurs occasionally to the capital femoral epiphysis in the head of the femur. This may occur in an adolescent athlete with an unfused capital femoral epiphysis. The signs and symptoms associated with this type of an injury normally resemble those of a hip dislocation.

A related condition athletic trainers must be aware of is a slipped capital femoral epiphysis. Displacement or slippage of the capital femoral epiphysis can be caused by apparently minor trauma. Frequently pain associated with this type of condition is referred to the knee. A slipped capital femoral epiphysis occurs in preadolescent or adolescent athletes, most frequently in endomorphic boys with delayed secondary sex characterisics. Be highly suspicious of this type of athlete complaining of hip or knee pain without an obvious cause. These athletes should be referred to a physician. Diagnosis is made from radiographic examination.

ATHLETIC INJURY ASSESSMENT PROCESS
Secondary survey

Evaluation of a majority of athletic injuries involving the thigh or hip consists of identifying the injured muscle or muscles and assessing the degree of severity. Athletic injuries to the thigh occur frequently and are a source of obvious concern. Unfortunately, this commonly injured area is often inadequately or poorly evaluated. Less painful thigh injuries are often ignored by both athlete and trainer, and participation continues. Quite frequently, injuries may not be apparent to the athlete or reported until after activity, and many times the significance of the injury is not known for 12 to 24 hours after the incident. In addition, many athletic trainers tend to push an athlete back into activity too quickly after a seemingly minor bruise or pull to the thigh muscles. All of these factors can lead to additional damage, increase the severity of the original injury, and promote chronic thigh injury problems.

History

The history phase of the assessment process will quickly determine if the injury is chronic or acute. Many thigh injuries have a high incidence of becoming chronic problems. Therefore question the athlete carefully concerning any previous injuries to the thigh or hip to determine if the current complaint is an aggravation or recurrence of a previous injury. If the area has been injured before, obtain as much information as possible about the nature of previous injuries, the treatment procedures used, and the extent of rehabilitation. Details are important. Are symptoms of the current injury similar to those of any previous injuries? Had symptoms completely subsided and full function been restored before the onset of the present injury? The more information gained concerning previous injuries, the better the evaluation will be of the nature and severity of the current problem. This type of information is also useful in establishing a treatment and rehabilitation program, if required.

Next question the athlete concerning the present injury. Was the onset gradual? Unfortunately, many thigh and hip injuries are not reported immediately. Injured athletes will often tolerate increasing soreness or tightness until, with continued activity, the symptoms become progressively worse and function is impaired. Only when the level of performance declines, or obvious symptoms such as limping or favoring an extremity are noted, is the injury reported and assessment initiated. Attempt to find out what has happened and how the symptoms have progressed since the athlete first noticed the injury. If the onset is sudden, the athlete will normally relate a sudden sharp pain and immediate loss of some functional ability. Have the athlete describe or demonstrate the mechanism of injury. Was there a direct blow delivered to the area, or did the injury result from forceful contraction or overstretching? This type of information is important in evaluating the nature of the injury and can indicate which anatomic structures may be involved.

Have the athlete describe any signs and symptoms associated with an injury to the thigh or hip as specifically as possible. Localization of pain is important. It is also important to determine when signs and symptoms occurred, if there has been any change, and what movements or motions affect them. The remainder of this section discusses the signs and symptoms that must be considered when evaluating thigh and hip injuries.

Ask the athlete to specifically locate and describe the pain. Are there any movements or activities that cause the pain to increase? This information will assist in identifying the structures involved and the actual extent of physical damage. It will also help differentiate among various injury types.

Is there a loss of motion, function, or strength associated with the thigh or hip injury? Loss in these three areas is normally caused by pain associated with the injury, swelling, or protective muscle spasms. Question the athlete about these areas because, later in the assessment process, each will be evaluated in more detail.

Also question the athlete about other sensations associated with the injury. Did he or she hear or feel anything at the time of injury, such as a popping or snapping sensation? When the injury results from a sudden explosive contraction of a muscle, the athlete may express the feeling of being kicked or hit at the time of injury. Ask if there are feelings of tightness or tension in the thigh, which may indicate swelling or muscle spasms. The athlete's descriptions of any sensations associated with the injury, as well as his or her impressions concerning the injury itself, should never be ignored. They often yield valuable information.

Observation

Observation begins as soon as you see the injured athlete. If the athlete is lying on the field or court, notice the alignment of the legs. Does the injured leg appear to be in an abnormal position? Is the athlete holding or rubbing a certain area of the hip or thigh? As you approach the injured athlete, notice his or her attitude and behavior concerning the injured area. If the athlete is moving around, notice the gait pattern. Does the athlete walk with a limp? Does the athlete seem to favor the thigh or hip? Does the athlete appear to have normal function at the hip and knee joints?

Fig. 16-16. Inspecting the thigh and hip area for obvious signs of injury.

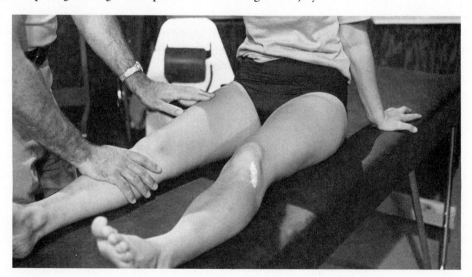

To conduct a complete inspection and continue the evaluation process, clothing and equipment should be removed from the thigh and hip area. Try to avoid causing any unnecessary embarrassment or discomfort. In most cases it is not necessary to remove the athlete's shorts or underwear. The individual should be sitting or lying with both legs supported in an attempt to relax the muscles.

Carefully inspect the thigh and hip area for obvious signs of injury (Fig. 16-16). Are there any signs of trauma, such as abrasions or contusions? Notice and compare the contours of both legs. Is there any sign of swelling, abnormal bumps, gaps, or loss of muscle definition or symmetry? Ask the athlete to contract both quadriceps muscles to compare the character of the muscle tone. Note any differences.

Palpation

Palpation is used to further identify specific structures involved in the injury and to locate pain and swelling. Palpation should also be conducted with both legs supported and the muscles as relaxed as possible. If the muscles are relaxed you have a better opportunity to feel any palpable masses or deficits within the thigh and will be able to recognize the presence of localized muscle spasms. This is also a more comfortable position for the injured athlete. Because most thigh and hip injuries involve muscles, it is important to determine which area of the muscle is injured. For example, injuries involving the muscle or tendinous attachments to bone may be avulsion injuries and may require further evaluation or referral.

When the injury is on the anterior aspect of the thigh or hip, the athlete should be supine. The quadriceps muscle unit can then be palpated along its entire course. Locate areas of point tenderness and feel for any masses that may indicate bleeding or swelling. If the injury is severe, you may be able to palpate a gap in the muscle definition, which may indicate a rupture of muscle fibers. Always remember to compare any palpable lumps or deficits with the uninjured leg to note differences or similarities. This can be accomplished by observing and palpating both thighs at the same time to compare symmetry.

Palpate the groin area to locate point tenderness associated with a groin strain or related injury. The groin is most effectively palpated when

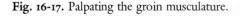

Fig. 16-17. Palpating the groin musculature.

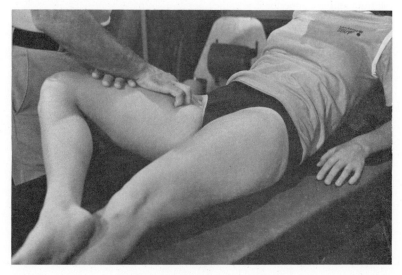

the heel of the injured leg is resting on the knee or shin of the uninjured leg (Fig. 16-17). This position places the hip in flexion, abduction, and external rotation. This position is also useful in palpating for enlarged lymph nodes in the groin, should infection be suspected, or in locating the femoral pulse. Muscles in the groin are difficult to palpate individually, and resistive movements, described later in this chapter, are used to distinguish specific muscle or muscle group involvement.

While the athlete is supine, you can also palpate the bony rim of the pelvis. Begin at the anterior superior iliac spine and continue to palpate along the crest of the ilium (Fig. 16-18). Remember, tenderness directly over the anterior superior iliac spine, especially in an adolescent athlete, may indicate an avulsion fracture. The iliac crest is subcutaneous and can be easily palpated along its entire length. Fig. 16-19 illustrates palpation along the iliac crest following a direct blow to the area. It is easier to palpate the posterior portion of the iliac crest as well as the posterior superior iliac spine with the athlete lying on the uninjured side.

To palpate for injuries on the posterior aspect of the thigh or hip, the athlete should be lying prone. In this position, the hamstrings can be palpated along their entire course. Remember, it is easier to feel the hamstring insertions during mild resistance to knee flexion (Fig. 16-20). Proceed to locate areas of tenderness as well as any palpable masses or deficits. Palpation can be continued to the origin of the hamstrings on the ischial tuberosity. If the injury involves the ischial tuberosity, the area can also be easily palpated with the athlete in the sidelying position. Tenderness directly over the ischial tuberosity may indicate ischial bursitis or possibly an avulsion fracture.

To place an injured athlete in a sidelying position, have him or her turn on to the uninjured side and bring the knee of the injured leg up toward the chest. In this position the posterior hip, including the gluteus maximus and medius, can easily be palpated. The greater trochanter of the femur can also be felt in this position (Fig. 16-21). Tenderness directly over the greater trochanter may be indicative of trochanteric bursitis or a localized contusion.

Stress

Because most athletic injuries to the thigh and hip involve the musculotendinous unit, those

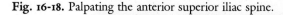

Fig. 16-18. Palpating the anterior superior iliac spine.

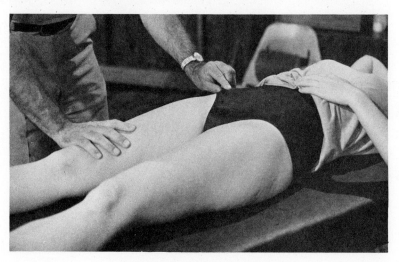

stress maneuvers used to evaluate the integrity of contractile elements are extremely important. Complete assessment of injuries to the thigh and hip requires accurate interpretation of active, resistive, and functional movement tests. Correct interpretation of the results of these tests depend on a knowledge of the muscles involved and the types of movement each muscle or muscle group produces. In short, an understanding of functional anatomy is essential for correct interpretation of stress procedures. You should review the major muscles or muscle groups in this area and the movements produced by each.

Active movements. Evaluation of active movements at the hip and knee joints is extremely useful in assessing range of motion. It is important to recognize any pain or discomfort with each movement. Instruct the athlete to perform each movement through as great a range of motion as possible and to express any sensations or feelings he or she may experience.

In the supine position, instruct the athlete to alternately pull each knee up to the chest (Fig. 16-22). This movement permits evaluation of both hip and knee flexion at the same time. Compare the motion of the injured leg to that of the uninjured. Is the range of motion limited or restricted? Does the athlete express any pain, discomfort, or other sensations during these movements? Evaluation of hip flexion with the knee extended is another active movement performed with the athlete in the supine position. This movement will give some indication of hamstring muscle flexibility. Remember to compare both sides.

Fig. 16-19. Palpating the iliac crest.

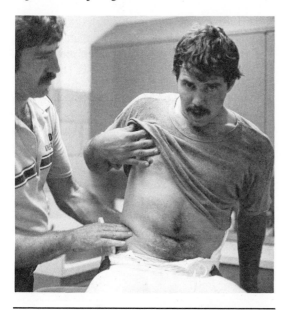

Fig. 16-20. Palpating hamstring insertions.

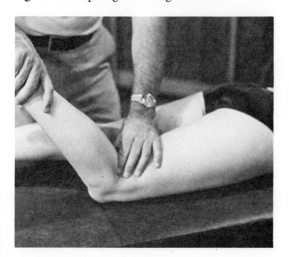

Fig. 16-21. Palpating the greater trochanter.

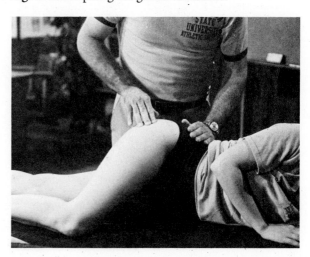

To more adequately evaluate the active range of movement of the knee joint, have the athlete lie in the prone position. Instruct the athlete to flex each knee, bringing the heel as close to the buttock as possible (Fig. 16-23, *A*). Again, compare the range of motion in each knee and ask the athlete to describe any pain or discomfort. The prone position is also used to evaluate hip extension. Instruct the athlete to lift each leg as high as possible, keeping the knee extended and fixed (Fig. 16-23, *B*).

To evaluate active abduction of the hip, have the athlete lie on his or her uninjured side and raise the injured leg as high as possible (Fig. 16-24). Instruct the athlete to keep the knee extended. To compare range of motion, have the athlete switch sides and complete the same movement with the uninjured leg.

Resistive movements. Resistive movements are used to further evaluate the integrity of contractile tissues. Manual resistance against active motion can accurately identify specific painful areas, allowing one muscle to be differentiated from another. Resistive movements are also used to compare muscular strength between extremities. Resistive procedures are potentially the most informative maneuvers used in assessing muscle injuries, and the knowledge gained during this part of the evaluation will indicate which muscles are involved.

When performing resistive movements, it is important that you explain exactly what you want the athlete to do as well as how and what you are going to do in applying resistance. The procedures can be performed with the uninjured side first to make sure the athlete understands. The exercises should be controlled and limited by the athlete's tolerance. Resistance should initially be applied gently and then the intensity increased according to the athlete's tolerance. If you begin the procedure using too much force or pressure, you may cause additional pain and discomfort, lose the athlete's cooperation, and possibly cause further damage.

When applying resistance, there should be just enough resistance against the movement to allow the athlete to complete the full range of motion. Some resistive procedures call for an

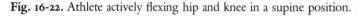

Fig. 16-22. Athlete actively flexing hip and knee in a supine position.

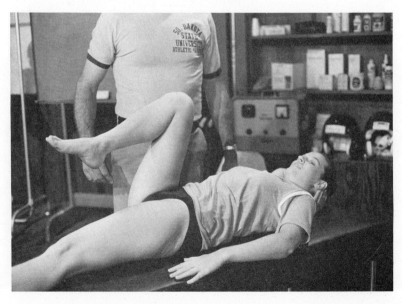

Fig. 16-23. Active motion in a prone position. **A,** Knee flexion; **B,** hip extension.

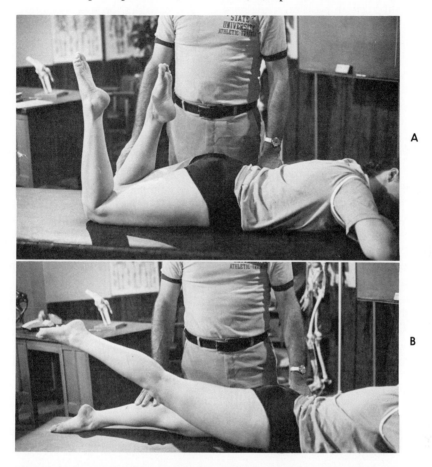

Fig. 16-24. Athlete actively abducting the hip in a sidelying position.

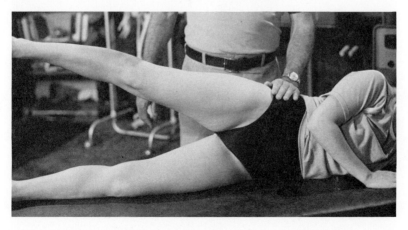

isometric exercise. In these cases the athlete is instructed to hold a certain position while resistance is applied. These maneuvers are probably less effective because the muscle is evaluated in only one position or length. Therefore whenever isometric resistive exercises are used, the involved joint should be placed in various positions to evaluate the muscles at different functional lengths.

To evaluate the integrity of the quadriceps, have the athlete in a sitting position with the legs hanging over the side or edge of a table. Instruct the athlete to extend the knee as you apply resistance against the anterior aspect of the ankle (Fig. 16-25). An alternate method would be to apply an isometric resistance against extension, or attempt to flex the knee while the athlete is instructed to keep the knee straight and fixed, as described in Chapter 15.

To evaluate the integrity of the hamstrings, instruct the athlete to flex the knee as resistance is applied against the back of the ankle (Fig. 16-26). An alternate method is to instruct the athlete to hold the knee in various degrees of flexion as you attempt to straighten the leg. Resistance can also be applied against the ham-

strings with the athlete lying prone. Instruct the athlete to flex the knee while resistance is applied to the back of the ankle.

The integrity of the hip flexors is easiest to evaluate in the sitting position. Instruct the athlete to bring the knee up toward his or her chest while resistance is applied on top of the knee (Fig. 16-27, A). Again, apply just enough resistance to allow slow movement. Resistance can also be applied against hip flexion while the athlete is lying supine, as described previously during active movements (Fig. 16-27, B).

To evaluate the integrity of hip adductors, ask the athlete to bring both legs together while resistance is applied against the medial side of both knees (Fig. 16-28). The hip abductors can be tested by instructing the athlete to spread both legs while resistance is applied against the lateral aspect of both knees (Fig. 16-29). Both of these procedures can be performed with the athlete supine or in a sitting position.

An alternate method of testing the abductors and adductors is to have the athlete in a sidelying position on the uninjured side. To evaluate the abductors in this position, ask the athlete to raise the leg upward while resistance is placed against

Fig. 16-25. Applying resistance to knee extension to assist in evaluating the integrity of the quadriceps.

Fig. 16-26. Applying resistance to knee flexion to assist in evaluating the integrity of the hamstrings.

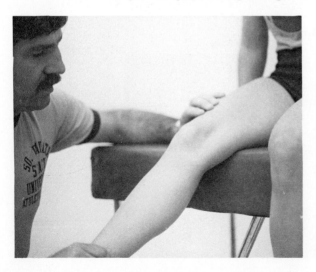

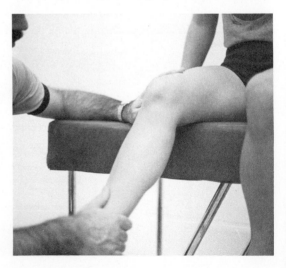

the lateral aspect of the knee (Fig. 16-30). If you are evaluating a hip pointer, pay particular attention to the exact location of pain caused by this movement. To test the hip adductors, have the athlete bring the legs together while resistance is applied to the medial aspect of both knees (Fig. 16-31).

To evaluate the integrity of the hip extensors, have the athlete assume the prone position. Instruct him or her to lift the leg as high as possible while resistance is applied against the posterior aspect of the thigh (Fig. 16-32). To decrease the action of the hamstrings, have the athlete flex the knee during hip extension. Be sure that mo-

Fig. 16-27. Applying resistance to hip flexion **A,** in a sitting position and **B,** in a supine position.

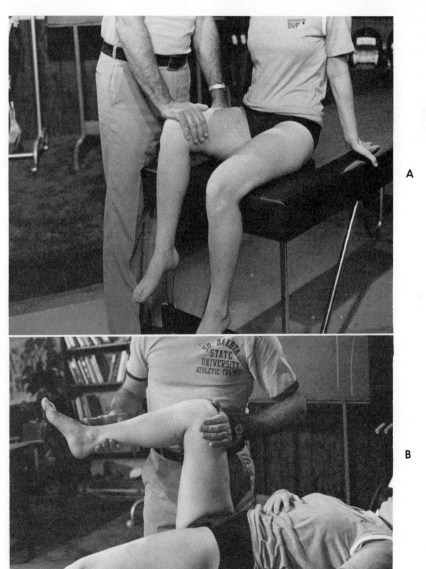

A

B

Fig. 16-28. Applying resistance to hip adductors.

Fig. 16-29. Applying resistance to hip abduction in a sitting position.

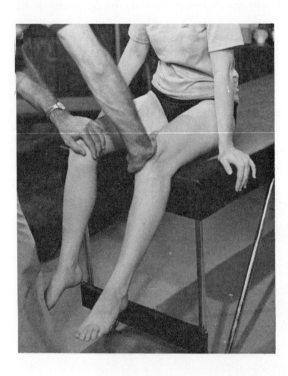

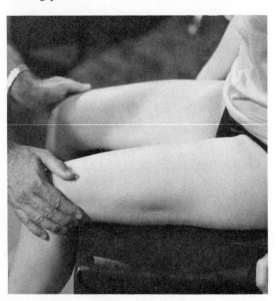

Fig. 16-30. Applying resistance to hip abduction in a sidelying position.

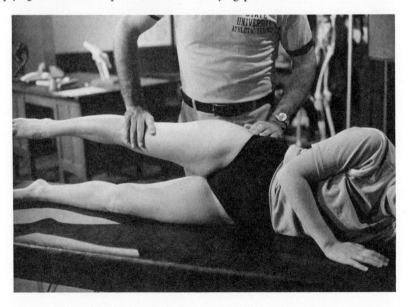

tion is taking place at the hip joint by stabilizing the pelvis. Occasionally an athlete will raise the pelvis using the lower back muscles in an attempt to substitute this motion for hip extension.

Passive movements. Passive movements are seldom necessary in evaluating thigh or hip injuries. Occasionally, the range of motion of the knee or hip is evaluated passively. These procedures involve the same positioning as described during active movements. The athlete is then instructed to relax the muscles, and all motion is performed by the athletic trainer. Caution must be exercised in performing these procedures, as the tolerance level is no longer controlled by the athlete and additional damage could result.

Functional movements. Functional movements are used mainly to determine when an athlete with a thigh or hip injury can return to full activity. As an athlete recovers from a thigh or hip

Fig. 16-31. Applying resistance to hip adduction in a sidelying position.

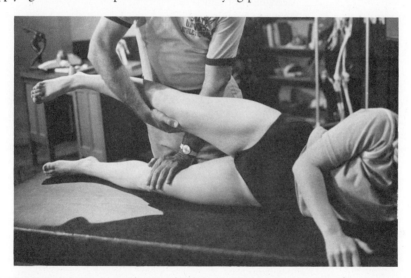

Fig. 16-32. Applying resistance to hip extension in a prone position.

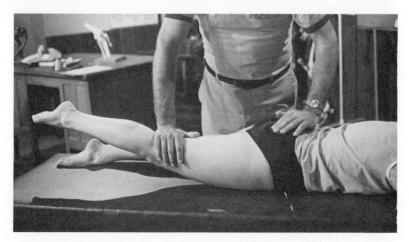

ATHLETIC INJURY ASSESSMENT CHECKLIST
THIGH AND HIP INJURIES

Secondary survey
_____ History
　　　_____ Previous injuries
　　　　　_____ Nature
　　　　　_____ Treatment
　　　　　_____ Rehabilitation
　　　_____ Present injury
　　　　　_____ Onset
　　　　　　　_____ Sudden
　　　　　　　_____ Gradual
　　　　　_____ Mechanism of injury
　　　　　_____ Signs and symptoms
　　　　　　　_____ Pain
　　　　　　　_____ Motion
　　　　　　　_____ Function
　　　　　　　_____ Strength
　　　　　　　_____ Sensations
_____ Observation
　　　_____ Gait pattern
　　　_____ Function
　　　_____ Alignment
　　　_____ Signs of trauma
　　　　　_____ Abrasions
　　　　　_____ Contusions
　　　　　_____ Contours
　　　　　_____ Swelling
　　　　　_____ Muscle definition or symmetry
_____ Palpation
　　　_____ Tenderness
　　　_____ Swelling
　　　_____ Masses or deficits
　　　_____ Muscle spasms
　　　_____ Muscle involved
　　　　　_____ Anterior thigh
　　　　　_____ Groin
　　　　　_____ Pelvic area
　　　　　_____ Posterior thigh
　　　　　_____ Posterior hip
_____ Stress
　　　_____ Active movements
　　　　　_____ Range of motion
　　　　　_____ Pain
　　　_____ Resistive movements
　　　　　_____ Pain
　　　　　_____ Strength
　　　_____ Passive movements
　　　　　_____ Range of motion
　　　_____ Functional movements
　　　　　_____ Functional activities

injury, information obtained from functional exercises becomes increasingly important on each re-evaluation. The intensity of functional activities should be continually increased within the pain tolerance level and range of motion limits. Limited athletic activities can be performed until functional performance of activities is at or near optimum capacity.

Evaluation of findings

Severe injuries, such as fractures of the femur or hip dislocations, are uncommon in athletic activities. These types of injuries can usually be identified readily and do not require extensive evaluative skills. Athletes with these injuries need immediate medical attention. Remember, young athletes may injure their epiphyseal plates or growth centers. These types of conditions must be recognized and the athletes referred to medical attention to avoid complications.

Most injuries involving the thigh and hip will require at least some of the preceding evaluative techniques for an accurate assessment. The responsibility of the athletic trainer is to determine which skeletal component, muscle, or muscle group is involved, as well as the severity of the injury. The athlete should be withheld from activity as long as he or she has a limited range of motion or pain with exercise. Thigh and hip injuries require almost daily evaluation in order to monitor progress and decide when the athlete can return to full activity. Once an athlete demonstrates full pain-free function of the injured area, he or she may return to activity.

When to refer the athlete

Many injuries to the thigh or hip may not require medical attention. Providing an accurate assessment has been carried out and standard guidelines are followed as to when an athlete can return to activity, many thigh or hip injuries can be cared for by the athletic trainer. Although severe injuries are uncommon, serious complications can arise from an improperly recognized and managed injury. Always keep a high index of suspicion when evaluating preadolescent and adolescent athletes. The following criteria can be used to determine if further medical attention is indicated.

---

1. Gross deformity or swelling
2. Significant loss of motion
3. Severe disability
4. Noticeable and palpable deficit in the muscle or tendon
5. Tenderness palpated at the bony attachments
6. Continued or severe pain in the hip
7. Thigh or hip injury that does not respond to treatment within 2 to 3 weeks
8. Any doubt regarding the severity or nature of the injury

KEY TERMS

acetabular labrum   Triangular ring of fibrocartilage attached to the rim of the acetabulum, increasing the depth of the cavity

charley horse   Term usually restricted to injuries of the quadriceps muscle group caused by a contusion or possibly a strain, producing soreness and stiffness

hip pointer   Contusion to the crest of the ilium

iliotibial band (iliotibial tract)   Strong lateral portion of the deep fascia of the thigh that is the insertion of the tensor fascia latae muscle

snapping hip   Chronic trochanteric bursitis with thickening of the bursal walls, causing an audible and palpable snap as the tensor fascia lata slides back and forth over the greater trochanter

SUGGESTED READINGS

Arnheim, D.D.: Modern principles of athletic training, ed. 6, St. Louis, 1985, Times Mirror/Mosby College Publishing.

Hoppenfeld, S.: Physical examination of the spine and extremities, New York, 1976, Appleton-Century-Crofts.

Kuland, D.N.: The injured athlete, Philadelphia, 1982, J.B. Lippincott Co.

O'Donoghue, D.H.: Treatment of injuries to athletes, ed. 4, Philadelphia, 1984, W.B. Saunders.

Sothmayd, W., and Hoffman, M.: Sports health, the complete book of athletic injuries, New York, 1981, Quick Fox.

UNIT

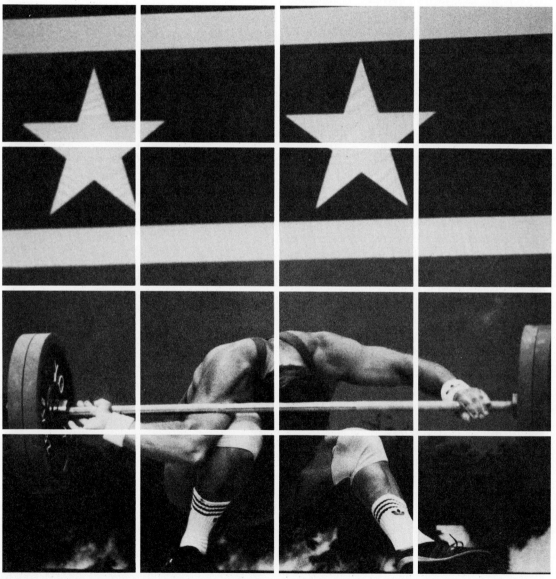

American weightlifter dislocating right elbow during 1984 Olympics in Los Angeles.
(UPI/Bettman Archive.)

S I X

Athletic injuries of the upper extremity

The final unit of this text is concerned with those athletic injuries or conditions involving the upper extremity. The upper extremity plays a vital role in athletic activity and presents a unique assessment challenge to the athletic trainer. Injuries to the upper extremity seldom involve a single anatomic structure or affect an isolated functional ability. As a result, complete and accurate assessment of injuries in this complex, highly mobile, and relatively unstable area will tax the skill and expertise of even the most seasoned athletic trainer. Upper extremity injuries occur less frequently than injuries to the knee, ankle, and foot. The result is a reduced frequency of assessment in this area compared to the high incidence of evaluations performed on the lower extremity. Because of the importance of the upper extremity in athletic activity, professional athletic trainers, and especially students of athletic training, must devote considerable time and effort to developing or retaining proficiency in evaluation procedures. Practice and frequent review of skills is essential.

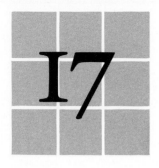

Shoulder injuries

The shoulder is more than simply the juncture of the arm and torso or the articulation between the humerus and the glenoid cavity. The shoulder encompasses all of the intricate arm-trunk mechanisms, including the elaborate anatomic and functional interrelationships between the thorax, clavicle, scapula, and humerus. This area is usually referred to as the shoulder girdle or complex. Each area or portion comprising the shoulder girdle plays an important role in the coordinated movements of the arm. Each of these areas must function properly, both separately and as a unit, for the shoulder complex to function smoothly. Because of the synchronous movements required for normal shoulder function, an athletic injury to any one area of the shoulder may cause impaired function of all areas. Therefore, to perform a comprehensive assessment of shoulder injuries, athletic trainers must possess a sound knowledge of the functional anatomy of the shoulder girdle and an understanding of its complex movements.

ANATOMY OF THE SHOULDER

To become proficient in the assessment of injuries to the shoulder and related areas, review of underlying anatomic structures is required. The major skeletal components of the shoulder are reviewed in Fig. 17-1. Pay particular attention to the bony landmarks. Understanding the complexities of the sternoclavicular, acromioclavicular, and glenohumeral joints, the bony components, and associated ligaments and muscles is particularly important. Along with the anatomy of each joint of the shoulder complex, a brief

discussion of the more common injuries and injury-causing mechanisms is reviewed in this chapter in order to provide the athletic trainer with greater insight during the evaluation process.

Sternoclavicular joint

Athletic injuries to the sternoclavicular joint occur infrequently. However, this synovial joint is critically important because it is the only bony attachment between the upper limb and the axial skeleton. The articulation between the clavicle and sternum is actually the pivot point about which movements of the shoulder as a whole occur. The type and freedom of movement is extensive.

The sternoclavicular joint is composed of the

Fig. 17-1. Skeletal components for right shoulder and arm. **A,** Anterior view; **B,** posterior view.

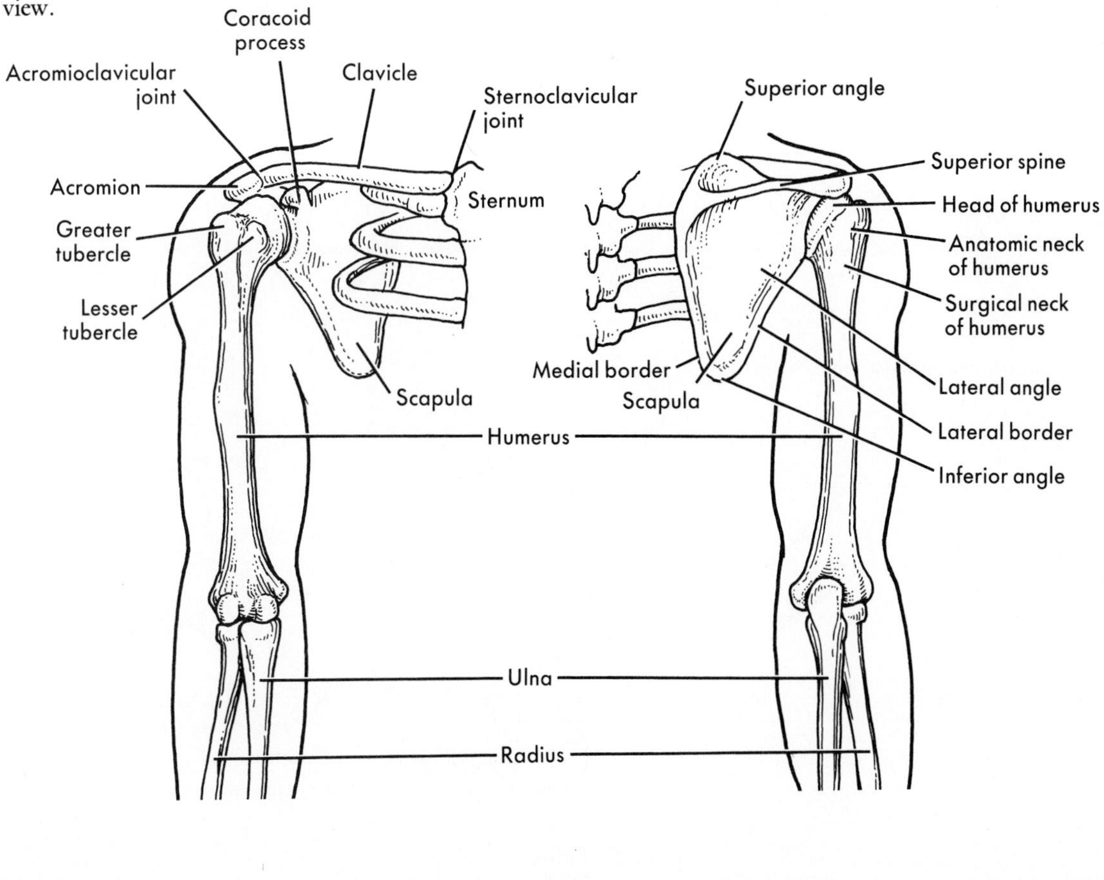

sternal end of the clavicle, the cartilage of the first rib, and the uppermost portion, or manubrium, of the sternum. The joint is surrounded by a loose articular capsule that is lined with a synovial membrane and attached to the margins of the articulating bones. This articular capsule is reinforced by the anterior and posterior *sternoclavicular ligaments*. An important accessory ligament that plays a role in limiting clavicular movements is the *costoclavicular ligament*. This dense band of fibers passes upward from the first rib to attach to the lower surface of the sternal end of the clavicle.

The thick *interclavicular ligament* (Fig. 17-2) strengthens the superior aspect of joint capsule. It stretches from clavicle to clavicle across the upper surface of the capsule, where it attaches to the suprasternal, or jugular, notch. Comparative anatomists often compare this ligamentous band to the wishbone of the bird. It plays an impor-

tant role in stabilizing both the right and left sternoclavicular joints. The sternoclavicular joint space is divided into two synovial cavities by a flat, circular articular disc of fibrocartilage. When the shoulder is elevated or depressed, the clavicle moves on the articular disc, which exerts a cushioning effect to the forces that are transmitted from the upper extremity.

Sternoclavicular injuries

The most common injuries to the sternoclavicular joint are sprains. These result when force is directed along the long axis of the clavicle toward the sternal end and stress is applied to the sternoclavicular and costoclavicular ligaments. When these supporting ligaments are stretched significantly or torn, the sternal end of the clavicle may dislocate. Dislocation of the sternoclavicular joint is almost always in an anterior direction, so that the sternal end of the clav-

Fig. 17-2. The sternoclavicular joints. Anterior aspect.

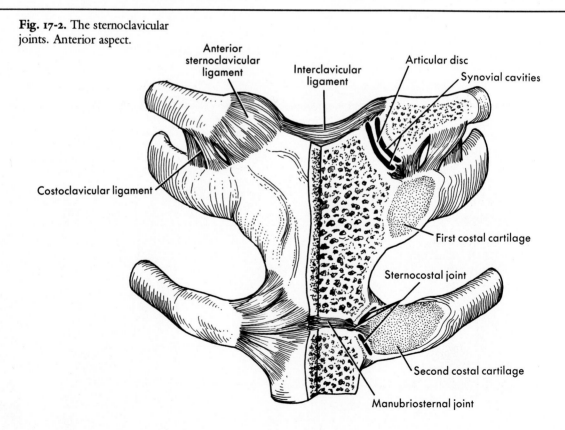

Anterior sternoclavicular ligament

Interclavicular ligament

Articular disc

Synovial cavities

Costoclavicular ligament

First costal cartilage

Sternocostal joint

Second costal cartilage

Manubriosternal joint

icle passes forward. The anterior sternoclavicular ligament is torn by the stress, and the clavicle passes upward to lie in the suprasternal notch. In a complete anterior dislocation, the costoclavicular ligament is ruptured, making reduction difficult. This injury commonly results in tenderness, swelling, and a visible prominence at the sternoclavicular joint. Discomfort and a limited range of shoulder motion are usually present.

A posterior dislocation of the sternoclavicular joint, although rare, is potentially much more serious than an anterior dislocation. With a posterior dislocation, the posterior sternoclavicular ligament is ruptured and the clavicle may compress the anterior structures of the neck. This may lead to dyspnea if the trachea is compressed. A posterior dislocation can also compress or rupture the innominate vein as it passes directly behind the sternoclavicular joint.

Clavicular injuries

Injuries involving the shaft of the clavicle are fairly common during athletic activity. Because this bone is subcutaneous, it is subject to contusions caused by any type of direct trauma to the area. Clavicular contusions will cause tenderness and swelling at the site of injury but normally little increase in pain with shoulder motion. The clavicle is also frequently fractured during athletic activity. This is especially true in preadolescent and adolescent athletes. In older athletes, ligament injuries to the sternoclavicular or acromioclavicular joints are more likely than fractures. Most fractured clavicles in young athletes are of the greenstick type. These can be difficult to detect because there may be no evident displacement of bone fragments or resulting angulation. Athletic trainers should suspect a greenstick fracture whenever there is tenderness di-

Fig. 17-3. Complete fracture of the clavicle as viewed from behind. Note the elevated medial fragment.
(Courtesy A.G. Edwards A.T.,C., University of Nevada–Las Vegas)

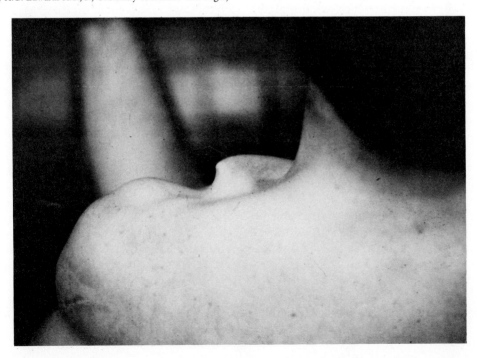

rectly over the shaft of the clavicle in a young athlete who has suffered trauma to the shoulder. Although the clavicle is fractured more frequently than any other major long bone in the body, serious complications are rare. The break is usually at the junction of the middle and outer thirds of the bone or where the clavicle changes direction. In older athletes, the medial fragment is normally pulled upward by the contractions of the sternocleidomastoid and trapezius muscles, whereas the lateral portion is displaced downward by the contraction of the pectoralis major muscle and the weight of the arm (Fig. 17-3).

Acromioclavicular joint

The acromioclavicular joint is the articulation between the lateral end of the clavicle and the medial margin of the acromion process of the scapula. This small synovial joint permits a limited amount of rotation and numerous gliding movements. The long axis of the joint lies in an anteroposterior direction. The placement of the clavicle is normally higher than the acromion at the point of articulation; as a result, a slope exists between the surfaces, which tends to predispose displacement of the acromion downward and under the clavicle when a blow is delivered to the tip of the shoulder.

The articular surfaces of the joint are covered with fibrocartilage. In addition, a wedge-shaped articular disc of shock-absorbing cartilage is found in the joint space. The disc does not, however, divide the space into two separate synovial cavities as in the sternoclavicular joint. A synovial membrane lines the relatively loose-fitting articular capsule, which completely surrounds the joint. The capsule is strengthened by the short *acromioclavicular ligament* extending between the lateral tip of the clavicle and the adjoining portion of the acromion over the superior aspect of the joint. The joint capsule and acromioclavicular ligament play only a minor role in holding the clavicle and scapula together. However, because they are richly supplied by sensory nerves, an injury to these structures is quite painful.

The *coracoclavicular ligament* plays the most important role in preventing separation of the clavicle from the scapula. This very strong ligament is divided into two components, the *trapezoid* and *conoid* ligaments. The flat, quadrilateral trapezoid ligament passes upward and laterally (in front) from the coracoid process to the clavicle. The triangular conoid ligament passes downward and medially (behind) from the clavicle to the base of the coracoid process. The conoid portion of the ligament restrains backward movement of the scapula, whereas the trapezoid portion prevents excessive forward displacement. If the coracoclavicular ligament is torn, displacing forces acting on the shoulder can cause the acromion to be forced down and away from the clavicle.

Acromioclavicular injuries

Injuries to the supporting ligaments of the acromioclavicular joint are not uncommon in athletics. They generally occur as a result of a blow to the tip of the shoulder or falling on an outstretched arm. When an athlete receives a direct blow to the point of the shoulder, which can occur during a fall, the acromion may be driven downward. During a sudden unexpected fall, an athlete may land on an outstretched hand or flexed elbow, which transmits force directly to the shoulder girdle and can drive the acromion backward and away from the clavicle. Either of these mechanisms can cause a sprain to the supporting ligaments, an injury commonly called a *shoulder separation.*

Sprains to the acromioclavicular joint are graded according to the degree of severity. A mild (first-degree) sprain is stretching or slight tearing of the ligament fibers. There is normally tenderness directly over the joint, mild swelling, and little or no disability of the shoulder. A moderate (second-degree) sprain is a partial disruption of the supporting ligaments. Such injuries will have pain and tenderness directly over and around the joint, local swelling, and an increase in pain on forced motion. This is accomplished by pulling downward or pushing upward on the arm in an attempt to separate the clavicle from the acromion, thereby applying stress to the supporting ligaments. A moderate sprain may or may not exhibit upward displacement of the clavicle. A severe (third-degree) sprain involves total disruption of one or more of the supporting ligaments. The athlete will generally exhibit varying degrees of tenderness, swelling, instability, and an increase in pain with any effort to stress the joint. The space between the acromion and clavicle may be widened and the coracoclavicular ligaments torn. When this occurs there is a characteristic upward riding of the clavicle (Fig. 17-4). This sign becomes more obvious when weight or downward traction is applied to the arm. A third-degree sprain of the acromioclavicular joint will often exhibit a *piano key sign;* that is, the clavicle can be pushed down but will spring back up when pressure is released. An upward riding of the clavicle in relation to the acromion has traditionally been called a *knocked-down shoulder.* Complete

acromioclavicular dislocations often require surgical intervention.

Complications that may accompany acromioclavicular sprains include pain, disability, and a decrease in shoulder range of motion. Degenerative changes often develop in this joint. Persons may have activity-limiting symptoms years later as a result of apparently "minor" injuries. The lateral end of the clavicle may also remain prominent, but this is often painless and may not interfere with shoulder function.

Shoulder complex

The shoulder (glenohumeral) joint is a synovial (diarthrotic) joint of the ball-and-socket variety. Recall from Chapter 4 that ball-and-socket type diarthroses are multiaxial joints that have two or more axes of rotation and permit movement in three or more planes. The shoulder, our most mobile joint, allows all types of movement and has three axes around which these actions occur: transverse (flexion and ex-

Fig. 17-4. Severe sprain of the right acromioclavicular joint exhibiting elevation of the clavicle. **A,** Anterior view and **B,** posterior view.
(Courtesy Bruce Johnson, A.T.,C., Orthopedic Clinic, Grand Forks, N.D.)

A   B

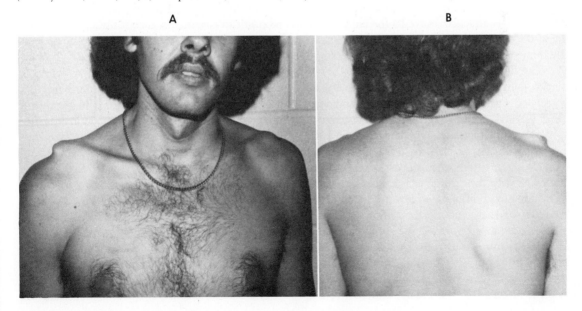

tension), anteroposterior (abduction and adduction), and vertical (medial and lateral rotation). The components of the shoulder joint include the large head of the humerus and the much smaller adjacent glenoidal surface of the scapula, the glenoid labrum, the fibrous articular capsule lined with synovial membrane, and the coracohumeral, glenohumeral, transverse, and coracoacromial ligaments.

The disparity in size between the large and nearly hemispheric head of the humerus and the much smaller and shallow glenoid cavity of the scapula is of great clinical significance to the athletic trainer. Because the head of the humerus is over two times larger than the shallow glenoid concavity that receives it, only part of the humeral head is in contact with the fossa in any given position of the joint. This anatomic fact helps explain the inherent instability of the shoulder joint. The *glenoid labrum* is a triangular ring of fibrocartilage attached to the margin of the glenoid cavity. Although the labrum helps deepen the concavity, its stabilizing effect on the joint is minimal. This ring of fibrocartilage can split or tear, giving rise to loose pieces within the joint that may cause clicking or locking with movement of the shoulder.

A thin articular capsule surrounds the shoulder joint. It is attached above to the edge of the glenoid fossa and below to the anatomic neck of the humerus. The capsule is extremely loose and does not function to keep the articulating bones of the joint in contact. This fact is obviously correlated with the great range of motion possible at this articulation. The tendons of the supraspinatus, infraspinatus, teres minor, and subscapularis muscles (called the SITS muscles) all blend with and strengthen the articular capsule. They fuse with the capsule near its distal margin. The musculotendinous cuff resulting from the blending of these muscle tendons with the fibrous joint capsule is called the ***rotator cuff*** because these muscles are also important in rotation at the shoulder. The supraspinatus, infraspinatus, and teres minor muscles are external rotators attached to the greater tuberosity; the

subscapularis is an internal rotator attached to the lesser tuberosity. The rotator cuff provides the necessary strength to help prevent anterior, superior, and posterior displacement of the humeral head during most types of activity. Review the placement and points of attachment of these muscles in Chapter 5 and in Figs. 17-7, 17-10, and 17-11 when you study the individual movements of the shoulder joint.

A unique relationship exists between the articular capsule of the shoulder joint, the tendon of the long head of the biceps muscle, and the synovial lining of the capsule. The tendon is within the substance of the capsule (intracapsular) but is outside of the actual joint cavity. The tendon invaginates the lining of the cavity until it is surrounded by the synovial membrane. The membrane then fuses over the tendon and encloses it in a tubular sheath, which surrounds it during its passage through the bicipital (intertubercular) groove of the humerus. The transverse ligament of the joint creates a canal for the tendon by bridging the groove between the greater and lesser tubercles. The distal segment of this ligament then arches over the tendon as it emerges from the capsule. The result is a continuous tubular sheath of synovial membrane that covers the long head of the biceps tendon from its point of origin and is continuous above with the general synovial lining of the joint and extends distally to the surgical neck of the humerus. It is important to understand that fusion of the synovial membrane "tube" around the tendon prevents infectious material, which can migrate along the surface of the tendon, from gaining access to the true joint space unless the membrane ruptures. This fact explains how a case of tenosynovitis can seemingly pass through the shoulder without infecting the joint space.

The *coracohumeral ligament* is a broad band that strengthens the upper portion of the joint capsule. Fibers from this ligament blend with the tendon of the supraspinatus muscle. As the name implies, it extends from the coracoid process of the scapula to the humerus.

The *glenohumeral ligament* is actually a

strengthening band within the joint capsule that can be separated into three components: the superior, middle, and inferior glenohumeral ligaments. All three extend from the anterior glenoid margin and radiate into the anterior wall of the capsule.

The *coracoacromial ligament* is in reality a ligament of the scapula. However, it is often described as a component of the shoulder joint and is classified as an accessory ligament of this joint. It is a strong triangular band that is attached to the whole length of the lateral border of the coracoid process and to the tip of the acromion. Together with the acromion and coracoid process this ligament forms an arch above the head of the humerus and helps to protect the joint. It is in contact with the deltoid muscle above and the infraspinatus muscle below. The subacromial bursa lies wedged between this ligament and the superior surface of the joint capsule below and the deltoid muscle above. Although the interior, or cavity, of this bursa may occasionally be connected with or open directly into the joint space, it usually does not. There are several additional bursae associated with muscles around the shoulder in addition to the subacromial. A bursa that does communicate with the joint space occurs deep to the subscapularis muscle. There is a bursa between the joint capsule and the infraspinatus muscle, whereas others are found between the coracoid process and the capsule, behind the coracobrachialis muscle, between the tendon of the subscapularis and the capsule, and one in front of and another behind the tendon of the latissimus dorsi muscle.

Any of these bursae can become inflamed and painful as a result of overuse or trauma to the area. The subacromial bursa is the most often affected. As it becomes aggravated, normally from friction, its lining often thickens, thus increasing pressure and in some cases creating a fold in the lining. This will cause rough movement and possibly a snap as the humerus moves. Symptoms include tenderness just distal to the acromion and pain on active motion of the shoulder, especially abduction and rotation.

Shoulder muscles and movements

The principal muscles of importance in moving the shoulder joint are listed in Table 17-1. Points of attachment and relationships between individual muscles in the shoulder girdle or joint are shown in Figs. 17-5 to 17-18.

Table 17-1. Movements of the shoulder joint

Movement	Principal muscles
Flexion	Biceps
	Coracobrachialis
	Deltoid (anterior fibers)
	Pectoralis major (clavicular fibers)
Extension	Latissimus dorsi
	Teres major
	Deltoid (posterior fibers)
	Triceps (long head)
Abduction	Supraspinatus
	Deltoid (middle fibers)
Adduction	Pectoralis major
	Latissimus dorsi
	Teres major
	Subscapularis
	Coracobrachialis
Medial rotation	Subscapularis
	Teres major
	Latissimus dorsi
	Pectoralis major
	Deltoid (anterior fibers)
Lateral rotation	Infraspinatus
	Teres minor
	Deltoid (posterior fibers)

Fig. 17-5. Deltoid (anterior fibers) and coracobrachialis muscles.

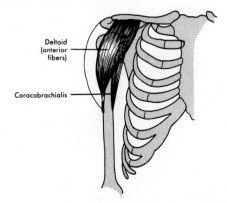

Deltoid
(anterior
fibers)

Coracobrachialis

Fig. 17-6. Teres major and latissimus dorsi muscles.

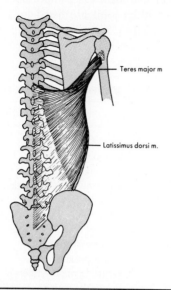

Fig. 17-7. Deltoid (middle fibers) and supraspinatus muscles.

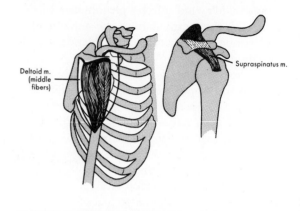

Fig. 17-8. Pectoralis major muscle.

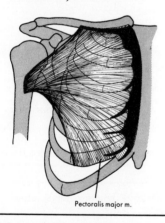

Fig. 17-9. Deltoid muscle (posterior fibers).

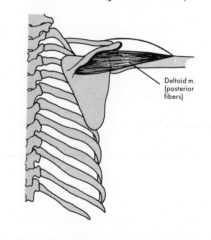

Fig. 17-10. Subscapularis muscle.

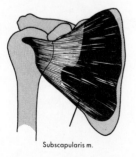

Fig. 17-11. Infraspinatus and teres minor muscles.

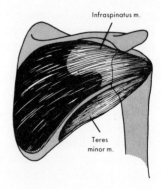

Fig. 17-12. Serratus anterior muscle.

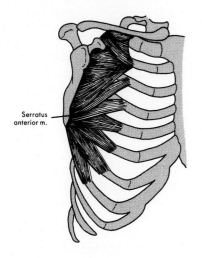

Serratus
anterior m.

Fig. 17-13. Trapezius muscle (middle fibers).

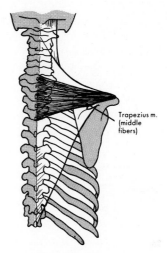

Trapezius m.
(middle
fibers)

Fig. 17-14. Trapezius (superior fiber) and levator scapulae muscles.

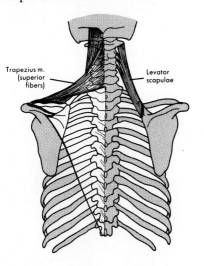

Trapezius m.
(superior
fibers)

Levator
scapulae

Fig. 17-15. Trapezius muscle (inferior fiber).

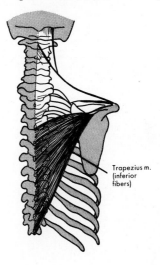

Trapezius m.
(inferior
fibers)

The muscles listed in Table 17-1 are grouped in a rather simplified way to indicate major function. It should be emphasized that if the position of the upper extremity is markedly changed or if the arm is held in a flexed, rotated, or extended position, points of reference would change and

additional muscles would assume important and in many cases differing functional roles. Further, still other muscles not specifically noted in Table 17-1 serve as fixators, synergists, or antagonists in the actions that are listed. A detailed explanation of the complex array of specialized movements possible at the shoulder girdle and joint is beyond the scope of this text. Interested students should refer to specialized texts in kinesiology and biomechanics.

Anatomic relationships

The principal anatomic structures in relation to the shoulder joint and articular capsule are illustrated in Fig. 17-19. They are, above, subacromial bursa, supraspinatus muscle, acromion and coracoacromial ligament; in front, subscapular bursa and subscapularis muscle; behind, teres minor muscle, infraspinatus muscle and its bursa; below, long head of the triceps brachii muscle, teres major muscle, and the inferior portion of the subscapularis muscle. Note how the supraspinatus, infraspinatus, teres minor, and subscapularis muscles serve to support the joint and help hold the articular surfaces of the joint against one another.

Fig. 17-16. Rhomboid major and minor muscles.

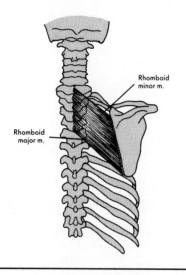

Fig. 17-17. Biceps brachii and brachialis muscles.

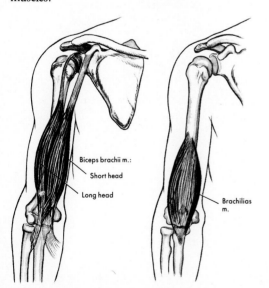

Fig. 17-18. Triceps brachii muscle.

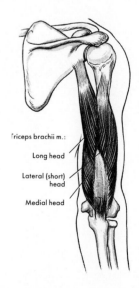

Injuries to the shoulder complex

A variety of athletic injuries can occur to the shoulder joint. Because of the extensive motion available and the inherent instability of the shoulder joint, this area of the body is very vulnerable to acute athletic injuries as well as chronic overuse conditions. The mechanisms causing most injuries to the shoulder are direct trauma, indirect trauma, or throwing movements. Direct trauma occurs because the shoulder is the portion of the anatomy best suited for forcible ramming, such as tackling in football or checking in ice hockey. This exposes the shoulder to direct contact. Athletes who are falling or being tackled may also land on their shoulder, which can result in direct trauma to the shoulder complex. Indirect trauma can occur as injurious forces are transmitted to the shoulder joint or the entire shoulder complex through the humerus as the result of direct trauma to the hand or elbow. Examples of indirect trauma to the shoulder girdle are athletes landing on an outstretched hand or the point of a flexed elbow (Fig. 17-20). Participants in all athletic activity are subject to falls that can cause an indirect insult to the shoulder. Attempts to break a fall frequently result in indirect shoulder trauma. Athletic injuries also occur frequently as a result of throwing movements. This includes all sports requiring throwing or swinging motions of the shoulder.

Fig. 17-19. Relations of the left shoulder joint: *(D)* deltoid, *(SU.)* supraspinatus, *(IN.)* infraspinatus, *(P.M.)* pectoralis major, *(SUB.)* subscapularis, *(T.MI.)* teres minor, *(T.MA.)* teres major, *(TRI.)* long head of triceps brachii, *(L.D.)* latissimus dorsi, *(1)* acromion, *(2)* subacromial bursa, *(3)* superior glenohumeral ligament, *(4)* coracoacromial ligament, *(5)* subscapular bursa, *(6)* coracoid process of scapula, *(7)* cephalic vein, *(8)* middle glenohumeral ligament, *(9)* inferior glenohumeral ligament, *(10)* parts of brachial plexus and its branches, *(11)* axillary nerve and posterior humeral circumflex vessels traversing quadrilateral space, *(12)* axillary vessels, *(13)* capsular ligament, *(14)* glenoid cavity, *(15)* biceps tendon and synovial sheaths.

(From Crafts, R.C.: A textbook of human anatomy, ed. 2, New York, 1979, Wiley Medical.)

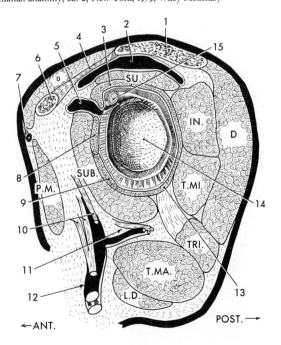

Injuries resulting from any of these mechanisms can be acute, including contusions, sprains, strains, dislocations, and occasionally fractures as well as chronic conditions. The athletic trainer must also consider the accessory structures that support the shoulder (that is, muscles that stabilize the scapula) when evaluating the shoulder complex because injury to any of these structures will influence range of motion.

Contusions. The most common contusion about the shoulder is to the tip of the shoulder or acromion process (Fig. 17-21). This is commonly called a *shoulder pointer*. A shoulder pointer implies a contusion with no ligamentous involvement. With this injury, the athletic trainer must be concerned with a more serious injury to the acromioclavicular joint. Accurately locate areas of tenderness and carefully examine the area to determine if there is any involvement of the acromioclavicular joint. The deltoid muscle is also susceptible to direct blows, which can result in contusions to the area. A possible complication of repeated contusions to the region of the deltoid attachment on the lateral humerus is a painful periostitis, which can develop into an irritative *exostosis* or spur formation sometimes referred to a *blocker's spur*.

Strains. A common injury about the shoulder joint is some type of muscular or musculotendinous strain. The glenohumeral joint relies on the surrounding musculature for most of its stability as well as its motion and power. Therefore the muscles and musculotendinous structures are involved in many types of athletic injuries. Various mechanisms can produce injuries to the musculotendinous units, including overstretching, violent contractions, and repetitive use.

Strains about the shoulder are especially common in athletic activities that require the arm to propel an object, such as pitching, or to over-

Fig. 17-20. Mechanism of injury to shoulder complex. Injurious forces are transferred to shoulder area as athlete falls on an outstretched arm.

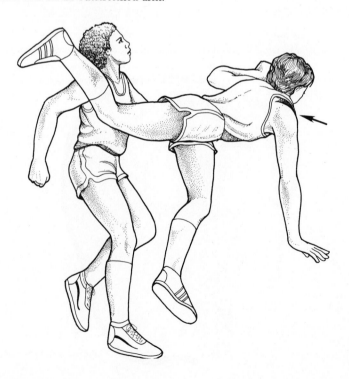

come a resistance, such as in swimming. During racquet sports the shoulder serves as the fulcrum for the arm, and major stresses are placed on the elbow and forearm. However, significant and often injurious forces are also placed on the shoulder joint. Each sport presents its own problems or situations for the shoulder, and the responses to stress vary in intensity and location. The nature of shoulder strains is influenced by many things, such as the age and maturity of the athlete; the type and weight of the object being propelled; the type of delivery; the presence of weakness, fatigue, or incoordination; fibrous scarring or degenerative changes from previous injuries; and microtrauma from repetitive activity. All of these factors must be considered during the assessment of shoulder injuries.

In evaluating an injury to the many muscles that attach and function about the shoulder, attempt to locate as precisely as possible the area

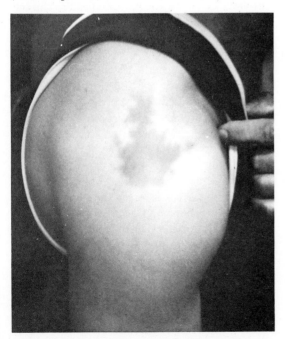

Fig. 17-21. Contusion injury. Note discoloration over tip of the shoulder (shoulder pointer).

of local tenderness and correlate this information with pain elicited on active contraction or passive stretching of the involved muscle. Because most muscles about the shoulder function during more than one movement, a basic knowledge of the functional anatomy of the area is necessary to isolate each muscle suspected of being injured. Evaluation techniques for the muscles most frequently injured are discussed during the assessment portion of this chapter. Strains to the rotator cuff and biceps tendon are more difficult to evaluate. They are briefly described in the following paragraphs.

Injuries involving the rotator cuff muscles are difficult to detect and isolate because these muscles, which reinforce the joint capsule, lie deep in the shoulder. Any of the mechanisms previously described can cause an injury to these muscles; however, when they occur in young athletes the problem is normally the result of direct trauma. As an athlete becomes older, he or she is more susceptible to rotator cuff injuries resulting from repeated stress. Repetitive use of the shoulder can result in microscopic damage to the rotator cuff muscles. A great deal of difficulty may be encountered in assessing these soft tissue lesions. Bursitis, tendinitis, partial rotator cuff tears, loose pieces of fibrocartilage, and calcific deposits are all capable of producing similar signs and symptoms. A variety of terms have been used to describe these conditions, such as supraspinatus syndrome, rotator cuff impingment, painful arc syndrome, and internal derangement of the subacromial joint. The supraspinatus muscle is most often involved. Secondary changes such as scarring, thickening of the involved tendon, chronic inflammation, and irritation of the overlying bursa frequently develop. These factors decrease the distance between the cuff and the overlying coracoacromial arch, which can cause pain and crepitus as the involved tissues are squeezed or impinged between the greater tuberosity of the humerus and the overlying arch. Activities involving repetitive use of the arm above the horizontal level, such as throwing, tennis, or swimming, may produce this overuse syndrome. The symptoms usually consist of continued discomfort, which is initially noticed after activity and progresses to pain during participation and eventually may affect the performance of the athlete. The pain may cause the athlete to restrict his or her movement and refrain from particular maneuvers that cause the impingement. Assessment procedures for evaluating impingment syndromes are discussed later with passive stress tests.

Another relatively common strain in the shoulder occurs to the long head of the biceps tendon. This is especially true in athletes who are skiing, throwing overhand, or playing tennis. As previously discussed, the long head of the biceps tendon lies in a tubular sheath as it passes through the bicipital groove. Repetitive motion of the shoulder causes this tendon to slide up and down through the tunnel. The irritation of constant motion can cause an inflammatory reaction. This bicipital tenosynovitis will cause tenderness along the bicipital groove and pain on active and resistive contraction or passive stretching of the biceps.

Dislocation or partial dislocation (subluxation) of the biceps tendon from its tunnel may occur with limited rupture or tears of the transverse ligament or the rotator cuff, especially the subscapularis tendon. In these cases, arm movement that involves external rotation of the humerus will cause sudden pain and a locking sensation accompanied by an audible click in the shoulder. The athletic trainer will usually be able to feel displacement or crepitus by applying finger pressure over the bicipital groove during external rotation of the humerus. Repeated or recurrent subluxation or dislocation requires surgical repair. Occasionally the biceps tendon ruptures as a result of degeneration caused by chronic tendinitis. The onset is normally sudden, with the athlete experiencing a sharp snap followed by pain and weakness of the arm. The evaluation is easily made by observing the abnormally large bulging muscle mass in the arm. Acute ruptures of the biceps tendon are more common in weight lifters and gymnasts.

Sprains. The most common sprains about the shoulder complex are to the acromioclavicular joint, which has been previously discussed. The ligaments and capsule about the glenohumeral joint contribute minimally to the stability of the shoulder joint. Therefore sprains of the shoulder joint seldom occur unless there is a subluxation or dislocation.

Dislocation. Because of its inherent instability, the shoulder joint has the highest incidence of dislocation of any major joint in the body. Shoulder dislocations are classified depending on the location of the head of the humerus. The anterior, or subcoracoid, dislocation is by far the most common. The mechanism of injury is forced abduction and external rotation. The athlete generally has the shoulder in an abducted, externally rotated position and receives a blow somewhere along the extremity. This force directs the humeral head toward the anterior portion of the joint capsule. This forward progression is checked by the coracoacromial ligament and diverted down toward the area of the capsule supported by the glenohumeral ligament. If the force is sufficient, the capsule and ligaments surrender and allow the humeral head to slip out of the glenoid fossa to lodge between the rim of the glenoid and coronoid process. A dislocated shoulder that remains displaced will usually be readily recognized, as is normally an associated deformity and the athlete is unable to or resists any movement of the arm. If the force is insufficient to cause a complete dislocation, the humeral head may sublux and then relocate, causing a sprain of the anterior capsule and supporting ligaments. The history of the injury then becomes more important. The athlete will often relate that the arm was forced into external rotation and abduction and he or she felt the humerus "slip out of place." This will be accompanied by pain in the anterior aspect of the joint, which is increased by any attempt to abduct and externally rotate the arm. The abduction and external rotation is the basis for the apprehension test described later.

A less common form of shoulder dislocation is

a posterior dislocation. The mechanism involves a posteriorly directed force against a flexed humerus. The humeral head slides posteriorly past the glenoid and posterior capsule to lodge against the rotator cuff musculature. Because of the tension of this musculature, posterior dislocations have a high incidence of spontaneous relocation, which makes the evaluation difficult. Symptoms are those of a strain or sprain of the posterior structures and an increase in pain when replicating the mechanism of injury.

Another seldomly encountered dislocation is an inferior dislocation in which the head of the humerus lies inferior to the lip of the glenoid. This type of dislocation can occur during forced abduction, when the capsule and supporting ligaments are torn and allow the humeral head to slip below the glenoid rim. An inferior dislocation that remains displaced may cause a *luxatio erecta,* in which the arm stands straight above the head and the athlete is unable to bring it down. An inferior subluxation will cause the arm to be held at the side because any attempt to abduct it will cause the athlete to feel as if the arm will slip out of place.

Dislocations of the shoulder have a high incidence of recurrence without a period of immobilization and a vigorous rehabilitation program. When a shoulder is not rehabilitated sufficiently following a dislocation, this joint is very susceptible to repeated episodes. Each successive dislocation requires less force to drive the humeral head out of the glenoid and also causes it to reduce more easily. Recurrent episodes can develop into a condition in which the shoulder will dislocate during abduction and external rotation without much additional trauma. This demonstrates the importance of early recognition and proper rehabilitation of all shoulder dislocations.

Fractures. Fractures about the shoulder joint are not common in athletic activity. When fractures do occur, they are often associated with subluxations or dislocations and appear as avulsion fractures of the rotator cuff tendons, supporting ligaments, or capsular attachments. This is a sound reason to refer all athletes with first-time shoulder dislocations to a physician for probable radiographic evaluation. Occasionally an athlete may suffer a fracture of the surgical neck of the humerus instead of a dislocation. In young athletes fractures may be through the proximal epiphysis.

One condition an athletic trainer must be alert to is development of *adhesive capsulitis.* This condition is commonly called a "frozen shoulder." It is an inflammation about the rotator cuff and capsular area and can develop because the athlete protects a painful shoulder by limiting movement. In some cases it may develop if the joint is immobilized after a serious injury. The main feature of adhesive capsulitis is lack of passive range of motion. If the athletic trainer cannot move an athlete's shoulder passively through a normal range of motion after the recovery period, adhesive capsulitis should be suspected and steps taken to correct the situation if it exists.

Brachial plexus

The most important nerves involved in the axilla and shoulder are components of the brachial plexus (Fig. 17-22) and its branches. The brachial plexus is a complex network consisting of nerves, trunks, divisions, and main branches that ultimately provide both motor and sensory innervation to the entire upper extremity. Pressure to this nerve plexus or its accompanying blood vessels can produce serious injury.

Brachial plexus injuries

Injuries to the brachial plexus normally involve the cervical spine, but the symptoms are exhibited in the shoulder and upper extremity. When an athlete's neck is violently forced into rotation or lateral flexion, especially while the opposite shoulder is depressed, considerable tension can be placed on the nerve branches of the brachial plexus. Occasionally part of the brachial plexus is compressed between the clavicle and first rib. Both of these mechanisms can result in transitory paralysis of the arm, with numbness or a burning sensation radiating down the arm and sometimes into the hand. This normally disappears in a matter of seconds to a few minutes. Occasionally recovery may take days. An injury to the brachial plexus is frequently called a "pinched nerve," "burner," "hot shot," or "stinger." Occasionally a persistent disability may result from this type of injury. Athletes experiencing repeated episodes of brachial plexus injuries or who complain of weakness or numbness in the arm that persists for an hour or more after the injury should be carefully evaluated and referred to a physician for a neurologic examination.

ATHLETIC INJURY ASSESSMENT PROCESS

The shoulder girdle is the most frequently injured area of the upper extremity. This complex is very vulnerable to acute athletic injuries as well as chronic overuse conditions because it

Fig. 17-22. The brachial plexus.

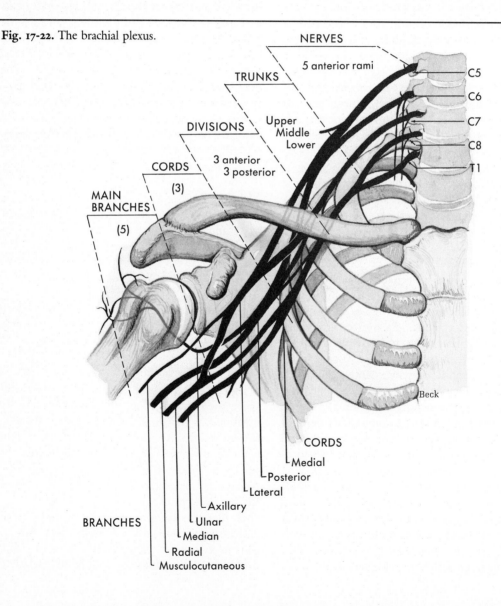

serves as the attachment and fulcrum for upper extremity action and is the portion of anatomy best suited for forcible ramming or butting. Although the glenohumeral joint has an extensive range of motion, it is relatively unstable compared to other major joints of the body. A wide variety of athletic injuries to the shoulder complex result from direct or indirect trauma as well as from activities requiring throwing movements. To complete a comprehensive assessment of injuries involving the shoulder girdle, athletic trainers must take many factors into consideration, such as: (1) unique anatomic features, (2) intricate functional characteristics, (3) various mechanisms of injury, and (4) associated signs and symptoms. A meticulous and systematic examination is often necessary to identify the anatomic structures involved and to determine the nature and severity of the injury. The initial assessment process is designed to generate a comprehensive data base for use in further evaluations, treatment, and rehabilitation programs.

Secondary survey

The evaluation procedures used during the assessment of shoulder injuries will initially depend on the position and status of the athlete at the time the injury is recognized or reported. Your initial observations and judgment will normally determine the direction in which you should proceed with the secondary survey. Most athletes with a shoulder injury will be sitting, standing, or moving around. It is unusual for an athlete with an isolated shoulder injury to remain lying on the field or court unless the injury is a dislocation or fracture. It is possible that an athlete involved in an injury, especially some type of collision, can sustain an injury to the head or neck as well as the shoulder. Whenever an athlete remains down after incurring what appears to be a shoulder injury, your suspicion level should remain high. Carefully check for a more serious injury to the head or neck or additional involvement such as internal thoracic injuries. Injuries to the head or neck must be ruled out before evaluating the shoulder. Another im-

portant consideration is the adequacy and integrity of circulation and neurologic pathways distal to a shoulder injury. These evaluative procedures may be incorporated into the physical assessment. Circulation is assessed by feeling for distal pulses, usually the radial. Neurologic involvement can be evaluated by checking skin sensations over the shoulder and arm as well as evaluating active motion of the shoulder and upper extremity as a whole. Remember, when a serious injury or circulatory or neurologic involvement is recognized, it is not necessary to continue with the assessment procedures. Emergency care, referral, or carefully supervised transportation techniques should be instituted as indicated. The specific assessment procedures used in evaluating shoulder injuries will vary depending on the signs and symptoms expressed as well as demonstrated by the athlete.

History

A comprehensive shoulder examination begins with a careful review of the history relevant to the shoulder injury (Fig. 17-23). Questioning should quickly determine if the injury is an acute

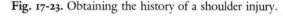

Fig. 17-23. Obtaining the history of a shoulder injury.

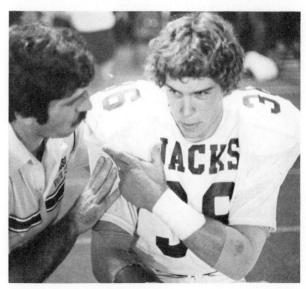

or a chronic problem. Many shoulder injuries are recurrent conditions or chronic overuse syndromes. If the area has been injured before, obtain as much information about the previous injury as possible. Question the athlete about the nature of previous injuries, the treatment procedures used, and the extent of rehabilitation. Had symptoms completely subsided and full function been restored before the onset of the current injury? Are symptoms of the current injury similar to those of any previous injuries? The more information gained concerning previous injuries, the better you can evaluate the nature and severity of the current problem.

Question the athlete concerning the present injury. When did the onset of symptoms occur? Chronic overuse syndromes normally begin slowly and insidiously with a low-grade ache. Symptoms gradually increase as the athlete continues to use and stress the shoulder. What has happened to the symptoms since the athlete first noticed the injury? If the onset is sudden, the athlete will usually relate a traumatic episode. Have the athlete describe the mechanism of injury in detail. Was there a direct blow delivered to the shoulder? What was the angle of the impact? Attempt to determine the amount of force at impact. Did the direct blow involve the side of the head or neck? Did the athlete fall and land on the shoulder or an outstretched arm? What was the position of the arm at the time of injury? Was the arm forced beyond normal limits? Did the injury result from a forceful muscular contraction? Obtain as much information as possible concerning the mechanism of injury because this knowledge is important in determining the nature of the injury and the structures involved.

Have the athlete describe the symptoms associated with the injury in as much detail as possible. Where is the pain? Ask the athlete to locate the pain or tender areas as precisely as possible and describe the characteristics of the pain. Is the pain sharply localized or dull and diffused? Is there any pain radiating down the arm? Are there any activities or movements that cause the pain to increase or decrease? Ask if there are any activities or movements that are difficult or impossible for the athlete to initiate. Is the pain severe enough to wake the athlete or prevent him or her from sleeping? Occasionally pain will only be present during certain movements or at a particular point in the range of motion. Ask the athlete to demonstrate the motion or movements that aggravate the shoulder. Remember, the shoulder is a classic area for referred and radiating pain. Therefore the chest, upper abdomen, neck, or spine may have to be carefully examined to determine if the pain is being referred or radiated to the shoulder.

Question the athlete about any other sensations associated with the injury. Did he or she hear or feel anything at the time of injury, such as a popping or snapping sensation? Does the athlete feel any tightness, tension, locking, or swelling associated with the injury? Is there or has there been any crepitation? Does the athlete complain of any numbness, burning, weakness or tingling in the upper extremity? Ask the athlete to describe his or her impressions concerning the injury and integrate this information into the assessment. If an athlete says a bone is broken or the shoulder is dislocated, believe it and proceed with the evaluation as if this is the problem until it is proved otherwise.

Observation

The statement "look before you touch" is one of the cardinal rules of assessment. The impact of your visual observations on the formal assessment process will diminish once you begin using other senses. It is important therefore that your initial assessment observations begin before you touch or even talk to the injured athlete. First note the overall position or posture of the athlete and the alignment of the upper extremities. Is the athlete moving or using the injured extremity? Is he or she holding, supporting, or favoring any area of the shoulder or arm? Does the shoulder or arm appear to be in an abnormal position, which may indicate a dislocation or fracture? Does the arm appear to be hanging limp at the athlete's side, which reflects the athlete's reluctance to move the arm? Always remember to observe the athlete's face. Does he or she appear to be uncomfortable or in a great deal of pain?

Many times, especially in contact sports, the injured shoulder will be covered with protective equipment and clothing. Do not disturb the shoulder girdle by removing the uniform and equipment until you are relatively sure of the nature and severity of the injury. Uniforms and protective equipment can be cut off as previously described, but in most cases the early stages of the assessment procedures can continue with the equipment in place. Palpation techniques are used at this time to further evaluate the injured shoulder. Gently slide your hand under the uniform or protective equipment to feel the entire shoulder complex (Fig. 17-24). Being firm but gentle, palpate the shoulder to locate any pain, tenderness or deformity. Continue questioning the athlete in a soft reassuring voice and watch his or her face to note any discomfort or reac-

tions. In this manner a preliminary evaluation of the injury can be performed without removing the uniform and causing any unnecessary movements of the shoulder. Remember to palpate the uninjured shoulder as well to compare symmetry. Of course, should a significant injury be found, the uniform and equipment can be cut off or the athlete referred to a physician or medical facility with the apparel left in place. Once you are relatively sure no serious injury exists, you can assist the athlete in removing the uniform and equipment and continue with a more thorough evaluation. Clothing and equipment should be removed from the uninjured extremity first and then slid off the involved side to prevent needless movement of the injured extremity. As the athlete disrobes, notice the shoulder movement. Does he or she favor the injured side? Look for any signs that may indicate neurologic involvement, such as paralysis or weakness.

Once clothing and equipment have been re-

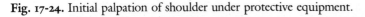

Fig. 17-24. Initial palpation of shoulder under protective equipment.

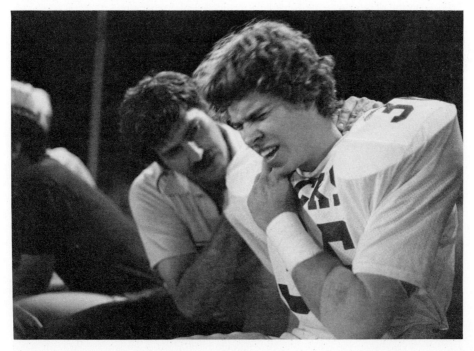

moved, observe the overall posture, muscular development, and alignment of both shoulders with the athlete standing or sitting and the arms at the sides. Compare the symmetry and appearance of the upper extremities from the anterior as well as the posterior position (Fig. 17-25). Note the contours. Are there any signs of deformities? Is there any marked swelling? Is there any definite atrophy of the muscles surrounding the shoulder girdle? Occasionally with a chronic condition there will be associated atrophy of muscle groups. Carefully inspect the injured shoulder for signs of trauma, such as abrasions or contusions. These signs can indicate what types of forces have been applied to the athlete's body and help establish the mechanism of injury.

Palpation

Thorough palpation techniques can be extremely beneficial in the assessment of athletic injuries of the shoulder. Palpation is used to investigate or confirm those findings or suspicions formulated during the history and observation procedures. The shoulder girdle is usually easily accessible to palpation because most of the structures are subcutaneous. However, palpation techniques may be more difficult in the overweight or highly muscular athlete. If the underlying anatomy is clearly understood, tenderness can normally be readily associated with those anatomic structures suspected of being injured.

Palpation of the shoulder girdle should be conducted with the area as relaxed as possible. Normally this is accomplished by having the athlete sit on a table or stand with the arms in a comfortable and relaxed position. The shoulder can also be palpated with the athlete supine and the arms supported by the table, ground or floor. This position should be used if the athlete is uncomfortable in an upright position or possibly suffering from the effects of shock. The

Fig. 17-25. Comparing symmetry and appearance of both shoulders. Note the prominence of the distal clavicle on the right side (second-degree acromioclavicular separation).

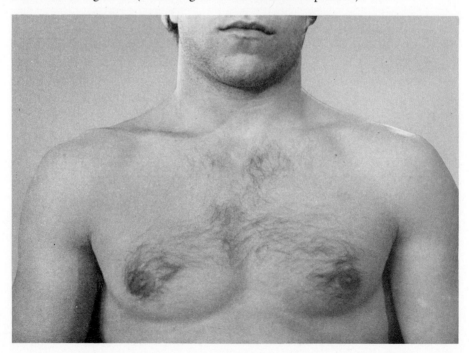

initial structures to be palpated will be determined by the suspicions raised during the preceeding phases of the assessment process. Remember, palpation techniques should be performed gently. Always begin away from the suspected area of injury to further promote cooperation from the athlete. Palpate both the injured and uninjured sides.

Bony anatomy. The integrity of the bony anatomy is normally evaluated first, followed by the assessment of any damage to the soft tissues. Carefully palpate the bones and bony landmarks about the suspected site of injury, noting any points of tenderness or crepitation. Palpate the various muscles and other soft tissue structures suspected of being involved in the injury, again noting specific areas of tenderness. Tenderness must be carefully localized and precisely identified in an attempt to accurately recognize the underlying structures that may be damaged. In the following paragraphs, the procedures used to palpate the various anatomic structures about the shoulder girdle are briefly discussed. In addition, the common athletic injuries that may be indicated by the physical signs noted during the assessment are reviewed.

The clavicle is a good point of reference to begin palpating the shoulder, as it is subcutaneous along its entire length. It is generally easier to palpate both clavicles simultaneously to note any differences in symmetry. Begin by placing your hands medially to feel the sternoclavicular joint (Fig. 17-26). This easily palpated joint is not commonly injured in athletic activity. A sprain of the sternoclavicular joint can be recognized by pain and point tenderness at this articulation, and depending on the severity, there may be varying degrees of visible and palpable deformity. The sternal end of the clavicle will normally be displaced forward and upward in a second- or third-degree sprain. Although rare, it must be remembered that posterior displacement of the clavicle or manubrium of the sternum can compress the trachea and occlude the airway. Displacement can occur with traumatic movements of the sternal portion of the clavicle or by a direct blow to the upper chest.

The anterior and superior surfaces of the clavicle can be palpated throughout its length. Slowly palpate this smooth S-shaped bone from its distal to proximal end, noting any tenderness, swelling, crepitation, or disruption of continuity. Fractures of the clavicle, one of the more frequent fractures in athletics, can normally be recognized by careful palpation. There may be no deformity associated with a clavicular fracture in a young athlete, as these are usually the greenstick type of fracture. Once an area of point tenderness is located along the clavicle, the possibility of a fracture should be considered. In the absence of deformity, an area of point tenderness can be further evaluated by applying stress to the clavicle away from the site of pain. Move away from the tender area an inch or two and very gently apply mild pressure to the clavicle. Remember to inform the athlete that you are going to press gently and to tell you if the procedure increases the pain. If this maneuver causes additional pain at the original site of tenderness, the athlete should be treated as if he or she has a fracture.

Continue palpating distally to the lateral end

Fig. 17-26. Palpating the sternoclavicular joint.

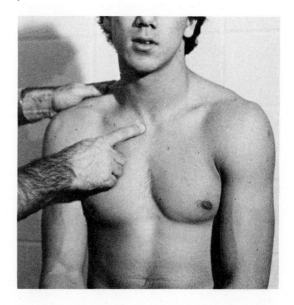

of the clavicle where it articulates with the acromion to form the acromioclavicular joint (Fig. 17-27). This is a frequently injured joint in the shoulder girdle. Tenderness expressed in this area indicates an injury to the acromioclavicular joint. The lateral end of the clavicle normally rides just slightly higher than the acromion. If the clavicle on the injured side is setting abnormally higher than the acromion when compared to the uninjured side, a second- or third-degree sprain of this joint should be suspected. A third-degree sprain will normally exhibit gross deformity, with the distal end of the clavicle being quite prominent. This type of injury should be readily recognized. Keep in mind that this athlete may have suffered a previous injury to the acromioclavicular joint, and the clavicle could have been higher before the current injury. Press down on the distal end of the clavicle. Is there an increase in pain? Is there an increase in mobility of the clavicle in its relationship to the acromion? Compare any hypermobility to the uninjured side. Remember, a second-degree sprain or partial separation will be indicated by in-creased tenderness and hypermobility of the acromioclavicular joint.

The acromion process of the scapula can be palpated at the tip of the shoulder. This flared projection is the lateral end of the scapular spine. Athletes landing on the tip of the shoulder may bruise this area; such an injury is commonly referred to as a "shoulder pointer."

The spine of the scapula is a sharp subcutaneous ridge running diagonally across the posterior surface of the shoulder blade. It can usually be palpated along its entire length (Fig. 17-28, A). Athletic injuries seldom occur to the scapular spine, but it is a good point of reference for palpating soft tissue structures about the scapula. The borders of the scapula can also be readily felt. Palpate along the vertebral or medial borders of both scapulae (Fig. 17-28, B) from the superior to the inferior angles. Normally the vertebral borders lie approximately 2 inches from the spinous processes of the thoracic vertebrae, and palpating both simultaneously can assist in determining if one of the scapulae is carried forward. The vertebral border is also the point of reference for the muscles attached along its length. From the inferior angle of the scapula, the lateral or axillary border can be palpated for a short distance before it is covered with muscles.

The head of the humerus can be palpated laterally and inferiorly to the acromion process. Although this area is covered by the deltoid muscle, careful palpation will reveal the greater and lesser tuberosities bordering the bicipital groove. The greater tuberosity forms the lateral border of the bicipital groove, whereas the lesser tuberosity comprises the medial lip. These structures are more easily recognized if the arm is rotated during palpation. With the humerus externally rotated, the bicipital groove and lesser tuberosity are in a more exposed position (Fig. 17-29, A). With internal rotation, the greater tuberosity becomes more prominent and easier to feel (Fig. 17-29, B). The long head of the biceps tendon lies in the bicipital groove, and point tenderness or crepitus in this area may indicate tenosynovitis or tendon subluxation. Pal-

Fig. 17-27. Palpating the acromioclavicular joint.

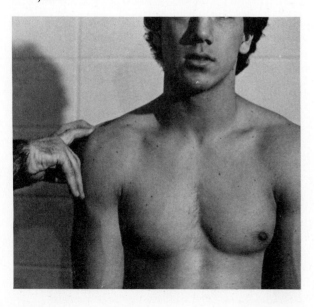

pation maneuvers of the bicipital groove should be performed gently so as not to cause unnecessary pain in the area, causing the athlete to become tense.

Two other bony landmarks that may be palpated in the shoulder girdle and serve as reference points are the deltoid tuberosity and the coracoid process of the scapula. The deltoid tuberosity is a V-shaped, roughened area midway down the lateral surface of the shaft of the humerus where the deltoid muscle inserts (Fig. 17-30). This is the site for the possible development of a blocker's spur. The coracoid process lies about 1 inch below the clavicle and may be

Fig. 17-28. Palpating the scapula: **A**, spine and **B**, vertebral border.

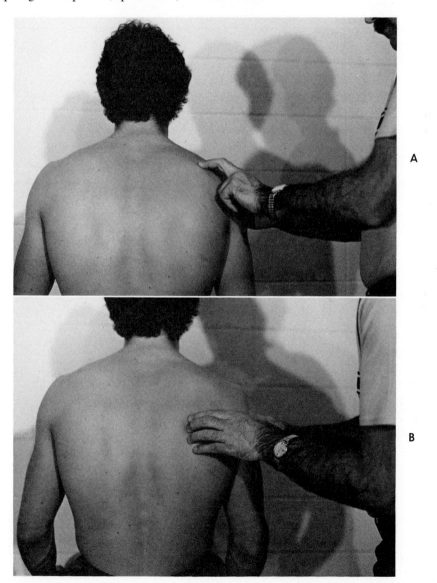

A

B

felt in the groove between the deltoid and pectoralis major muscles. Because this structure lies beneath muscle, firm pressure is necessary to feel the tip of the coracoid process (Fig. 17-31).

Soft tissue anatomy. The majority of soft tissue structures about the shoulder girdle can be palpated to evaluate their involvement in an athletic injury. Knowledge of the underlying anatomy combined with careful palpation techniques provides the athletic trainer the opportunity to rec-ognize any areas of tenderness, swelling, or anatomic inconsistencies. This information, combined with various stress procedures, is valuable in assessing soft tissue injuries. Although palpation of bony and soft tissue structures is discussed separately, they are normally performed in conjunction with one another during a shoulder assessment.

The prominent muscles of the shoulder girdle can be palpated individually. Anteriorly, the pec-

Fig. 17-29. Palpating **A,** the bicipital groove during external rotation of the arm and **B,** the greater tuberosity during internal rotation of the arm.

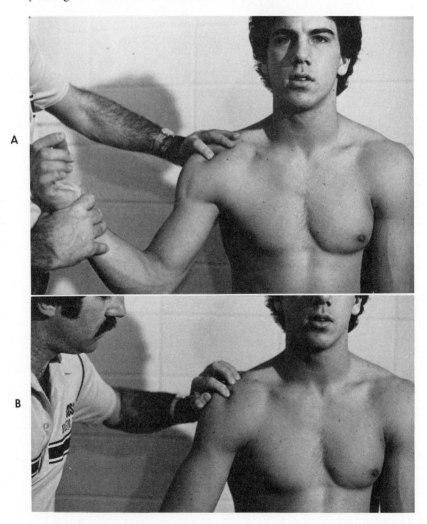

toralis major muscle can be palpated from its origins on the chest wall and clavicle to its insertion on the greater tuberosity of the humerus. This muscle forms the anterior wall of the axilla when the arm is abducted (Fig. 17-32).

The deltoid muscle covers the lateral aspect of the shoulder, and each of the three portions can

Fig. 17-30. Palpating the deltoid tuberosity.

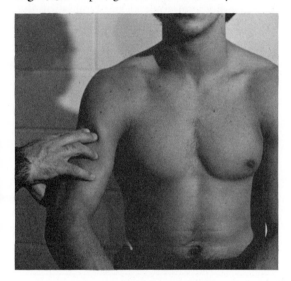

be easily palpated. This muscle must be carefully palpated, as it covers several structures that are often involved in athletic injuries; thus tenderness elicited by touch may be common to one of several different structures. For example, tenderness over the bicipital groove may indicate a tenosynovitis of the biceps tendon or an injury to the deltoid muscle. Tenderness deep to the deltoid muscle is also frequently associated with subdeltoid bursitis or rotator cuff problems.

The large subacromial (subdeltoid) bursa, wedged between the superior surface of the joint capsule and the inferior surface of the deltoid muscle, may be tender to touch just below the edge of the acromion process if bursitis is present. Passively hyperextending the arm exposes a greater portion of the bursa as well as the insertion of the supraspinatus muscle from beneath the acromion process. Palpate just below the anterior border of the acromion. Tenderness elicited during this maneuver may indicate an injury to the rotator cuff or bursitis. To distinguish between these conditions, stress techniques described on p. 506 must be employed.

Several muscles on the posterior surface of the shoulder girdle can be palpated. The most super-

Fig. 17-31. Palpating the coracoid process.

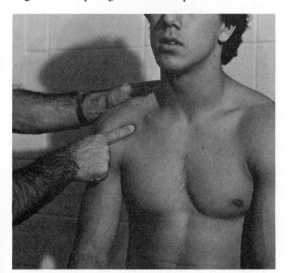

Fig. 17-32. Palpating the pectoralis major muscle.

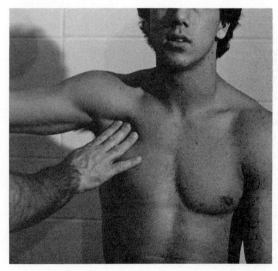

ficial and readily felt of these is the trapezius, which originates on the occipital bone and the cervical and thoracic spinous processes and inserts on the scapular spine, acromion, and clavicle. The superior portion of the trapezius is frequently involved in neck strains, which may be recognized by point tenderness and increased pain on active and resistive motion. The latissimus dorsi muscle forms the lateral border of the axilla and can be readily palpated when the arm is abducted, making this muscle more prominent and easier to locate (Fig. 17-33). Additional muscles can be palpated on the posterior surface of the shoulder; however, they are not subcutaneous or readily distinguishable and are seldom involved in athletic injury. When these muscles are strained, they are identified by local tenderness and pain when the particular muscle is contracted.

The major muscles of the upper arm are occasionally injured as the result of athletic activity. Palpate the biceps on the anterior aspect of the humerus. This muscle becomes more prominent when the elbow is flexed (Fig. 17-34, *A*), and we

have already discussed finding the tendon of the long head of the biceps as it lies in the bicipital groove. The triceps can be palpated on the posterior surface of the humerus (Fig. 17-34, *B*).

Stress

Stress procedures are often used to facilitate the assessment of athletic injuries occurring to the shoulder girdle, especially those involving the glenohumeral joint. The stability of this highly mobile joint is almost totally dependent on combined muscular and ligamentous structures. Because of the anatomic characteristics of this area, a comprehensive examination of the shoulder will normally include a progressive series of functional tests.

Active movements. Active movements are performed to evaluate the relationships between movements of the clavicle, scapula, and humerus, to determine the range of motion of the entire arm-trunk mechanism, and to begin assessing the integrity of the contractile units. It is important to remember, because of the anatomic features of the shoulder girdle, that active move-

Fig. 17-33. Palpating the latissimus dorsi muscle.

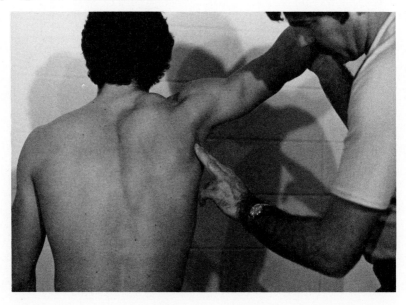

ments will also stress some noncontractile structures. For example, the acromioclavicular and sternoclavicular joints are stressed during active motions of the shoulder. Active movements can best be performed with the athlete sitting or standing. Instruct the athlete to execute each movement through as great a range of motion as possible and to express any sensations or symptoms that are experienced.

A phenomenon that must be kept in mind as you observe an athlete performing a range of active movements is what is described as a *painful arc*. This means that motion is pain free at the beginning of the range but develops near the

Fig. 17-34. Palpating major muscles of the upper arm: **A,** biceps and **B,** triceps.

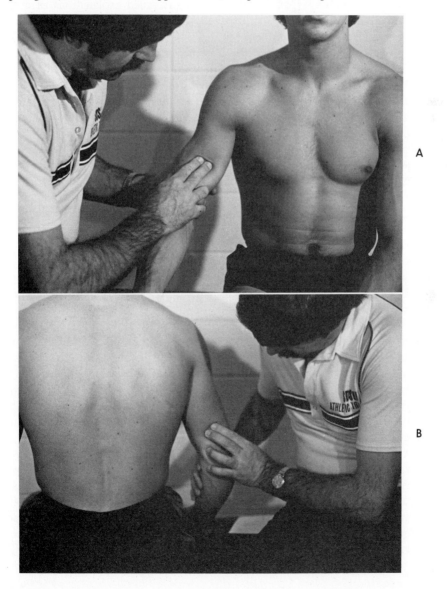

A

B

midrange of a movement and then ceases as this point is passed. This pain is caused by a tender tissue being painfully squeezed when passing a certain point during the range of motion. A painful arc is best evoked by active movements and appears most commonly in shoulder injuries; however, a painful arc can be recognized in injuries involving other joints. This phenomenon may appear only during the upward or downward movement of the arm or during movement in both directions. A painful arc at the shoulder normally indicates an impingement syndrome, as tender tissue is pinched between the acromion process and one of the humeral tuberosities. This finding usually implicates the subacromial bursa or the supraspinatus tendon.

When evaluating active motion always remember that the shoulder girdle functions in complex movement patterns. For example, to abduct the arm to 180°, an athlete must also elevate the shoulder girdle, upwardly rotate the scapula, and externally rotate the arm. Without this combination of movements, an athlete could not abduct the arm through a normal range of motion. Although it is not necessary in every case to separately evaluate motions available at each joint in the shoulder girdle, such observations can provide useful information. In most cases it is sufficient to instruct the athlete to perform active motions of the arm and observe the gross movement patterns. While observing these gross movement patterns, look for similarity in the relationship and ratio of movements between the scapula, clavicle, and humerus on both sides of the body. For example, during the first 30° of abduction the scapula will move on the trunk to a point of maximum stability. It is interesting to note that arm abduction to this point can be accomplished without the use of the deltoid muscle. Movement can occur simply by "shrugging the shoulders," that is, by moving the scapula and fixing the glenohumeral joint. However, from 30° to 180° of abduction there is a unique "rhythm" that normally exists between movements of the scapula and humerus. Kinesiologists often refer to a "scapulohumeral rhythm" that results in a 2 to 1 ratio of movement between the humerus and scapula during abduction. Look for this ratio of movement as the athlete abducts the arm beyond 30°. For every 30° of additional abduction, 20° of movement will normally occur at the glenohumeral joint and 10° results from rotation of the scapula on the trunk. In cases of acute paralysis of the deltoid muscle, abduction beyond 30° (accomplished by scapular movement) is impossible. Detailed explanations of arm-trunk movement rhythms are beyond the scope of this text. Interested students will find ample information in most advanced kinesiology texts.

Ask the athlete to flex and extend the arm through as great a range of motion as possible (Fig. 17-35, *A*). Normally an athlete should be able to flex the arm 180°, bringing the arm up even with the ear. An athlete should be able to backward extend or hyperextend the arm approximately 60°. Can the athlete complete a normal range of motion? Was the motion comfortable without any complaints of pain or weakness? Is the motion available in both shoulders equal? Ask the athlete to flex both arms at the same time to provide a bilateral comparison.

In evaluating shoulder abduction and adduction, an athlete can normally abduct the arm 180° and adduct the arm approximately 45° across the front of the body (Fig. 17-35, *B*). Can the athlete perform these motions? Is the range of motion equal on both sides? Does the athlete express any pain or weakness? Determine the site of any pain elicited with this active motion. Horizontal abduction and adduction can also be evaluated as the athlete is asked to move the arm in the horizontal plane (Fig. 17-35, *C*).

Rotation of the humerus is essential for normal elevation of the upper extremity. Internal and external rotation of the arm can be evaluated with the arm at the side and the elbow flexed to 90° (Fig. 17-35, *D*). Keeping the arm next to the body, instruct to athlete to rotate the arm outwardly and inwardly. Normally an athlete should be able to externally rotate the arm about

45° and internally rotate until the forearm touches the body. Rotation can also be tested with the arm in 90° of abduction and the elbow in 90° of flexion (Fig. 17-35, *E*). Instruct the athlete to rotate the arm up and down and compare to the uninjured side. Rotation in this position normally has less range than with the arm at the side of the body. The rotator cuff muscles together with the pectoralis major and latissimus dorsi muscles aid in arm rotation.

A quick and easy method to evaluate active range of motion in the shoulder is the ***Apley scratch test.*** The athlete is instructed to place each hand in two different places to determine the active range of motion of the shoulder and compare bilaterally. Ask the athlete to reach behind his or her back as high as possible (Fig. 17-36, *A*). Notice the distance the fingertips reach in relation to the scapula or thoracic spine. This movement involves internal rotation and

adduction of the shoulder. Then have the athlete reach behind the head and down the back as far as possible (Fig. 17-36, *B*). Again note the distance the fingertips can reach. This involves external rotation and abduction. Is the athlete able to complete these maneuvers? Can the athlete reach as far with the injured side as the uninjured? Was there any limitation of motion, weakness, or pain expressed?

Depending on the injury suspected, additional active motion tests can be used to evaluate scapulothoracic movements specifically. Scapular elevation and rotation is accomplished by asking the athlete to shrug both shoulders (Fig. 17-37, *A*). Scapular protraction and retraction is evaluated by having the athlete bring both shoulders forward and then backward as far as possible (Fig. 17-37, *B* and *C*). Note any pain, weakness, or limitation of motion between the shoulders. Watch for any winging of the scapu-

Fig. 17-35. Range of motion of the shoulder. **A,** Flexion and extension, **B,** abduction and adduction, **C,** horizontal abduction and adduction, **D,** internal and external rotation with the arm at the side of the body, and **E,** internal and external rotation with the arm abducted to 90°.

(From Malasanos, L., et al.: Health assessment, ed. 2, St. Louis, 1981, The C.V. Mosby Co.)

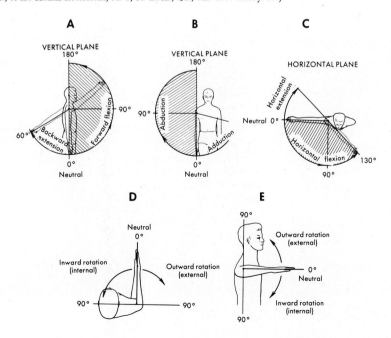

Fig. 17-36. Apley scratch test. **A,** Athlete reaching behind back; **B,** athlete reaching behind head and down the back.

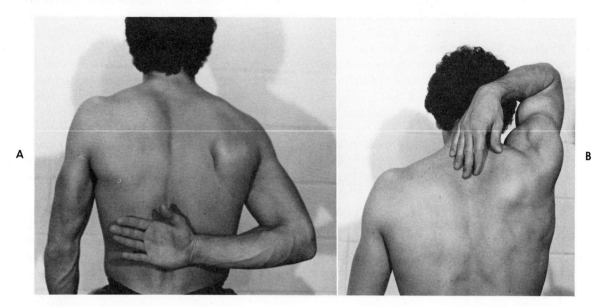

A   B

Fig. 17-37. Active scapulothoracic movements. **A,** Elevation, **B,** protraction, and **C,** retraction.

A   B   C

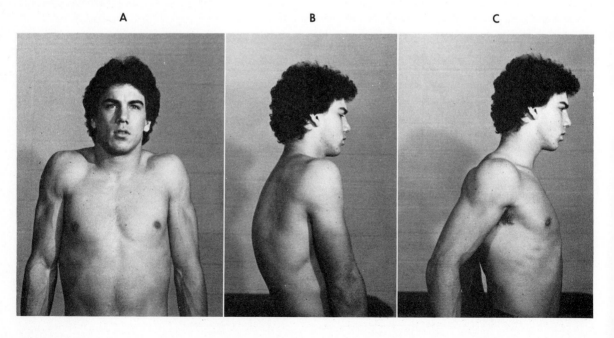

la, which may indicate a weakness of the serratus anterior muscle. Remember, performing these motions also puts mild stress on the sternoclavicular and acromioclavicular joints and may be used to assess their integrity when moving the arm is too painful.

Resistive movements. Following the evaluation of the active range of motion, resistance can be applied against these same movements to further assess the integrity of the contractile units. Whenever a muscle injury is suspected or indicated, resistive movements can assist in identifying specific tender areas as well as assessing and comparing muscular strengths. Once again, manual resistance can be applied throughout the range of motion or isometrically in various positions. Resistive movements can be performed with the athlete sitting, standing, or lying down. Remember, because shoulder motions are complex patterns, several muscles are being evaluated with each movement. For example, resistance against shoulder flexion may also cause pain in muscles responsible for shoulder elevation or upward rotation of the scapula. To be effective in assessment the athletic trainer must possess a sound knowledge of functional shoulder anatomy. Refer to Table 17-1 for a listing of the prime movers and accessory muscles for selected shoulder movements.

To apply resistance against shoulder flexion, place one hand on the athlete's shoulder for stability and the other just proximal and anterior to the elbow (Fig. 17-38, *A*). The stabilizing hand can also palpate the muscles primarily responsible for the action during each movement. Have the athlete flex the elbow to reduce the effects of the biceps muscle. Instruct the athlete to flex the shoulder or move the arm forward and up as you apply resistance. Gradually increase your resistance until you can determine the maximum resistance the athlete can overcome.

Those muscles involved with shoulder extension can be stressed by applying resistance to the posterior distal portion of the humerus (Fig. 17-38, *B*). This test should follow the evaluation of

shoulder flexion without interruption. Moving your resistive hand from the anterior surface of the athlete's arm to the posterior surface will ensure a smooth transition from testing flexion to extension.

Shoulder abduction and adduction can also be evaluated during the same cycle of motion. Again place one hand on the point of the shoulder to stabilize the shoulder girdle and to palpate the involved muscles. To test shoulder abduction, place the other hand on the distal and lateral aspect of the humerus (Fig. 17-38, *C*). Instruct the athlete to abduct the arm, lifting it away from the side of the body. To test shoulder adduction, move your resistance hand to the medial side of the humerus and apply resistance as the athlete adducts the arm (Fig. 17-38, *D*).

Horizontal adduction and abduction are additional motions commonly evaluated using resistive techniques. For horizontal adduction, begin with the arm abducted to 90° and apply resistance on the medial side of the arm proximal to the elbow (Fig. 17-38, *E*). Instruct the athlete to bring his or her arm straight across the chest. Moving your resistive hand to the posterior surface of the arm, ask the athlete to move the arm straight back to test horizontal abduction (Fig. 17-38, *F*).

Internal and external rotation are normally tested with the arm at the side of the body and elbow flexed to 90°. Stabilize the flexed elbow to the body to ensure the athlete does not substitute abduction for rotation. Instruct the athlete to outwardly and inwardly rotate the arm as you apply resistance at the athlete's wrist with the other hand (Fig. 17-38, *G* and *H*).

Resistance can also be applied to scapulothoracic movements. Resist scapular elevation by placing your hands on each shoulder and pressing down as the athlete shrugs both shoulders (Fig. 17-39, *A*). Normally an athlete can still shrug his or her shoulders against your maximum resistance. Scapular protraction and retraction are best evaluated unilaterally so the thorax can be stabilized to prevent substitute motions.

Fig. 17-38. Applying manual resistance against shoulder motion: **A**, flexion, **B**, extension, **C**, abduction, **D**, adduction, **E**, horizontal adduction, **F**, horizontal abduction.

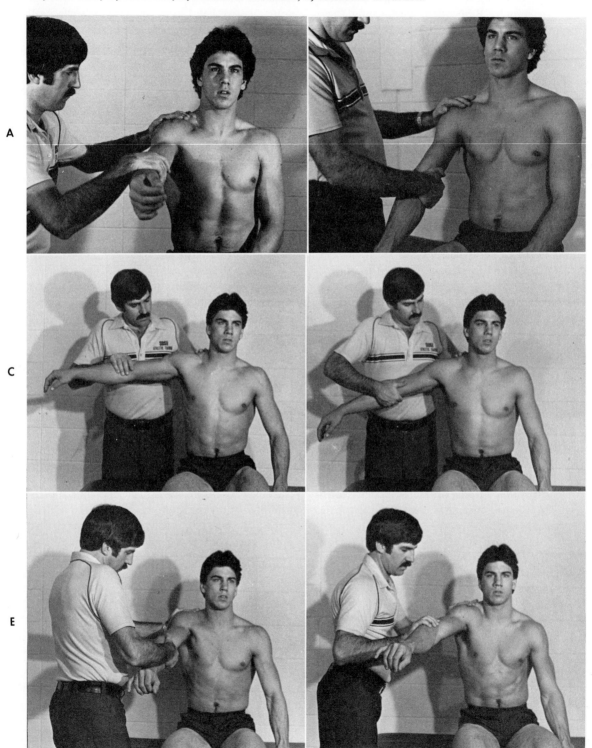

Fig. 17-38, cont'd. G, internal rotation and **H,** external rotation.

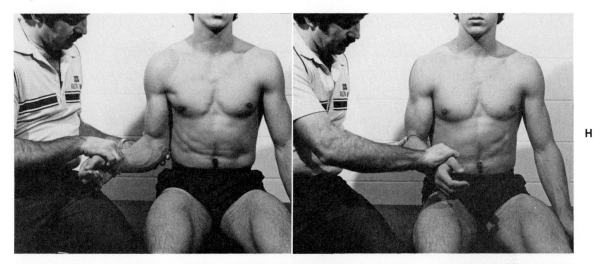

Fig. 17-39. Applying manual resistance against scapulothoracic movements. **A,** Shoulder elevation; **B,** shoulder protraction; **C,** shoulder retraction.

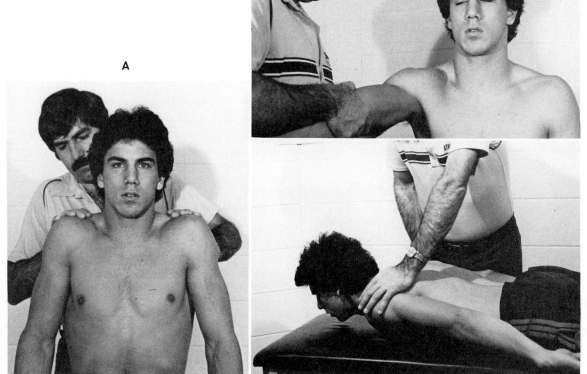

With the athlete sitting and the shoulder flexed to 90°, place one hand along the spine to stabilize the thorax and apply resistance to protration with the other (Fig. 17-39, *B*). Note any winging of the scapula. Winging may also be demonstrated when an athlete performs a push-up or pushes against a wall (Fig. 17-40). Scapular retraction is probably best performed with the athlete lying in a prone position. Resistance is applied to the lateral angle of the scapula as the athlete is instructed to lift the shoulder or bring the shoulder blades together (Fig. 17-39, *C*).

Special resistive tests are used to evaluate specific anatomic structures when they are suspected of being injured. One such maneuver is called the ***drop arm test***. This test is used to evaluate the status of the supraspinatus tendon of the rotator cuff. Instruct the athlete to position the arm in 90° abduction, 30° horizontal adduction, and internal rotation. Have the athlete maintain that position as you press down on the forearm (Fig. 17-41). If there is involvement of the supraspinatus tendon, the arm will drop because of weakness or pain. This test should follow active abduction of the arm, especially when a painful arc is exhibited.

Another specific evaluative maneuver is known as the ***Yergason test***. This test determines if the tendon of the long head of the biceps is stable in the bicipital groove or if a tenosynovitis exists. Have the athlete flex the elbow on the involved side to 90°. Support the elbow with one hand and grasp the athlete's wrist with the other. Instruct the athlete to maintain this position as you attempt to extend the elbow and externally rotate the arm (Fig. 17-42). This places

Fig. 17-40. Winging of the left scapula. (From Prior, J.A., Silberstein, J.S., and Stang, J.M.: Physical diagnosis, ed. 5, St. Louis, 1977, The C.V. Mosby Co.)

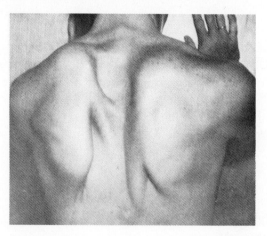

Fig. 17-41. Drop arm test to evaluate the status of the supraspinatus muscle. Applying manual resistance to shoulder abducted 90°, horizontally adducted 30°, and internally rotated.

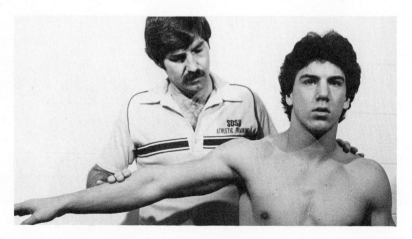

Fig. 17-42. Yergason test to evaluate the stability of the tendon of long head of the biceps. With the arm held in a 90° flexed position, attempt to extend the elbow and externally rotate the arm.

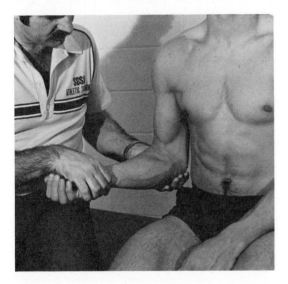

stress on the biceps tendon and will normally produce pain in the bicipital groove if there is a tenosynovitis. A painful snap along the bicipital groove may be caused by subluxation of the tendon because of a tear of the transverse humeral ligament. If the tendon is not injured or involved in an injury, this test will produce no discomfort in the bicipital groove.

Passive movements. Passive movements are often used to facilitate the assessment of shoulder injuries. The specific maneuvers used depend on the type of injury suspected or indicated by the evaluation up to this point.

Occasionally, the range of motion of the shoulder will be evaluated passively. In order to obtain the most useful information, the shoulder must be relaxed during these maneuvers. It is best to have the athlete lying down and in a comfortable position. Passive range of motion may be especially informative when active motion appears limited. Is motion limited by pain

Fig. 17-43. Evaluating the presence of an impingment syndrome. **A,** forcibly flexing arm to drive the greater tuberosity against the anteroinferior surface of the acromion; **B,** forced internal rotation of the proximal humerus with the arm flexed to 90° to drive the greater tuberosity under the coracoacromial ligament.

A

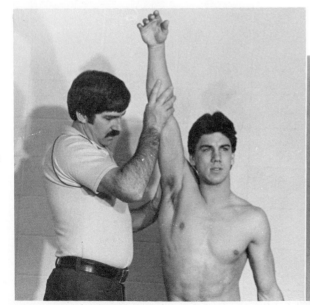

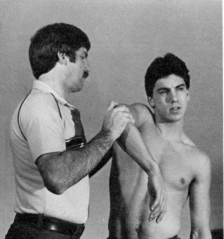

B

or muscular weakness or restricted by a frozen shoulder syndrome? Athletes exhibiting restricted active motion but a normal range of motion when the contractile units are relaxed probably have muscular involvement resulting in pain and weakness. Passive range of motion procedures must be done *cautiously* so as not to cause further damage.

Passive movements are also used to evaluate impingment syndromes of the shoulder. Remember, these conditions are caused as soft tissue structures are impinged (squeezed) between the unyielding coracoacromial arch and the greater tuberosity of the humerus. Two procedures are commonly used in an attempt to reproduce the symptoms associated with an impingment syndrome. One is to passively bring the arm into complete flexion, driving the greater tuberosity against the anteroinferior surface of the acromion (Fig. 17-43, *A*). An alternate method is to forcibly rotate the proximal humerus internally when the arm is flexed 90° (Fig. 17-43, *B*). This maneuver drives the greater tuberosity under the coracoacromial ligament, which may reproduce the impingment pain.

Passive procedures can also be used to assess the integrity of the articulations of the shoulder girdle. These procedures would be used to assess the severity of the injury and would not be attempted until you are relatively sure of the nature of the injury. Passive maneuvers should be

Fig. 17-45. Passively stressing the acromioclavicular joint by **A,** squeezing the clavicle towards the scapula and **B,** pulling down on the arm to stress the joint.

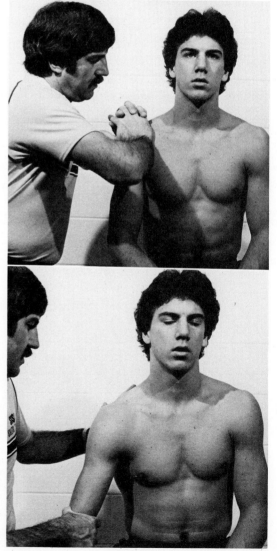

A

B

Fig. 17-44. Applying passive stress to the clavicle to evaluate the sternoclavicular and acromioclavicular joints.

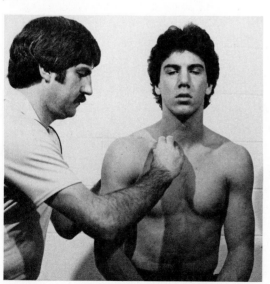

performed gently to begin with, so as not to aggravate the injury and lose the athlete's cooperation. The force used with each of these maneuvers can then be increased, depending on the athlete's tolerance and the severity of the injury.

To passively stress the sternoclavicular and acromioclavicular joints, attempt to manually move the clavicle. This can be accomplished by grasping the clavicle between the thumb and fingers and attempting to move it up and down or simply pressing down (Fig. 17-44). An alternative method of passively stressing the acromioclavicular joint is to place your hands over the shoulder, the heel of one hand on the clavicle and the other on the scapular spine. Then squeeze the heels of the hands together (Fig. 17-45, *A*). This causes a shearing movement, especially at the acromioclavicular joint, and may elicit abnormal mobility or pain. Another procedure that may be used to stress the acromioclavicular joint is to attempt to separate the acromion and clavicle by pulling down on the arm (Fig. 17-45, *B*). Pain and mobility may be increased by this maneuver if the athlete has suffered a partial separation. Another passive test

(or active, if the athlete does it) for assessment of abnormalities within either the acromioclavicular or sternoclavicular joint is to bring the abducted arm across the front of the body, thus compressing both of these joints.

To passively evaluate the integrity of the glenohumeral joint, the athletic trainer commonly uses the *apprehension test*. This test is best performed with the athlete in a supine position so the muscles about the shoulder are as relaxed as possible. Passively move the arm into 90° of abduction and then gently externally rotate (Fig. 17-46). This puts the glenohumeral joint in a compromising position; if there is a history of subluxations or dislocations, the athlete will normally express apprehension in this position and resist any further motion. If the movement to this position is tolerated, pressure may be applied to the posterior aspect of the shoulder, pushing the humeral head anteriorly. Apprehension may be increased and the humeral head may actually sublux if the athlete has a chronic subluxing shoulder.

Functional movements. Functional movements or activities can be very beneficial to the comprehensive assessment of shoulder injuries. Because

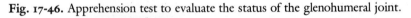

Fig. 17-46. Apprehension test to evaluate the status of the glenohumeral joint.

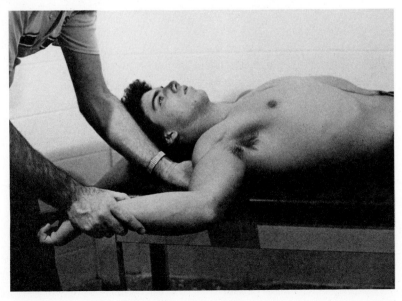

ATHLETIC INJURY ASSESSMENT CHECKLIST
SHOULDER INJURIES

Secondary survey

———— History
       ———— Primary complaint
       ———— Previous injuries
       ———— Mechanism of injury
       ———— Onset of symptoms
       ———— Pain
       ———— Sensations
———— Observation
       ———— Overall position and posture
       ———— Compare symmetry and appearance
       ———— Deformities
       ———— Swelling
       ———— Signs of trauma
———— Palpation
       ———— Tenderness
       ———— Swelling
       ———— Deformity
       ———— Crepitation
       ———— Distal pulses
       ———— Neurologic pathways
———— Stress
       ———— Active movements
             ———— Range of motion
             ———— Painful arc
             ———— Pain
             ———— Scapulohumeral rhythm
       ———— Resistive movements
             ———— Pain
             ———— Strength
                   ———— Drop-arm test
                   ———— Yergason test
       ———— Passive movements
             ———— Range of motion
             ———— Integrity of joints
                   ———— Apprehension test
       ———— Functional movements
             ———— Functional abilities

many injuries involving the shoulder result from repetitive throwing or swinging activities, those same activities may be required to replicate the injury-causing movements and demonstrate the signs and symptoms associated with the injury. Occasionally, this is the only type of activity that will reproduce the signs and symptoms. The action of throwing or swinging involves complex, coordinated movements, and athletic trainers must possess a fundamental knowledge of these important skills to accurately assess associated injuries.

When the assessment process completed to this point has produced few definitive signs and symptoms, functional activities can be very helpful in evaluation. Instruct the athlete to perform functional activities of the shoulder that are required for his or her particular sport. These activities will vary greatly, depending on the sport, the equipment used, the age and maturity of the athlete, any history of previous injuries, or the presence of weakness, fatigue, or incoordination of motion. Swinging activities are in many ways similar to the throwing motion. Can the athlete perform the activity normally and without pain or other symptoms? During which phase of the motion are signs and symptoms expressed? Correlating the precise location of pain with the specific function will greatly assist in identifying the anatomic structures involved in the injury.

Functional movements are always used to determine when an athlete can return to activity. As an athlete recovers from a shoulder injury, functional activities become increasingly important on each re-evaluation. Keep accurate and dated records of each evaluation. The intensity of functional movements should be progressively increased within the limits of pain and range of motion.

Evaluation of findings

The shoulder is one of the most frequently injured areas of the upper extremity. The extensive range of motion and the inherent instability of the shoulder joint make this area of the body vulnerable to acute athletic injuries as well as chronic overuse conditions. Because of the complex movement patterns of the shoulder girdle, an injury to one segment can involve the others; in addition, many different shoulder structures can be involved in a single injury. The nature and severity of shoulder injuries can therefore be extremely difficult to accurately assess.

This chapter has presented basic evaluative procedures used to isolate the various structures about the shoulder to either implicate or rule out their involvement following injury. All of these procedures will not be applicable to any one shoulder injury. Whenever a serious injury is indicated or suspected, the athlete should be promptly referred to a physician. In the interim, the arm should be maintained in a position that provides optimum comfort and should be supported by the use of a pillow or sling. The athlete should be withheld from full activity as long as he or she has a limited range of motion or pain with exercise. Shoulder injuries require frequent re-evaluations to monitor progress and determine when the athlete can return to activity.

When to refer the athlete

Because of the complexity of this body area and the importance of early care, many shoulder injuries should be evaluated by a physician. The following list of conditions or findings can be used to determine if medical referral is indicated.

1. Suspected fracture, separation, or dislocation
2. Gross deformity
3. Significant loss of motion
4. Significant or continued pain
5. Joint instability
6. Abnormal sensations that do not quickly go away, such as weakness or numbness
7. Absent or weak pulse distal to the point of injury
8. Any doubt regarding the severity or nature of the injury

KEY TERMS

adhesive capsulitis (frozen shoulder) Inflammation of the rotator cuff and capsular area, which develops because of immobility resulting in loss of range of motion

Apley scratch test Method to evaluate active range of motion of the shoulder by asking athlete to place hand behind the back and neck

blocker's spur Irritative exostosis that develops near the deltoid muscle insertion caused by repeated blows to the area, and most frequently seen in football players

drop arm test Test to evaluate the status of the supraspinatus tendon—athlete abducts arm to 90°, horizontally adducts it 30°, internally rotates it, and maintains against resistance

exostosis Bony growth projecting outward from the surface of a bone

knocked-down shoulder Separation of the acromioclavicular joint, resulting in obvious deformity, with the clavicle displaced upward and the acromion remaining down

luxatio erecta Inferior dislocation of the shoulder in which the arm stands straight above the head

painful arc Pain caused by tender tissue being squeezed as a joint passes the midpoint during the range of motion

piano key sign High-riding clavicle resulting from a third-degree sprain of the acromioclavicular joint; it can be pushed down but will spring back up when pressure is released, much like a piano key

rotator cuff Four muscles whose tendons surround and attach about the head of humerus and are primarily responsible for the integrity of the shoulder joint; that is, maintaining the head of the humerus within the glenoid labrum

shoulder pointer Contusion to the tip of the shoulder (over acromion process)

shoulder separation Sprain of the acromioclavicular joint

Yergason test Test that evaluates the status of the long head of the biceps tendon—athlete flexes elbow at side of body as resistance is applied against elbow flexion and external rotation

SUGGESTED READINGS

Arnheim, D.D.: Modern principles of athletic training, ed. 6, St. Louis, 1985, Times Mirror/Mosby College Publishing.

Booth, R.E., and Marvel, J.P.: Differential diagnosis of shoulder pain, Orthop. Clin. North Am. 6:353-379, 1975.

Clinics in Sports Medicine: Symposium on injuries to the shoulder in the athlete. In Jobe, F.W., editor: vol. 2, Philadelphia, 1983, W.B. Saunders Co.

Hoppenfeld, S.: Physical examination of the spine and extremities, New York, 1976, Appleton-Century Crofts.

Mercier, L.R.: Practical orthopedics, Chicago, 1980, Year Book Medical Publishers, Inc.

Moseley, H.F.: Shoulder lesions, ed. 3, London, 1979, E & S Livingstone, Ltd.

Neviaser, J.S.: Injuries of the clavicle and its articulations, Orthop. Clin. North Am. 11:233-237, 1980.

Neviaser, R.J.: Anatomic considerations and examination of the shoulder, Orthop. Clin. North Am. 11:187-195, 1980.

O'Donoghue, D.H.: Treatment of injuries to athletes, ed. 4, Philadelphia, 1984, W.B. Saunders Co.

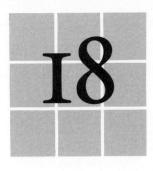

18 Elbow and forearm injuries

The elbow and forearm are important functional links between the shoulder and the intricate mechanisms of the hand. The elbow joint allows the arm to flex and extend, whereas the articulations between the radius and ulna permit the forearm to rotate, that is, pronate and supinate. In addition, all the extrinsic muscles of the hand originate about the elbow or forearm. Therefore the ability to perform athletic skills involving the upper extremities is dependent on the integrity of the bones, ligaments, and muscles of the elbow and forearm.

ANATOMY OF THE ELBOW

The elbow is sometimes described as "three joints in one capsule." One joint exists between the humerus and ulna, a second between the humerus and radius, and the third between the proximal ends of the ulna and radius. These components of the elbow share a common articular capsule, and their joint spaces are continuous. Although movements at the elbow joint proper should not be confused with those that occur at the superior radioulnar joint, it would be unwise from a functional standpoint for the athletic trainer to only consider one and not the others when assessing an elbow injury.

The elbow joint is often subdivided into two points of articulation: (1) the humero-ulnar, between the trochlea of the humerus and the ulna, and (2) the humeroradial, between the capitulum of the humerus and the radius.

Begin your review of elbow anatomy by identifying the four bony projections on the distal end of the humerus—the medial and lateral epi-condyles, the capitulum, and the trochlea—and two depressions—the olecranon and coronoid fossae in Fig. 18-1. The epicondyles and their supracondylar ridges can be palpated as rough projections on both the medial and lateral sides of the distal humerus. These bony prominences are the points of attachment for the shared tendons called the common flexor and extensor tendons of the forearm, which are frequent sites of athletic-related injuries. The capitulum and the trochlea are located just distal to the lateral and medial epicondyles of the humerus, respectively. The capitulum is a rounded knob that articulates with the head of the radius, whereas the trochlea is a pulley or spool-shaped projection that fits into the trochlear notch of the ulna.

In the anatomic position the ulna is located on

Fig. 18-1. Bony anatomy of the elbow and forearm. **A,** Anterior view and **B,** posterior view.

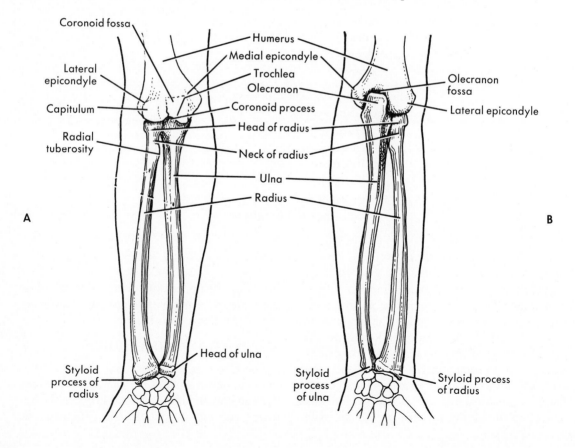

Coronoid fossa

Lateral epicondyle

Capitulum

Radial tuberosity

Humerus

Medial epicondyle

Trochlea

Olecranon

Coronoid process

Head of radius

Neck of radius

Ulna

Radius

Olecranon fossa

Lateral epicondyle

Styloid process of radius

Head of ulna

Styloid process of ulna

Styloid process of radius

A

B

the medial (little finger) side and the radius on the lateral (thumb) side of the forearm. In this position both bones are approximately parallel and the forearm and hand are said to be in supination. The palm of the hand is turned forward (anteriorly) when the forearm is supinated. In the position of pronation the palm is turned backward (posteriorly) as the radius crosses in front of the ulna.

The upper (proximal) end of the ulna is easily identified by a large concavity called the semilunar (trochlear) notch. As indicated previously, this notch serves as a point for articulation with the trochlea of the humerus. This deep notch lies between two bony projections, the large proximal and posteriorly projecting olecranon process and the less massive, distal and anteriorly projecting coronoid process. These processes are the points of attachment for the triceps brachii and the brachialis, respectively. Just below the notch on the lateral side of the coronoid process there is a small concave depression, the radial notch, which receives the head of the radius. During pronation and supination of the forearm the head of the radius rotates within this notch.

The proximal end of the radius has three prominent bony features: a round head, which has a smooth, slightly concave upper surface; a narrow neck; and just below the neck, on the ulnar (medial) side of the body, the radial tuberosity, which is the insertion of the biceps brachii.

Articular capsule and collateral ligaments

The elbow joint proper and the superior radioulnar joint share a common fibrous articular capsule and have a continuous joint space—an anatomic fact of considerable clinical significance. The capsule is lined by a synovial membrane that reflects onto the bones of the joint and attaches to the edges of the articulating surfaces. This capsule is thin and rather loose on the anterior and posterior surfaces of the joint to permit flexion and extension and thick and strong on the medial and lateral surfaces to enhance joint stability. The capsule is subdivided into four ligaments, the ulnar (medial) collateral ligament, the radial (lateral) collateral ligament, the anterior ligament, and the posterior ligament (Fig. 18-2).

The *ulnar (medial) collateral ligament* consists of three bands passing between the medial epicondyle and the medial edge of the trochlear

Fig. 18-2. Major ligaments of elbow joint: **A,** medial view and **B,** lateral view.

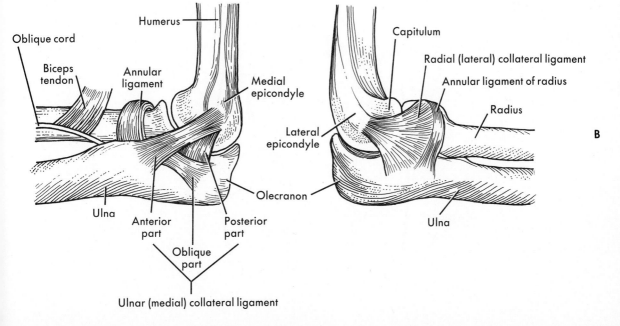

notch. The oblique portion of the ligament helps to deepen the socket for articulation of the trochlea of the humerus. The anterior part of the ligament becomes taut in extension and the weak, fan-shaped posterior portion becomes taut in flexion. The ulnar nerve lies on this ligament as it passes behind the medial epicondyle into the forearm. The strong fan-shaped *radial (lateral) collateral ligament* extends from the outer surface of the lateral epicondyle of the humerus to the outer edge of the annular ligament. The thin *anterior ligament* is attached to the medial epicondyle and to the humerus above the coronoid fossa. The distal portion of this ligament is continuous with the collateral ligaments. The medially placed *posterior ligament* is thin and weak. Proximally it is attached to the epicondyles and margins of the olecranon fossa, whereas distally it is attached to the olecranon process of the ulna.

Synovial membrane and subcutaneous bursae

The synovial membrane that lines the articular capsule of the elbow is extensive. It projects into the recesses of the common joint space and extends into both the coronoid and olecranon fossae. A redundant fold of synovial membrane also extends under the annular ligament (Fig. 18-3). This fold provides a cushion for rotation of the head of the radius during pronation and supination of the forearm.

Pads of fat are often found between the synovial membrane and fibrous capsule over or near the articular fossae. The largest of these fatty accumulations is found over the olecranon fossa. It is pressed into the fossa during extension by the tendon of the triceps.

The subtendinous olecranon bursa is located between the tendon of the triceps, the outer, or posterior, surface of the olecranon process, and

Fig. 18-3. The elbow joint, posterior view. Note the fold of synovial membrane passing below the annular ligament.

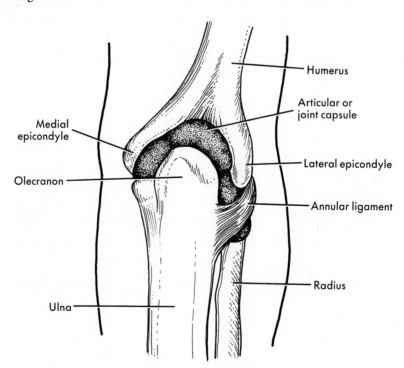

the skin. It is most frequently found just proximal to (above) the insertion of the triceps tendon. The olecranon is the most commonly injured bursa of the elbow, as is discussed later in this chapter. Numerous other subcutaneous bursae are also found (inconsistently) over the medial and lateral epicondyles of the humerus.

Elbow muscles and movements

The reciprocally concave-to-convex articular surface between the trochlea of the humerus and the wrenchlike upper end of the ulna permits only flexion and extension. The result is a typical uniaxial, or hinge-type, joint. Flexion (Fig. 18-4) is produced primarily by the biceps, brachialis, and brachioradialis muscles. In addition, in strongly resisted flexion, muscles arising from the medial epicondyle of the humerus act as weak accessory flexors. During flexion, the coronoid fossa on the anterior surface of the humerus receives the coronoid process of the ulna. The degree of flexion that is permitted varies between persons and is limited by contact of soft tissues between the forearm and arm. The prime mover in elbow extension is the triceps muscle (Fig. 18-5). The tiny anconeus muscle arising from the lateral epicondyle and attaching to the ulna may act as a weak accessory extensor. The olecranon fossa, a depression on the posterior surface of the humerus just above the trochlea, receives the olecranon process of the ulna during extension of the forearm. Extension is limited by actual contact of the olecranon with the floor of the olecranon fossa.

When considered as a total functional unit, the elbow complex permits not only flexion and extension but also supination and pronation of the forearm and hand. These movements are possible because of the uniaxial pivot-type articulation between the head of the radius and the ulna, called the superior radioulnar joint. The superior radioulnar joint is supported by a strong *annular ligament* that encircles the head of the radius and forms a collar, holding it in close contact with the articular surface (radial notch) of the ulna. Pronation and supination movements produce rotation of the forearm along its long axis, with the radius "crossing

Fig. 18-4. Muscles of elbow flexion. (From Malasanos, L., et al.: Health assessment, ed. 2, St. Louis, 1981, The C.V. Mosby Co.)

Fig. 18-5. Muscles of elbow extension. (From Malasanos, L., et al.: Health assessment, ed. 2, St. Louis, 1981, The C.V. Mosby Co.)

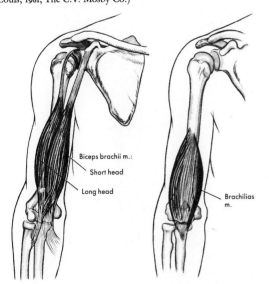

Biceps brachii m.:

Short head

Long head

Brachilias m.

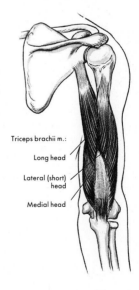

Triceps brachii m.:

Long head

Lateral (short) head

Medial head

over" the ulna. Pronation is produced primarily by the pronator teres and pronator quadratus muscles (Fig. 18-6) and supination by the biceps and supinator muscles (Fig. 18-7).

Muscles of the forearm

The muscles of the forearm can be divided into flexor and extensor groups and act on the elbow, wrist, and digits. The flexor muscles arise in large part from the medial epicondyle from a shared tendon called the *common flexor tendon*. Muscles involved in pronation also originate in this area. The flexor and pronator muscles occupy the medial border and anterior surface of the forearm. The extensor muscles arise in large part from the lateral epicondyle from a shared tendon called the *common extensor tendon*. Muscles involved in supination also originate in this area. The extensor and supinator muscles occupy the lateral border and posterior surface of the forearm. In the upper part of the forearm, the flexor and extensor muscles form fleshy masses below the medial and lateral epicondyles. The hollow triangular area lying just distal to the elbow joint

and formed between these two muscle masses is called the cubital fossa. The muscle mass of the forearm rapidly tapers off towards the wrist, where the long tendons of these muscles continue into the hand.

Interosseous membrane

The interosseous membrane is a strong fibrous sheet of connective tissue that connects the shafts of the radius and ulna. Its fibers run downward and medially from radius to ulna.

The proximal (superior) end of the ulna is heavy and firmly articulated at the elbow, whereas the radius is strong and broadened at the wrist. Therefore, for practical purposes, the athletic trainer should think of the ulna as the distal extension of the humerus, which is associated with elbow strength and motion, and the radius as an upward, or proximal, extension of the hand, which is associated with motions of the hand and wrist.

Forces placed against the hand must be transmitted from the radius to the ulna and then to the humerus. When this occurs, the radius is

Fig. 18-6. Muscles of elbow pronation.
(From Malasanos, L., et al.: Health assessment, ed. 2, St. Louis, 1981, The C.V. Mosby Co.)

Fig. 18-7. Muscles of elbow supination.
(From Malasanos, L., et al.: Health assessment, ed. 2, St. Louis, 1981, The C.V. Mosby Co.)

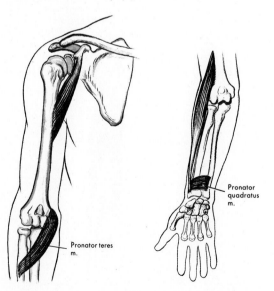

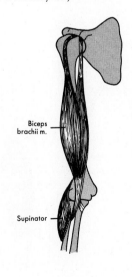

forced superiorly and the ulna inferiorly. The arrangement of fibers in the interosseous membrane transmits to the ulna, and then to the humerus, forces acting upward through the hand. The membrane also prevents the displacement that these forces would otherwise create between ulna and radius.

An understanding of the direction of fibers in the interosseous membrane (downward and medially from radius to ulna) explains the difficulty and forearm pain often associated with carrying or lifting, such as deadlifting a heavy weight. In this type of activity the weight is pulling the two forearm bones apart, and the interosseous membrane is constructed so that it can provide only very limited help in preventing displacement. Heavy loads can be carried more easily on the palm of the hand with the elbow flexed, as a powerlifter holds a weighted bar during a squat lift or deep knee bend. In this position the interosseous membrane helps prevent displacement of the forearm bones. A waiter takes advantage of this same principal by carrying a heavy tray of dishes on the palm of the hand with the elbow flexed. The interosseous membrane, in addition to binding the forearm bones together, serves as a point for attachment of muscles and helps separate the forearm into two anatomic compartments. The interosseous membrane joins with the radius, ulna, and a strong aponeurotic-like sheet of fascia (antebrachial fascia) to separate the forearm into dorsal (extensor) and volar (flexor) compartments. The result is an anatomic separation of the flexor muscles arising from the medial epicondyle and anterior surface of the forearm from those extensors arising from the lateral epicondyle and posterior surface of this area. Anatomists group the forearm muscles according to their location in either the dorsal (extensor) or volar (flexor) compartment. Note in the following box that muscles in each group are classified as either superficial or deep. To acquire a working knowledge of the location, points of attachment, innervation, blood supply, and discrete action of the individual forearm muscles requires the expenditure of considerable time

and effort. Most athletic trainers evaluate injury in this area by functional grouping of involved muscles.

INJURIES TO THE ELBOW AND FOREARM

Injuries involving the elbow and forearm are common in athletic activity. Many different types of force and stress are applied about the elbow during the various activities involved in different sports. A variety of athletic injuries can result from direct trauma to the area, indirect trauma such as falling on an outstretched hand, or acute and chronic stresses associated with throwing and swinging activities. These mech-

---

MUSCLES OF THE FOREARM

Volar (flexor) muscles

Superficial group
  Pronator teres
  Flexor carpi radialis
  Flexor carpi ulnaris
  Flexor digitorum sublimis
  Palmaris longus
Deep group
  Flexor digitorum profundus
  Flexor pollicis longus
  Pronator quadratus

Dorsal (extensor) group

Superficial group
  Brachioradialis
  Extensor carpi radialis longus
  Extensor carpi radialis brevis
  Extensor digitorum communis
  Extensor digiti minimi
  Extensor carpi ulnaris
  Anconeus
Deep group
  Supinator
  Abductor pollicis longus
  Extensor pollicis brevis
  Extensor pollicis longus
  Extensor indicis proprius

anisms of injury can result in contusions, sprains, strains, dislocations, and fractures.

Contusions

Contusions are common injuries to this area of the body and may involve the muscles of the forearm or the subcutaneous bony prominences of the elbow. An athlete's forearms absorb the brunt of many impacts during athletic activity, especially during contact sports. Direct blows to these muscular areas can result in bruising and subsequent bleeding, producing stiffness during function and active range-of-motion. The direct blow that caused the contusion may also be responsible for additional trauma such as a fracture; therefore care must be taken during the evaluation of contusions to determine if there is any additional injury. Proper management must also be exercised during the treatment of contusions, to ensure the area is protected from additional trauma and to guard against the possible development of myositis ossificans.

Direct blows to the subcutaneous olecranon process of the ulna or epicondyles of the humerus can also result in contusions. A common in-

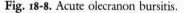

Fig. 18-8. Acute olecranon bursitis.

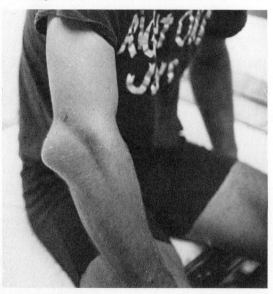

jury resulting from a blow to the tip of the elbow is olecranon bursitis. This can produce an acute hemorrhagic bursitis or a more common chronic form in which the bursal sac is distended with additional fluid. Acute bursitis occurs when a blow to the tip of the elbow results in hemorrhaging into the olecranon bursa (Fig. 18-8). This can cause immediate dramatic swelling, pain, and restriction of motion. Often an acute olecranon bursitis will spontaneously subside. Improper initial care and repeated irritation of this area may allow this condition to develop into a chronic bursitis. Chronic trauma or repeated bruising to the tip of the elbow can result in synovial membrane irritation and thickening, a gradual distention of the bursal sac, and the formation of excess bursal fluid. The olecranon bursa is also one of the more frequently infected bursae. This is partially a result of the frequency of abrasions occurring over the tip of the elbow.

An injury that almost everyone has suffered at one time or another is a contusion to the ulnar nerve. As this nerve passes behind the medial epicondyle of the humerus, it lies subcutaneously and is vulnerable to trauma. A direct blow to this area may cause immediate pain and burning sensations shooting down the ulnar side of the forearm to the ring and little fingers. This paresthesia, commonly referred to as "hitting the crazy bone," is normally transient and disappears in a few minutes depending upon the severity of the blow.

Strains

Strains to the muscular and musculotendinous structures about the elbow are common athletic injuries. These normally occur as a result of tremendous stresses being placed on the elbow joint, especially in those sports requiring throwing or swinging motions. Strains are divided into acute and chronic types. Acute strains occur when a sudden overload is applied to the contractile units of the elbow joint. The resulting injury is a strain to muscles, musculotendinous junctions, or points of tendinous attachment in the area. The most common areas for acute strains are the common flexor tendon around the medial epicondyle and the common extensor tendon over the lateral epicondyle. There may also be an avulsion of muscle with a fragment of bone present. The biceps or triceps muscular unit may also be strained and occasionally the tendon of one of these muscles is ruptured. The symptoms of an acute strain to the musculature supporting the elbow include the history of an incident of sudden excessive overload followed by tenderness over the involved area and pain on function or resisted motion. If the injury results in a rupture of the tendon, there may also be a palpable gap, a bunching of the injured muscle, and a loss of efficient function of the involved muscle.

Chronic strains commonly occur about the elbow as the result of continued overuse of a musculotendinous unit, with ultimate failure or impairment of function. Overuse, especially in sports requiring throwing or swinging, may cause irritation of the muscle fibers, resulting in microscopic tears of the contractile unit. Continued trauma to this area can develop into overuse syndromes and chronic degenerative processes. The process is one of progressive attritional wear and tear.

Chronic strains commonly occur in the region of the medial and lateral epicondyles of the humerus, depending on the muscle groups irritated. For example, overuse of the wrist flexor-pronator muscles may cause symptoms over the medial epicondyle, whereas chronic irritation of the wrist extensor-supinator muscles may result in symptoms over the lateral epicondyle (Fig. 18-9). Names are frequently given to these overuse conditions, depending on the location of symptoms or the athletic activity involved in at the time of their development. For example, "tennis elbow" is a name commonly given to pain on the lateral side of the elbow because it frequently occurs in tennis players. However, tennis players

Fig. 18-9. Mechanism of injury that may result in tennis elbow (chronic irritation of the extensor-supinator muscles).

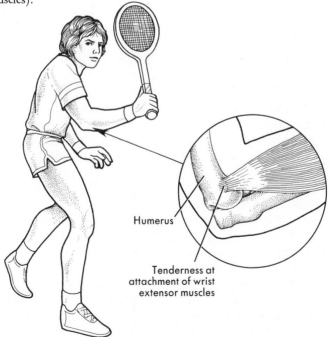

Humerus

Tenderness at attachment of wrist extensor muscles

can develop pain on the medial side of the elbow, depending on which muscle groups are irritated. "Little league elbow" is a term used to describe elbow lesions that result from the repetitive act of throwing in immature athletes. The most common problem of the little leaguer is an injury to the epiphysis of the medial epicondyle of the humerus. This epiphysis is normally the last epiphyseal center to close around the elbow and one of the weakest. The symptoms may be of acute or gradual onset. When the onset is sudden, the injury is more likely to involve an avulsion of the epicondyle. Acute pain and tenderness over the epicondyle indicates that an immature athlete should be referred to a physician for further assessment. More commonly, little league elbow is a chronic condition, and the symptoms are usually those of persistent discomfort and stiffness about the elbow and are aggravated by use of the arm. "Pitcher's elbow" or "javelin thrower's elbow" are other names given to painful elbow conditions that develop because of the sport in which the athlete is involved. These are overuse conditions and are often attributed to chronic strains.

Early and accurate recognition is very important in the proper care of these overuse conditions. Initial symptoms of chronic strains are local tenderness, pain on use of the involved muscles, and perhaps swelling. Without proper treatment, these conditions may develop into prolonged degenerative changes resulting in chronic epicondylitis, contractures of the elbow, reduced function, and possibly rupture of the muscle tendon unit.

Sprains

Sprains of the elbow joint are uncommon. Because of the configuration of the ulna in the trochlear notch, this is a relatively stable joint. Injuries involving the ligamentous system of the elbow most commonly result from partial dislocations or subluxations. The mechanism of injury is frequently forced hyperextension or lateral motion. Athletes with this type of history will often describe a "click" or "pop" along with sharp pain at the time of injury. In addition to tenderness at the site of injury, there is normally localized swelling and pain on any attempt to reproduce the mechanism of injury. Pain is usually relieved by bending the elbow, and athletes will normally hold their injured extremity in some degree of flexion. Swelling and muscle spasms will often limit complete extension. It may be difficult to determine significant instability of the elbow joint unless there has been a complete dislocation and rupture of ligaments. There may also be an avulsion of the ligament with a fragment of bone present. It is important to recognize significant ligamentous injuries to the elbow and initiate proper treatment procedures to prevent the development of residual contractures with resultant loss of motion and chronic disability.

Dislocations

Dislocations involving the elbow joint are moderately common in athletic activity. The most common type of dislocation is the posterior displacement of the ulna and radius in relationship to the humerus. This normally occurs because of a fall on an outstretched hand with the elbow in extension. As the elbow is forced into hyperextension, the olecranon process is levered against the humerus, which can force the ulna backward (posteriorly) (Fig. 18-10). The collateral ligaments are severely stretched or ruptured but the annular ligament often remains intact so that the head of the radius usually accompanies the ulna in its posterior displacement. In addition, there may be an associated lateral displacement, with either a varus or valgus deformity of the forearm. Elbow dislocations that remain displaced appear deformed, with the olecranon process abnormally prominent and the athlete expressing considerable pain. The initial examination of these injuries must include an evaluation of the circulation and nerve function to the distal portion of the extremity. Determine the presence or absence of a radial pulse as well as sensory and motor functions of the hand. All elbow dislocations should be properly immobilized and referred to a physician immediately.

Fractures

Fractures about the elbow and forearm can result from any of the injury-producing mechanisms described in this chapter. Normally fractures occur as the result of either direct trauma to the forearm or elbow or indirect stresses transmitted through the upper extremity as the result of falling on an outstretched arm. In addition, excessive forces associated with throwing and swinging activities may cause an interruption in bony continuity. Fractures about the elbow are among the most frequent involving children and skeletally immature athletes. Many of these involve the epiphysis because the ligamentous structures in young athletes are much stronger than the bony and cartilaginous components of the growth plate. Therefore athletic trainers should maintain a high level of suspicion concerning fractures whenever evaluating an acute elbow injury in a young athlete. Fortunately, fractures of the elbow are not common in skeletally mature athletes. All epiphyses at the elbow are fused by 18 years of age.

The most common fracture of the elbow is the humeral supracondylar fracture, or fracture proximal to the growth plate. This fracture is caused by falling on an outstretched hand or by forced hyperextension and frequently occurs in children. The distal fragment is usually pushed upward and backward by the fracturing force and is maintained in that position by spasm of the triceps. Athletic trainers should be aware of the fact that a supracondylar fracture of the distal humerus may appear to be a posterior dislocation. However, the epicondyles of the humerus and the olecranon process maintain their normal anatomic relationship in a supracondylar fracture.

There are a wide variety of fractures that may occur about the elbow. These may involve the distal humerus, proximal ulna, or radius. These can range from simple avulsions with a small flake of bone to serious and complicated fractures. The signs and symptoms associated with these injuries are directly related to the degree of severity. There may or may not be any visible or palpable deformity. Point tenderness is normally present at the site of injury, and varying amounts of hemorrhaging or swelling are common. The athlete may also demonstrate a limited range of motion, disability at the elbow or hand, and an increase in pain at the fracture site with attempted movements. Potential complications resulting from fractures about the elbow or from improper management of the injuries include neurovascular compromise and faulty bony union with deformity. Direct disruption of an artery or arterial occlusion as a result of swelling in the closed relatively inelastic compartment of the forearm may result in an impairment of the distal circulation. This can cause a compartment syndrome, which may in turn result in irreparable damage to the forearm and hand musculature, a condition called ***Volkmann's ischemic contracture.*** Volkmann's contracture is now considered the result of a vascular disturbance that may arise in a number of different ways. We know, for example, that trauma inflicted on any body area will have significant effects on the functioning of the sympathetic nervous system in the area involved. Sympathetic stimulation

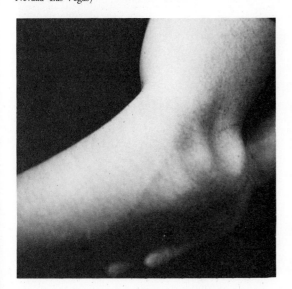

Fig. 18-10. Posterior dislocation of an elbow. (Courtesy A.G. Edwards. A.T.,C., University of Nevada–Las Vegas)

caused by elbow trauma can cause very sudden and serious changes to occur in forearm blood vessels. Vasoconstriction and segmental arterial spasm can result in paralysis and widespread degeneration of the flexor compartment forearm muscles. If this should occur, replacement of muscle by fibrous tissue results in a disabling "claw hand" syndrome. In addition to sympathetic stimulation, increased compartment pressure caused by internal swelling as a result of hemorrhage or external pressure caused by tight bandages or splints can also result in ischemic contracture. This tragic condition may develop insidiously for 6 to 12 hours after the injury. The classic signs of a compartment syndrome and impending Volkmann's contracture include pain, pallor, paralysis, and absence of pulse. The most important of these findings is deep, unremitting, and poorly localized pain, particularly when pain increases with finger motion. Always be suspicious in cases in which pain is disproportionate to the apparent seriousness of the injury. Remember, fractures about the elbow can be extremely serious and require early recognition and prompt referral so that they can be reduced early.

Fractures of the forearm are common in young athletes. They are usually caused by a direct blow or falling on an outstretched hand (Fig. 18-11). The signs and symptoms of forearm

Fig. 18-11. Wrestler with a fractured radius. (X-ray shows fracture near midpoint of diaphysis)

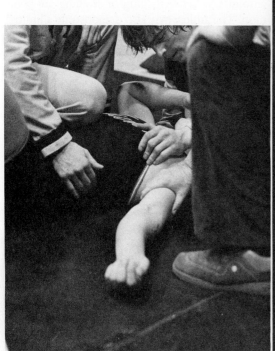
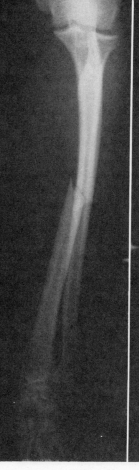
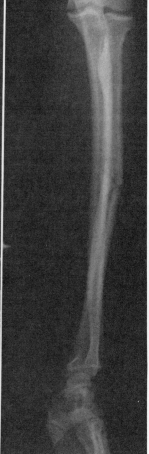

fractures may include point tenderness, swelling, angulation of the bone, pain on motion, disability, and crepitation. Whenever a fracture is suspected, the athlete should be referred to a physician.

ATHLETIC INJURY ASSESSMENT PROCESS

The elbow and forearm are frequently injured during athletic participation. Most athletic injuries in this area result from some type of direct blow such as falling on an outstretched arm, or by overload forces associated with throwing or swinging activities. As a group, athletic injuries to the elbow are potentially serious because inadequate evaluation and inappropriate treatment may lead to functional impairment or permanent disability. Of all the large joints in the body, the elbow is the most susceptible to loss of motion after injury or insult. Therefore proper care of elbow injuries is dependent on accurate assessment and closely supervised treatment and rehabilitation programs.

Secondary survey

Accurate determination of the severity of injury is the first step in assessment of elbow injuries. Unrecognized, a serious injury in this area can result in catastrophic complications, especially in children. Fractures and dislocations involving the elbow can cause circulatory or neural impairment that can result in irreparable damage to the forearm and hand. This is especially true in children and skeletally immature athletes. Athletic trainers must consider the age of the athlete and be cognizant of the possibility that these elbow injuries may involve the epiphysis or growth centers in young athletes. Any suspected fracture or elbow dislocation should not be manipulated in any manner. These injuries must be protected from further damage by gently splinting them in the position found and referring the athlete to medical assistance for further diagnosis and proper care. Therefore the assessment of all acute elbow injuries, especially in children and those who express much pain or remain lying on the court or field, should include an evaluation of circulation to the hand and an investigation of nerve function distal to the site of injury. Adequacy of hand circulation can be evaluated by checking for the radial pulse and compressing the nail beds and noting the return of normal color. Nerve impairment can be assessed by evaluating sensations over the palm, thumb, and fingers and noting the ability to contract the extrinsic and intrinsic muscles of the hand. Once the presence of adequate circulation and nerve functions has been established, the athletic injury assessment process can continue. Significant injuries to the elbow should also be reevaluated frequently after the injury to recognize the development of any circulatory or nerve impairment.

History

The comprehensive assessment of injuries to the elbow and forearm includes a careful history. Begin by inquiring about the primary complaint. What happened to the elbow or forearm? Question the athlete about the mechanism of injury to determine exactly how the injury occurred. Was there a direct blow delivered to the elbow or forearm? If a blow was delivered, was the elbow joint forced in an abnormal direction? Did the athlete fall and land on the elbow, forearm, or outstretched hand? What was the position of the elbow at the time of injury? Did the injury result from throwing or swinging activities? Did the symptoms of this injury, including onset of pain, come on very suddenly or did they develop over a period of time? The more information gained concerning the mechanism of injury and the onset of symptoms, the easier it is to accurately assess the nature and severity of the injury and determine those structures that may be involved.

Allow the athlete to describe the symptoms associated with the injury. Exactly where are the painful or tender areas? Ask the athlete to locate and describe the pain. Pain about the elbow and forearm is normally easy to localize and is seldom diffuse or radiating unless there is neural involvement. On those occasions when a nerve is compressed, a burning pain may travel the length of the nerve pathway, such as occurs when the ulnar nerve is hit. Is pain only present during activity? If so, what types of activities or movements cause the pain? The athlete may be asked to demonstrate the painful motions.

Question the athlete about any unusual sensations associated with the injury. Did he or she feel anything at the time of injury, such as a popping, clicking, or snapping sensation? Does the athlete feel any crepitation? Is there any tightness, tension, or swelling associated with the injury? Does the athlete complain of any numbness, burning, tingling, or weakness in the forearm or hand? Ask the athlete to describe his or her impressions concerning the injury.

Also inquire about previous injuries. Has the athlete suffered an injury to this area of the body before? If so, obtain as much information as possible concerning the circumstances surrounding previous injuries. When was the athlete injured? What was the nature and severity of previous injuries? Had the athlete fully recovered from prior injuries or did he or she still experience symptoms? What types of activities could the athlete participate in before the current injury? Was the athlete's elbow able to function normally? Does this injury appear to be the same or very similar to previous injuries?

Observation

The initial observations regarding injuries about the elbow must be concerned with recognizing obvious deformity. As previously discussed, it is critically important for the athletic trainer to recognize elbow dislocations and fractures early in the assessment process in order to initiate proper handling and treatment procedures. Early identification of serious injury reduces the possibility of complications. If clothing or protective equipment covers the elbow, it can generally be removed easily from this area of the body without causing additional trauma or pain to the athlete. Remember, if the athlete is unable or unwilling to move the elbow, visual inspection should be accomplished in whatever position the injured elbow is held. Begin the observation by noting the contours of the elbow and forearm. Is there any obvious deformity? Dislocations that remain displaced are normally easy to visually recognize due to the associated deformity. Note in Fig. 18-10 the posterior displacement of the ulna in relation to the humerus. Remember, to the untrained observer, a supracondylar fracture may look like a posterior dislocation. However, the epicondyles and the olecranon process maintain their normal anatomic relationship in a supracondylar fracture. This would not be the case in a posterior dislocation. In this type of fracture the median nerve and blood vessels in the cubital fossa are easily injured and the possibility of Volkmann's contracture must be considered. Supracondylar or fractures of the distal humerus occur most frequently in young athletes. In addition to the presence of a growth plate, in the years before skeletal maturity the anteroposterior diameter of the humerus is quite narrow just above the condyles. Fractures about the elbow and forearm may be less obvious than a dislocation and may require close visual inspection combined with various signs and symptoms recognized and expressed during the assessment process.

Whenever confronted with an injured elbow, inspect and compare both elbows to note any differences in symmetry. Is there any swelling? If so, note exactly where the swelling is located. Swelling about the elbow or forearm may be localized to the olecranon bursa or diffused throughout the joint. Athletes with diffuse swelling will normally hold the elbow in a flexed position to accommodate the swelling with minimal pain. Whenever you suspect bleeding into the elbow of a young athlete, consider the possibility of development of Volkmann's ischemic contracture and refer the athlete to medical assistance. In addition to swelling, carefully inspect the injured area for signs of trauma that can indicate what type of force has been applied and assist in establishing or confirming the mechanism of injury.

Note the alignment of both arms. Normally with the arm in complete extension the forearm forms a slight valgus (lateral) angle at the elbow joint in relation to the upper arm. This is called the *carrying angle* and normally ranges from approximately 5° in men to 10° to 15° in women. If the forearm bones were in straight alignment with the humerus in the anatomic postion, a 180° line would result. Instead, the carrying angle reduces the 180° straight line to 175° in men and less than 170° in women. As a result, the hand is normally carried away from the sides of the body when the elbow is extended and the forearm supinated.

Compare the carrying angle of both arms. Are they equal? An increase *(cubitus valgus)* or decrease *(cubitus varus)* in the carrying angle of the injured elbow may be caused by a fracture or epiphyseal separation. Fig. 18-12 shows a cubitus varus, sometimes called a *gunstock deformity,* resulting from a malunion of a fracture to the dis-

tal end of the humerus. This type of deformity is seen more frequently than an increase in the carrying angle.

Palpation

Palpation of the injured elbow or forearm is used to identify specific structures that may be involved in the injury. This is accomplished by accurately locating all areas of associated tenderness and swelling as well as any other physical signs that may assist in recognizing the injury. The specific structures or areas to be palpated will be determined by the information gained during the history and inspection phases in the assessment process.

As with any area of the body, palpation procedures should be conducted with the injured area as relaxed as possible. This is best accomplished by supporting the athlete's injured arm with one hand and palpating the suspected area of injury with the other hand. The athlete may be sitting, standing or lying. Gently feel those areas suspected of being injured and correlate this information with the underlying anatomy. Procedures used to palpate the various anatomical structures of the elbow and forearm will be discussed briefly as will the common athletic injuries which may be indicated by positive findings.

The olecranon process of the ulna is a good point of reference to begin palpating the elbow (Fig. 18-13). This bony tip of the elbow feels subcutaneous although it is covered by the olecranon bursa and the insertion of the triceps. When an olecranon bursitis is present there will be varying amounts of swelling and tenderness over the olecranon. Occasionally there will be a small palpable mass in this area. This is normally a fibrinous or cartilaginous mass but may be mistaken for a chip of bone. A physician may order radiographs to rule out a bone chip or other fracture.

Just proximal to the olecranon is the olecranon fossa of the humerus. This depression can best be felt with the elbow in about 45° of flexion and the triceps completely relaxed (Fig. 18-14). If

---

Fig. 18-12. Gunstock deformity resulting from malunion of a fractured humerus.

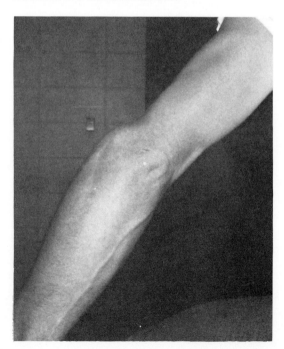

Fig. 18-13. Palpating the olecranon process of the ulna.

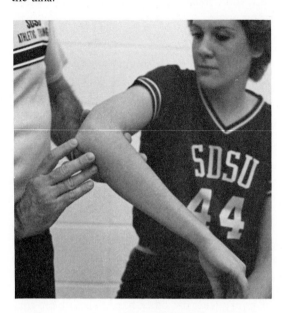

Fig. 18-14. Palpating the olecranon fossa of the humerus.

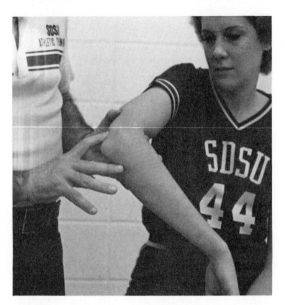

Fig. 18-15. Palpating styloid process of ulna.

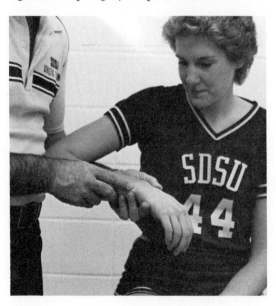

Fig. 18-16. Palpating and noting the geometric alignment of the olecranon process, the medial epicondyle and the lateral epicondyle.

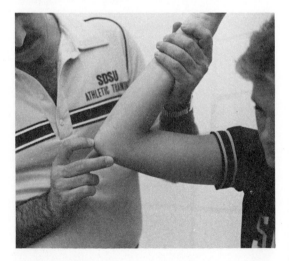

the triceps is not relaxed, the tendon of this muscle will be palpated covering the fossa. With the elbow in extension, the olecranon process will fill this depression. Distal to the olecranon process, the subcutaneous border of the ulna can be palpated along its entire length to the styloid process at the wrist (Fig. 18-15).

On either side of the olecranon the epicondyles of the humerus can be palpated. The medial epicondyle, the lateral epicondyle, and the olecranon process should lie in a straight line when the elbow is completely extended. With the elbow in flexion, these three bony prominences should form an isosceles triangle. The geometric alignment of these bony prominences can best be appreciated by placing your index finger on the olecranon process and your thumb and middle finger on either epicondyle (Fig. 18-16). A noticeable deviation in this alignment when compared to the uninjured elbow may indicate a structural problem such as a condylar fracture.

The medial epicondyle of the humerus is larger and more easily palpated than its lateral counterpart. Gently palpate about this bony prominence (Fig. 18-17, *A*). Various athletic injuries can cause pain or tenderness when palpating on and around the medial epicondyle. Remember, this medial epicondyle is the part of the elbow most frequently fractured, especially in young athletes whose epiphyses are not yet united. Palpating proximal to this eminence, you can feel the medial supracondylar ridge for a short distance. Lying just posterior to the medial epicondyle is the groove through which the ulnar nerve passes into the forearm (Fig. 18-17, *B*). Palpating just distal to the medial epicondyle, you can feel the common flexor tendon, which is the shared origin of four muscles (Fig. 18-18, *A*). Pain in this area frequently represents an acute or chronic strain resulting from activities requiring acute or chronic pronation and wrist flexion.

The less prominent lateral epicondyle of the humerus is palpated on the outside of the elbow. The lateral supracondylar ridge can be felt running proximal to the lateral epicondyle. The common extensor tendon, which is the shared origin for supinator and wrist extensor muscles, arises along this ridge and the lateral epicondyle (Fig. 18-18, *B*). Pain in this area frequently repre-

Fig. 18-17. Palpating the: **A,** medial epicondyle and **B,** ulnar nerve.

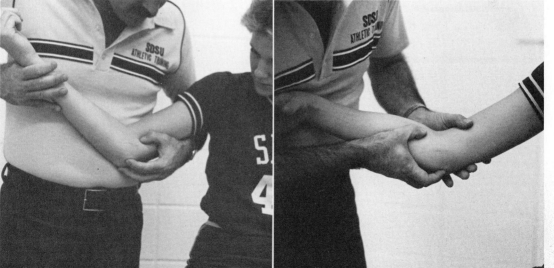

Fig. 18-18. Palpating the: **A,** common flexor tendon and **B,** common extensor tendon.

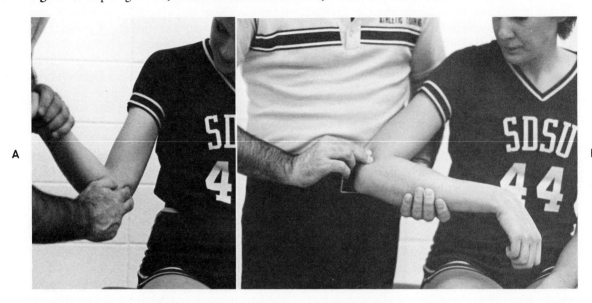

A   B

Fig. 18-19. Palpating the radius: **A,** head of the radius and **B,** the styloid process.

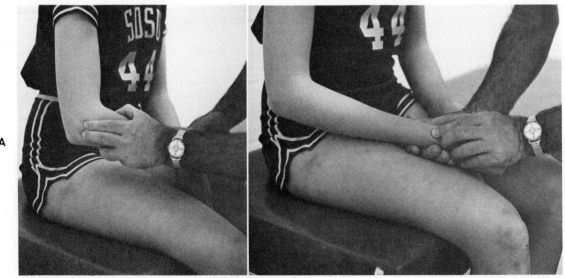

A   B

sents an acute or chronic strain resulting from activities requiring supination and wrist extension. Just distal to the lateral epicondyle, palpate the head of the radius (Fig. 18-19, *A*). This is most easily felt when the elbow is in approximately 90° of flexion with the surrounding muscles relaxed. Instruct the athlete to pronate and supinate the forearm as you palpate the radial head. Just distal to the head of the radius lies the annular ligament, which cannot be directly palpated. The proximal half of the radius then becomes obscured by the overlying muscles of the forearm. The distal shaft of the radius can be palpated from the radial styloid at the wrist to a point approximately half way up the forearm (Fig. 18-19, *B*).

Soft tissue structures can be palpated over the anterior surface of the elbow. The hollow triangular area in front of the elbow is called the *cubital fossa* and is formed by the pronator teres muscle medially and the brachioradialis laterally. The base of the cubital triangle is formed by a line drawn between the humeral condyles. At the apex of the fossa the brachioradialis muscle overlaps the pronator teres. Within this space are two structures that are usually easily palpable, the biceps tendon and the brachial artery. The biceps tendon with its strong expansion, the **bicipital aponeurosis,** is readily palpated during mild resistance to elbow flexion (Fig. 18-20, *A*). The brachial artery lies directly medial to the biceps tendon (Fig. 18-20, *B*). This pulse is normally used when taking blood pressure.

The muscles of the forearm should be palpated as a unit, that is, the wrist flexors and extensors as two separate groups. Support the forearm to ensure the muscles are as relaxed as possible. Attempt to locate areas of tenderness, swelling, muscle spasm, deficits, or masses. Not all of the muscles of the forearm are distinguishable by palpation, and resistive motion is normally required to complete the evaluation of muscle integrity.

Stress

Stress procedures should never be used during the assessment of elbow injuries until you are sure there is no associated fracture or disloca-

Fig. 18-20. A, Palpating the biceps tendon during mild resistance to elbow flexion. **B,** Locating the brachial pulse.

A

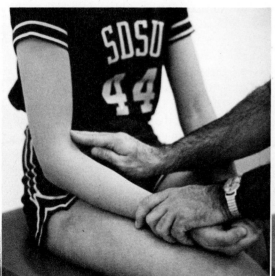

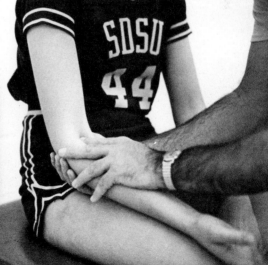

B

tion. Manipulation of the elbow when these types of injuries are present may cause additional damage and perhaps permanent disability. Therefore, all elbow injuries suspected of involving a fracture or dislocation should be protected from any movements and referred to a qualified physician.

Active movements. Active movements are normally performed to evaluate range of motion and begin assessing the integrity of contractile structures in the area of injury. A classic symptom involving the elbow, which may indicate the development of a severe complication, is an increase in pain at the elbow with finger motion. This is especially true when the fingers are actively or passively moved into extension (Fig. 18-21). Therefore the initial active movements used to evaluate an injured elbow should be finger motions. These movements require no motion of the elbow joint and may be extremely important in recognizing the development of anterior compartment syndrome or Volkmann's ischemic contracture. Athletes suffering an el-

bow injury and not referred to medical attention should also be instructed to be alert for the development of increased swelling or tightness and pain about the elbow, especially pain increasing on finger extension.

To evaluate active range of motion at the elbow, instruct the athlete to flex and extend at the elbow as far as possible. Normally a person can flex approximately 150°, being limited by the muscle mass of the front of the arm, and extend the arm straight out to 0° (Fig. 18-22). Many athletes, especially women, can hyperextend at the elbow as much as 5° to 15° beyond the straight position (Fig. 18-23). The active range of motion of both elbows should be examined simultaneously to detect any differences. Remember, pain, swelling, muscle spasms, and previous injuries can all limit the range of motion available at the elbow joint.

Active supination and pronation should also be evaluated in one continuous motion. Instruct the athlete to flex the elbow to 90° to avoid shoulder motion, and then turn the palm up and down. Normally the forearm can be rotated approximately 90° in each direction or until the palm is facing directly upward or downward (Fig. 18-24). Small differences in the range of motion between both forearms may be more easily noticed if the athlete is asked to hold something, such as tape scissors, in each fist as he or she supinates and pronates both forearms simultaneously (Fig. 18-25).

Resistive movements. Resistive movements are used to further evaluate the integrity of contractile structures. Applying manual resistance against each of the active motions of the elbow and forearm can assist in accurately locating specific painful areas. A knowledge of the functional anatomy allows you to differentiate one muscle from another. Resistive movements are also used to compare muscular strength between extremities.

To apply resistance against elbow flexion, stabilize the arm or elbow with one hand and apply resistance to the movement proximal to the wrist with the other hand (Fig. 18-26). Note any

Fig. 18-21. Instructing athlete to actively extend fingers to recognize increased pain at the elbow.

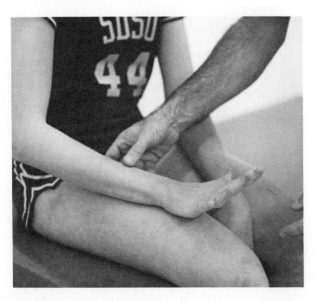

Fig. 18-22. Range of motion of the elbow: flexion, extension, and hyperextension. **A,** Flexion and hyperextension. *Flexion:* zero to 150 degrees. *Extension:* 150 degrees to zero. *Hyperextension:* measured in degrees beyond the zero starting point. This motion is not present in all persons. When it is present, it may vary from 5 to 15 degrees. **B,** Measurement of limited motion. (The unshaded area indicates the range of limited motion.) Limited motion may be expressed in the following ways: (1) the elbow flexes from 30 to 90 degrees (30° → 90°); (2) the elbow has a flexion deformity of 30 degrees with further flexion to 90 degrees.
(From Malasanos, L., et al.: Health assessment, ed. 2, St. Louis, 1981, The C.V. Mosby Co.)

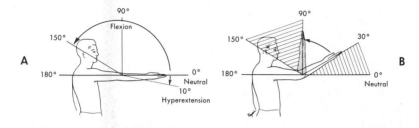

Fig. 18-23. Athlete exhibiting hyperextension at the elbow joint.

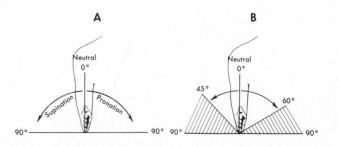

Fig. 18-24. Range of motion of the elbow: pronation and supination. **A,** Pronation and supination. *Pronation:* zero to 80 or 90 degrees. *Supination:* zero to 80 or 90 degrees. *Total forearm motion:* 160 to 180 degrees. Persons may vary in the range of supination and pronation. Some persons may reach the 90-degree arc, whereas others may have only 70 degrees plus. **B,** Limited motion. *Supination:* 45 degrees (0 → 45°). *Pronation:* 60 degrees (0 → 60°). *Total joint motion:* 105 degrees.
(From Malasanos, L., et al.: Health assessment, ed. 2, St. Louis, 1981, The C.V. Mosby Co.)

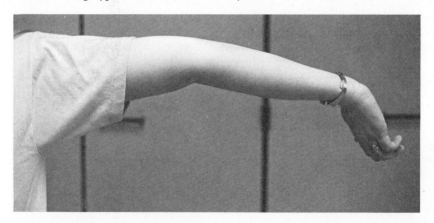

areas of pain. While this is primarily a test for the biceps and brachialis muscles, other accessory muscles may assist elbow flexion and exhibit pain if injured. For example, those muscles originating high in the common flexor and common extensor tendons may also weakly assist elbow flexion. To evaluate these muscles, further resistance must be applied against their primary action.

Maintain the same position to apply resistance against elbow extension. Instruct the athlete to slowly extend his or her arm while you increase the resistance against extension. Again note any areas of pain on resisted movement and evaluate the relative strength of both triceps.

It is difficult as well as unnecessary to differentiate individual muscles of the forearm during the assessment process. These muscles act in groups and are primarily responsible for supination and pronation as well as wrist flexion and extension. Therefore resistance should be ap-

plied against each of these movements to evaluate the integrity of each functional muscle group. To resist supination, maintain the same positioning, with the athlete's forearm pronated, and instruct the athlete to supinate as you apply resistance against the dorsal surface of the distal end of the radius. Resistance to pronation is accomplished by applying resistance on the volar surface of the distal end of the radius as the athlete pronates. To test wrist flexion and extension, stabilize the athlete's forearm and apply resistance to the hand during each movement (Fig. 18-27). To rule out the finger flexors and extensors assisting during each movement, instruct the athlete to keep the thumb and fingers relaxed.

Passive movements. Generally the only passive movements or maneuvers that are performed in conjunction with elbow injuries are those that evaluate the integrity of the medial and lateral collateral ligaments. The range of motion of an

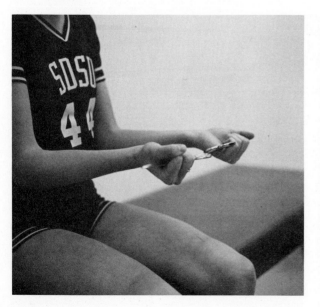

Fig. 18-25. Active supination and pronation with athlete grasping bandage scissors in an attempt to note small differences in range of motion.

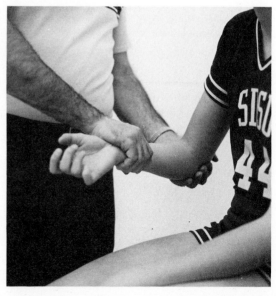

Fig. 18-26. Applying manual resistance against elbow flexion.

injured elbow should always be evaluated actively. Passive procedures can cause further damage and must be used with caution and restraint.

To assess the integrity of the collateral ligaments, cup the injured elbow in one hand and grasp the wrist with the other. Flex the elbow approximately 15° to 20° in order to "unlock" the olecranon process from the olecranon fossa. Instruct the athlete to relax the muscles of the upper extremity. To evaluate the medial (ulnar) collateral ligament, apply a valgus stress to the elbow (Fig. 18-28, *A*). Remember to begin this type of maneuver very gently and then increase intensity depending on the athlete's tolerance. To evaluate the lateral (radial) collateral ligament, apply a varus stress to the elbow joint (Fig. 18-28, *B*). Does the athlete express any pain with these stress procedures? Note any gapping or instability with either of these movements and compare to the uninjured elbow.

Another method of demonstrating medial instability is with a ***gravity stress test.*** Have the athlete lie supine, externally rotate the shoulder, and flex the elbow approximately 20° (Fig. 18-29). If the elbow is unstable, the weight of the forearm and hand will normally exert enough valgus stress to open the medial side. In a muscular athlete, a 1- or 2-pound weight may be placed on the hand to increase the stress or a manual valgus force can be applied by the athletic trainer. A physician may use this procedure in conjunction with radiography to determine the extent of medial instability.

Passive stress procedures may also be used to assess the integrity of the two long bones of the forearm. If the signs and symptoms exhibited to this point in the assessment process cause you to suspect a possible fracture of the shaft of the radius or ulna, stress can be applied to these two bones. This can be accomplished by applying longitudinal or transverse stress. This stress

Fig. 18-27. Applying manual resistance against wrist flexion **(A)** and wrist extension **(B)**.

A   B

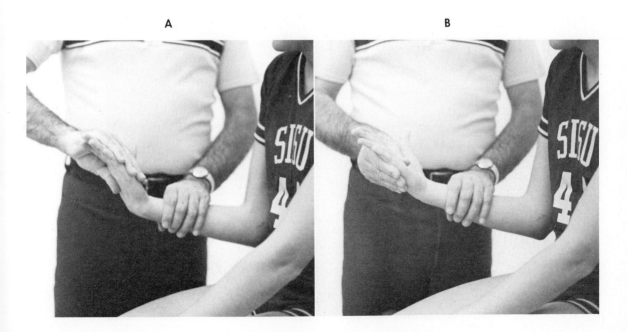

should be very gentle initially and increased depending on the athlete's tolerance. Longitudinal stress can be accomplished by stabilizing the elbow with one hand and applying force or pressure directly along the long axis of both bones (Fig. 18-30, *A*). Transverse stress is applied away from the site of pain and can be accomplished by squeezing the ulna and radius together (Fig. 18-30, *B*) or applying a medial or lateral force. Locate the point tenderness and move away from this area to apply the transverse pressure. If the bone integrity is intact, there should be no pain

Fig. 18-28. Stressing collateral ligaments. **A,** Valgus stress to evaluate the integrity of the ulnar collateral ligament and **B,** varus stress to evaluate the integrity of the radial collateral ligament.

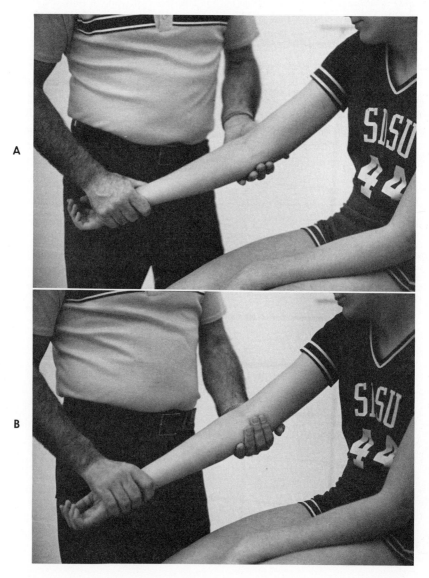

or crepitation with these stress procedures. However, if these maneuvers cause additional pain at the original site of tenderness, the athlete should be treated as if there is a fracture.

Functional movements. As with shoulder injuries, functional movements or activities can prove helpful in the assessment of elbow injuries. Many injuries involving the elbow also result from repetitive throwing or swinging activities, and these same movements may be required to replicate the associated symptoms. Instruct the athlete to perform those activities that

Fig. 18-29. Gravity stress test to evaluate medial collateral instability.

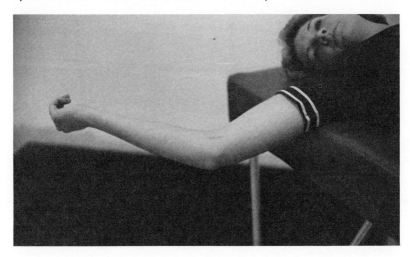

Fig. 18-30. Applying passive stress to evaluate the integrity of the radius and ulna: **A,** longitudinal compression stress and **B,** transverse stress by squeezing radius and ulna.

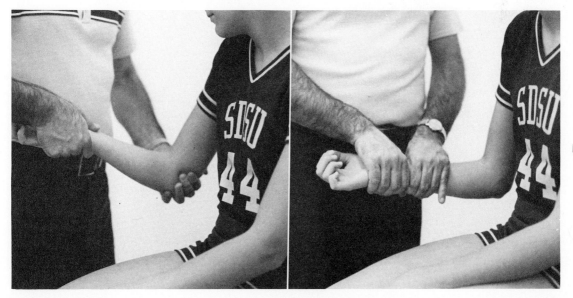

A

B

produce the symptoms in an effort to identify the mechanism of injury as well as those anatomic structures that may be involved.

Functional movements are normally used to assist in determining when an athlete can return to athletic activity, especially those requiring throwing or swinging. During each reevaluation, question the athlete directly or observe his or her functional abilities concerning the elbow. The intensity of these activities should be progressively increased within the athlete's tolerance.

Evaluation of findings

The elbow can be subjected to tremendous forces or stresses during many types of athletic activity. This area of the body is frequently involved in athletic injuries occuring as acute traumatic episodes (direct or muscular violence) or chronic overuse syndromes. Acute fractures and dislocations must be promptly recognized and adequately managed to avoid serious and possibly catastrophic complications. Early recognition of circulatory impairment or nerve compression syndromes is essential to preventing

---

ATHLETIC INJURY ASSESSMENT CHECKLIST
ELBOW AND FOREARM INJURIES

Secondary survey

———— History
———— Primary complaint
———— Position of the elbow
———— Pain
———— Sensations
———— Previous injuries
———— Observation
———— Obvious deformity
———— Compare symmetry of both elbows
———— Swelling
———— Signs of trauma
———— Carrying angle
———— Palpation
———— Tenderness
———— Swelling
———— Deformities
———— Crepitation
———— Stress
———— Active movements
———— Range of motion
———— Pain
———— Resistive movements
———— Pain
———— Strength
———— Passive movements
———— Ligament instability
———— Integrity of long bones
———— Functional movements
———— Functional abilities

permanent impairment. Overuse syndromes resulting from the cumulative harmful effects associated with throwing or swinging activities must also be accurately recognized and properly treated to promote healing and allow the athlete to return to participation. Inadequate treatment may result in permanent functional disability, chronic problems, or possibly early retirement from athletic activity.

When to refer the athlete

Elbow injuries, especially acute traumatic episodes should be evaluated and managed with caution and a high index of suspicion. You must be cognizant of epiphyseal injuries in skeletally immature athletes. With all elbow injuries, you must be concerned with circulation and nerve function to the forearm and hand. Following is a list of conditions or findings that can be used to determine if medical referral is indicated:

1. Gross deformity about the elbow or forearm
2. Significant swelling about the elbow joint
3. Considerable pain, especially on finger extension
4. Significant loss of motion
5. Audible "click" or "pop" at time of injury
6. Loss of sensation below the elbow
7. Abnormal sensations that do not quickly subside, such as numbness, tingling, or weakness
8. Joint instability
9. Suspected fracture or dislocation
10. Any doubt regarding the severity or nature of the elbow or forearm injury

KEY TERMS

bicipital aponeurosis Strong expansion of the biceps tendon, which blends with the fascia over the flexor muscles of the forearm

carrying angle Angle formed by the axes of the arm and forearm when the elbow is extended

cubitus valgus Increase in the carrying angle

cubitus varus Decrease in the carrying angle; also known as a *gunstock deformity*

gravity stress test Passive test using gravity and the weight of the hand and forearm to stress the medial side of the elbow: to perform the test, place the athlete supine, externally rotate the shoulder, and flex the elbow approximately 20° (Weights can be added to increase the stress)

Volkmann's ischemic contracture Condition that may develop after a severe injury in the region of the elbow and is caused by the loss of blood supply to the musculature of the forearm; this catastrophic complication is characterized by permanent flexion of the fingers and sometimes of the wrist

SUGGESTED READINGS

Arnheim, D.D.: Modern principles of athletic training, ed. 6, St. Louis, 1985, Times Mirror/Mosby College Publishing.

Conwell, H.E.: Injuries to the elbow, CIBA Clinical Symposia, 21:2, 1969.

DeHaven, K.E., and Evart, E.M.: Throwing injuries of the elbow in athletics, Orthop. Clin. North Am. 3:801-808, 1973.

Hoppenfeld, S.: Physical examination of the spine and extremities, New York, 1976, Appleton-Century-Crofts.

Mercier, L.R., and Pettid, F.J.: Practical orthopedics, Chicago, 1980, Year Book Medical Publishers, Inc.

Midgley, R.D.: Volkmann's ischemic contracture of the forearm, Orthop. Clin. North Am. 4:983-986, 1973.

O'Donoghue, D.H.: Treatment of injuries to athletes, ed. 4, Philadelphia, 1984, W.B. Saunders Co.

Roy, S., and Irvin, R.: Sports medicine: prevention, evaluation, management, and rehabilitation, Englewood Cliffs, N.J., 1983, Prentice-Hall, Inc.

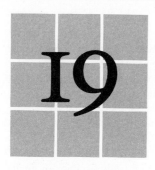

19 Hand and wrist injuries

The hand, which includes the fingers and thumb, is a functionally intricate and complex anatomic structure located at the distal end of our upper extremity. The wrist is that area of articulation between the forearm and hand. Precise functioning of the hand and wrist is essential to almost every type of athletic activity. The primary function of the proximal portion of the upper extremity is to position the hand where it can best perform its designated tasks. Functional anatomists sometimes refer to the hand and

wrist as the "reason for the upper extremity." Both structures are frequently used during athletic activity and often function as a single unit. Together they permit an incredible array of intricate movements and also serve to absorb or transmit forces caused by falls or traumatic contact. Because the hand and wrist normally do not bear weight and because injuries to this area are not usually totally disabling, there is a tendency by some athletes to underestimate the severity and importance of these injuries. Many injuries to the hand and wrist are relatively minor and do not require extensive care. However, if neglected or unrecognized, they can develop into long-term impairment and possibly permanent disability and disfigurement. Hand and wrist injuries may require expert treatment to avoid these complications. It is imperative therefore that athletic trainers be able to accurately assess athletic injuries to this important area of the body, initiate proper treatment, and recognize when referral is necessary. The comprehensive evaluation of injuries to the hand and wrist begins with a well-founded knowledge of gross and functional anatomy of the area as well as an understanding of the common athletic injuries and how they may occur.

ANATOMY OF THE WRIST

The term *wrist* is used to describe the anatomic and functional link between forearm and hand. It contains the carpal bones, the distal ends of the radius and ulna, and the proximal ends (bases) of the metacarpals together with the surrounding soft tissues. The wrist actually contains three sets of joints: (1) the radiocarpal, (2) the midcarpal, and (3) the carpometacarpal joints.

Carpals

The eight carpal bones of the wrist (Fig. 19-1) are named according to their general appearance and shape. They are arranged in two rows, proximal and distal, each consisting of four bones.

Fig. 19-1. Bones of the right hand and wrist: **A,** dorsal view; **B,** palmar view.

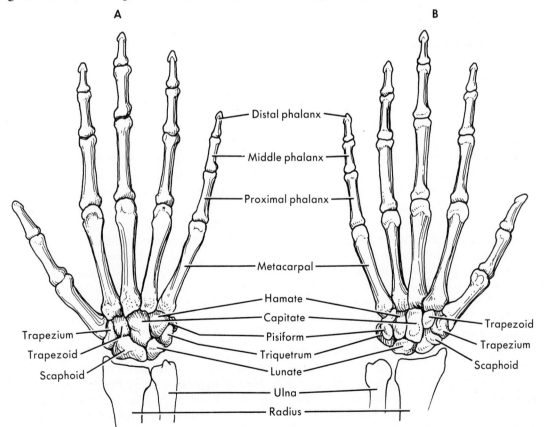

A

B

- Distal phalanx -
- Middle phalanx -
- Proximal phalanx -
- Metacarpal -
- Hamate -
- Capitate -
- Pisiform -
- Triquetrum -
- Lunate -
- Ulna -
- Radius -

Trapezium
Trapezoid
Scaphoid

Trapezoid
Trapezium
Scaphoid

The proximal row of four carpals, from thumb (radial) side to little finger (ulnar) side, is composed of the navicular or scaphoid (boat-shaped), the lunate (moon-shaped), the triquetrum (three-cornered), and the pisiform (pea-shaped) bones. The distal row, from thumb side to little finger side, is made up of the trapezium (greater multangular), trapezoid (lesser multangular), capitate (head-shaped), and hamate (hooked) bones.

The navicular, lunate, and capitate carpals are of particular significance in the assessment of athletic injuries. The navicular is the most commonly fractured of all the carpals. The lunate (moon-shaped) carpal is the middle bone of the proximal row and is the one most frequently dislocated. The capitate is the largest of the carpals and is the most prominent bone in the central wrist. The capitate transmits the force of a fall on the hand, through the navicular and lunate bones, to the radius. The interval between the pisiform and hamate carpal bones permits the passage of the ulnar artery and nerve into the hand, which is of considerable clinical significance. The pisiform is easily located on the little finger (ulnar) side of the wrist. Anatomists consider this carpal as a sesamoid bone in the tendon of the flexor carpi ulnaris (a major flexor of the wrist). When this tendon is relaxed the pisiform can be moved about on the adjacent carpal. As a result, it is sometimes erroneously identified as a bone fragment if a fracture is suspected after some type of wrist trauma.

The carpal bones are often injured as a result of trauma produced by a fall on the outstretched hand. As stated previously, the most common carpal injury is fracture of the navicular, and the next most frequent is dislocation of the lunate. Both injuries are good examples of how the anatomy of a structure can influence the mechanism of injury or progression of pathology after trauma.

As a group, the posterior surfaces of the carpal bones are larger than the anterior surfaces. They resemble wedges with the bases behind (posterior). The navicular and lunate bones are exceptions. Both have anterior surfaces that are more extensive than the posterior. This explains why, when dislocations occur, the navicular and lunate almost always dislocate anteriorly whereas the other carpals dislocate posteriorly. Fracture of the navicular carpal occurs when it is brought directly under the radius as a result of a fall on the outstretched hand and is pinched between it and the capitate bone.

Distal radio-ulnar articulation

The distal, or inferior, radio-ulnar joint is the articulation between the head of the ulna and the ulnar notch on the lower end of the radius. A triangular fibrocartilaginous disc (articular disc) is located between the distal end of the ulna and the carpal bones of the wrist and also serves as the chief uniting structure at the distal radio-ulnar joint. This distal radio-ulnar joint is covered by a thin, lax fibrous capsule that is lined by a synovial membrane.

Radiocarpal articulation

The radiocarpal (wrist) joint (Fig. 19-2) is the articulation between the concave distal end of the radius and its intervening articular disc with the convex proximal surfaces of the navicular, lunate, and triquetrum bones. The navicular and lunate form the primary articular surface. The proximal surfaces of these bones form the carpal articular surface in the radiocarpal (wrist) joint. The concave to convex surfaces form an elipsoid articulation. It is a true synovial (diarthrotic) joint. The movements available are flexion and extension around the transverse axis, abduction (radial deviation) and adduction (ulnar deviation) around the anteroposterior axis, and circumduction.

Midcarpal articulations

The principal midcarpal (intercarpal) joint is located between the bones of the proximal and distal rows of the wrist as the two rows articulate with each other. In addition, discrete articulations also exist between adjacent carpals in both the proximal and distal rows of bones. A small joint also exists between the pisiform and triquetrum bones. The cavity of this joint is independent of all others in the wrist. Combined movements at the midcarpal articulations increase the range of movements of the hand and supplement movements at the radiocarpal joint. Limited gliding movements also occur between adjacent carpals in both the proximal and distal rows.

Carpometacarpal articulations

The articulation between the trapezium and the first metacarpal (of the thumb) is unique in that the joint cavity formed by this articulation is separate from all others in the area. The joint cavities of the four other carpometacarpal joints (of the fingers) communicate with the large midcarpal joint cavity.

The second metacarpal articulates with the trapezoid, the capitate with the third metacarpal, and the hamate with the fourth and fifth metacarpals. The bases of the four metacarpal bones of the fingers are united by strong ligaments in an intermetacarpal joint. No joint or direct bony articulation exists between the first and second metacarpals.

The separate carpometacarpal joint of the thumb is a saddle-shaped articulation with reciprocally concavoconvex surfaces between the trapezium and first metacarpal. This "thumb joint" is surrounded by a strong but loose articular capsule that permits opposition, flexion, extension, abduction, adduction, and circumduction. In contrast, only slight gliding movements are possible between the carpals and the metacarpals of the four fingers.

Ligaments

A fibrous capsule formed by a complex series of ligaments binds the carpals firmly together into a functional unit (Fig. 19-3). A large and complex intercarpal synovial cavity extends between the carpals and communicates with the joint cavities of the four medial carpometacarpal and intermetacarpal joints. It does not communicate with the wrist joint. The dense ligamentous mass on the palmar surface of the wrist is much stronger than the dorsal ligaments. Also located on the palmar surface of the wrist is the osseofibrous carpal canal, or *carpal tunnel,* which is formed by the arched carpal bones, the transverse carpal, and the volar carpal ligaments. Except for the flexor carpi ulnaris and the palmaris longus muscle tendons, all of the flexor tendons and the median nerve pass through this confined tunnel. This gives rise to the possibilities of *carpal tunnel syndrome* developing as a result of constriction within the tunnel and pres-

Fig. 19-2. Joints articulating the bones of the wrist and hand.
(From Malasanos, L., et al.: Health assessment, ed. 2, St. Louis, 1981, The C.V. Mosby Co.)

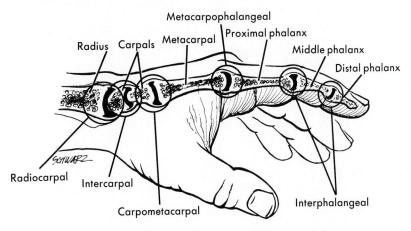

sure on the median nerve. Crossing the dorsal surface of the wrist are the extensor tendons of the fingers, which are surrounded by tendon sheaths as they pass between the extensor retinaculum and the underlying bones of the wrist. This dorsal retinaculum is attached to the underlying bones in such a manner to form six separate compartments for the extensor tendons.

Anatomic snuffbox

Of particular importance to the athletic trainer is a landmark called the *anatomic snuffbox,* which is formed by three dorsal tendons. The radial border of the snuffbox is formed by the abductor pollicis longus and the extensor pollicis brevis tendons, and the ulnar border is formed by the extensor pollicis longus tendon. The tendons forming the anatomic snuffbox become prominent when the thumb is extended (Fig.

19-4). The navicular lies just below the anatomic snuffbox and this surface landmark is used to locate and palpate this most frequently fractured carpal. The tip of the styloid process of the radius can also be palpated at the proximal end of the snuffbox.

INJURIES TO THE WRIST

The wrist is a frequently injured area of the body. Athletic injuries often result from a direct blow to the wrist or stresses that force the wrist beyond its normal range of motion. The wide range of mobility available at the wrist contributes a great deal to overall hand function. The wide use of the hands in athletics, such as breaking a fall, warding off another player, grasping, catching, throwing, or hitting, frequently force the wrist beyond its normal range of motion (Fig. 19-5). Structures in the wrist can also be

Fig. 19-3. The wrist joint. **A,** Palmar view. **B,** Dorsal view.

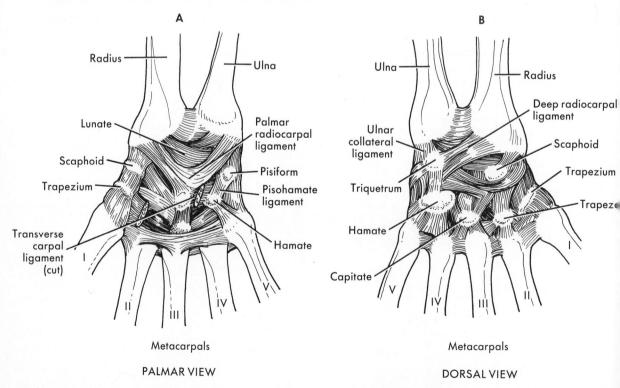

A

Radius — Ulna

Lunate

Scaphoid

Trapezium

Palmar radiocarpal ligament

Pisiform

Pisohamate ligament

Transverse carpal ligament (cut)

I

Hamate

II

III

IV

V

Metacarpals

PALMAR VIEW

B

Ulna — Radius

Ulnar collateral ligament

Triquetrum

Hamate

Capitate

Deep radiocarpal ligament

Scaphoid

Trapezium

Trapeze

I

V

IV

III

II

Metacarpals

DORSAL VIEW

Fig. 19-4. Anatomic snuffbox formed by dorsal tendons of the thumb.

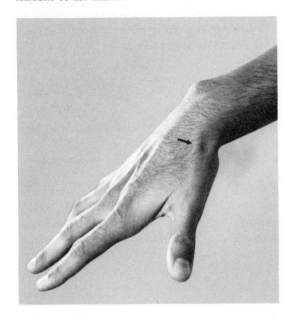

injured as the result of chronic overuse. These mechanisms of injury can result in contusions, sprains, strains, dislocations, and fractures.

Contusions

Contusions of the wrist frequently occur as the result of a direct blow. The result is a bruise involving underlying structures such as the bones, tendons, nerves or blood vessels. For one of the carpals to be fractured in this manner, the blow would have to be a severe crushing type. A more common injury associated with contusions is involvement of one of the many tendons that cross the wrist. A tenosynovitis may result from a direct blow to the wrist or repeated trauma to this area. Occasionally a nerve compression or vascular injury may develop from repeated trauma about the wrist. Therefore athletic trainers must carefully examine all wrist contusions for associated injuries to underlying structures. Athletes exhibiting sharp localized pain over a bony

Fig. 19-5. Common mechanism of injury to the wrist or hand as athlete breaks a fall with an outstretched arm.

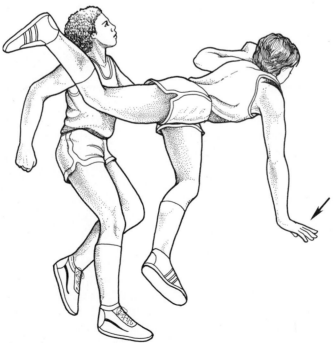

prominence, or pain, tingling, or numbness radiating into the fingers, should be referred to medical assistance.

Strains

Each of the many tendons that cross the wrist may be strained. This is especially true of the wrist flexors and extensors. Strains can result from a violent muscular contraction against resistance, an overstretching such as that associated with hyperflexion or hyperextension, or chronic overuse. These injuries can also be confused with a wrist sprain or carpal fracture. Strains, however, will cause increased pain on active and resistive contraction of the muscle or muscles involved.

The tendon and its synovial sheath may also become inflamed as a result of a strain and progress to a tenosynovitis. As this condition develops the tendon swells and the synovial sheath thickens, causing discomfort and pain as the tendon slides within the tubelike sheath. As this constriction progresses, palpable and audible sensations may be exhibited in the area, such as clicking or grating. Tenosynovitis of the flexor tendons may predispose an athlete to carpal tunnel syndrome. This condition may progress until the tendons are no longer able to move through these tunnels. This condition may also be caused by an active violent contraction, passive stretching, or contusion to the area.

Another condition that can involve the tendinous sheath or synovial joint capsule is a synovial hernia or knotlike mass called a *wrist ganglion,* which occurs most often on the back of the wrist. It is believed that a ganglion of this type results from a defect in the fibrous sheath of a tendon or joint, which permits a portion of the underlying synovium to herniate through it. This herniated sac forms a cystic enlargement that gradually fills with fluid and may become quite large. In athletics, this condition usually follows a strain or sprain of the wrist but can occur without any trauma. A ganglion generally appears as a small nodule over the dorsum of the wrist, but can also occur on the palmar aspect. Its cysticlike mass may vary in consistency from very soft to firm and is generally not painful. A ganglion that is painful or limits motion should be examined by a physician.

Sprains

Many athletic injuries to the wrist are sprains. The most common mechanism of injury is forced hyperextension. Isolated injury to the large and very strong volar ligaments seldom occurs. Instead injuries in this area will involve the volar tendons or bones of the wrist. Forced hyperflexion may injure the weaker dorsal ligaments as well as involve the tendons or bones. Therefore wrist sprains should be approached assuming an associated fracture until proved otherwise. Tenderness over the carpals or styloid processes of the radius or ulna should be referred to a physician for x-ray. If initial radiographs are negative, the athlete should be treated as if there is a sprain. In the presence of persistent pain and swelling lasting for 2 to 3 weeks a second radiograph should be requested.

Dislocations

Because of the strong ligamentous structures about the articulations of the wrist, dislocations are not common injuries and occur far less often than fractures. Dislocations of the radiocarpal, midcarpal or carpometacarpal joints are extremely uncommon in athletic activity, although they may occur as the result of violent trauma and associated fractures. These types of injuries are normally indicated by obvious disability and deformity and are readily recognized.

The most commonly dislocated carpal of the wrist is the lunate. This bone may be displaced by forced hyperextension because of its shape and relationship to the surrounding carpals. Dislocation of the lunate is usually caused by a self-reduced backward dislocation of the carpals and often occurs in two steps. The ligaments of the lunate attach it much more firmly to the distal radius and ulna than are the other carpal bones.

As a result of its shape and this strong attachment, the lunate does not dislocate backward with the wrist after trauma. Instead, ligaments connecting it with adjacent carpals are torn. The second step in the dislocation occurs as a result of spontaneous reduction of the other displaced carpals. When they return to their normal position they push the lunate forward and tend to rotate it around its dorsal ligamentous attachment to the radius. This ligament carries the most important nutrient vessel to the bone. If it is torn as a result of the dislocation, the reduced blood supply may cause progressive degeneration or necrosis *(Kienboch's disease)*. Despite an impaired blood supply, early reduction of a dislocated lunate may prevent necrosis if other nutrient vessels remain uninjured.

Dislocation of the lunate may not be readily recognized. Symptoms usually include tenderness and swelling over the lunate. Palpation may detect the displaced lunate under the flexor tendons. Movements of the wrist are often painful and limited. On making a fist, the knuckle formed by the head of the third metacarpal moves proximally, so that it is on a level with the adjoining knuckles and does not project distally to them as it normally should. This is known as *Murphy's sign*. The medial nerve is normally some distance anterior to the lunate; however, forward displacement of the lunate may compress the carpal tunnel, causing pain and paresthesia in the median nerve distribution of the hand.

Fractures

Fractures about the wrist most commonly result from forced hyperextension such as falling on an outstretched hand. This mechanism transmits the force of the fall, through the capitate, lunate, and navicular bones, to the radius. As previously mentioned, the carpal most often fractured is the navicular. This is a result of its shape and location. The navicular is an oval, elongated bone that extends the most distally of those in the proximal row of carpals. The center portion, or waist, of the navicular is narrowed,

making this area most vulnerable to fracture. During forced hyperextension, the navicular may be impinged between the capitate and radius, resulting in a fracture. Normally there is no displacement of fragments, and such an injury may be erroneously evaluated as a wrist sprain. A fractured navicular will cause pain just distal to the radius, and point tenderness will be elicited during palpation of the anatomic snuffbox. Therefore all wrist injuries exhibiting these symptoms should be referred for radiographic examination. If initial x-ray films are negative, the wrist should be handled as if the athlete has suffered a sprain. The wrist should be radiographed again if pain and disability should persist for 2 weeks because a navicular fracture is notorious for not being readily visible on initial x-ray films. Navicular fractures frequently result in complications, such as nonunion or avascular necrosis *(Preiser's disease)*, because the blood supply to the fracture fragments is not always adequate.

This same mechanism of injury may cause a fracture to the distal end of the radius. This type of fracture will cause tenderness over the lower end of the radius and pain on hand movement. Complete fracture of the distal radius, in which the fragment is displaced dorsally, is known as *Colles' fracture* (Fig. 19-6). With this type of fracture, movement of the hand and fingers is markedly limited or absent. In Colles' fracture a so-called *silver fork deformity* results, in which there is a prominence on the back of the wrist and a lateral or radial displacement or deviation of the hand. Dislocations of the wrist are rare. If a dorsal dislocation does occur, the deformity will resemble a Colles' fracture but will be closer to the hand. The reverse of Colles' fracture, produced by a fall on the back of the hand with the wrist flexed, is called *Smith's fracture* in which the fragment is forwardly displaced. In preadolescent and adolescent athletes, these same mechanisms may cause an epiphyseal displacement rather than a fracture. These are normally more difficult to recognize; therefore young athletes with tenderness around the wrist after trauma to the area should be referred to medical assistance.

ANATOMY OF THE HAND

The hand is an organ capable of a great variety of discrete and complicated movements. These movements, so important in numerous sports and athletic activities, are possible because of the coordinated actions of its many joints and muscles. Remember from Chapter 3 that the metacarpals form the skeleton of the major part of the hand and the phalanges are the bones of the digits. Anatomically, the hand can be divided into the (1) palmar region, (2) dorsal region, and (3) phalanges.

Metacarpals

The metacarpals of the hand are identified by numbers from 1 to 5, beginning on the lateral side with the metacarpal of the thumb. Each metacarpal has a slightly curved shaft and two extremities—(1) a *base,* which articulates proximally with the carpals, and (2) a *head,* which articulates distally with the proximal phalanx in the thumb or one of the digits. The heads of the metacarpals form the knuckles on the back of the hand.

Phalanges

The phalanges form the bony framework of the digits. There are 14 phalanges in each hand: two for the thumb and three for each of the remaining four fingers. The bony anatomy of all five fingers is essentially the same. Starting proximally the phalanges are identified by name or number as the proximal, middle, and distal phalanges, or as the first, second, and third phalanges. They resemble the metacarpals in shape and appearance.

Metacarpophalangeal articulations

The metacarpophalangeal joints are synovial articulations between the head of a metacarpal and the base of a proximal phalanx. With the digits clenched into a fist the metacarpophalan-

geal joint is about 1/2 inch distal to the prominence of the knuckle on the dorsum of the hand. Each joint is maintained by a joint capsule that is thin posteriorly (dorsally) but thickened by a palmar ligament anteriorly and by collateral ligaments laterally. Movements available at these joints include flexion, extension, adduction, abduction, and circumduction. No rotation occurs at these joints. Metacarpophalangeal joint dislocations resulting from athletic activity do occur, particularly in the thumb. In dislocations at these joints the base of the first phalanx will usually pass posteriorly (backward). Small sesamoid bones, which may be mistaken for bone fragments, are sometimes present near the metacarpophalangeal joint of the thumb. Although such bones may be found around the other metacarpophalangeal joints, they are not common.

Interphalangeal articulations

The interphalangeal joints are similar in structure to metacarpophalangeal joints. Both are classified as diarthrotic (synovial) joints and both have a thin capsule and a pair of strong collateral ligaments that pass around onto the palmar aspect to fuse with the sides of the *palmar (volar) plate.* This plate is a fibrocartilaginous structure that covers the palmar aspect of the metacarpophalangeal and proximal interphalangeal joints. Each palmar plate has a distal fibrous portion and a proximal membranous portion that shortens during digital flexion. In prolonged flexion of a finger, this proximal membranous portion can passively shorten by fibrosis, resulting in stiffness and a limiting of complete extension. Interphalangeal articulations join the head of one phalanx and the base of the more distal one. They do not permit abduction or adduction, only flexion and extension.

Of the two palmar skin creases between the first and second phalanges, the proximal crease identifies the joint. The crease between the second and third phalanges marks the distal joint. The skin creases of the proximal interphalangeal joints are closely bound to the underlying flexor sheaths. Even superficial cuts in these proximal creases can cause serious infections. Such injuries, although they appear to be minor, should be monitored very carefully for signs of developing infection.

Palmar region

The palmar region of the hand is quadrilateral in shape and contains the soft tissues, which are located anteriorly to the metacarpals. A triangular "hollow" central portion of this region is bounded on the lateral or radial side by the ***thenar eminence*** and on the medial or ulnar side by the ***hypothenar eminence***. The thenar eminence at the base of the thumb contains the short intrinsic muscles of the hand involved in moving the thumb, whereas the hypothenar eminence consists of muscles involved in moving the little finger. The two eminences almost approximate each other proximally as they approach the wrist. The skin of the palm is thick and coarse, especially over the heads of the metacarpals. It is firmly bound to the underlying palmar aponeurosis and is well supplied with sweat glands. No hairs or sebaceous glands are present in the skin of the palm. In most persons two transverse skin creases, proximal and distal, are present in the palm. Movements of the index finger are accommodated by the proximal crease, whereas the distal crease permits movements of the medial

three digits and serves as a surface landmark for the heads of the third, fourth, and fifth metacarpals.

Dorsal region

The dorsal region of the hand, in contrast with the palmar surface, is covered with loose skin containing numerous sweat and sebaceous glands. The skin has a fine texture and in men contains a variable number of short but visible hairs. The extensor tendons are both visible and palpable over the dorsum of the hand. They are united by oblique bands and form a thin aponeurotic sheet that attaches to the sides of the second and fifth metacarpal bones. The dorsal subcutaneous space is an extensive area of loose areolar tissue just below the skin over the dorsum of the hand. It permits dramatic swelling to occur over the back of the hand during infection or after trauma.

Fingers

The skin of the flexor surface of all the digits is thick, only slightly mobile, and devoid of hair. Some subcutaneous fat is present. Over the dorsum of the digits the skin is thinner and more mobile. Subcutaneous fat is extremely limited or absent. Transverse flexor skin creases approximate the positions of the underlying joints. The skin creases are closely bound to the underly-

Fig. 19-6. Colles' fracture of the wrist.

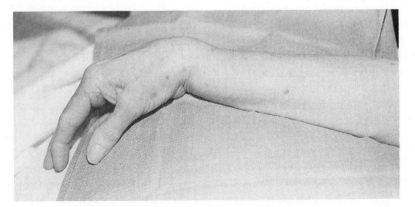

ing flexor tendon sheaths, and any penetrating wound at the crease is likely to penetrate the synovial sheath beneath it.

Sensory innervation of the hand

The sensory innervation of the hand involves the median, ulnar, and radial nerves. Sensory branches of the median nerve supply the median (central) palmar area and the palmar surfaces of the lateral three and one-half fingers. It also supplies the skin over the dorsum (top) of the distal two phalanges of the thumb, index, and middle fingers. The ulnar nerve supplies sensory nerves to the palmar and dorsal surfaces of the medial third of the hand and to both surfaces of the little finger and half of the ring finger. The radial nerve transmits sensory impulses from the thenar eminence and from the lateral two thirds of the dorsum of the proximal hand and dorsal aspects of the proximal phalanges of the thumb, index, middle, and one half of the ring finger. It is important to remember the peripheral nerve supply of the hand when performing a sensory neurologic evaluation.

Motor innervation of the hand

Motor control of the intrinsic hand muscles is furnished by the ulnar and median nerves. However, since these intrinsic muscles are not the sole manipulators of the hand, the radial nerve, which supplies motor control to a number of important extrinsic muscles, must also be considered when discussing control of voluntary hand movements.

The ulnar nerve supplies motor control to those muscles that abduct and adduct (spread and approximate) the fingers, whereas functioning of the median nerve is required to approximate successively the tip of the thumb to the tips of the fingers. Damage to the radial nerve results in *wristdrop,* which is caused by paralysis of the wrist extensor muscles.

INJURIES TO THE HAND

There are few sports in which the hands are not used in some manner. An athlete's hands are constantly exposed to various types of forced movements and direct trauma. As a result, a wide variety of athletic injuries to the hands can occur. Many injuries to the hands are relatively minor and are never reported to the athletic trainer. In addition, there is a tendency by many athletes to underestimate or minimize injuries to this area of the body. Injuries to the hands can develop into long-term impairment and permanent disability if not recognized and cared for properly. Therefore it is important for athletic trainers to be aware of signs and symptoms associated with the various injuries to the hand to avoid possible complications.

Contusions and abrasions

These types of injuries are normally of little consequence; however, whenever the skin is broken about the hand, infection becomes a concern. All abrasions must be thoroughly cleaned and properly cared for in an attempt to prevent contamination and subsequent infection. Contusion injuries resulting in hematoma formation about the hand are uncommon. The firmly fixed skin on the palmar surface allows little room for the pooling of blood. The loose mobile skin on the dorsum of the hand, however, permits very marked swelling (Fig. 19-7), even if the initial trauma or focus of infection is located on the palm of the hand or on the fingers. This type of dorsal hand swelling, which may be marked and spectacular in appearance soon after an injury, normally subsides quickly and seldom develops into a fixed or pooled hematoma. On the palmar surface, the fleshy thenar and hypothenar eminences can be contused because of some type of direct blow. These injuries can be quite bothersome to an athlete, as swelling in the confined area can produce tightness and pain, which limits hand function. Occasionally subcutaneous structures may be compressed and damaged in conjunction with contusing trauma. A careful evaluation of contused or abraded areas can generally determine if there is any associated involvement of underlying structures.

Direct trauma to the tips of the fingers or fingernails can cause blood to accumulate under the nail *(subungual hematoma)*. As the blood pools under the fingernail, a painful, throbbing pressure develops that is usually relieved by drilling a hole in the nail and releasing the blood. Every athletic trainer has a favorite method of drilling a hole in the fingernail to relieve a subungual hematoma. The most common methods involve use of a nail drill designed for that purpose, drilling with a sharp-pointed scapel blade, or applying a red-hot paper clip to the nail.

Lacerations and punctures

Although open wounds such as lacerations or punctures are generally not serious, the potential for significant and serious consequences exists, and such wounds should never be taken lightly. An athlete wearing a ring during activity is at risk in the event of localized finger trauma. Fig. 19-8 shows a finger injury caused by wearing a ring. Open wounds may damage subcutaneous structures such as tendons or nerves, which are often close to the surface. Therefore, following

Fig. 19-7. Marked swelling of the dorsal surface of the hand following trauma.

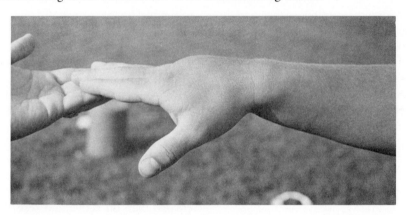

Fig. 19-8. Example of a "ring injury."
(Courtesy Gregg Voigt, A.T.,C., Dakota Wesleyan University.)

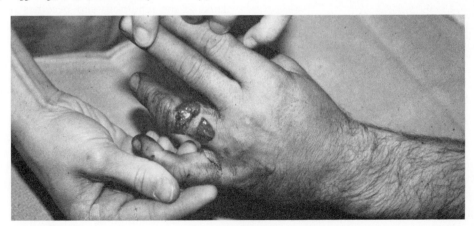

athletic injuries of this nature, a complete and careful evaluation of hand and finger function should be performed.

Infections

Another important consideration of all open injuries about the hand is infection, because this too may have serious consequences. Infection about the hand can impair performance and develop into permanent disability. Therefore all open injuries about the hands must be thoroughly cleaned, debrided, and protected from further injury and contamination in an attempt to avoid infections. In addition, athletes should be instructed to report any symptoms that may indicate a developing infection such as an increase in aching, soreness, or throbbing in the hand, the presence of pus, or an increase in body temperature.

A *felon,* or *whitlow,* is an extremely painful infection located in the soft tissues surrounding the terminal phalanx of a finger. Accumulation of pus or fluid in the confined tissue spaces of the fingertip produces marked pressure that can shut off the blood supply and cause early necro-sis of bone. Suppurative felons are common and dangerous and should always be referred to a physician for treatment and drainage.

Paronychia is an infection involving the subepithelial folds of tissue surrounding the fingernail. It can be acute or chronic and is usually caused by staphylococci. The infection is frequently introduced as a result of picking at a hangnail or rough manicuring. In the early stages there is pain, redness, and swelling of the tissues at the side of the nail (Fig. 19-9). If incised and drained early, no ill effects result. However, if neglected the infection may spread along the sides and base of the nail, forming what is called a "run around." Occasionally a subungual abscess can result.

Strains

Injuries involving the vast complex of tendons in the hand are not uncommon in athletics and are often missed on examination. The most common cause of these strains is overstretching or forcing the musculotendinous unit beyond its normal range of motion. The long flexor and extensor tendons are those most often strained. Symptomatically, these tendinous strains will present tenderness at the site of injury and increased pain on active and resistive contraction or passive stretching of the musculotendinous unit. Occasionally there will be a tendon rupture or avulsion of the tendinous attachment to the bone. This occurs most often at the distal phalanx, as the tendinous slip becomes narrow at the point of attachment. The extensor tendon may be injured by a blow to the tip of finger, forcing the distal interphalangeal joint into flexion and rupturing or partially rupturing the extensor tendon slip at the point of its insertion into the base of the terminal phalanx. This injury, commonly called a *mallet finger,* is characterized by the athlete being unable to extend the distal phalanx. The distal attachment of the flexor digitorum profundus muscle can also be ruptured or avulsed. This type of injury occurs more often in a contact sport in which an actively flexed finger is violently extended. If the extend-

Fig. 19-9. Infection involving the subepithelial folds of tissue around a thumbnail (paronychia).

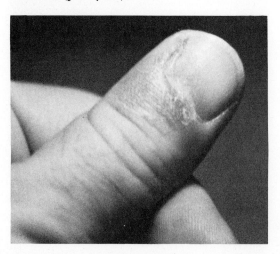

ing force is too great, the flexor digitorum profundus may be avulsed from its insertion into the distal phalanx. This injury is characterized by pain, swelling, and tenderness at the distal interphalangeal joint as well as the inability of the athlete to actively flex at this joint while the proximal and middle finger joints are held straight.

Another tendon injury that athletic trainers should be familiar with involves the central slip of the extensor tendon. This tendon can be avulsed from its insertion in the dorsal lip of the middle phalanx by a severe flexion force or crushed by a direct blow to the proximal interphalangeal (PIP) joint. Initially the athlete may be able to extend the PIP joint and straighten this finger. However, this extension is very weak when tested against resistance. Without proper recognition and adequate care, the soft tissues surrounding the joint or the central slip itself begin to stretch, and the finger may gradually stiffen in a flexed position. Finally, like a button going through a buttonhole, the PIP joint will extrude through the defect in the tendon, forming the *boutonnière deformity* (Fig. 19-10). This classic deformity is characterized by hyperextension of the metacarpophalangeal joint, flexion of the proximal interphalangeal joint, and hyperextension of the distal interphalangeal joint.

Fig. 19-10. Boutonnière deformity of a finger. (Courtesy Bruce Johnson, A.T.,C., Orthopedic Clinic, Grand Forks, N.D.)

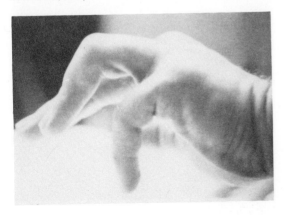

The tendon of the extensor pollicis longus muscle inserts into the terminal phalanx of the thumb. This muscle, which originates from the ulna and interosseus membrane, not only extends the terminal phalanx of the thumb but also assists in extending the hand at the wrist. It is this tendon that is most often ruptured in a Colles' type fracture. The rupture may occur at the time of the fracture or 6 to 7 weeks after the injury. Anytime an athlete cannot fully and strongly flex and extend at each joint of the finger, tendon rupture should be suspected and the athlete referred to a physician.

Strains may occur to the intrinsic muscles of the hand because of excessive overuse. This happens more often in sports requiring constant gripping such as gymnastics or rowing. Symptomatically, these injuries present cramping and fatigue of the involved muscles and an increase in pain against resistive movements. Symptoms normally subside when activity is reduced or discontinued.

Sprains

Injuries involving the ligaments or ligamentous capsules surrounding the various joints of the hand are very common in athletic activity. This is especially true of the interphalangeal joints and the metacarpophalangeal joint of the thumb. Sprains are normally the result of forced motion at a joint that stresses the supporting ligaments, causing varying degrees of damage. This forced motion is usually lateral motion, which stresses the collateral ligaments, or hyperextension, which stresses the anterior capsule. If this displacing force is strong enough or continuous, the joint will sublux (dislocate).

Symptomatically, sprains about the hand or digits will present tenderness at the site of injury and an increase in pain on reproduction of the stress that caused the injury. In addition, there are normally varying amounts of swelling, stiffness, and soreness surrounding the articulation that may take months to resolve. Depending on the amount of ligamentous damage, there may be varying amounts of instability associated with sprain injuries. If instability is recognized, the athlete should be referred to medical assistance.

The most common sprain of the hand is to the proximal interphalangeal joints. When a finger is pulled or forced to the side, the supporting collateral ligaments or volar plate may be injured. This type of injury will exhibit tenderness over the collateral ligament involved, rapid swelling, and pain on passive stressing. Instability will be present on severe sprains. Inadequate evaluation and treatment of these injuries may lead to prolonged swelling, stiffness, pain, and loss of motion.

A sprain of the ulnar collateral ligament of the metacarpophalangeal joint of the thumb is called a *gamekeeper's thumb.* This commonly sprained ligament provides the stability necessary for normal grip and pinch. This type of injury is often overlooked or dismissed as a sprained thumb. If the ulnar collateral ligament is torn and inadequately cared for, continued instability, weakness of pinch, and recurrent effusion will probably occur. Characteristically this injury exhibits local tenderness over the ligament, joint effusion, and increased pain on attempted abduction of the thumb. Instability will be present if the ligament is torn (Fig. 19-11).

Dislocations

The same mechanisms causing sprains may result in dislocations of the many joints of the hand. Dislocations involving the fingers occur more commonly than those in any other area of the body (Fig. 19-12). These dislocations may remain displaced or may reduce spontaneously and appear as sprains on assessment. Finger dislocations are often readily reduced by the player, coach, or athletic trainer. It is a good practice to refer all athletes with dislocations, no matter how minor the injury may seem, to medical assistance. Radiographic studies may be necessary to evaluate the presence of gross instability, ligament avulsion, or articular fracture. All too often athletes suffering dislocated fingers are treated casually and never seen by a physician. Inadequate treatment can lead to permanent instability and deformity of the joint.

Complete dislocations of the metacarpophalangeal joint of the thumb presents another problem in that the flexor tendons may loop around the metacarpal head, making closed reduction impossible. Dislocation of the thumb most often results from a fall that produces

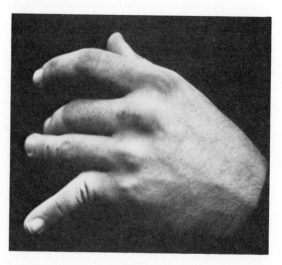

Fig. 19-12. Finger dislocation.
(Courtesy A.G. Edwards, A.T.,C., University of Nevada–Las Vegas)

Fig. 19-11. Torn ulnar collateral ligament of the metacarpophalangeal joint of the thumb. Note abnormal abduction of the joint.

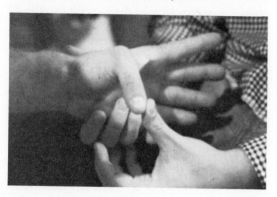

forceful hyperextension of the thumb on an extended hand. The usual deformity permits the phalanx to pass backward and rest upon the dorsal aspect of the thumb metacarpal. Dislocated thumbs should be reduced by a physician.

Fractures

Fractures of the hand frequently occur in athletics and result from the same mechanisms of injury previously described. Because these fractures involve small bones, they are sometimes felt to be minor injuries and thus treated casually. However, finger stiffness, malunion, and functional disability may be disturbing consequences of hand fractures. Fractures of the metacarpals, which are more common than phalangeal fractures, usually result from a direct blow to the area or to the metacarpal head, which transmits the force down the shaft of the bone. In metacarpal fractures exclusive of the thumb, the typical deformity is characterized by bowing of the fragments and shortening of the bone. The result is an inverted V-type deformity with a dorsal projection at the fracture site and a palmar or volar displacement of the metacarpal head (Fig. 19-13). A fracture of the proximal end (base) of the first metacarpal is often complicated by an associated subluxation of the carpometacarpal joint of the thumb *(Bennett fracture)*.

Fractures of the proximal and middle phalanges can result from a direct blow or the same mechanisms that cause dislocations, that is, forced lateral motion or hyperextension. A fracture of the shaft of a proximal phalanx, which is more commonly fractured than the other two phalanges, may result in a V-shaped deformity or angulation (Fig. 19-14). A fracture at the base of a proximal phalanx may be a combination fracture-dislocation. The distal phalanx is fractured most often by a crushing-type of mechanism.

Fig. 19-13. Midshaft fracture of a metacarpal with deformity.
(From Flatt, A.E.: Care of minor injuries, ed. 4, St. Louis, 1979, The C.V. Mosby Co.)

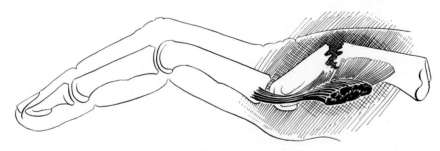

Fig. 19-14. Fracture of proximal phalanx with deformity.
(From Flatt, A.E.: Care of minor injuries, ed. 4, St. Louis, 1979, The C.V. Mosby Co.)

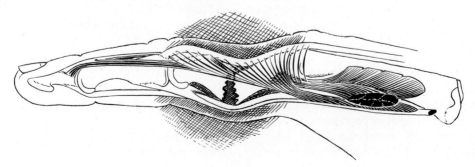

Because of the subcutaneous nature of the long bones of the hand, athletic trainers should be able to readily recognize the presence of a fracture. Remember, it is a good practice to approach significant hand injuries as if there is a fracture until proved otherwise. Symptomatically, fractures will present tenderness at the site of injury, with pain elicited at the fracture site during longitudinal or transverse stress. In addition, deformity, crepitation, and a false joint may be present. All suspected fractures should be examined by a physician.

ATHLETIC INJURY ASSESSMENT PROCESS

The hands and wrists are exceedingly vulnerable to athletic injuries. There are few sports in which the fingers, hands, and wrists are not used in some manner, thereby exposing them to a wide variety of possible injuries. Many of these injuries are relatively minor and do not require extensive treatment; unfortunately, too many potentially serious injuries to the hands, wrists, and especially the fingers are regarded as insignificant and neglected by the athlete, coach or athletic trainer. It must also be remembered that even seemingly minor injuries can be extremely disabling to certain athletes, depending on their sport. For example, finger injuries on the throwing hand of a pitcher can prevent the athlete from competing, whereas such an injury may be only a minor annoyance to athletes in other sports. Injuries to the hand and wrist can develop into long-term impairment and permanent disability or disfigurement. The key to proper care of injuries to this area of the body is an early, accurate assessment followed by proper care and referral as indicated.

Secondary survey

Evaluation procedures used during the assessment of hand and wrist injuries are concerned with recognizing an injury that has the potential to result in dysfunction or permanent deformity. Athletic trainers must maintain a high level of suspicion during the assessment process so an injury is not neglected or dismissed as minor when in fact a more serious injury is involved. The significant role of the intricate movements performed by the hands and wrists in regular daily functions as well as in many athletic activities makes the accurate evaluation of these injuries extremely important. Therefore careful attention must be exercised by the athletic trainer to ensure that a proper and thorough evaluation is performed.

Circulatory and neurologic assessment

An important consideration that has been mentioned throughout this unit is the value of assessing circulation and neurologic involvement with any significant injury involving the upper extremities. These evaluations are normally performed about the wrist, hand, and fingers and must be considered with any upper extremity injury. Circulation can be evaluated by feeling for a radial or ulnar pulse. The nail beds can also be temporarily compressed to check the return of normal color. To evaluate sensations, it is important to remember the sensory distribution of each nerve. The radial nerve supplies sensation mainly to the radial side of the dorsum of the hand, and the median nerve supplies sensation to the radial side of the palm and fingers. The ulnar nerve supplies sensation mainly to the ulnar side of the hand, little finger, and half of the ring finger. To evaluate motor function, it is again important to remember nerve distribution. The radial nerve supplies motor function to the extrinsic wrist and finger extensors. The median nerve supplies the thenar muscles; its function is evaluated by resisting opposition or abduction of the thumb. The ulnar nerve provides motor supply to most of the intrinsic muscles of the hand, with the exception of the thenar muscles. Its function is easily evaluated by resisting finger abduction. Once the presence of adequate circulation and nerve functions has been established, the athletic injury assessment process can continue.

Most athletic injuries to the hand and wrist result from acute trauma or direct impact. This can occur during any athletic activity as an athlete hits another athlete or object or falls on an outstretched hand. The instinctive reaction to any fall is to thrust out the hand in an attempt to break the fall. When this occurs, the outstretched hand may receive the entire stress or force of the fall. This can result in injury to the hand or wrist and can transmit injurious forces throughout the upper extremity, as described in the previous two chapters. An accurate assessment of hand and wrist injuries includes a detailed history of the causative trauma accompanied by systematic physical examination.

History

Because most athletic injuries to the hand and wrist result from direct trauma, the initial history procedures should be concerned with the primary complaint and mechanisms of injury. Question the athlete to get a detailed description of how the injury occurred. Did the athlete fall and land on the hand? If so, what was the position of the wrist and fingers at the time of impact? Was the wrist forced into flexion or extension? Were the fingers extended or flexed into a fist? Was there a direct blow delivered to the hand? If so, exactly where on the hand and by what? Attempt to determine the severity of the blow or force. Were the fingers forced through an excessive range of motion or in an abnormal direction? Was there a blow delivered to the tip of a finger? Occasionally injuries to the hand or wrist result from overuse or repetitive trauma. In other instances an athlete will consider the injury trivial and not report it for a period of time or until it begins to impair function. When these situations occur, inquire about the onset of symptoms. Attempt to find out what happened and how the symptoms have progressed since the athlete first noticed the injury. The more information gained concerning the mechanisms of injury, the better you can assess the nature and determine those structures that may be involved.

Instruct the athlete to describe the symptoms associated with the injury. Where exactly are the painful or tender areas? Pain is not referred appreciably from tissues lying at the distal extent of a limb; therefore the tenderness is usually felt exactly at the site of the lesion. Ask the athlete to locate and describe the pain. Is there pain present only during movement of the fingers, thumb, or wrist? If so, ask the athlete to demonstrate these movements. The athlete should also be asked about any other sensations associated with the injury. Did he or she feel anything at the time of the injury, such as a popping or snapping sensation? Does the athlete experience any crepitation? The athlete's descriptions of any sensations and impressions concerning the injury should never be ignored, as they often yield valuable information.

Question the athlete carefully concerning any previous injuries to the hand or wrist in an attempt to determine if the current complaint is an aggravation or recurrence of a previous injury. If the area has been injured before, obtain as much information as possible concerning the circumstances surrounding previous injuries. Are symptoms of the current injury similar to those of any previous injuries? Had symptoms completely subsided and full function been restored before the onset of the present injury? The more information gained concerning previous injuries, the better you can evaluate the nature and severity of the current complaint.

Observation

Observations concerning hand and wrist injuries should commence with looking for obvious deformity. This area of the body is primarily subcutaneous, which very often allows for the visual recognition of any irregularities such as those associated with an unreduced dislocation or angulated fracture. Note the contours of the hand and wrist. Is there any obvious deformity? If so, note the exact location of the deformity and plan your strategies for caring for the injury.

Notice the positioning and functioning of the injured hand as you talk with the athlete. Is the athlete holding or supporting the hand in such a manner as to protect the area and guard against any movements? If so, note the position of the wrist, hand, fingers, and thumb. Do they all appear to be held in a normal position of function, that is, slight extension or dorsiflexion of the wrist, all joints of the fingers partially flexed and the thumb lying parallel to the forearm? Are all fingers parallel to each other, or is one finger held in an abnormal position? Does the hand appear to be hanging limp? Is the athlete voluntarily moving the wrist, thumb, and fingers? If so, do the movements appear to be normal and performed freely, or unnatural and guarded? Is there any indication of pain on movement?

Carefully inspect the injured hand for signs of trauma which can indicate what type of force has been applied and assist in establishing or confirming the mechanism of injury. Is there any bleeding? Since this area is mainly subcutaneous, fractures and dislocations may split the skin, especially on the volar surface (Fig. 19-15). Because this area commonly is subjected to direct impact, lacerations, abrasions and contusions are common. Injuries involving the fingertips may cause tearing of the fingernail or blood pooling under the nail *(subungual hematoma)*.

In the absence of obvious deformity, inspect and compare the injured hand or wrist to the uninjured side to note any differences in symmetry. Do the metacarpophalangeal joints (knuckles) appear to line up normally and symmetrically on both hands? Is there an obvious difference between corresponding knuckles? Is there any swelling? If so, note exactly where the swelling is located. As previously explained, the loose skin over the back of the hand allows this area to swell quickly. Blood accumulated in the dorsum of the hand also readily infiltrates out of the area; thus hematoma formation is not common. On the palmar surface of the hand there is not much room for the accumulation of fluid, therefore any bleeding into the front of the hand readily shows up as an ecchymosis. Periarticular swelling around the joints of the fingers can impair function and take months to be absorbed. It may never completely disappear.

Palpation

In the absence of obvious deformity, the assessment of injuries to the hand and wrist should include palpation techniques. The subcutaneous nature of this area makes underlying structures readily accessible to palpation. Athletic trainers should always approach hand and wrist injuries as if there is a fracture until indicated otherwise.

Fig. 19-15. Skin is split on the volar surface of a finger after a proximal interphalangeal joint dislocation.
(Courtesy A.G. Edwards, A.T.,C., University of Nevada–Las Vegas)

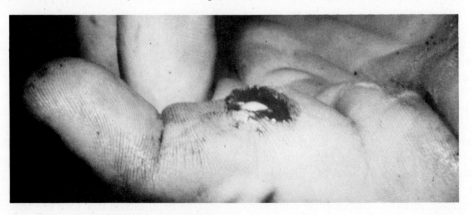

Frequently, fractures can be recognized by careful palpation and gentle manipulation described later in this chapter. Gently palpate those areas suspected of being injured to accurately locate such physical signs as tenderness, deformity, swelling, or crepitation. Correlate this information with the underlying anatomy. Procedures used to palpate the various anatomic structures of the hand and wrist are discussed briefly, as are the common athletic injuries that may be indicated by positive signs. Specific structures to be palpated are determined by the information gained up to this point during the assessment process.

The radial and ulnar styloid processes are good points of reference to begin palpating the wrist. Place your thumb on one of these processes and your index finger on the other (Fig. 19-16). Note that the radial styloid process is located more distally than the ulnar. The two rows of small carpal bones lie just distal to these points of reference. With careful palpation techniques, athletic trainers can palpate each of the carpals individually. However, in most athletic injuries involving the wrist, it is not necessary to be able

to distinguish by touch each carpal bone. When evaluating wrist injuries, signs and symptoms that indicate the athlete should be referred to medical assistance include point tenderness over a carpal bone, pain on forced motion, and local swelling. These signs and symptoms can be confusing because they may indicate a sprain, strain, fracture, or dislocation.

Athletic trainers should be able to locate and palpate the two primary carpals that articulate with the radius and are the most commonly injured, the navicular and the lunate. The navicular, which is the carpal most frequently fractured, is situated just distal to the radial styloid process. When the wrist is ulnarly deviated, this bone will slide out from beneath the radial styloid, making it easily palpable. The navicular also forms the floor of the anatomic snuffbox and can be felt by pressing into this depression during ulnar deviation (Fig. 19-17). Any time point tenderness is elicited during palpation of the navicular, the athlete should be referred to a physician. The lunate, which is the carpal most frequently dislocated, lies next to the navicular and distal to the radius. It can be palpated just

Fig. 19-16. Palpating the radial and ulnar styloid processes. Note the radial styloid is more distal.

Fig. 19-17. Palpating the navicular bone during ulnar deviation.

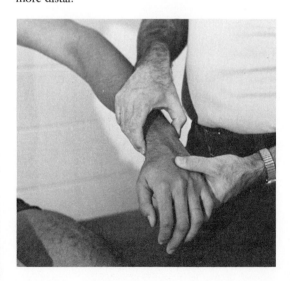

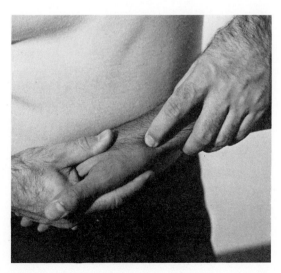

distal to the radial tubercle, which is the bony prominence lying approximately one third of the way across the dorsum of the wrist from the radial styloid process. Palpating just distal to the radial tubercle, a slight depression can be felt. Ask the athlete to flex his or her wrist and feel the lunate as it becomes more prominent on sliding out from under the radius (Fig. 19-18).

The full length of the metacarpals can be palpated because these bones are mainly subcutaneous, especially on the dorsum of the hand. Gently palpate from the base of each of these bones to their distal ends or heads (Fig. 19-19). Note the areas of pain. Point tenderness along the shaft of one of these bones suggests a possible fracture. Tenderness expressed around the articulations suggests a possible sprain. Additional stress maneuvers discussed later will assist in differentiating these symptoms.

Each of the phalanges can also be palpated individuallly and along their entire length. Gently palpate each digit, including the shaft of the phalanges, the metacarpophalangeal joints, the proximal interphalangeal joints, and the distal interphalangeal joints. Note areas of tenderness, swelling, deformity, or crepitation. Are physical defects felt along the shaft of one of the phalanges or about an articulation? Additional stress procedures may be indicated to complete the assessment.

Palpating soft tissues about the wrist and hand is generally not as extensive as in other areas of the body. The numerous tiny ligaments surrounding the various joints are palpated in conjunction with the bony anatomy. The intrinsic muscles are for the most part indistinguishable from each other through palpation techniques. These muscles and the structures within the palm are palpated as a group in an attempt to localize the injured area. The extrinsic muscles of the hand are tendons of attachment by the time they cross the wrist. Each of these tendons can be palpated should they be suspected of being injured. These tendons become more pronounced and easier to palpate during active and resistive movements of the hand and digits. To palpate individual tendons about the hand and wrist, review the location of the muscle and the action each performs.

Fig. 19-18. Palpating the lunate bone during wrist flexion.

Fig. 19-19. Palpating the second metacarpal bone.

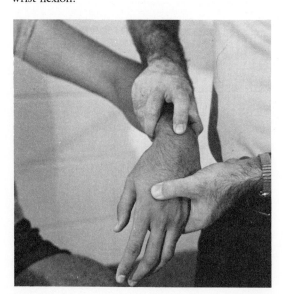

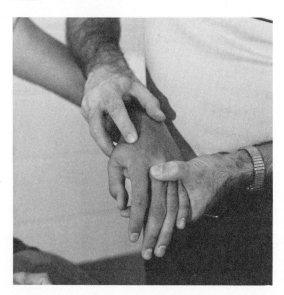

Stress

Stress procedures are often used to facilitate the assessment of athletic injuries of the wrist and hand. Because of the delicate and intricate makeup of this area of the body, various types of stress techniques are usually necessary to complete the assessment process. These techniques are used to apply stress to various structures in and around the injury site in an attempt to implicate or rule out involvement of specific anatomic structures. Remember, these stressful procedures should be performed gently to begin with so as not to cause additional trauma or unnecessary pain.

Active movements. Active movements are performed first to evaluate the range of motion as well as to begin assessing the integrity of specific contractile units. These movements can be performed with the athlete sitting, standing, or supine. Instruct the athlete to execute each movement through as great a range of motion as possible and to express any sensations or symptoms that are experienced. It is very helpful to have the athlete perform each movement on both sides simultaneously for a bilateral comparison.

To evaluate the active range of motion available at the wrist, instruct the athlete to flex and extend as well as radially and ulnarly deviate as far as possible. Normally a person can flex (palmar flexion) approximately 80° and extend (dorsiflexion) approximately 70° (Fig. 19-20, *A*). An athlete can normally deviate the wrist farther toward the ulnar side than the radial because the ulna does not extend distally as far as the radius

and does not articulate directly with the carpals. Normally a person can ulnar deviate approximately 30°, whereas radial deviation is limited to about 20° (Fig. 19-20, *B*).

The active range of finger motion is usually evaluated en masse, that is, each finger and all joints collectively in continuous motion. For example, ask the injured athlete to make a tight fist and then straighten the fingers. Notice whether each digit is able to move easily through a complete range of motion at each joint. If one of the fingers does not appear to move through a complete range of motion, that digit can be evaluated separately. Particular attention must be paid to the distal phalanx where the narrow flexor and extensor tendons insert. Make sure the athlete can actively and strongly flex and extend the distal phalanx. Abduction and adduction can be evaluated by instructing the athlete to spread his or her fingers apart and then bring them back together again. Observe if the fingers move consistently in comparison to the uninjured hand. Each of the digits and each motion of the finger can be evaluated separately if necessary. Refer to Fig. 19-21 for a description of the range of motion for the fingers.

The active range of motion for the thumb consists of flexion and extension, abduction and adduction, and opposition. Instruct the athlete to perform each of these motions and observe the movement. Refer to Fig. 19-22 for a description of the range of motion for the thumb.

Resistive movements. After evaluating the active range of motion, apply resistance against

Fig. 19-20. Range of motion of the wrist. **A,** Flexion and extension. *Flexion* (palmar flexion): zero to ±80 degrees. *Extension* (dorsiflexion): zero to ±70 degrees. **B,** Radial and ulnar deviation. *Radial deviation:* zero to 20 degrees. *Ulnar deviation:* zero to 30 degrees. Ulnar deviation is usually measured with the wrist in pronation. When measured in supination, ulnar deviation will be somewhat increased.
(From Malasanos, L., et al.: Health assessment, ed. 2, St. Louis, 1981, The C.V. Mosby Co.)

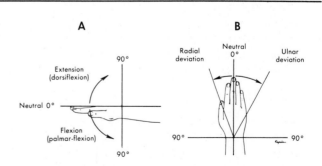

these same movements to further assess the integrity of the contractile units. Manual resistance against each of these motions can assist in accurately identifying specific painful areas and in comparing muscular strengths between extremities. Remember, various muscles can enter into different actions about the wrist and hand, which can make it difficult to evaluate each muscle separately.

To apply resistance against wrist flexion, stabilize the athlete's forearm with one hand and apply resistance to movement against the palm of the athlete's hand with your other hand (Fig. 19-23, *A*). Instruct the athlete to keep the muscles of the thumb and fingers relaxed to ensure they do not assist wrist flexion. To evaluate wrist extension, apply resistance against the dorsum of the athlete's hand (Fig. 19-23, *B*). Again, the muscles of the thumb and fingers should remain relaxed. It is not necessary to resist radial and ulnar deviation because these muscles are evaluated during flexion or extension. However, spe-

---

Fig. 19-21. Range of motion of the fingers. **A,** Flexion. *1,* This motion can be estimated in degrees or in centimeters. Flexion is a natural motion in all joints of the fingers. *2,* Composition motion of flexion. This motion can be estimated by a ruler as the distance from the tip of the finger (indicate midpoint of pad and nail edge) to the distal palmar crease *(left)* (this measures flexion of the middle and distal joints) and the proximal palmar crease *(right)* (this measures the distal, middle, and proximal joints of the fingers).
B, Extension, abduction, and adduction. *1,* Extension and hyperextension. Extension is a natural motion at the metacarpophalangeal joint, but an unnatural one in the proximal interphalangeal joint and in the distal interphalangeal joint. *2,* Abduction and adduction. These motions take place in the plane of the palm away from and to the long or middle finger of the hand. This can be indicated in centimeters or inches. The spread of fingers can be measured from the tip of the index finger to the tip of the little finger *(right).* Individual fingers spread from tip to tip of indicated fingers *(left).*
(From Malasanos, L., et al.: Health assessment, ed. 2, St. Louis, 1981, The C.V. Mosby Co.)

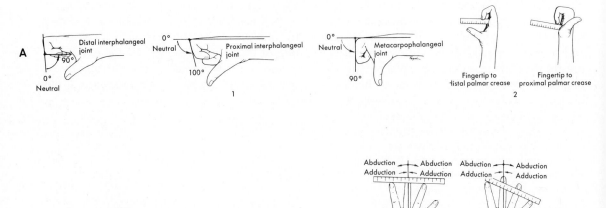

cific muscles may be isolated and evaluated by adding radial or ulnar deviation to the resistance sequence. For example, to specifically test the flexor carpi radialis muscle, apply resistance in the direction of wrist flexion and radial deviation.

Finger flexion is often resisted as a functional unit. Instruct the athlete to flex all fingers into a fist as you curl and lock your fingers into his or hers and attempt to pull the fingers into extension (Fig. 19-24). Can the athlete resist your at-tempt to straighten the fingers? Each joint can also be resisted separately. The motion at the metacarpophalangeal joints is resisted by having the athlete flex these joints while keeping the interphalangeal joints extended as resistance is applied to the proximal row of phalanges (Fig. 19-25). Resistance can also be applied to each finger if strength appears to be unequal. Flexion of the proximal interphalangeal joints can be re-sisted by stabilizing the proximal phalanges and instructing the athlete to flex these joints while

Fig. 19-22. Range of motion of the thumb. **A,** Abduction. *1,* Zero starting position: the extended thumb alongside the index finger, which is in line with the radius. *Abduction* is the angle created between the metacarpal bones of the thumb and index finger. This motion may take place in two planes. *2,* Abduction parallel to the plane of the palm (extension). **B,** Flexion. *1,* Zero starting position: the extended thumb. *2,* Flexion of the interphalangeal joint: zero to ±80 degrees. *3,* Flexion of the metacarpophalangeal joint: zero to ±50 degrees. *4,* Flexion of the carpometacarpal joint: zero to ±15 degrees. **C,** Opposition. Zero starting position *(far left):* the extended thumb in line with the index fingers. *Opposition* is a composite motion consisting of three elements: *1,* abduction, *2,* rotation, and *3,* flexion. This motion is usually considered complete when the tip, or pulp, of the thumb touches the tip of the fifth finger. Some surgeons, however, consider the arc of opposition complete when the tip of the thumb touches the base of the fifth finger. Both methods are illustrated. (From Malasanos, L., et al.: Health assessment, ed. 2, St. Louis, 1981, The C.V. Mosby Co.)

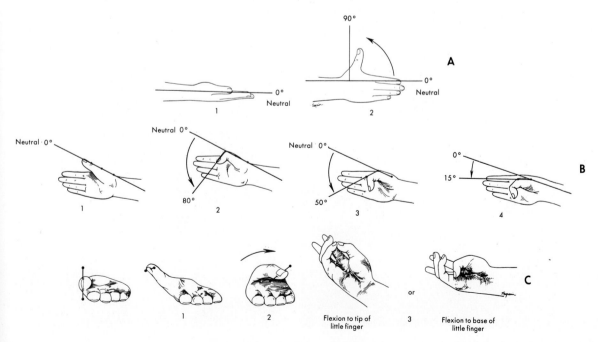

Fig. 19-23. Applying manual resistance against wrist motion: **A,** flexion and **B,** extension.

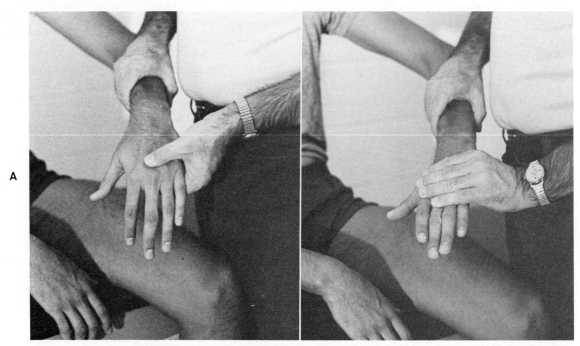

A   B

Fig. 19-24. Applying manual resistance against flexion of the fingers as a functional unit.

Fig. 19-25. Applying manual resistance against flexion of the metacarpophalangeal joints.

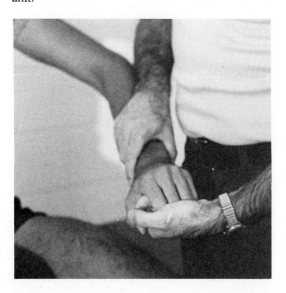

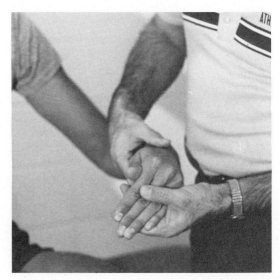

resistance is applied to the middle phalanges. The distal interphalangeal joints should remain extended. Flexion of the distal interphalangeal joints can be resisted by stabilizing the middle phalanges and asking the athlete to flex the tips of the fingers while resistance is applied to the distal phalanges. It may be easier to perform these last two resistive procedures on the fingers individually (Fig. 19-26).

The muscles involved with finger extension can be resisted in the same manner as the flexors, that is, all at one time, each separate joint or each individual finger. A quick and easy method to resist gross finger extension is to have the athlete make a fist, curl your fingers over his or hers, and instruct the athlete to extend the fingers as you apply resistance (Fig. 19-27). Note any differences in strength or increases in pain. To resist metacarpophalangeal extension, stabilize the metacarpals and apply resistance against the proximal row of phalanges (Fig. 19-28). Resistance can be applied in a similar manner to each individual joint.

To resist finger abduction, instruct the athlete to spread the fingers as far apart as possible. Resistance is then applied to the outside surfaces of those fingers being tested (Fig. 19-29, *A*). To test finger adduction, instruct the athlete to keep the fingers together as you attempt to pull them apart (Fig. 19-29, *B*).

Resistance is applied against thumb movement similar to those techniques used on the fingers. To test thumb flexion at the metacarpophalangeal joint, stabilize the first metacarpal and apply resistance to the volar surface of the proximal phalanx (Fig. 19-30, *A*). To test the interphalangeal joint of the thumb, stabilize the proximal phalanx and resist flexion on the distal phalanx (Fig. 19-30, *B*). Resisting thumb extension is performed in the same manner, with the resisting force applied on the dorsal surface of the thumb.

Thumb abduction is accomplished by stabilizing the hand and wrist with your hand and applying resistance against the lateral border of the proximal phalanx of the thumb during abduc-

Fig. 19-26. Applying manual resistance against flexion of an individual finger: **A,** proximal interphalangeal joint and **B,** distal interphalangeal joint.

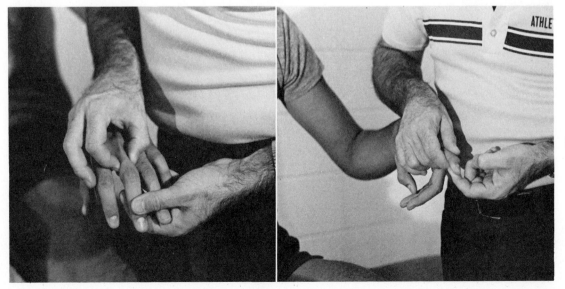

A

B

Fig. 19-27. Applying manual resistance against extension of all the fingers.

Fig. 19-28. Applying manual resistance against extension of the metacarpophalangeal joints.

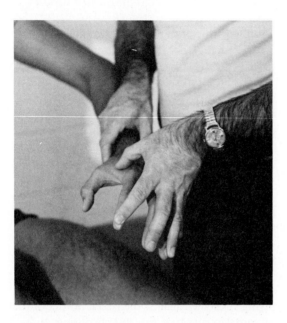

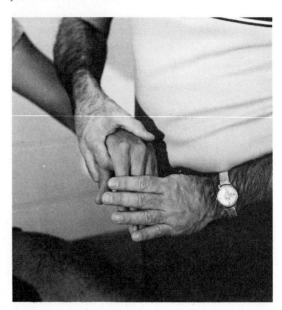

Fig. 19-29. Applying manual resistance against **A,** finger abduction and **B,** finger adduction.

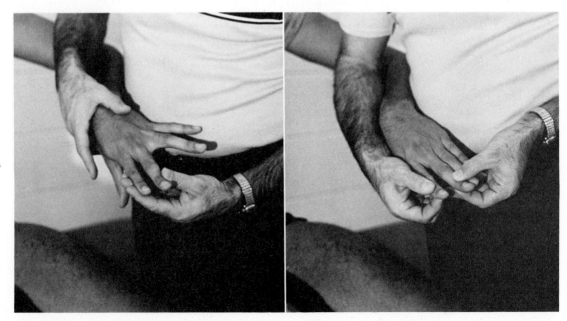

A

B

Fig. 19-30. Applying manual resistance against thumb flexion: **A,** metacarpophalangeal joint and **B,** interphalangeal joint.

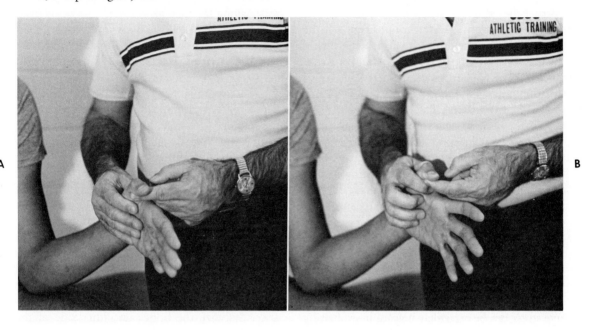

Fig. 19-31. Applying manual resistance against thumb **A,** abduction and adduction and **B,** opposition.

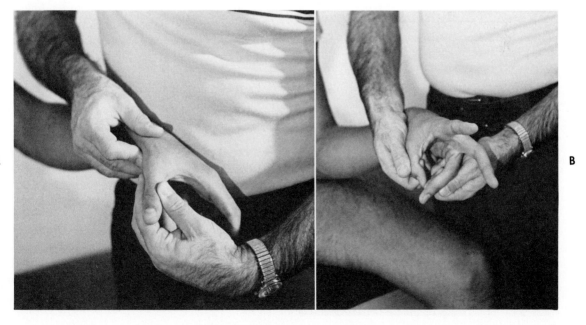

tion (Fig. 19-31, *A*). Reverse your resistance to the medial border of the proximal phalanx and instruct the athlete to adduct the thumb to test thumb adduction. To test opposition of the thumb, instruct the athlete to touch the top of the little finger with the tip of the thumb. Resistance is then applied to the palmar surfaces of the thumb and little finger (Fig. 19-31, *B*).

Passive movements. Passive movements are frequently used to facilitate the assessment of hand and wrist injuries. These include evaluating the bony integrity, assessing the integrity of the supporting ligaments, and performing passive range of motion tests. The specific maneuvers used depend on the type of injury suspected or indicated up to this point in the assessment process.

When the signs and symptoms exhibited to this point cause you to suspect a possible fracture in the hand or fingers, passive stress can be applied to each bone. Applying this type of passive stress can be extremely helpful in evaluating bony integrity. The metacarpals and phalanges are all long bones and mainly subcutaneous. Longitudinal stress can be applied, beginning very gently and then gradually increased de-

Fig. 19-32. Applying passive longitudinal compression stress to evaluate the bony integrity of the second metacarpal.

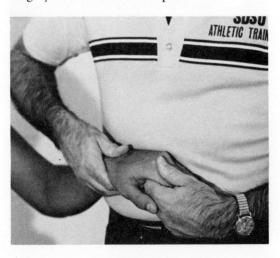

pending on the athlete's tolerance. This stress is accomplished by applying force or pressure directly along the long axis of the bone being evaluated (Fig. 19-32). If the bony integrity is intact, there should be no increase in pain. When the pain is located about a joint, this same longitudinal stress can be used to assess the bony integrity at the articulation. Stabilize both bones involved and apply longitudinal pressure directly along the long axis of these bones (Fig. 19-33). Again, if the bony integrity is intact, there should be no increase in pain. If this longitudinal stress causes additional pain or crepitation at the original site of tenderness, the athlete should be treated as if there is a fracture.

Once the bony integrity is assured, the athletic trainer should evaluate the supporting ligaments believed damaged. This is accomplished by applying transverse stress to those joints suspected of being injured. Again, begin very gently and increase pressure according to the athlete's tolerance. Stabilize the bones on either side of the injured joint and apply lateral, medial, or hyperextensive stress to the articulation. For example, Fig. 19-34 shows a method for testing the stability of the supporting ligaments around the proximal interphalangeal joint of the index finger. Note any increase in pain or instability with these passive maneuvers. Note in Fig. 19-35 the instability of the index finger during passive transverse stress.

Passive range of motion can also be used to evaluate the integrity of a joint. Whenever active range of motion is limited or restricted in a joint or joints, passive motion may be implemented to evaluate the available range. As with all areas of the body, passive range of motion must be performed gently and cautiously so no further damage results. All motions described under active movements can be evaluated passively.

Functional movements. Occasionally functional movements or activities can be beneficial to the comprehensive assessment of wrist and hand injuries. There will be times when observing an athlete perform those activities that reproduce

Fig. 19-33. Applying passive longitudinal compression stress to evaluate the bony integrity of **A,** metacarpophalangeal joint and **B,** proximal interphalangeal joint.

A

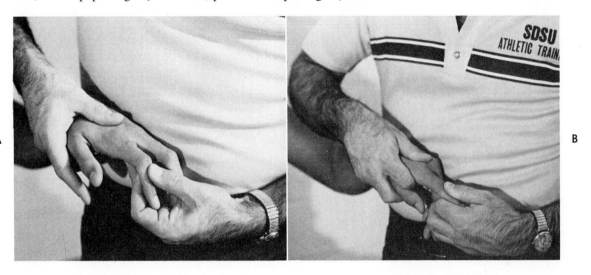

B

Fig. 19-34. Applying passive transverse stress to evaluate the supporting ligaments around the proximal interphalangeal joint of the index finger.

Fig. 19-35. Subluxation of metacarpophalangeal joint of index finger during transverse stress.

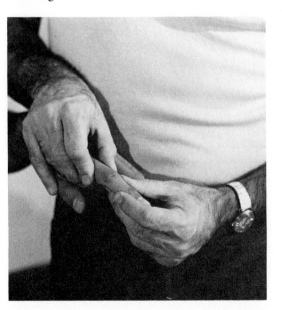

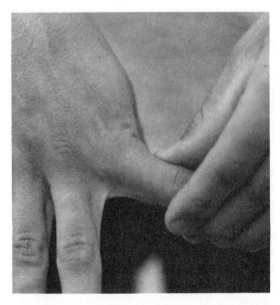

ATHLETIC INJURY ASSESSMENT CHECKLIST
HAND AND WRIST INJURIES

Secondary survey

_____ History
        _____ Primary complaint
        _____ Mechanism of injury
        _____ Pain
        _____ Sensations
        _____ Previous injuries
_____ Observation
        _____ Obvious deformity
        _____ Positioning and functioning of injured hand
        _____ Signs of trauma
        _____ Compare symmetry
        _____ Swelling
_____ Palpation
        _____ Tenderness
        _____ Deformity
        _____ Swelling
        _____ Crepitation
_____ Stress
        _____ Active movements
                _____ Range of motion
                _____ Associated symptoms
        _____ Resistive movements
                _____ Pain
                _____ Strength
        _____ Passive movement
                _____ Bony integrity
                _____ Ligament instability
                _____ Range of motion
        _____ Functional movements
                _____ Functional abilities

---

painful symptoms will be helpful. Observing such activities assists the athletic trainer in identifying the mechanism of injury and the anatomic structures that may be involved. However, for the most part, functional movements are used to determine when an athlete with a wrist or hand injury can return to full activity. As an athlete recovers from an injury to this area of the body, assessment of functional activity becomes increasingly important on each reevaluation. Can the athlete perform skills required of his or her

sport effectively and without an increase in injury symptoms? The intensity of functional activities should be continually increased within tolerable levels until the athlete is functioning at or near optimum capacity.

Evaluation of findings

Injuries involving the wrist and hand commonly occur in athletics. Most of these injuries occur because of direct trauma to the exposed area or overload forces associated with absorbing direct impacts. The many small bones and articulations may not be able to withstand the numerous and accumulative stresses that can be associated with all the various functions of the hand in athletic activity. Many athletic injuries to the hand and wrist are relatively minor and do not require extensive treatment. However, because even potentially serious injuries to this area of the body are usually not disabling to an athlete, there is a tendency to underestimate the severity and importance of injuries to the hand and wrist. If neglected or unrecognized, these injuries can develop into long-term impairment and possibly result in permanent disability and disfigurement. It is therefore important that athletic trainers not ignore injuries involving the hand and wrist and be able to accurately assess injuries to this important area of the body.

When to refer the athlete

Many hand and wrist injuries can be accurately evaluated and properly managed without seeking additional medical assistance. However, these injuries also have the potential of resulting in dysfunction or permanent deformity. Hand and wrist injuries may require expert medical attention to avoid these complications. The following list of conditions or findings can be used to determine if medical referral is indicated.

---

1. Gross deformity
2. Suspected fracture or dislocation
3. Significant swelling about any of the joints
4. Significant pain
5. Joint instability
6. Loss of motion
7. Anytime the resting position of the hand appears abnormal
8. Any doubt regarding the severity or nature of the injury

KEY TERMS

Bennett fracture Fracture of the proximal end or base of the first metacarpal, often associated with subluxation of the carpometacarpal joint

boutonnière deformity Deformity that results from an injury to the central slip of the extensor tendon where the proximal interphalangeal joint is flexed and the distal interphalangeal and metacarpophalangeal joints are in a hyperextended position

carpal tunnel Passageway for the median nerve and flexor tendons, formed by the arched carpal bones, the transverse carpal, and the volar carpal ligaments

carpal tunnel syndrome Symptoms resulting from constriction in the carpal tunnel and pressure on the median nerve

Colles' fracture Fracture of the distal end of the radius in which the fragment is displaced dorsally

extrinsic muscles Long flexor and extensor muscles that take origin within the forearm and are entirely tendinous in the hand

felon (whitlow) Painful infection located in the soft tissues surrounding the terminal phalanx of a finger

gamekeeper's thumb Sprain of the ulnar collateral ligament of the metacarpophalangeal joint of the thumb

hypothenar eminence Prominence at the base of the little finger containing the intrinsic muscles involved in moving the little finger

intrinsic muscles Musculotendinous units contained within the hand and responsible for the delicate movements of the fingers

Kienbock's disease Slow progressive avascular necrosis of the carpal lunate bone resulting from a circulatory disturbance

mallet finger (dropped finger) Deformity resulting from rupture of the extensor tendon slip at the point of its attachment into the base of the distal phalanx

Murphy's sign Condition observable on dislocation of the lunate—the head of the third metacarpal moves proximally so that it is on a level with adjoining knuckles and does not project distally to them

palmar (volar) plate Fibrocartilaginous structure that covers the flexor aspect of the metacarpophalangeal and proximal interphalangeal joints

paronychia Acute infection involving the subepithelial folds of tissue surrounding a fingernail

Preiser's disease Avascular necrosis of the carpal navicular (scaphoid) caused by trauma or a fracture that has not been kept immobilized

silver fork deformity   Particular deformity associated with a Colles' fracture, in which the distal fragment of the radius is displaced dorsally

Smith's fracture   Fracture of the distal end of the radius in which the fragment is displaced forward; also called reversed Colles' fracture

subungual hematoma   Accumulation of blood under the fingernail

thenar eminence   Prominence at the base of the thumb containing the intrinsic muscles involved in moving the thumb

wrist drop   A condition resulting from paralysis of the wrist extensor muscles

wrist ganglion   Cystic enlargement or knotlike mass formed by the synovial herniation of a tendon sheath on the back of the wrist

SUGGESTED READINGS

Birnbaum, J.S.: The musculoskeletal manual, New York, 1982, Acadmic Press, Inc.

Burton, R.I., and Eaton, R.G.: Common hand injuries in the athlete, Orthop. Clin. North Am. 4:809-839, 1973.

Conwell, H.E.: Injuries to the wrist, CIBA Clinical Symposia 22:1, 1970.

Flatt, A.E.: The care of minor hand injuries, ed. 4, St. Louis, 1979, The C.V. Mosby Co.

Hoppenfeld, S.: Physical examination of the spine and extremities, New York, 1976, Appleton-Century-Crofts.

McCue, F.C., and others: Hand and wrist injuries in the athlete, Am. J. Sports Medicine 7:275-286, 1979.

Mercier, L.R.: Practical orthopedics, Chicago, 1980, Year Book Medical Publishers.

O'Donoghue, D.H.: Treatment of injuries to athletes, ed. 4, Philadelphia, 1984, W.B. Saunders Co.

Ruby, L.K.: Common hand injuries in the athlete, symposium on sports injuries, Orthop. Clin. North Am. 11:819-839, 1980.

GLOSSARY

abdomen Body area between the diaphragm and pelvis

abducted scapulae Condition in which the scapulae are held a greater distance from the vertebral column than is considered normal

abduction Movement of a body part away from the midline of the body

abduction stress test Passive procedure used to evaluate medial stability of the knee

abrasion Break in skin continuity occurring when the epidermis and a portion of the dermis is scrapped or rubbed away

acetabular labrum Triangular ring of fibrocartilage attached to the rim of the acetabulum, increasing the depth of the cavity

acetabulum Socket in the hip bone into which the head of the femur fits

acromion Bony projection of the scapula, forming point of shoulder

active movements Those movements that can be initiated and completed by the athlete without assistance of any kind

acute Of short duration

acute traumatic injury Injury occurring instantaneously as a result of some type of trauma

adduction Movement of a body part toward the midline of the body

adduction stress test Passive procedure used to evaluate lateral stability of the knee

adhesions Fibrous bands that may connect or unite two adjacent surfaces or parts

adhesive capsulitis (frozen shoulder) Inflammation of the rotator cuff and capsular area, which develops because of immobility and results in loss of range of motion

agonists (prime movers) Muscles whose contraction produces movement

amphiarthroses Slightly movable joints having a pad of either hyaline or fibrocartilage located between adjoining bony surfaces

anatomic position Position in which the body is upright, the feet are parallel, and the palms of the hands face forward

anesthesia Loss of feeling or sensation

angiography Radiographic study of the vascular system, using a contrast medium injected either intra-arterially *(arteriogram)* or intravenously *(venogram)*

annulus fibrosus Circumferential portion of an intervertebral disk, composed of fibrocartilage and fibrous tissue

antagonists Muscle or muscles that oppose action of other muscles or gravity

anterior (ventral) Front

anterior compartment syndrome Pain and tenderness in the anterior compartment caused by swelling within this tightly closed space—in later stages, numbness and the inability to dorsiflex the foot will develop

anterior drawer test (ankle) Test to evaluate the integrity of the anterior talofibular ligament—with the athlete's ankle in a relaxed position, the athletic trainer stabilizes the leg with one hand and lifts anteriorly with the other while cupping the calcaneus

anterior drawer test (knee) Test to evaluate the anterior cruciate ligament—with hip flexed approximately 45° and the knee flexed 90°, the tibia is lifted anteriorly

anterograde amnesia Loss of memory for events occurring immediately after awakening

anterolateral rotatory instability Instability represented by anterior displacement of the lateral tibial plateau with respect to the femur during testing of the knee

anteromedial rotatory instability Instability represented by anterior displacement of the medial tibial plateau with respect to the femur during testing of the knee

aphasia Loss of speech, writing, or comprehension of spoken or written language

Apley's compression test Test to evaluate the integrity of the menisci—with the athlete lying prone and the injured knee flexed 90°, pressure is applied to the heel in an attempt to entrap a torn meniscus between the articular surfaces

Apley's distraction test Test to differentiate between a meniscal and ligamentous injury—with the athlete lying prone and the injured knee flexed 90°, pull up and rotate on the tibia in an attempt to distract the knee joint; in case of a ligamentous injury, this maneuver should elicit pain, whereas if it is a meniscal injury, there should be no increase in pain

Apley's scratch test Method to evaluate active range of motion of the shoulder by asking athlete to place hand behind the back and neck

apnea Temporary cessation of breathing

appendicular Pertaining to the appendages of a structure; in the body this refers to the upper and lower extremities

apprehension test Test to evaluate possible subluxations—often used in the assessment of patellofemoral and glenohumeral integrity

arcuate complex An anatomic complex that consists of the arcuate ligament, the popliteal tendon, the lateral collateral ligament, and the posterior third of the capsular ligament of the knee

arthrography Radiographic study of joints using a contrast medium to outline the soft tissue structures; the resulting radiograph is called an *arthrogram*

arthroscopy Surgical procedure that allows the surgeon to view the interior of a joint through a series of small lenses with a fiberoptic light source

articular Refers to a joint

articulation Joint

ataxia Failure of muscular coordination or irregularity of muscular action

athletic injury Disruption in tissue continuity that results from athletic activity and causes a cessation of participation or restriction of usual activity

athletic injury assessment Comprehensive evaluation of an athletic injury beginning when the injury occurs and continuing through the healing process until the injured area has been rehabilitated to its fullest extent

athletic trainer Provider of athletic training services, which can be divided into six major functions: (1) prevention, (2) assessment, (3) management and treatment, (4) rehabilitation, (5) organization and administration, and (6) education and counseling

athletic training Sports medicine subspecialty that provides a wide array of health care support services for athletes

atrophy Wasting away or deterioration of a tissue, organ, or part

avascular Without blood vessels

avulsion Tearing away of part of a structure, which may be torn completely free or remain partially attached, hanging as a flap

avulsion fracture Fracture in which a piece of bone is pulled loose at the attachment of a tendon, ligament or muscle, normally occurring with a sudden violent contraction or stress

axial Pertaining to the axis of a structure; in the body this refers to the head, neck, and trunk

ballotable patella Palpatory procedure for evaluating marked effusion of the knee; when the patella is pressed down and released quickly, the large amount of fluid under it causes the knee cap to rebound or appear to be floating

battle's sign Discoloration appearing over the mastoid area

Bennett fracture Fracture of the proximal end or base of the first metacarpal, often associated with subluxation of the carpometacarpal joint

bicipital aponeurosis A strong expansion of the biceps tendon, which blends with the fascia over the flexor muscles of the forearm

blocker's spur Name given to an irritative exostosis that develops near the deltoid muscle insertion caused by repeated blows to the area; it is most frequently seen in football players

blood pressure Pressure caused by blood exerting force on the walls of blood vessels

bone scan Nuclear imaging technique used to detect particular areas of abnormal metabolic activity within a bone

boutonnière deformity Deformity that results from an injury to the central slip of the extensor tendon; the proximal interphalangeal joint is flexed and the distal interphalangeal and metacarpophalangeal joints are in a hyperextended position

brachial Pertaining to the arm

bunion Abnormal enlargement of the metatarsophalangeal joint of the great toe; it usually is the result of chronic irritation and pressure from poorly fitted shoes and is characterized by soreness, swelling, and lateral displacement of the great toe

bunionette Bunionlike enlargement of the metatarsophalangeal joint of the little toe (also called a *tailor's bunion*)

bursa Fluid-containing sac lined with synovial membrane

carpal Pertaining to the wrist

carpal tunnel Passageway for the median nerve and flexor tendons, formed by the arched carpal bones, the transverse carpal, and the volar carpal ligaments

carpal tunnel syndrome Symptoms resulting from constriction in the carpal tunnel and pressure on the median nerve

carrying angle Angle formed by the axes of the arm and forearm when the elbow is extended

cauda equina Latin equivalent for horses' tail; the lower spinal nerve roots descending in the spinal canal from their point of attachment to the spinal cord to the site of their emergence between the vertebrae

cavities Depressions, openings, and grooves within bones

cavus foot (pes cavus) Inflexible high-arched foot that does not adequately absorb shock or easily adapt to various surfaces

celiac Pertaining to the abdomen

celiac plexus (solar plexus) Largest of the abdominal plexuses, it supplies the viscera in the abdominal cavity and lies in the upper middle region of the abdomen

cervical lordosis Increased concavity in the curvature of the cervical spine

charley horse Term usually restricted to injuries of the quadriceps muscle group caused by a contusion or possibly a strain producing soreness and stiffness

chondral fracture Break involving the articular cartilage

chondrocytes Cartilage cells

chondromalacia patellae Degenerative process that results in a softening or degeneration of the articular surface of the patella

chronic Of long duration

chronic overuse syndrome Athletic injury resulting from forces or stresses applied to a structure or tissues over a considerable period of time

circumduction Composite movement that combines flexion, abduction, extension, and adduction in which the body segment describes a cone

closed (simple) fracture Fracture that does not break the skin

collagen Main supportive protein in skin, tendon, bone, cartilage, and connective tissue

Colles' fracture Fracture of the distal end of the radius in which the fragment is displaced dorsally

coma State of unconsciousness from which the athlete cannot be aroused, even by powerful stimulus

communited fracture Break in which three or more bone fragments are produced

compartment syndromes Conditions in which increased tissue pressure compromises the circulation of the muscles and nerves within one of the osseofascial compartments; these may be acute or chronic in nature

compression fracture Impacted break characterized by crushed bone tissue such as to the body of a vertebra

computerized tomography (CT Scan) Sophisticated procedure using computerized radiographic equipment to get a three-dimensional image of the area

concussion Syndrome involving an immediate and transient impairment in the ability of the brain to function properly

condyle Rounded projection at the end of a bone

conduction Process of transfer by direct contact

contralateral Pertaining to the opposite side

contrecoup (counterblow) Injury resulting from a blow on the opposite side, such as an intercranial injury

contrecoup fracture Break of the skull at a distance away from the point of impact

contusion (bruise) Skin or soft tissue injury that usually results from a direct blow or impact delivered to some area of the body

convection Transfer of heat from one place to another by motion or circulation

coronal or frontal plane Runs from side to side and divides the body into front and back

costal Pertaining to the ribs

crepitation Grating, grinding, or sticking sensations that may be produced by various conditions

cubital Pertaining to the forearm

cubitus valgus Increase in the carrying angle of the elbow

cubitus varus Decrease in the carrying angle of the elbow (also known as a *gunstock deformity*)

cyanosis Bluish discoloration of skin caused by poor oxygenation of the circulating blood

---

decerebrate rigidity Postural attitude characterized by extension of all four extremities

decorticate rigidity Postural attitude characterized by extension of the legs and marked flexion of the elbows, wrists, and fingers

deep Away form the body surface

deep fascia Sheet of fibrous connective tissue investing the trunk, limbs, and various muscles

deep frostbite Freezing of the entire tissue depth, including muscles and bone

delayed union fracture Fracture that has not united successfully within expected period of time although the healing process continues

dens Conical pivot process that projects from the superior surface of the axis

depression Return of movement from an elevated position

depressed fracture Fracture in which part of a flat bone, such as the skull or cheek bone, is depressed inward or below the surface

dermatome Segment or strip of skin supplied by a given spinal nerve

dermis Inner and thicker layer of the skin

diapedesis Movement or migration of blood or its elements through the intact vessel wall

diaphysis Long shaftlike portion of the bone

diarthroses Freely movable joints, often called synovial joints

diastolic blood pressure Force with which the blood is pushing against the artery walls when the ventricles are relaxed

diplopia Double vision

discography Radiographic study of the spine using a contrast medium injected into an intervertebral disc; the resulting radiograph is called a *discogram*

dislocation Luxation, or displacement, of contiguous surfaces of bones, thus comprising a joint

displaced fracture Fracture in which a bone fragment is out of normal alignment

distal Farther from the point of attachment of an extremity to the trunk or the point of origin of a part

distended Inflated, swollen, or stretched

diuresis Increased urine production

dorsal Posterior; pertaining to the back

dorsiflexion Movement of the top of the foot upward

drawer test Passive procedure used to evaluate anterior and posterior stability of the knee and ankle

drop arm test Test that evaluates the status of the supraspinatus tendon—athlete abducts arm to 90°, horizontally adducts 30°, internally rotates, and maintains against resistance

dura mater Outermost layer of the meninges

dysphagia Difficulty in swallowing

dyspnea Difficult or labored breathing

dysuria Sensation of pain, burning, or itching on urination

---

ecchymosis Discharge or escape of blood into the tissues under the skin (black & blue mark)

echocardiography Technique that uses echoes or reflected high-frequency sound waves to visualize the heart

ectomorphy Type of body build in which there is a relative predominance of linearity over fat and muscle

edema Accumulation of excessive amounts of body fluids in the tissue spaces

electrocardiography Study of electrical activity of the heart; the graphic recordings are called an *electrocardiogram* (ECG or EKG)

electromyography Study of electrical potentials generated in muscles; the graphic recordings are called an *electromyogram* (EMG)

electronencephalography Study of electrical currents developed by the brain; the graphic recordings are called an *electroencephalogram* (EEG)

elevation Upward movement of the shoulder girdle

emesis Vomiting

encephalon Brain

endomorphy Type of body build in which there is a relative predominance of roundness and softness of the body

endomysium Connective tissue between individual muscle fibers

endosterm Fibrous membrane that lines the marrow cavity of long bones

epidermis Outer and thinner layer of the skin

epidural hematoma Hematoma outside the dura

epilepsy Disorder of the brain characterized by a tendency for recurrent seizures

epimysium Connective tissue sheath that envelops a skeletal muscle

epiphyseal fracture Break at the growth plate of long bones that occurs in growing children, as this is the weakest link along the bone

epiphyseal (growth) plate Thin plate of cartilage separating the diaphysis from each epiphysis in growing bones

epiphyses Extremities, or ends, of long bones

epistaxis (nosebleed) Hemorrhage from the nose

evaporation To dissipate in the form of vapor

eversion Sole of the foot is turned outward

exostosis Bony growth projecting outward from the surface of a bone

exposed injury Athletic injuries or conditions that disrupt the continuity of the skin

extension Return from the flexed position

external otitis (swimmer's ear) Common infection of the external ear in swimmers

external rotational recurvatum test Test for posterolateral rotatory instability in which both legs are held extended by the heels; a positive test results in the tibia showing excessive hyperextension and external rotation

extravasate Process of escaping or passing out of a vessel into the tissues

extrinsic muscles Long flexor and extensor muscles that take origin within the forearm or leg and are entirely tendinous in the hand or foot

exudate Fluid that has escaped from a tissue or its vessels

fascia Sheet of connective tissue

fasciculi Groups of individual muscle fibers bound into discrete bundles

felon (whitlow) Painful infection located in the soft tissues surrounding the terminal phalanx of a finger

fibroblasts Connective tissue cells that form collagen fibers

fibroplasia Production of fibrous tissue

fibroplastic phase Initial phase of the healing process in which fibrous tissue is produced

fissure Groove

fixators Muscles that fix or stabilize joints to assist prime movers

flexion Decreasing the size of the angle between the anterior or posterior surfaces of articulated bones

footdrop A condition in which the foot hangs in a plantarflexed position because of a lesion of the peroneal nerve

forefoot Area of the foot composed of the metatarsals and phalanges

forward head Deviation from normal alignment in which the head is carried in an abnormal anterior position

forward shoulders Deviation from normal alignment in which the shoulders are carried in an abnormal forward position

fossa Cavity or hollow

fracture Disruption in the continuity of bone

fracture-dislocation Fracture near a joint that occurs simultaneously with a dislocation

frostbite Localized freezing of a part of the body

frostnip Initial stage of frostbite involving only the surface of the skin

functional movements Series of active movements or activities performed by the athlete that simulate the type of activity required in a particular sport

gamekeeper's thumb Sprain of the ulnar collateral ligament of the metacarpophalangeal joint of the thumb

ganglion Cluster of nerve cell bodies outside the central nervous system

gaster Central fleshy or "meaty" contractile portion of a muscle

gastric Pertaining to the stomach

genu Pertaining to the knee

genu recurvatum (knee hyperextension) Angulation of leg is posterior, or backward, from the midline of the body

genu valgus (knock knees) Angulation of lower leg is away from the midline of the body

genu varum (bowlegs) Angulation of lower leg is toward the midline of the body

gomphosis Type of synarthrotic joint in which a conical peg or projection fits into a socket

grand mal seizure Classic type of seizure in which the person will fall down and display uncontrollable jerking or shaking movements of the extremities

gravity stress test Passive test using gravity and the weight of the hand and forearm to stress the medial side of the elbow; place the athlete supine, externally rotate the shoulder, and flex the elbow approximately 20° (weights can be added to increase the stress)

greenstick fracture Incomplete break of a long bone that occurs in adolescent athletes whose bones are still pliable; a common example would be a greenstick fracture of the clavicle in children

gunstock deformity (cubitus varus) Decrease in the carrying angle of the arm

hammertoe Toe permanently flexed at midphalangeal joint, resulting in clawlike appearance

healing by first intention Primary union by fibrous adhesions without the formation of infection and pus

healing by second intention Secondary union accompanied by infection and delayed healing

heat acclimation Process of becoming accustomed to athletic activity in hot weather

heat cramps Painful muscle spasms resulting from a fluid volume problem

heat exhaustion Heat stress condition characterized by profuse sweating, which makes the skin cool and clammy

heatstroke Heat stress condition characterized by lack of sweating, resulting in hot dry skin and a rising body temperature

heel spur Bony projection at the plantar aspect of the calcaneal tuberosity, which may accompany or result from severe cases of plantar fasciitis

hemarthrosis Accumulation of blood in joint cavity

hematemesis Vomiting of blood

hematoma Accumulation of extravasated blood that becomes organized into a localized mass

hematoma auris (cauliflower ear) End result of keloid formation between the skin and underlying cartilage of an injured external ear

hematuria Blood in the urine

hemopneumothorax Presence of both blood and air in the pleural cavity

hemopoiesis Process of blood cell formation

hemoptysis Coughing up blood or blood-stained sputum

hemorrhage Internal or external bleeding

hemothorax Blood in the pleural cavity

hernia Protrusion of abdominal viscera through a portion of the abdominal wall

hindfoot Area of the foot composed of the calcaneus and talus, including the ankle joint

hip pointer Contusion to the crest of the ilium

history procedures Process of finding out as much information as possible about the injury itself and the circumstances surrounding its occurrence

horizontal abduction Movement of the upper limb through the transverse plane at shoulder level away from the midline of the body

horizontal adduction Movement of the upper limb through the transverse plane at shoulder level toward the midline of the body

hyaline (articular) cartilage Thin layer of gristle-like material firmly fixed to the layer of compact bone covering the joint surfaces of the epiphyses

hyperextension Continuation of extension beyond the anatomic position

hypertrophy Increased size of a part caused by an increase in the size of the cells

hyperthermia Greatly increased body temperature

hyperventilation Overbreathing or very rapid deep breathing, resulting in abnormally lowered carbon dioxide levels in the blood

hyphema Hemorrhage into anterior chamber of eye

hypothenar eminence Prominence at the base of the little finger containing the intrinsic muscles involved in moving the little finger

hypothermia Systemic condition in which the core temperature falls below 95° F (35° C)

hypotonia Condition of abnormally diminished tone, tension, or activity

hypoxia Inadequate or reduced oxygen content

iliotibial band or tract Strong lateral portion of the deep fascia of the thigh that is the insertion of the tensor fascia latae muscle

impacted fracture Fracture in which one fragment of bone has been driven into and embedded in another fragment

incision Open wound caused by cutting the skin with a sharp object such as a knife

inflammation Basic response of vascularized tissues to an injurious agent, whether the source is physical, bacterial, thermal, or chemical

inferior Away from the head; lower

inguinal Of the groin

insertion More movable end of a muscle attachment

intracerebral hematoma Hematoma within the cerebrum

intrinsic muscles Entire musculotendinous units contained within the hand

inversion Sole of the foot turned inward

ipsilateral Pertaining to the same side

ischemia Local anemia; temporary lack of blood supply to an area

isometric Muscle contraction that produces no change in length of muscle

jerk test   Test for anterolateral rotatory instability in which the knee is flexed to 90°, the tibia internally rotated, and a valgus stress is applied to the knee; if positive, as the knee is passively extended the lateral tibial plateau will audibly and palpably sublux at approximately 30° to 40° and relocate as it approaches complete extension

joint effusion   The accumulation of fluid in a joint cavity

jumper's knee (patellar tendinitis)   Inflammatory response to repeated stress or irritation at the patellar tendon insertion

---

Kehr's sign   Referred pain to the left shoulder and upper arm resulting from an injury to the spleen

keloid   New growth or tumor of the skin, consisting of whitish ridges, nodules, and plates of tense tissue

Kienbock's disease   Slow progressive avascular necrosis of the carpal lunate bone resulting from a circulatory disturbance

knocked-down shoulder   Separation of the acromioclavicular joint resulting in obvious deformity, with the clavicle displaced upward and the acromion remaining down

kyphosis   Increased convexity in the curvature of the thoracic spine

---

laceration   Open wound or cut made by tearing the skin, which usually results from some type of direct blow to the skin; lacerations are especially common over bony prominences

Lachman's test   Passive procedure used to evaluate anterior and posterior stability with the knee flexed 10° to 15°

lacunae   Small cavity or space in cartilage or bone

laryngitis   Inflammation or irritation of the larynx indicated by hoarseness, dryness, soreness, and difficulty in swallowing

larynx (voice box)   Anatomic structure between the root of the tongue and the upper end of the trachea

lateral   Away from the midline of the body

lateral pivot shift test   Test for anterolateral rotatory instability that begins with the leg extended, the tibia internally rotated, and a valgus stress at the knee; as the knee is passively flexed, the lateral tibial plateau subluxes immediately and relocates again at approximately 30° to 40° if the test is positive

lethargic   Condition of drowsiness

lever   Mechanical device consisting of a bone (force arm), fulcrum (joint), weight arm (resistance), and force or effort movement (muscle contraction)—*first-class lever,* lever system in which the fulcrum lies between the effort and resistance; *second-class lever,* lever system in which the resistance lies between a long force and a short weight arm; *third-class lever,* lever system in which the effort is exerted between the fulcrum and resistance

ligament   Band of fibrous tissue that connects bone to bone

locomotion   Movement of the body as a whole

lumbar lordosis   Increased concavity in the curvature of the lumbar spine

lumbar puncture   Piercing of the subarachnoid space in the lumbar region, usually between the third and fourth lumbar vertebrae, for the purpose of withdrawing cerebrospinal fluid

luxatio erecta   Inferior dislocation of the shoulder in which the arm stands straight above the head

luxation   Complete dislocation

---

malleolus   Projection at the distal end of the tibia and fibula

mallet finger (dropped finger)   Deformity resulting from rupture of the extensor tendon slip at the point of its attachment into the base of the distal phalanx

malunion   Fracture that has united with faulty alignment of the fragments

manual muscle testing   Subjective grading of muscle strength by applying resistance against active movements

manubrium   Upper part of the sternum

march fracture   Stress fracture of one of the metatarsals; this name caught on during World War II, when many soldiers unaccustomed to being on their feet received fatigue fractures after walking long distances

margination   Accumulation of white blood cells on the inner surface of blood vessels near the site of an injury

marrow (medullar) cavity   Tubelike hollow in the diaphysis of long bones

maturation phase   Final phase of the repair process, in which the newly formed fibrous connective tissue matures and becomes stronger

McMurray test   Test to evaluate the integrity of the menisci; the athlete's hip and knee are flexed maximally, and as the leg is passively extended the tibia is rotated and valgus or varus force is applied to the knee

mechanism of injury Manner and location by which excess forces or stresses are applied to the body, resulting in athletic injuries

medial Toward the midline of the body

mediastinum Central portion of chest cavity containing the heart, its great vessels, part of the esophagus, and part of the trachea

meninges Three membranes surrounding the brain and spinal cord

menisci Crescent-shaped discs of fibrocartilage

mesomorphy Type of body build in which there is a relative predominance of muscle, bone, and connective tissue

metabolism Chemical process by which energy is produced

metatarsalgia Pain or tenderness beneath the metatarsal head, more commonly the second and occasionally the third

metatarsus Consists of the five metatarsal bones

midfoot Area of the foot composed of the navicular, cuboid, and three cuneiform bones

Morton's foot Characterized by a short first metatarsal and a longer second metatarsal

Morton's neuroma Swelling of one of the digital nerves, which is squeezed or pinched between the metatarsal heads; the nerve between the third and fourth metatarsal heads is involved most often

motoneuron Nerve fiber that transmits nerve impulses away from the brain or spinal cord (to a muscle)

motor unit One neuron plus the muscle fibers it innervates

Murphy's sign Sign evident on a dislocation of the lunate; the third metacarpal moves proximally so that it is on a level with adjoining knuckles and does not project distally to them

myelography Radiographic study of the spinal cord and canal, using a contrast medium injected into the spinal canal; the resulting radiograph is called a *myelogram*

myology Study of muscles

myositis ossificans Formation of bone within or around a muscle (commonly called calcium deposits)

---

necrosis Death of one or more cells or of a portion of tissue or organ

neuromuscular junction Area of contact between a nerve and muscle fiber

nondisplaced fracture Fracture in which pieces of bone lie in relatively normal alignment; occasionally this type of break may be difficult to see on x-ray films

nonunion Failure of the ends of a fracture to unite

nuclear imaging Radiographic study using short-term radioactive substances injected into the body and recorded on a scanner

nucleus pulposus Semifluid mass of fine white and elastic fibers that forms the central portion of an intervertebral disc

nystagmus Involuntary rapid movement of the eyeball

---

oblique fracture Fracture in which the break line crosses the bone at an oblique angle to its long axis

observation procedures Process that involves the recognizing, noticing, and inspecting an injured area and the circumstances associated with its occurrence

olecranon Proximal bony projection of the ulna at the elbow

olfactory Pertaining to the sense of smell

open (compound) fracture Fracture in which a bone is broken and the fragments cut through the skin

open wound Wound in which the skin is broken

ophthalmic Pertaining to the eyes

optimum angle of pull Right angle to the long axis of a bone to which a muscle is attached

origin More fixed end of a muscle attachment

Osgood-Schlatter syndrome Condition involving the epiphysis of the tibial tuberosity in adolescents

osteochondral fracture Break involving the articular cartilage and underlying bone

osteochondritis dissecans Condition of unknown cause in which a segment of subchondral bone undergoes avascular necrosis

otorrhea Discharge from the ear

overriding fracture Fracture in which bony fragments overlap, resulting in shortening of the bone

---

painful arc Pain caused by tender tissue being squeezed as a joint passes midpoint during the range of motion

pallor Paleness or absence of skin coloration

palmar (volar) plate Fibrocartilaginous structure that covers the flexor aspect of the metacarpophalangeal and proximal interphalangeal joints

palpation procedures Process of examination by touch

paralysis Loss or impairment of motor function

paraplegia Paralysis of the lower extremities

paresis Slight or incomplete paralysis

paresthesia An abnormal sensation such as burning, itching, or prickling

paronychia Acute infection involving the subepithelial folds of tissue surrounding a fingernail

passive movements Procedures performed entirely by the athletic trainer

patella femoral grinding test Test to evaluate the integrity of the underside of the knee cap; the patella is pushed manually against the femoral condyles and the athlete is asked to contract the quadriceps as pressure is maintained

pectoral Pertaining to the chest or breast

pedal pulse Foot pulse

periodontal membrane Fibrous membrane located between the root of a tooth and its socket

perimysium Connective tissue between bundles of muscle fibers

periosteum Dense fibrous membrane covering the outer surface of long bones except at the joint surfaces

peripheral Pertaining to the outside surface

peritoneum Membrane that lines the abdominal cavity

pes planus (flat foot) Static structural abnormality in which the relative position of the foot bones have been altered, resulting in a lowering of the longitudinal arch

petechiae Small, nonelevated, pinpoint purplish or red discolorations resulting from localized hemorrhage into the skin or mucous membranes

phagocytosis Ingesting and disposing of unwanted substances such as elements of a hematoma

pharyngitis Inflammation of the pharynx, or throat, indicated by pain on swallowing, dryness, burning, and hoarseness

pharynx Throat

pia mater Vascular innermost covering (meninges) of the brain or spinal cord

piano key sign High-riding clavicle resulting from a third-degree sprain of the acromioclavicular joint; it can be pushed down but will spring back up when pressure is released, much as a piano key

pigment labile Area of the body that may show abnormal changes in skin color

plain-film radiography Procedure that uses no contrast materal to enhance the various structures of the body; these are the most common types of radiographic procedures used in sports medicine

plantar Pertaining to the sole of the foot

plantar aponeurosis Strong band of fibrous connective tissue originating on the calcaneal tuberosity and inserting near the metatarsal heads which acts as one of the primary supports for the longitudinal arch; also called *plantar fascia*

plantar fasciitis Overuse syndrome that involves an inflammatory reaction at the insertion of the plantar fascia or aponeurosis into the calcaneus

plantar flexion Movement of the sole of the foot downward

pleura Double membrane sac; the outer layer lines the chest wall and the inner layer covers the outside of the lungs

plexus Network

pneumocephalus Presence of air in the intracranial cavity

pneumothorax Air in the pleural cavity

ponderal index Height/weight index in which height in inches is divided by the cube root of the weight in pounds $\frac{\text{ht (in)}}{\sqrt[3]{\text{wt (lbs)}}}$

popliteal Behind the knee

posterior (distal) Back

posterolateral rotatory instability Instability represented when the lateral tibial plateau displaces backward in relation to the lateral femoral condyle

posture Position or attitude of the body

Pott's fracture Fracture of the lower fibula that involves the tibial articulation and usually a chipping off of a portion of the medial malleolus or a rupture of the deltoid ligament; also called *Dupruytren's fracture*

Preiser's disease Avascular necrosis of the carpal navicular (scaphoid) caused by trauma or a fracture that has not been kept immobilized

primary injury Initial insult or injury resulting directly from the trauma

primary lesions Those lesions that appear initially in response to some changes in the internal or external environment of the skin

primary survey Portion of the athletic injury assessment process concerned with evaluation of the basic life support mechanisms of airway, breathing, and circulation

processes Prominences and projections on bones

pronated foot Flexible foot that exhibits excessive pronation, which is a combination of dorsiflexion, eversion, and abduction at the subtalar joint

pronation Palms-downward position

prone Lying face down

protraction Motion moving a body part forward

proximal Nearer the point of attachment of an extremity to the trunk or the point of origin of a part

pulse Alternate expansion and contraction of arterial walls as the heart pumps blood

puncture wound Open lesion occurring as a result of direct penetration of the skin with a pointed object

pupillary reflex Contraction of the pupil on exposure of the retina to light

---

Q angle Angle formed by a line from the anterior superior iliac spine to the midpatella and another line from midpatella to the tibial tuberosity; an angle of 15° or less is considered normal

quadriplegia Paralysis of all four extremities

---

racoon eyes Discoloration around the eyes, indicative of a skull fracture

radial flexion Movement at the wrist of the thumb side of the hand toward the forearm

radiation Process of emitting radiant energy in the form of waves

referred pain Pain felt in a part of the body other than where the source or cause of the pain is located

reflex Involuntary action

rehabilitation Restoration of optimum form and function following an injury in the shortest possible time

renal Pertaining to the kidney

resistive movements Resistance applied against active movements

retraction Return of a protracted body part

retrograde amnesia Loss of memory for events leading up to the injury

rhinorrhea Discharge from the nose

Romberg's sign Sign elicited by having the athlete stand with his or her feet together, arms at the side and eyes closed; normally a person can stand still in this position

rotated fracture Fracture in which one of the bony fragments has rotated in relation to the other

rotation Pivoting of a body part on its own central or longitudinal axis

rotator cuff Group of four muscles whose tendons surround and attach about the head of humerus and are primarily responsible for the integrity of the shoulder joint, that is, maintaining the head of the humerus within the glenoid labrum

rubor Redness of the skin

---

sagittal plane Plane that runs from front to back and divides the body into right and left

sarcomere Contractile unit of muscle tissue

sciatica Pain along the course of the sciatic nerve, with possible associated paresthesia of the thigh and leg and atrophy of calf muscles

scoliosis Lateral curvature or deviation of the spine

secondary injury Additional responses or damage occurring secondary to the primary injury

secondary lesion Lesions that do not appear initially but result from a primary lesion

secondary survey Portion of the athletic injury assessment process that examines the athlete in an attempt to recognize and evaluate all athletic injuries and conditions; it consists of an ordered sequence of procedures used to assess the nature, site, and severity of an athletic injury

shin splints Catch-all term for chronic pain and discomfort in the leg, generally limited to musculotendinous involvement

shock State of collapse or depression of the cardiovascular system

shoulder pointer Contusion to the tip of the shoulder or over acromion process

shoulder separation Sprain of the acromioclavicular joint

sign Objective evidence of an injury, something the athletic trainer can see, hear or feel

silver-fork deformity Particular deformity associated with a Colles' fracture in which the distal fragment of the radius is displaced dorsally

sinus tarsi Concavity or space between the calcaneus and talus

Slocum test Test for anterolateral rotatory instability similar to the pivot shift test except the athlete is placed on his or her uninjured side

Smith's fracture Fracture of the distal end of the radius in which the fragment is displaced forward; also called *reversed Colles' fracture*

snapping hip Chronic trochanteric bursitis with

thickening of the bursal walls, causing an audible and palpable snap as the tensor fascia lata slides back and forth over the greater trochanter

somatotype Particular category of body build, determined on the basis of certain morphologic traits

somatotyping System of objectively classifying body build or physique

spina bifida occulta Defect in the bony spinal without involvement of the spinal cord or meninges

spiral fracture Fracture in which the break twists around and through the bone and is usually caused by a twisting injury

spondylolisthesis Forward displacement or slippage of one vertebra on another, usually occurring between L_4 and L_5 or L_5 and the sacrum

spondylolysis Defect in the pars interarticularis, or that part of the vertebra between the superior and inferior articular processes

spontaneous pneumothorax Pneumothorax occurring without apparent cause

sports medicine Multifaceted term encompassing all phases of medical concerns as they relate to the biomechanical, psychologic, nutritional, environmental, pathologic, and physiologic nature of the athlete

sprain Athletic injury involving a ligament

squinting patellae Patellae that appear to face inward when the feet are pointed straight ahead

status epilepticus Successive seizures occurring within a short period of time

stone bruise Persistent contusion on the plantar aspect of the foot; also called a *heel bruise* when located under the calcaneus

strains Athletic injuries involving a musculotendinous unit

strangulated hernia Herniated portion of viscera that has become incarcerated or tightly constricted and is likely to become gangrenous

stress fracture Incomplete break in a bone occurring after prolonged repetitive activity

stress procedures Involves the use of manipulative techniques to locate and define the structures involved in the injury

stress radiograph Radiographic procedure performed while stress is being applied to the joint; these are normally performed with the athlete under anesthesia

stupor Partial or nearly complete unconsciousness

sty Localized, painful infection of the small glands or hair follicles around the eyelash

subconjunctival hemorrhage (red eye) Rupture of the tiny blood vessels in the conjunctiva

subcutaneous Beneath the skin; usually refers to the fatty and connective tissue layer found beneath the dermis

subdural hematoma Hematoma beneath the dura

subluxation Incomplete dislocation

substrate phase Initial phase of the acute inflammatory response characterized by localized vascular changes

subungual hematoma Accumulation of blood under the fingernail

superficial Near the surface

superficial fascia Sheet of fibrous connective tissue just below the skin

superficial frostbite Freezing of the skin and subcutaneous tissue

superior Toward the head end of the body

supination Palms-upward position

supine Lying on the back

sustentaculum tali Medially projecting ledge on the upper surface of the calcaneus; it is the largest articular facet for the talus

sutures Type of synarthrotic joint united into rigid, immovable joints by a series of jagged, interlocking processes

symphyses Type of amphiarthrotic joint in which a pad of fibrocartilage joins one bone to another

symptom Subjective evidence of an injury or something the athlete relates

synarthroses Immovable joints

synchondroses Type of amphiarthrotic joint in which a pad of hyaline cartilage joins one bone to another

syndesmosis Type of synarthrotic joint characterized by the presence of a dense fibrous membrane that binds the articular surfaces together

synergists Muscles that assist prime movers

synovial joint Diarthrotic, or freely movable, joint

systole Contraction of the heart muscle

systolic blood pressure Force with which the blood is pushing against the artery walls when the ventricles are contracting

---

tachypnea Abnormally rapid shallow breathing

tarry stool Blood in the fecal discharge from the bowels

tarsus Collective term used to describe the seven bones that constitute the mid- and rear foot: talus, calcaneus, navicular, cuboid, and the three cunei-forms

tendon Band or cord of fibrous connective tissue that attaches a muscle to a bone or other structure

tension pneumothorax Condition in which air continues to be drawn into the pleural cavity and cannot escape; pressure continues to rise on the affected side, pushing the collapsed lung against the heart and unaffected lung

thenar eminence Prominence at the base of the thumb containing the intrinsic muscles involved in moving the thumb

Thompson test Test to indicate the integrity of the Achilles tendon; with the athlete's legs extended and feet hanging over the table, each calf muscle is squeezed, and normally, the foot will react by plantar flexing; if the Achilles tendon is ruptured, there will be no movement of the foot

thoracic cavity Body cavity above the diaphragm

thorax Chest

tinnitus Ringing in the ears

tomography Radiographic technique using a specialized computer to give a view of one particular area of tissue at any depth; the resulting radiograph is called a *tomogram*

torticollis (wryneck) Contracted state of the cervical muscles, producing an unnatural position of the head

trachea Windpipe

transverse (horizontal) plane Crosswise section that divides the body into upper and lower portions

transverse fracture Fracture in which the break is across the bone at a right angle to its long axis and is often caused by a direct blow

trauma Injury

triceps surae Name given to the gastrocnemius and soleus muscles, which share the same tendon of insertion

trochlea Pulley-shaped surface of the talus that articulates with the tibia and fibula

turf toe Sprain of the metatarsophalangeal joint of the great toe normally caused by extreme dorsiflexion or plantar flexion

---

ulnar flexion Movement at the wrist of the little finger side of the hand toward the forearm

unconsciousness Unresponsiveness, or the inability to respond to any sensory stimuli, with the possible exception of those causing pain

unexposed injury Internal athletic injuries with no associated disruption or break in the continuity of the skin

urography Radiographic study of the urinary tract using a contrast medium injected intravenously; the resulting radiograph is called an *intravenous pyelogram* (IVP)

---

valgus Bent outward; denoting a deformity in which the angulation of the distal part is away from the midline of the body

vaporization Conversion of a liquid or solid into a vapor

varus Bent inward; denoting a deformity in which the angulation of the distal part is toward the midline of the body

vastus Wide, of great size

ventral Front or anterior

vertigo Sensations of movements

viscera Internal organs; usually refers to the abdominal organs

volar Pertaining to the palm of the hand or the sole of the foot; palmer; plantar

Volkmann's ischemic contracture Condition that may develop after a severe injury in the region of the elbow and is caused by the loss of blood supply to the musculature of the forearm; this catastrophic complication is characterized by permanent flexion of the fingers and sometimes of the wrist

---

wen Sebaceous cyst

wheeze Whistling sound made during breathing

winged scapula Marked projection and upward tilt of the lower angle of the scapula

wristdrop Condition resulting from paralysis of the wrist extensor muscles

wrist ganglion Cystic enlargement or knotlike mass formed by the synovial herniation of a tendon sheath on the back of the wrist

---

xiphoid Inferior process of the sternum

Yergason test Evaluates the status of the long head of the biceps tendon; athlete flexes elbow at side of body as resistance is applied against elbow flexion and external rotation

---

zygomatic bone Cheek bone

INDEX